The
Holistic
Health
Lifebook

The Holistic Health Lifebook

A Guide to Personal and Planetary Well-Being

A COMPANION VOLUME TO THE
HOLISTIC HEALTH HANDBOOK

Compiled by the Berkeley Holistic Health Center

Edward Bauman   **Lorin Piper**
Armand Ian Brint   **Amelia Wright**

Published by
AND/OR PRESS, INC.
Berkeley, California

Library of Congress Cataloging in Publication Data
Main entry under title:

The Holistic health lifebook.
    "A companion volume to the Holistic health handbook."
    Includes bibliographies and index.
    1. Health—Addresses, essays, lectures. 2. Holistic medicine—
Addresses, essays, lectures. 3. Human ecology—Addresses,
essays, lectures. I. Bauman, Edward, 1946-   II. Berkeley
Holistic Health Center.
RA776.5.H633   613   81-2846
ISBN 0-915904-53-5   AACR2

Published and Distributed by: And/Or Press, Inc.
                            P.O. Box 2246
                            Berkeley, CA 94702

Printed in the United States of America
First Printing: October 1981

12   11   10   9   8   7   6   5   4   3   2   1   *(current printing)*

Project Co-ordinators: Sebastian Orfali, Carlene
    Schnabel

Developmental Editors: Sebastian Orfali, Alta Picchi
    Kelly, Peter Beren, Leslie Strauss, Jim Schreiber,
    Jean-Louis Brindamour

Manuscript Editors: Aidan A. Kelly, Anita O. Miller,
    Jim Schreiber

Additional Editorial Assistance: Bebe Bertolét, Leslie
    Carr, Dzintar Dravnieks, Linda Gibbs, Jean
    Haseltine, Sayre Van Young

Typing: Leslie Strauss, Bebe Bertolét, Iris Miller

Typesetting: Marti Craig of prePrint, Funky Hollow
    Typesetting, Richard Ellington, Aurora Type,
    Accent and Alphabet, Petrographics

Proofreading: Martha Benson, Bebe Bertolét, Bennett
    Cohen, Dzintar Dravnieks, Ron Fielder, Jean
    Haseltine, Alan Klein, Jim Schreiber, Sayre Van
    Young

Bibliography and Index: Sayre Van Young

Book Design; Art and Production Direction: Carlene
    Schnabel

Pasteup and Production: supervisor—Phil Gardner
                        staff—Catherine Conner,
                            Marian O'Brien,
                            Sally Taback

Cover: Artwork—Deborah Cotter
    Art Direction—Carlene Schnabel
    Mechanicals—Marlyn Amann
    Color Separation—Color Tech

Camerawork: Circus Litho, Custom Process, Ed
    Kirwan Graphic Arts, Graphic Impressions

Printing: Delta Lithograph Company

Illustrations:

Marlyn Amann: pp. 115, 173.

Ross Carlton: pp. 4, 209, 361, 364, 377.

Cata Carney: pp. 33, 69, 72, 125-26.

R. Casley: p. 387.

Deborah Cotter: pp. 113, 114, 117, 141-44, 206, 217, 219-20, 233-34, 238-39, 275, 284, 287, 294, 313, 328-33.

Marti Craig: pp. 98, 336, 338.

Phil Gardner: pp. 177, 344.

Matt A. Gouig: pp. 37, 43, 59-60, 62-63, 75-79, 120, 155-57, 181, 199, 200-201, 244-45, 249, 252-53, 360.

Cathy Greene: pp. xii, 8, 84, 151, 193, 272, 296-97, 304, 309, 311, 344-45, 348.

Pamela Myers Rhodes: pp. 86, 106-107, 108-109, 134-35, 146-48, 179, 194, 204, 327.

Tobi: pp. 187, 190, 227-28.

Bill Wells: pp. 339, 341-42.

Ingo Werk: pp. 28, 29, 41-42, 47, 49, 162, 167.

Strephon Kaplan Williams: pp. 161, 165.

Illuminated Letters:

Deborah Cotter: pp. 38, 44, 52, 58, 67, 74, 87, 94, 97, 101, 105, 111, 118, 124, 127, 140, 145.

Phil Gardner: pp. xi, xiii, 3, 7, 9, 12, 17, 21, 26, 151, 154, 160, 176, 180, 186, 193, 197, 205, 344.

Matt Gouig: pp. 33, 36, 213, 216, 226, 231, 237, 243, 247, 251, 256, 261, 265, 369.

Cathy Greene: pp. 131, 351, 354, 359, 365, 375, 378, 388, 391.

Adrian Tubio: pp. 271, 274, 282, 295, 303, 308, 314, 319, 326.

Photographs:

Anne Dorfman, p. 16; Earth photo courtesy of NASA, p. 39; Bob Knighton and Roger Russell, pp. 53-56; Patrick Woods, p. 65; Diane Padis, p. 66; Jason Mundstuk, p. 84; Peter E. Harris, p. 100; Susan Storch, p. 104; Terry Guyer, p. 110; Mark Stephenson, p. 123; Phil Smith, p. 201; Betty Freeman, p. 204; James Ketsdever, p. 225; Ruth Gilmore, p. 242; George Post, p. 257; Karen Preuss, pp. 261-64; Photo courtesy of University of the Trees Press, p. 291; Lee Foster, pp. 321, 323, 325; Judy Jackl, p. 371; Bruce Gorman, p. 371; Robert Kirck, pp. 379-80; Chris Clay, pp. 380-81; Paul Bauman, p. 398; Jill Snoa, p. 398; Wiley Reed, p. 399; Lisa Toby, p. 399.

Dedication

This book is dedicated to the earth, all sentient beings that derive nourishment from her, and the spirit of unity that guides our collective evolution.

Table of Contents

SECTION VI
EVOLUTION OF HOLISTIC HEALTH: Concepts,
Networking, Legal Issues, The Future

Foreword

C. Norman Shealy, M.D., Ph.D., and
Patricia L. Midboe, R.N., M.S.N.

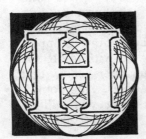olistic health is comprehensive. It utilizes the best of both worlds—the old and the new—the East and the West. This book demonstrates this comprehensiveness as it provides historical perspectives and images of the future, words of Eastern philosophers, and medicine of Western practitioners. Holistic health is an integrated approach to wellness. It implies that there is a cooperative relationship among participating systems. At the Pain and Health Rehabilitation Center, we apply this comprehensive approach to clients who choose to participate in our 12-day patient sessions and five-day Self-Health Awareness sessions. We have titled our approach Biogenics®. Biogenics® includes positive attitude, belief in self and possibility of health, relaxation, balancing body and autonomic nervous system, balancing emotions, programming goals, words and images, biofeedback for reinforcement, and spiritual attunement.

We see that in order to have long lasting benefits, the clients must understand and practice self-regulation. Our intent as staff is to act as tour guides. We provide information and share the maps or tools that can lead to high level wellness. When clients open up and accept the information and the tools and *willfully apply* Biogenics® within all aspects of their lives, then the transformation occurs. Holistic health is about what we as individuals can do for ourselves, not what someone can do to us or for us. We are the creator and we can create anything imaginable.

The Holistic Health Lifebook is an extension of our work at the Pain and Health Rehabilitation Center. It provides information and maps and tools for those individuals who willingly and joyfully accept self-responsibility. That acceptance extends beyond self and can become universal in perspective. This book is a fine blend of the work of tour guides who represent a wide variety of cultures as well as expertise. As tour guides it is important for us to recognize and utilize the integrated, interdisciplinary approach which is available to us. This book is a reminder to all of us that we can and do complement each other's work. I am particularly impressed with the cookbook approach of this work as it supplies the recipes for sound health and a sane environment. It is both practical and theoretical. It recognizes the needs of individuals, families and communities, large and small. As I reflect upon Abraham Maslow's hierarchy of needs, I see that the editors of this book have addressed themselves to each of these categories. In so doing, *The Holistic Health Lifebook* is a guide for what Abraham Maslow calls "self-actualization."

It is always a pleasure to see individuals, groups, and communities transforming disorder into order, disharmony into harmony, and manifesting the love, the peace, and the joy that is available when one controls thoughts and emotions as opposed to being controlled by them. I look forward with joy to the continuous unfoldment of inner wisdom and inner beauty that awaits discovery within each and every one of us. This book is a reflection of several great and magnificent beings who willingly and joyfully share their thoughts and their feelings that others might SEE and BE.

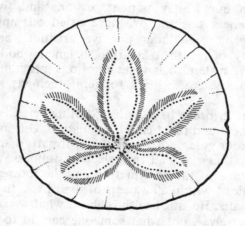

Prelude: What I Learned from 3000 Doctors
Norman Cousins

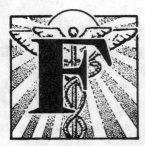

For the past year, I have been the beneficiary of some 3,000 letters from doctors in about a dozen countries. The letters were in response to the article "Anatomy of an Illness (As Perceived by the Patient)," published in *The New England Journal of Medicine* on Dec. 23, 1976, and reprinted in *Saturday Review* on May 28, 1977. The article described a recovery from a crippling illness that specialists believed at the time (1964) to be irreversible.

What is most remarkable and gratifying about these letters is the evidence of an open attitude by doctors to new or unconventional approaches to the treatment of serious disease. There was abundant support for the measures that had figured in my own recovery—a well-developed will to live, laughter, and large intravenous doses of sodium ascorbate (vitamin C). Far from resenting the intrusion of a layman into problems of diagnosis and therapy, the doctors who wrote in response to the article warmly endorsed the idea of a patient's partnership with his physician in the search for a cure.

The letters reflected the view that one of the main functions of the doctor is to engage to the fullest the patient's own ability to mobilize the forces of mind and body in turning back disease. There was general agreement in the letters that modern medication is becoming increasingly dangerous and that, to the fullest possible extent, the careful physician should attempt to educate the patient away from reliance on exotic drugs. The new trend favors an understanding of the powerful recuperative and regenerative forces possessed by the human body under conditions of proper nourishment and reasonable freedom from stress.

A CASE IN POINT

Not all the communications came from doctors. One episode involving a layman underlines many of the key points raised by physicians. A New York lawyer telephoned to say that his 4-year old daughter was in critical condition in Lenox Hill Hospital. She was stricken by viral encephalitis against which antibiotics have no record of success. The lawyer wanted to know whether, in the light of my own recovery from a severe collagen disease after taking large doses of ascorbic acid, the same treatment might be useful for his daughter.

I told the lawyer that it would be highly irresponsible of me, a layman like himself, to attempt to give medical advice, which in any case I was unqualified to offer. Moreover, there was no way of determining what part of my recovery was due to the intravenous infusion of ascorbate and what part to a full mobilization of the salutary emotions, not excluding laughter and a robust will to live. I suggested that the lawyer consult his daughter's doctor about the possible use of ascorbic acid.

The lawyer said he feared the child's doctor would be scornful of anything as unsophisticated and overpopularized as vitamin C. I then told him of the large number of medical tracts I had received from doctors, in response to my article, supporting the use of ascorbate in a wide range of disorders beyond the reach of antibiotics or other medication.

In particular, I spoke of the work of Irwin Stone, a biochemist in San Jose, Calif., who is among the country's leading authorities on the efficacy of ascorbic acid in the treatment of serious disease. I offered to send the lawyer reprints of articles from medical journals about the work of Stone and others on the functions of ascorbate in body chemistry. What seemed impressive to me about these papers was the data on the ability of ascorbate to activate and enhance the body's own healing mechanism. I suggested that the lawyer might wish to review this material with his child's doctor in the event he had not already seen it.

The next day I left for a new round of the Dartmouth Conferences in Latvia, U.S.S.R. While abroad, I made inquiries at various medical centers and learned that intravenous infusions of ascorbic acid had been effectively used in a number of cases of viral encephalitis.

ICE CREAM CURE

On my return to New York, I telephoned the lawyer to ask about his daughter. He said he had spoken with Stone, who told him about recent experiences in which serious cases of viral encephalitis have been reversed through large doses of ascorbate. Armed with this information and with reprints from medical journals I had sent him, the lawyer had spoken to the child's specialist, only to be rebuffed. When he had offered the materials from the professional journals, the doctor had said he didn't need to be instructed by a layman in medical matters.

The lawyer then decided on a plan of action. Several days later he asked the specialist whether the next time his child came out of the coma he might offer her some ice cream. The specialist encouraged the lawyer to do so. The lawyer bought a pound of powdered sodium ascorbate, which is more soluble and less bitter then the ascorbic acid form. He mixed at least 10 grams of the powder into the ice cream, which the child eagerly devoured. The next day the lawyer again gave her ice cream, enriched this time with an even larger dose of sodium ascorbate.

He continued the process day after day. After two weeks the child was taken out of the oxygen tent altogether. The improvement continued steadily in the following days, during which the lawyer gave his daughter an average of 25 grams of sodium ascorbate daily.

The lawyer's voice vibrated with elation as he described the child's complete recovery and the prospect of having her home again. I asked if he had told the specialist what he had done.

"Certainly not," he replied. "Why should I make trouble for myself?"

DOCTOR AND PATIENT

Obviously, it is poor—and dangerous—policy for any layman to act behind a doctor's back. Yet there may be something about the specialist's attitude that warrants scrutiny. Was there a hardening of the categories that caused him to shut himself off from a serious consideration of alternatives? Was he over-reacting to what he regarded as an intrusion? One of the most striking features that emerged from the letters I received from doctors is the evidence of a new respect for the ideas of non-professionals.

"Nothing is more out of date than the notion that doctors can't learn from their patients," wrote Dr. Gerald Looney, of the Medical College of the University of Southern California. "People today are far

better educated in medical matters than they were only a quarter of a century ago. The entire field of nutrition, for example, is one in which many patients can hold their own, to say the least, with their doctors. Maybe the new spirit of consumerism has at last reached medicine. I teach my students to listen very carefully to their patients and to concerned and informed laymen. That's what good medical practice is all about."

One of the attractive characteristics of ascorbate is that it does no harm even if it may do little good. Under these circumstances, was there any justification for the total refusal of the child's specialist to give serious consideration to the lawyer's request? Is the obligation of the doctor confined only to the patient? What about the legitimate emotional needs of those very close to the patient? The specialist's relationship with the child was limited in chronology and circumstance; the father had a lifetime commitment.

Another example of a problem arising from a doctor's dealing with a relative and patient concerns the wife of a man dying from cancer in Boston, Mass. She telephoned to say her husband had been through standard treatment—radiation, surgery and chemotherapy—and she was despairing about the future. She had read that Linus Pauling, the Nobel prize-winning chemist, had said that vitamin C is a cure for cancer. Her hopes had been raised by the prospect, and she wanted to know if, on the basis of my own experience with a supposedly irreversible illness, I thought ascorbic acid ought to be tried.

CANCER TREATMENT

As in the case of my conversation with the lawyer, I told the woman that it would be highly improper for me to attempt to give advice. I did, however, call her attention to the fact that Pauling's conclusions were based largely on the research of Dr. Ewan Cameron, of the Vale of Leven Hospital of Loch Lomondside, Scotland.

Cameron has published reports telling of his studies involving patients suffering from advanced malignancies who were given large doses of sodium ascorbate over a period of many weeks. The results were compared with the experiences of 1,000 cancer patients of similar condition who were given no ascorbate. The average survival time of the patients in the first group was substantially longer than that of the second group. (It is important to note that "substantially" refers to weeks or months, rather than to years.) Cameron makes no claim that sodium ascorbate is a cure for cancer. The significance of his research is tied to the clear indication of an agent in ascorbate that retards cancer.

Cancer cells, Cameron says, release hyaluronidase, an enzyme that attacks intercellular cement. "Proliferation will continue as long as hyaluronidase is released; proliferation will stop when the release of hyaluronidase stops." Ascorbic acid, according to Cameron, strengthens tissue-grounding and therefore counteracts hyaluronidase activity.

Such, at least, was the gist of the material that I offered to send to the woman in Boston whose husband was dying of cancer. I emphasized that ascorbic acid could not be regarded as a sure cure for cancer or other advanced diseases. She asked whether I would be willing to discuss these matters with her husband's doctor. I told her I thought this would be inappropriate but suggested that her doctor might like to talk to my own physician, Dr. William Hitzig, who had provided full support for my decision to discontinue aspirin, Butazolidin, colchicine, and sleeping pills—all of which were toxic in varying degrees—and to seek to reverse my condition through a comprehensive regimen, only one part of which was regular intravenous doses of ascorbate.

The woman telephoned two days later to say she had attempted to discuss the possible efficacy of ascorbate for her husband, only to have the doctor cut her short by chanting "quack, quack," and describing the whole business as "b.s."

The woman and her husband decided to discontinue the doctor's services, although he had been a longtime family friend. They also decided to leave the hospital and to return home, where the atmosphere made for a less stressful environment and where a local doctor was glad to administer the sodium ascorbate.

Their course of action produced results similar to the findings reported by Cameron. The husband has gained some ground. His appetite has improved; and so has his will to live. He is still doomed to die from cancer, but he already has had a few more months of life than seemed possible only a short time ago. Most important, perhaps, he is able to spend his remaining time in congenial surroundings in the company of his wife.

Death is not the ultimate tragedy of life. The ultimate tragedy is depersonalization—dying in an alien and sterile arena, separated from the spiritual nourishment that comes from being able to reach out to a loving hand.

The trend in modern medicine is to move away from the notion that it is always mandatory to hospitalize seriously ill patients. The great technological advances in electronic equipment, typified by the hospital intensive-care unit, are not without their built-in penalities. A patient in the center of an exotic Buck Rogers medical wonderworld is provided with everything diagnostically necessary in an emergency—everything, that is, except the sense of security and ease that the body needs even more than pinpointed and clicking surveillance. A mood of panic can trigger a cardiac disaster. Today, doctors are increasingly aware of the circular paradox of the intensive-care unit. It provides better electronic aids than ever before for dealing with emergencies that are often made all the more intensive because they communicate a sense of imminent disaster to the patient.

Dr. Jerome D. Frank, of the John Hopkins University School of Medicine, told students at the graduating exercises of John Hopkins in 1975 that any treatment of an illness that does not also minister to the human spirit is grossly deficient. He cited a 1974 British study showing that the survival rate of patients with heart disease being treated in an intensive-care unit was no higher than the survival rate of similar patients being treated at home. His interpretation was that the emotional strain of being surrounded by emergency electronic gadgets in an atmosphere of crisis offsets any theoretical technological gain.

In that same commencement talk, he referred to 176 cases of cancer that remitted without surgery, x-rays, or chemotherapy. One wonders whether a powerful factor in those remissions may have been the deep belief by the patients that they were going to recover and their equally deep conviction that their doctors also believed they were going to recover. Treatment works best when the patient has faith in it. More than 76 years ago, the great Canadian physician-philosopher William Osler referred to faith as the physician's greatest aid.

STATE OF MIND

Hundreds of letters from doctors about the *New England Journal of Medicine* article reflected the view that no medication they could give their patients is as potent as the state of mind that a patient brings to his or her own illness. In this sense, they said, the most valuable service a physician can provide to a patient is helping him mobilize all the resources of mind and body in order to maximize his own recuperative and healing potentialities.

With respect to my own illness, several doctors expressed the view that my will to live represented the primary therapy and that the ascorbate may have been secondary. In my article I allowed for the possibility that I might have been all wrong about the efficacy of ascorbate in my case, and that I could have been the beneficiary of a self-administered placebo.

Dr. Bernard Ecanow and Dr. Bernard H. Gold, of the University of Illinois at the Medical Center, wrote to say that it was a serious error for me to believe that the improvements in my condition after the systemic use of ascorbate was merely a placebo effect. They had done extensive research on the subject, and enclosed papers showing that ascorbate has a dispersal effect on clusters of red blood cells (RBCs). The reason my sedimentation rate had dropped after each intravenous dose of ascorbate, they said, was because it "produced dispersal of aggregated RBCs through its water structure breaking (hydrophobic bond-breaking) effect, breaking up the structural water macromolecular matrix so that the RBCs are no longer held together by it."

I interpreted this explanation to mean that ascorbate was useful in restoring the chemical balance in the blood, or what the famous Walter Cannon termed "homeostasis" some thirty years ago.

Additional supporting data on the improvement in my condition after taking ascorbic acid came from the Lederle Research Laboratories. Drs. Arnold Oronsky and Suresh Keway reported that ascorbic acid is essential for the proper functioning of prolylhydroxylase, which in turn is essential for the synthesis of collagen. The significance of ascorbate in the treatment of collagen diseases such as arthritis, therefore, seems compelling.

GENETIC DEFECT

Earlier in this article, I referred to the work of Irwin Stone. With the possible exception of Albert Szent-Gyorgi, Stone probably has probed more deeply into the phenomenon of ascorbic acid than any other medical researcher in the country.

Stone has attempted to account for the fact that the human species is unable to manufacture or store ascorbic acid, a vital ingredient in the immunological system installed by nature in all members of the animal kingdom except man and several other mammals.

Fascinated by this fact, Stone has pursued his study of the subject both anthropologically and biochemically. He has developed the theory that a genetic defect took place very early in the course of evolution: Human beings lost their ability to make ascorbic acid and have had to depend on food containing the substance that plays so large a part in the

immunological system. In areas where citrus fruits and certain vegetables abound, the regular diet has compensated, to a certain extent, for the natural deficiency. In northern climes, however, the absence of citrus fruits has resulted not just in scurvy but in increased susceptibility to a wide range of illnesses, minor and major.

Stone emphasizes that ascorbic acid strictly speaking, is not a vitamin but a liver metabolite. Its primary reputation as a vitamin, however, has made it heir to the negative feelings of doctors because of the public's tendency to be attracted to miracle vitamin cures. Stone is hopeful that the medical profession will make a distinction between ascorbic acid and other vitamins not because he undervalues the need for adequate intake of vitamins but because the therapeutic properties of ascorbic acid play such a vital role in the healing process. With respect not just to poor diet but to an environment becoming increasingly burdened with air and water pollution, congestion, noise, and stress, the antitoxic role of ascorbic acid cannot be underestimated.

One can understand the apprehensions of the medical profession about the absurd notion that vitamins are the answer to any illness. Yet it is also true that some doctors have fostered the equally erroneous idea that the average supermarket shopping basket is insurance against any nutritional deficiency. Considering the preservatives, coloring agents, additives, and sugar overload in many processed foods, the pronouncement of the White House Conference on Food, Nutrition, and Health in 1969, seems highly pertinent; namely, that one of the great failures in the education of medical students is the absence of adequate instruction in nutrition.

BALANCED ATTITUDE

In any event, it is encouraging to me, in going through the mail from doctors, to see the growing evidence of a balanced attitude about nutrition in general and ascorbic acid in particular. The negative views that many doctors held only a few years ago are now being replaced by a willingness to examine new findings and to apply them in proper proportion.

It is also encouraging to know that the medical profession is giving increased emphasis to immunology and to the natural drive of the human body to heal itself. Considerable mystery still surrounds this process. As indicated earlier in this article, one of the interesting clues now being pursued is the function of ascorbic acid in serving both the immunological and healing processes. In this connection, it is worth calling attention to the current practice of many British hosptials of administering intravenous doses of ascorbic acid instead of antibiotics as a routine post-operative procedure in guarding against infection.

A number of doctors felt that my emphasis on the positive emotions was in accord with an important new trend in medicine. They said it was scientifically correct for me to state in the *New England Journal of Medicine* article that, just as the negative emotions produce negative chemical changes in the body, so the positive emotions are connected to positive chemical changes. My attention was called to a paper by Dr. O. Carl Simonton on emotional stress as a cause of cancer and to a paper by Dr. J.B. Imboden and Dr. A. Canter showing that moods of depression impair the body's immunological functions.

The emphasis I had placed on laughter as therapy drew perhaps two dozen supportive letters. Dr. Walter E. O'Connell, a clinic director at the Veterans Administration hospital in Houston, Texas, sent voluminous materials on the physiological benefits of laughter. These materials indicated that it was no accident that hearty laughter has reduced the pain in my joints and improved the quality of my sleep. O'Connell referred to the importance placed by Sigmund Freud on humor as a factor in good health. He cited two papers by Freud: "Wit and Its Relationship to the Unconscious" (1905) and "Humour," which was included in a collection of Freud's writings published in 1928.

EARLY EXPERIENCE

Several doctors wrote to ask whether I had been influenced in my decision to use large doses of ascorbic acid by the statements and writings of Linus Pauling. My experience with ascorbic acid occurred in 1964. Pauling's first major work on ascorbic acid *(Vitamin C and the Common Cold)* appeared in 1970. After the publication of that work, I wrote to Pauling about the episode.

Some of the letters from doctors asked whether there had been anything in my medical history to prepare me psychologically and philosophically for "partnership" with Dr. Hitzig in the diagnosis and treatment of my illness in 1964. There are two such episodes.

My first experience in coping with a bleak medical diagnosis came at the age of 10, when I was sent to a tuberculosis sanitarium. I was terribly frail and underweight, and it seemed logical to suppose that I was in the grip of a serious malady. Later it was discovered that the doctors had mistakenly interpreted normal calcification as TB markings. X-rays at that time were

not yet a totally reliable basis for complex diagnosis. In any case, I spent six months at the sanitarium.

What was most interesting to me about that early experience was that the patients divided themselves into two groups: Those who were confident they would beat back the disease and be able to resume normal lives, and those who resigned themselves to a prolonged and even fatal illness. Those of us who held to the optimistic view became good friends, involved ourselves in creative activities, and had little to do with the patients who had resigned themselves to the worst. When newcomers arrived at the hospital, we did our best to recruit them before the bleak brigade went to work.

I couldn't help being impressed with the fact that the boys in my group had a far higher percentage of "discharged as cured" outcomes than the kids in the other group. Even at the age of 10, I was being philosophically conditioned; I became aware of the power of the mind in overcoming disease. The lessons I learned about hope at that time played an important part in my complete recovery and in the feelings I have had since about the preciousness of life.

By the time I was 17, I had completely overcome that early frailty. I had fallen in love with vigorous sports; year by year, even in adulthood, my body continued to grow and harden. I also have had the advantage of being married to a woman who has a positive outlook on life and believes deeply in the advantages of good nutrition.

TWO ROADS

The second major episode occurred during 1954, my 39th year. With increased family responsibilities, I thought it prudent to apply for additional insurance. The company doctors turned me down, saying the cardiograms showed evidence of a serious coronary occlusion. My aunt, who was the insurance agent, was completely frank about the findings of the doctors. She said they urgently advised me to give up almost everything by their report. It was inconceivable that I would have to give up my job, my travels, and an active sports life. But here was my aunt telling me that the insurance doctors said that if I became completely inactive, I might be able to stretch my life out for a year and a half.

I decided to say nothing to my wife about the verdict of the insurance doctors. When I came home that night, my little daughters came running to me. They like to be thrown high in the air and to dive from my shoulders onto the couch. For one second I looked down two roads. One was marked cardiac alley. If I accepted the advice of the specialists, I would never throw my girls in the air again.

The second road would find me working full tilt at *Saturday Review* and doing all the other things that spell life to me, especially throwing my little girls in the air. It was an easy decision. The second road might carry me for a few months or a few weeks or a few minutes; but it was my road. I threw the little girls higher than I had ever thrown them before. The next day I played in a singles tennis tournament for perhaps a total of 45 or 50 games.

The following Monday I telephoned Hitzig and informed him of the melancholy verdict of the insurance doctors. He ordered me to his office immediately, then took me to the chief of cardiology at Mt. Sinai Hospital. The hospital cardiograms confirmed the insurance reports. I went back to Hitzig's office. We had a good talk. I told him I intended to do exactly what I had been doing all along and that I didn't think there was any cardiograph in the world that was smart enough to know what made my heart tick. Hitzig patted me on the back and said he was behind me all the way.

Three years later I met Paul Dudley White, the famed heart specialist. He listened carefully to the account of what had happened, then told me that I had done the only thing that could have saved my life. He believed that sustained and vigorous exercise is necessary for the health of the human heart, even when there is evidence of the kind of cardiac inefficiency that had been diagnosed in my case. He said that if I had accepted the verdict of the specialists in 1954, I probably would have confirmed it.

EXPERT ADVICE

The meeting with White was something of a landmark in my life. It gave me confidence in my rapport with my own body. It reinforced me in my conviction that the human mind can discipline the body, can set goals for itself, can somehow comprehend its own potentiality and move resolutely forward.

In recounting this episode, I certainly do not intend to suggest that patients with heart disease should ignore the advice of their doctors. What worked for me may not work for others.

Has my respect for the medical profession diminished as the result of the three episodes? Just the opposite. The thousands of letters I have received from doctors have demolished any notion that physicians are universally resistant to psychological, moral, or spiritual factors in the healing process. Most doctors recognized that medicine is just as much an art as it is a science and that the most important knowledge in medicine to be learned or taught is the way the human mind and body can summon innermost resources to meet extraordinary challenges.

Some of the letters asked whether I would be able, in the event of another serious illness, to mount the kind of total response I did 14 years ago.

My answer was that I honestly don't know. I don't know how many such efforts are possible in a single lifetime. But I know I would certainly try.

I know I have been lucky. My body has already carried me far beyond the point where the medical experts in 1954 thought it would go. According to my calculations, my heart has furnished me with 871,946,280 more heartbeats than were thought possible by the insurance doctors 24 years ago. I dare not even estimate the number of games of tennis or rounds of golf I have played, or the miles I have sprinted, since then.

It was the sheerest of coincidences that, on the 10th anniversary of what was supposed to have been an irreversible crippling illness, I should happen to meet on the street in New York one of the specialists who in 1964 had made the melancholy diagnosis of progressive paralysis. He was clearly surprised to see me. I held out my hand. He took it. I had a point I wanted to make, and I thought the best way to do so was through a greeting firm enough to make an impression. I actually increased the pressure until he winced and asked to be released. He said he could tell from my handshake that he didn't have to ask about my health, but he was eager to hear about my recovery.

It all began, I said, when I decided that some experts don't really know enough to make a pronouncement of doom on a human being. And I said I hoped they would be careful about what they said to others; they might be believed and that could be the beginning of the end.

The
Holistic
Health
Lifebook

Preface
Amelia Wright and Lorin Piper

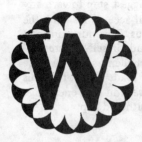e are happy and proud to be presenting you with this book. It represents the natural evolution of the holistic health movement. In our first book, the *Holistic Health Handbook,* we presented information and education about many healing practices and techniques used throughout the world. Our intent was to provide tools and an awareness that would enable you to assume responsibility for your health. In this companion volume, we offer a broader perspective on what it means to live holistically. We offer tools and models to help you assume responsibility for your whole lifestyle.

To live a full natural and positive life is to be happy. Real health can be measured in terms of vitality, growth, and self-actualization. Healing begins to take place when we allow ourselves to touch and be touched by life. It is the friendly and concerned conversation, the smile, and the knowledge that we are not alone, separated, or isolated that contribute to health and happiness.

With this in mind, we have presented approaches to help you integrate and enhance the various aspects of yourself and your world.

The book is divided into six sections.

1. *Overview of Holistic Health.* The articles here cover some of the roots of holistic health.
2. *Body/Mind.* The articles here concern the health of mind and body, and how they are intricately connected.
3. *Mind/Spirit.* We believe that a reverence for life gives a person a richer and fuller experience in day-to-day living. Spiritual expressions are as diverse as people are. We have presented articles offering perspectives and experiences that may be a springboard for your own spiritual expression.
4. *Relationships.* How we relate to people, how capable we are of giving and receiving love, are good gauges for measuring how healthy and happy we can be. How deeply can you touch and be touched? We have presented articles about male/female relationships, gay relationships, parent/child relationships, elderly relationships, sexuality, and love. We all need to love and to be loved. Unfortunately many of us have internal blocks that keep us from experiencing the love and intimacy we want and are capable of. The articles in this section are frank and sincere, and were written with the reader in mind, as contributions to their quest for true intimacy and love.

5. *Society/Environment.* The environment and society we live in affects us significantly. Finding meaningful work, a good education for your children, a clean environment to live in: these are concerns we all share. In this section we cover these topics and more.

6. *Evolution of Holistic Health.* This last section outlines the growth and maturing of the holistic health movement. There is a massive surge toward holistic living, and many people have worked together to provide humanistic, economical health services. We present profiles on these people and the services they offer, as well as a picture of the current policies concerning the national health plan.

Some chapters will mean more to you than others. This is a natural result of our diversity as human beings, and further illustrates that we are all unique entities contributing to a many-faceted whole.

This book, like the last, is not designed to be read from cover to cover. Rather, read what you are attracted to, curious about, and interested in. At the beginning of each section, you will find a set of questions concerning the subject matter of the chapter. These questions are intended to allow you to assess the quality and frequency of your individual patterns of thought and action, so that you might better understand yourself and decide which areas of yourself you might want to develop, change, or bring more to the surface. We encourage you to establish some personal goals in the areas you feel appropriate. Setting goals and observing your progress is a rewarding way to acknowledge your constant growth and evolution.

The field of holistic health is not isolated. It is directly laced into our social, political, economic, spiritual, and personal evolutions. We believe that positive growth in all of these areas is happening. In presenting the information and tools in this book, we have not been unaware of the seriousness of the problems we face as a civilization and of the decisions we must make, both individually and collectively. We have chosen not to criticize, but instead to offer positive forms suitable for the attainment of our healthy future evolution.

Many people have spent the past decade working on individual growth. Although it has sometimes been criticized as an era of self-centeredness and narcissism, it has brought about a new clarity of purpose, a mass examination of what motivates us and what we really want. Along with this clarity comes the strength necessary to put these ideals into action; we realized that we are responsible for ourselves and our surroundings. With this inner direction, we can trust in our vision of a better world.

Although there are many thought-provoking subjects included in this volume, some more charged than others, we feel that the biggest step toward any transformation begins with self-acceptance and the love and care of those around us. This nurturing at a ground level promotes the kind of self-directed individuals needed to face the challenges that we are now presented with. And so, reader, we offer this book in hopes that it will serve you and encourage you in your journey toward health and happiness.

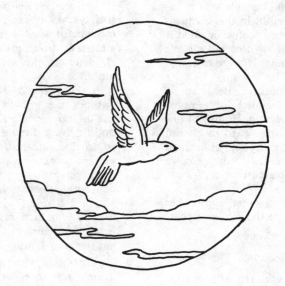

Section I:
Overview of Holistic Health

"It's supposed to be a professional secret, but I'll tell you anyway. We doctors do nothing. We only help and encourage the doctor within."

Dr. Albert Schweitzer

"People talk about this crisis or that, but actually the world has only one crisis—a crisis of consciousness. There reside within the higher human consciousness at this moment clear and happy solutions to all the problems that confront mankind—energy, food, population, pollution, atomic genocide, and all the rest. The only thing that holds us back is the fact that the general level of consciousness operates at so low a level that it is impossible to gain a large enough consensus to put into effect the known solutions. The primary job, then, is consciousness raising."

Jerome Ellison

"It's more important to know what kind of a patient has a disease, than what kind of disease the patient has."

Sir William Osler, M.D.

"The real purpose of attaining better physical health and longer life is not just the enjoyment of a pain and disease-free existence, but a higher divine purpose for which life was given to us."

Dr. Paavo Airola

"When we propose holistic health today, we are attempting to recontact, at the same time, the physical basis of our being, the origin of human science, and the planetary nature which gives us our own natures. This so called 'new medicine' was not born yesterday, but comes to us again and again as a primordial thing. We may give him/her a holistic name, but she gives us back a far more valuable and incorruptible thing."

Richard Grossinger

Introduction
OVERVIEW OF HOLISTIC HEALTH

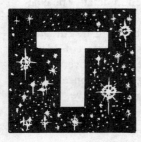

The holistic health way is broad. It includes all paths that encourage humankind to cooperate in the peaceful and creative habitation of our planet. As we grow in experience, we naturally enlarge and deepen in insight and outlook. The material in this section presents an evolving, multidimensional picture of holistic health. Underlying the importance and efficacy of health therapies, providers, and facilities is the core belief that individuals have an innate but neglected capacity for self-healing. Holistic health suggests self-responsibility as a way to tap this powerful, natural human resource.

Ours is an era of terrific growth and decay. Each of us orchestrates myraid influences in our lives, and responds to life-promoting and life-destroying stimuli. Our society and many others are undergoing a massive transformation. The old models for organizing and directing our lives no longer serve the majority of the people. Holistic health is creating a bridge of support that our sick society can cross to heal itself. Our small-minded, stubborn belief in the ethic of individualism no longer provides us with the security we seek, the solutions to the problems we face, or the room to grow, not necessarily bigger, but better. A broader, nonideological spirit of cooperation and revitalization is clearly needed. Amidst the decay of outworn values, seeds of change have germinated and are beginning to grow.

We have much to learn from the lessons of the past. Both healing and history are concerned with process. An important aspect of holistic living is to reconnect with our roots. Overemphasis on material technology has cluttered our inner and outer world. We no longer value intuition, an instinct our ancestors practiced as second nature. We have forgotten the simple natural laws of the universe. Holistic health has a relevance for this time as it teaches us to value and trust ourselves, and make one the duality that separates past and future, inner and outer, thinking and feeling.

William Blake suggested that "Everything that lives is holy." Hippocrates understood that medicine, science, and philosophy were not separate disciplines, but one great discourse on life. Our twentieth-century beliefs, conceived largely in the eighteenth-century Age of Reason, have dichotomized body and mind, and virtually exiled spirit altogether. The coming age portends a rebirth of our integral wholeness, unity, and flow.

Holistic health offers basic life-education tools for increased self-care and social responsibility. It is a movement of like-minded and heartful individuals, who may or may not express themselves in the explicit field of health care. In it there is a unifying spirit of good will, and an appreciation of the growth potential of all living beings. Holistic health is an attitude and a discipline that deepens and is realized through practice.

One of the grand illusions of modern life is that we can abuse our vehicle (our body/mind), and it can be serviced and repaired by specialized medical "mechanics." After much suffering and indignation, we are acknowledging that this extravagance is an unreliable method of health maintenance. As we begin to follow the time-honored counsel, "Know thyself," we automatically engage the mechanism to "heal ourselves" by making healthy lifestyle changes. To get well, we have to stop making ourselves sick. Our whole situation will shift with the reactivated commitment to grow.

Healing is a naturally occurring phenomenon within human beings. Much healing goes on without our being aware of exactly how it is happening. We do know that we all have a cellular and systemic intelligence that responds to the needs of the organism. When stress and pollutants enter the body, immunological defenses are triggered. When tissue has decayed or been damaged, regenerative activity increases. This healing impulse is greatly encouraged by sufficient rest, relaxation, nutrition, and the desire to be well, or whole again.

Chemical medicine, intended to ease the suffering of the individual and to promote healing, often undermines the body's ability to rid itself of the cause of dis-ease. "Heroic" medicine, invaluable in emergency situations, does not concern itself with the multiple factors that wed an individual to his or her situation. Self-abuse patterns resulting from unmet emotional needs must be acknowledged and responded to while a physical complaint is treated. As treatment proceeds, health is restored gradually, as body,

mind, and spirit regain a positive relationship to one another and to the environment.

The articles that constitute this overview present a mosaic of past, present, and future considerations of the emerging holistic health movement. Natural healing and social and political organizing around the issues of health care are discussed in detail. The challenge to bring holistic health into the mainstream, and to educate the general public and health practitioners about its relevance, is likewise considered and deliberated. We are reminded in this overview of our common concern for living well, a concern that galvanizes our ability to respond, to evolve, and to endure.

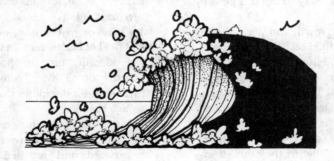

A Holistic View of Health:
The Search for Systemic Harmony

Dick Andersen, M.A.

A revolution is going on in the field of health. More and more health professionals are discovering that there are dimensions of health care that have been given little attention by Western medicine. A new theory of health and health maintenance is emerging that is both more holistic and more committed to "humanistic" values. This essay is an attempt to articulate the fundamental components of this emerging theory.

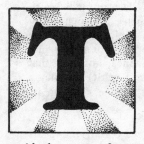

he holistic view sees a human life as a total system, composed of both a subjective and an objective component. The subjective component of the human system has two aspects. First is the psyche, which belongs to the individual center of consciousness. Within the psyche, several distinctions can be made, though such distinctions are not clear-cut. One can, however, distinguish the mind (the thinking aspect) from the emotions (the affective aspect); and, within the mind, the active (analytic) function from the receptive (intuitive) function.

The other subjective component of the human system is the spirit, the "farther reaches of human nature" that transcend the limitations of the isolated center of consciousness. It may be called the aspect of the being that thirsts for an ultimate value and a universal meaning, transcending the limitations of selfhood.

The subjective component of the human system is not self-sustaining; it has certain needs that must be

This article originally appeared in the University of California Extension Media Center publication *Audiotapes and 16mm Films on Medicine and Health Care, Lifelong Learning*, Vol. XLV, No. 42, January 16, 1976, copyright © 1976 by the Regents of the University of California. This article is reprinted here by kind permission of the University of California Extension Media Center, 2223 Fulton Street, Berkeley, CA 94720.

satisfied if it is to function properly. The need of the mind is primarily for exercise, including a need for the analytic and intuitive functions to be exercised in the proper balance. The emotional need is for caring human relationships. The spiritual need is to experience oneself as having a meaningful role in a human and cosmic community. Finally, the system as a whole has a need for the proper balance between activity and repose.

The body (soma) may be considered as either objective or subjective. It is perhaps most correct to view the soma *per se* (apart from the neuroendocrine system) as objective, i.e., as part of the physical environment. The neuroendocrine system can then be looked upon as the mediator between psyche and soma, and between the subjective and objective systems.

The objective component of the human system has four aspects: one's relationship to one's own soma; one's relationship to other human beings (both "intimate" and "public"); one's relationship to nonhuman life; and one's relationship to the "nonliving" environment. The total human system consists of the aggregate of all the very complex interactions among both the subjective and objective aspects.

TOWARD A HOLISTIC VIEW OF HEALTH

Western medicine and psychology have made great strides in treating the symptoms of various states of "un-health" of the human system. They have not yet, however, developed a coherent theory of systemic health, integrated with a program for health maintenance. In this respect, some other cultures are far ahead of us. Chinese medicine, for instance, is based on a theory of health as the balancing of polarized energies in the total system. For several thousand years, Chinese physicians have had programs for the maintenance of this balance. As is well-known, traditionally the physician was paid on a regular basis for helping to carry out the health-maintenance program. If the client became ill, the program was considered a temporary failure and the payments were stopped until health was regained.

The word "health" is etymologically related to the word "wholeness." It implies that all aspects of the total system are in balance with one another—that physical, emotional, mental, and spiritual needs are being met in the proper proportion. If the needs of each aspect of being are satisfied, then each will be properly tuned to the others, like instruments in an orchestra. In fact, the analogy between music and health is very close. "Harmony" originally meant "articulation," and referred to the proper fitting together of all the parts of the body. The term will be used here to refer to the balanced, rhythmic functioning of the total system. Thus, a state of health is a state of *systemic harmony*. Again, for a state of systemic harmony to exist, all the needs of the system (physical, emotional, mental, and spiritual) must be satisfied at a certain minimum level. Each person is a delicately balanced spiritual-psychophysical system. If one section of the orchestra is out of tune, then the harmony of the whole is disturbed.

The human system is not closed, but is open to the environment through the mediation of the neuroendocrine system, including its extensions, the sensory apparatus. This openness to the environment allows for the various needs of the system to be met. It also leaves the subjective system open to disturbance by disharmonious influences in the environment. There are physical "poisons" that can disturb the physical system. In addition, there are mental, emotional, and spiritual "poisons" that can disturb the subjective system. These "subjective poisons" include such things as uncaring thoughts, feelings, and actions, as well as unaesthetic aspects of the environment (e.g., noise pollution).

The neuroendocrine system serves as a double-sided mirror, or feedback mechanism, which reflects the state of the psyche in itself and then reflects that same state "downward" into the soma. Similarly, it reflects the state of the soma into itself and then reflects that same state "upward" into the psyche. It can thus be seen that every phenomenon in the human system, whether harmonious or disharmonious in character, is psychosomatic.

MORE EMPHASIS ON "HUMANISTIC" VALUES

In addition to viewing human life as a total system, the new theory of health commits itself explicitly to certain beliefs. The first is that the essence of the individual is spirit; that is, that each individual can be and needs to be part of an increasingly caring community that includes all other life, and especially other human beings.

Another vital belief is that one is responsible for one's condition and has the power to change it. Thinking of man as a total system implies that one can always change one's condition by changing one's attitude of mind; therefore, one is always responsible for one's condition. To combine this belief with the first is to realize that we can and must help one another discover our responsibility. To discover one's responsibility is to discover one's power. Helping others discover their power can be referred to as empowerment.

THE ETIOLOGY AND DURATION OF SYSTEMIC DISHARMONY

It has been the tendency of Western medicine to think that physical illness is caused primarily by physical factors. Consequently, treatment has been primarily by physical means, i.e., surgery and chemotherapy. There is increasing evidence, however, that the subjective system (psyche and spirit) can play a dominant role in the etiology of illness and in its duration.

There is evidence, for example, that the fast, competitive pace of life in industrialized countries appears to induce a general state of stress in the psychic system. This stress reflects itself into the somatic system, creating a general "alarm state" that predisposes it to certain "diseases of civilization." When this general level of stress in the environment is reinforced by events in life that are particularly stressful, the predisposition to disease is then even stronger, and may combine with physical conditions to produce disease. On the other hand, if the predisposing psychic stress remains below a certain threshold, one may fill oneself full of cigarette smoke and cholesterol and never develop either lung cancer or arteriosclerosis.

Furthermore, certain diseases may be associated with a particular psychological profile or with a particular life history that constitutes a psychological predisposition to the disease. There is much evidence, for instance, that cancer is associated with emotional deprivation and difficulties in relationships throughout life, a high capacity for control and for suppressing anger and resentment, and a traumatic crisis in a close relationship in the 6 to 18 months preceding the onset of the illness. The association of the "Type A" personality with cardiovascular disease is already well-known. Other apparently "purely somatic" diseases, such as arthritis, may turn out to be associated with predisposing psychological conditions.

Certain aspects of the belief system of the society and of health professionals as a group may also contribute to the continuation of certain illnesses and militate against a cure. Emphasis on chemotherapy and surgery, and the minimization of the role of psychic factors, encourage patients to feel powerless to affect their outcome. If one does not try to exercise one's power, then, of course, this becomes a self-fulfilling prophecy. In addition, the relative impersonality of the usual relationship between patient and health professional, together with the impersonal nature of the environment in most health-care facilities, repeats the conditions of emotional deprivation that are suspected to be behind certain forms of mental as well as physical illness (e.g., cancer). This impersonal atmosphere may actually contribute to the continuation of the illness. Furthermore, the generally accepted belief that illness is something completely negative may create a negative mind set, which is reflected in the physical system, and thereby contributes to the continuation of the illness.

THE REESTABLISHMENT AND MAINTENANCE OF SYSTEMIC HARMONY

New ways are being discovered to help fulfill previously neglected needs of the total system. Among these are the fulfillment of the systemic need for repose by various relaxation techniques, the fulfillment of emotional needs by the creation of a more personal environment in the health-care facility, and a more personal relationship between the health professional and the patient. There is also a growing awareness of the patient's spiritual need to see meaning both in the illness and in the total pattern of life. Moreover, health professionals are learning to encourage patients to consider themselves the primary agents in the healing process, with the health professionals taking the role of facilitator in what is essentially a self-healing process. The patient can become the principal agent in several ways: by looking at the illness as a message from the total system that

one has not been paying enough attention to systemic harmony; by making the decision to use the illness as an opportunity for self-renewal; by using the active visualization of health, together with the control of autonomic processes (e.g., biofeedback), to directly affect the somatic system; and by acting to create more harmonious human relationships and more harmonious physical environments in both the private and the public (e.g., work) spheres.

All these curative approaches should, of course, be integrated with more traditional techniques of chemotherapy and surgery when appropriate, and can also be used in a program of health maintenance. Obviously, the continuous "tuning" of all the subjective and environmental factors that make up a human life is a complex job. Much more attention needs to be given to how this can be done in an integrated manner.

In order to regain or maintain total systemic harmony, one may need the services of various kinds of medical professionals—a psychologist, a career counselor, a financial planner, a spiritual teacher, etc. What is needed is a total approach to life that can integrate all these services and that is tailored to the individual. This is what the Greeks referred to as *diaita* (from which comes our too-restricted word "diet"): a plan for the maintenance of systemic harmony that integrates all factors. There may indeed be a need for a "systemic harmonist," a new kind of professional who could assist in this overall integration and planning.

Dick Andersen holds a master's degree in philosophy and religion; is an educational planner for the University of California; and is a partner in a consulting firm that teaches life-work planning, a framework for harmonious integration of all aspects of life. His interest in new trends in medicine is part of his interest in the harmony of the total life system.

For an extensive, free bibliography that Mr. Andersen has made available, send a stamped, legal-size, self-addressed envelope to:
Holistic Medicine Bibliography
University of California Extension Media Center
Berkeley, CA 94720.

The Roots of Holistic Healing

Barbara Einzig

The roots of holistic healing reach deep into the body of knowledge and experience of world culture, from antiquity to the present day. Ms. Einzig examines the cultural, philosophic, and socioeconomic precedents of the holistic health movement. With the rise of the Industrial Revolution and scientific medicine, rich natural healing traditions were plowed under. Today, the perennial seeds of noninvasive, nontoxic healing are germinating. The healthy beliefs and practices of our ancestors offer us a valuable resource to draw upon to address our modern manifestations of dis-ease.

"We wanted
more of our life to live in us.
To imagine each other."

Denise Levertov[1]

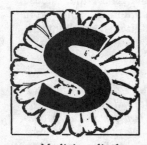 ometimes one dreams of being in a familiar house and discovering for the first time a room which had always been there. Tracing some broad outlines of holistic healing and following these back in time is a similar experience.

Medicine displays a serpent coiled about a staff—the emblem of Asclepius, the Greek god of medicine. Asclepius' teacher was the centaur Cheiron ("hand"), who is, appropriately, linked with the skills of surgery. But the high visibility of the Asclepian tradition in waiting rooms eclipses the fact that all the Greek gods possessed healing attributes. Artemis, protector of women and children; Hygeia, goddess of health; Panacea, healer of all ills; Aphrodite, protector of sexual life—all had places in the pantheon. Pan, Juno, Neptune, Bacchus, Hecate, the Fates—they all caused and averted disease, but have become invisible or survive only in distorted reputations. Although to tell their stories would be beyond the scope of this article, the evocation of their names may metaphoric-ally suggest the wealth of healing traditions it is possible for us to recover.

Holistic health is not a change in what is being prescribed, but a more radical change in attitudes and perceptions. As such, it is part of a larger recognition of the underlying relatedness of all life. This recognition develops as we come to sense a spiritual impoverishment in the so-called "developed nations," and come to see the limitations of industrial and scientific models. Relative to the beginning of the human species, these models are quite recent—of seventeenth- and eighteenth-century vintage. To many of us, thinking about it for the first time, holistic health appears to be a new field. The kind of treatment received at a doctor's office or at a hospital is often thought of as "traditional medicine." But from the historical point of view, holistic health is actually a very old field which is being plowed anew, and it is "traditional medicine" that is startlingly young. (The latter is often called "modern medicine," "Western medicine," or "scientific medicine," terms which are misleading for reasons well-stated by the medical anthropologist Charles Leslie, whose alternative term, "cosmopolitan medicine," we will be using in this article.[2])

Today almost all systems of health care in the world are based on holistic concepts that integrate body, mind, and environment. These systems continue traditions that evolved during antiquity. At the end of the Middle Ages, the rise of the experimental method and of forms of professional association led to a break with ancient traditions and to the eventual formation of cosmopolitan medicine as we know it today. In the United States this system of medicine won its victory over other therapeutic approaches at the turn of this century. The triumph was so complete that alternative approaches were relegated to categories which then appeared irregular, superstitious—"quack."

But the body politic can also be viewed holistically. Our many ways of imagining the human body find natural expression in different health systems. There are benefits to be gained from pluralism, and in other countries cosmopolitan medicine coexists and cooperates with alternative therapies. For example, Kanpo medicine, Chinese traditional medicine in Japan, has gained increasing strength parallel with the development of modern medicine. Holistic health recognizes the valid contributions of cosmopolitan medicine, particularly in the treatment of accidents (broken bones, burns) and infectious diseases, situations in which medicine's philosophy of fast, heroic intervention is appropriate. The nineteenth-century advances in the germ-theory of disease and in surgical techniques were certainly impressive, but even then the limitations of the scientific model were recognized by those with larger vision. As the poet Walt Whitman wrote:

"Hurray for positive science! long live exact
　　demonstration!
. . . This is the geologist, this works with the
　　scalpel,
and this is a mathematician.

Gentlemen, to you the first honors always!
Your facts are useful, and yet they are not my
　　dwelling,
I but enter by them to an area of my
　　dwelling."[3]

The field of holistic health encompasses many viewpoints and procedures which have been cast out by cosmopolitan medicine in the last 150 years. We will suggest the relevance of a few of these historical orientations by giving four characteristics of holistic healing and then looking at their historic precedents. The relevance of poetic traditions to wholism will be suggested by quotations.

HOLISTIC HEALTH FOCUSES ON WELL-BEING RATHER THAN DISEASE

"As stone suffers of stoniness,
As light of its shiningness,
As birds of their wingedness,
So I of my whoness.

And what the cure of all this?
What the not and not suffering?
What the better and later of this?
What the more me of me?

How for the pain-world to be
More world and no pain?"

Laura Riding[4]

The word "health" is itself formed from the Anglo-Saxon hal, whole, and is defined as a "flourishing condition: well-being, vitality, prosperity."

Medicine, on the other hand, is something given as a remedy for disease. In the system of cosmopolitan medicine, disease is something foreign, a discrete clinical entity to be conquered and driven out, along with its pain. Sometimes this approach works, but more than half of those who seek physicians' services do not have medical disorders but bring their inevitable human suffering as a disease for medicine to cure.[5] The already overworked medical doctor has nothing in his or her black bag for these people. Nevertheless, their histories are taken—a strange, cold place for our culture's storytelling!—and they are "treated," perhaps prompting Immanuel Kant's statement: "Physicians think they are doing something for you by labeling what you have as a disease."[6] But what else can we do when "it hurts"?

Natural childbirth is a familiar illustration of a different approach to pain. By working with her pains, the mother tries to breathe rhythmically through them instead of screaming against them. If we are sensitive to the life within us, pain and diseased states can be viewed as manifestations of that life. In Japanese traditional medicine, ki is the "essence which sustains the body, which causes it to move and to live."[7] This power works invisibly and exists within everything in the universe. Ki can be translated as "nature," "spirit," or "feeling." Genki means cheerful, vigorous; kichigai, crazy, mad, of a different and disturbed spirit; ki no doku, pitiful or regrettable, literally, "the spirit is poisoned." So Japanese traditional medicine hears the same syllable, the same force, informing both positive and negative states. (The French poet Jean Cocteau recognized this unity of living/dying processes in his Orpheus. In this film, the angel Heurtebise says: "Spend your life looking at yourself in a mirror, and you'll see Death at work like a swarm of bees storing up honey in a hive of glass.")

The same dualistic philosophy is reflected in a Chinese proverb that tells us that the ancient sages did not treat those who were already ill; they instructed those who were not ill. According to the theoretical texts of Chinese traditional medicine, curing is not the ideal of medical practice. The good physician prevents his or her patients from becoming ill in the first place. The theories of the Five Evolutive Phases (wu shing) and of yin-yang are applied to the body. Complementary and mutually destructive powers are to be kept in equilibrium, and in this way disease is prevented. The Chinese system of healing embraces the patient's whole way of life. Diet, regular sleep, sex, and physical exercise are a comprehensive system of health practices.

HOLISTIC HEALING VIEWS NATURE AS A FRIEND, NOT AN ADVERSARY, AND IMAGINES THE BODY AS ONE WITH THE MIND AND SOUL

"He went from house to house dragging two metal ingots and everybody was amazed to see pots, pans, tongs, and braziers tumble down from their places and beams creak from the desperation of nails and screws trying to emerge, and even objects that had been lost for a long time appeared from where they had been searched for most and went dragging along in turbulent confusion behind Melquiades' magical irons. 'Things have a life of their own' the gypsy proclaimed with a harsh accent. 'It's simply a matter of waking up their souls.'"
Gabriel Garcia Marquez[8]

"Behold, the body includes and is the meaning, the main concern, and includes and is the soul. Whoever you are, how superb and how divine is your body, or any part of it!"
Walt Whitman[9]

Body, mind, and soul were conceived of as integral until seventeenth-century Cartesian philosophy created a division between mental and physical states. This division eventually led to the creation of separate physical- and mental-health systems in cosmopolitan medicine. Such a division of body and mind was paralleled by a division of the material and spiritual worlds. But the very first natural philosophers, although recognizing mind and matter, did not regard them as mutually exclusive and did not attempt to "conquer nature" (mind over matter). There was gross matter that could be grasped and handled, and then a series of grades of ever-subtler matter, ranging from mists, clouds, and smoke through exhalations, air, ether, and the animal spirits, to the soul and spiritual beings.

History is rich with images of an ensouled universe. Thales said that all things are full of gods; Empedocles witnessed that "effluences flow from all things that come into being"; more recently, Blake exults, "Everything that lives is holy." When Hippocrates states in *De nutrimento* that "All things conspire together as one, all flow together in a single confluence, all suffer in sympathy, each with the other," his statement is a window into a world view which saw the Earth echoing the sky, faces reflected in stars, and plants holding secrets of healing. This was (and is!) a world of correspondences.

With Beauty Before Me
Traditional Navajo Prayer

With beauty before me may I walk
With beauty behind me may I walk
With beauty above me may I walk
With beauty below me may I walk
With beauty all around me may I walk
As one who is for long life and happiness
May I walk
In beauty it is finished
In beauty it is finished
Traditional Navajo prayer

"Let it not be said: this is cold, this warm, this moist, this dry, but rather let it be said: This is Saturn, this Mars, this Venus, this the Pole-star." This is a statement of the extraordinary Paracelsus, a physician who wandered about in the Western and Arabic worlds of the sixteenth century. His writings on alchemy instruct us that the duty of the physician is to discover the inner virtues of things and to extract from them the vital elixirs of alchemy and occult botany. Microcosm and macrocosm (the theory of the two worlds) are in constant relation. Paracelsus called the universe "exterior man" and saw in the body processes corresponding to metallic sublimation, combustion, and reduction to ashes. It is very difficult to give a brief summary of the complex, ancient, and varied traditions of alchemy, but alchemy may be roughly described as an attempt to get at the soul of things.[10] The famous attempts to turn lead into gold were less efforts to strike it rich than metaphysical refinements of the golden essence within the basest metal. Thus, out of the tradition of alchemical refinement we inherit not only the practical art of distilling alcohol, but also the more metaphoric art of bringing things into right relationship.

HOLISTIC HEALING IMAGINES THE BODY IN RELATION TO EVERY-BODY AND TO THE ENVIRONMENT

If all life is related, then everybody must be seen in relation to one another and to the man-made, as well as natural, world. States of illness and of health must be viewed in this "context" (a telling word, coming from the root "to weave together," i.e., to make whole). This means that some sense of what is now bracketed off as "sociology" and "ecology" enters our health thinking. The contextual view enables us to perceive imbalanced relationships (such as asbestos/cancer) and also gives positive texture to our lives. Such a texture is suggested in the Pythagorean tradition. Aristotle speaks of a Pythagorean doctrine which maintains that an intimate relationship unites all living beings on the Earth. Pythagoras mentions particularly the passage of the soul into animals of different species in various periods, and the relationships of all animal beings.

Looking at the study of health care as a discipline gives us some idea of how recently cosmopolitan medicine has subdivided the corpus of knowledge. The time of Hippocrates (fifth to fourth century, B.C.) was one in which medicine, science, philosophy, and history were not viewed as separate disciplines, but as one great discourse. One of the central themes of this discourse was healing and wholeness.

In contrast, the schism between body and environment is reflected in the training of cosmopolitan medical practitioners. In 1910, Abraham Flexner published his highly influential findings on all existing medical schools. Until that time economics and sociology had often been included in the medical curriculum, continuing the Hippocratic inclusiveness. But Flexner declared biochemistry and physiology to be the only "basic sciences." So it was that cosmopolitan medicine became a medicine of the individual, and population medicine, which deals with whole communities, was relegated to schools of public health. Some researchers have speculated that this move arose from commercial motivations: a community may suffer from disease but, in our cultural arrangement, have no immediate way of purchasing its health. Individual medicine, however, has a ready market, and is currently referred to by hospital administrators as an industry.

HOLISTIC HEALING RESPECTS AND CULTIVATES THE PATIENT'S KNOWLEDGE OF HIS OR HER OWN BODY

Hippocrates wrote, in *On Aliment,* that "Nature acts without masters." Because holistic healing recognizes the basic authority of the patient over his or her own body, the health worker becomes less an expert and more a facilitator or educator. The knowledge of the health/disease of the body comes not only from so-called "objective" data (physical examination, laboratory tests, etc.), but also directly from the patient's experience. For example, in the modern Chinese sanatorium, the patient keeps a diary in writing, including a description of each phase of his or her illness, and notes on any progress or signs of relapse; this diary takes its place among the medical findings and clinical histories compiled by the doctors and nurses.[11]

Such a cooperative relationship between patient and healer hearkens back to Plato, who tells us that the physician talks with the patient and with the patient's friends and in this manner learns from the sufferer while he gives instruction. Respect for the patient's knowledge of his or her own body has been the dominant healing tradition. The eminence of "doctor's orders" in our times belies their newness. Where do they come from, these orders based on a hermetic knowledge which we as patients cannot hope to understand, but must, for the sake of our lives, obey? They come from a view of disease as verifiable entity or object. Diagnosis fits the dark chaos of what is happening in the body into a disease idea amenable to "standard operating procedure," often losing sight of the fact that no two diseases are ever identical.

This overcoming of the body's darkness by means of classification arose from that same Cartesian philosophy of the seventeenth century that was responsible for the mind/body split, a philosophy which Rene Dubos identifies as the philosophical base for modern science. He points out that its method is to subdivide anatomic structures, physiological functions, and biological processes into small and smaller subunits in order to study each of them separately and in greater detail.[12]

The French philosopher Michel Foucault links this "great break in the history of Western medicine" with the opening of the dark body to the light of day.[13] Autopsy is a fundamental change in the method of knowing disease. It became important at the beginning of the nineteenth century. Before that time, a physician's knowledge of disease always came from the living, as Plato had advised. A medical history, heard holistically, is a physical, psychological, and spiritual report. It is a complex document which yields the kind of powerful but uncertain knowledge that careful listening and sympathy evoke. But when knowledge comes from a dead body, we have less feeling but a more certain image of disease. In 1803, Bichat wrote:

"For twenty years, from morning to night, you have taken notes at patients' bedsides on affections of the heart, the lungs, and the gastric viscera, and all is confusion for you in the symptoms which, refusing to yield up their meaning, offer you a succession of incoherent phenomena. Open up a few corpses: you will dissipate at once the darkness that observation alone could not dissipate."[14]

The privilege of violating the dead (and the power violation of such a taboo confers) is at the base of the M.D.'s status as "expert."

CONCLUSION

History is a process of inquiry and reinterpretation. Classical sources usually linked to cosmopolitan medicine also may be seen as sources of holistic healing. For example, Hippocrates is known as the Father of Medicine, but could just as well be known as the Father of Holistic Healing. Such a contradiction is hardly surprising, when we consider that Hippocrates was claimed and invoked by many historic schools of medicine which differed markedly from each other— the Dogmatics, Empirics, Skeptics, and Galen.

Neglected or reviled sources may have been cast out of conventional history because of a fairly recent political or philosophical prejudice. The lost members of the Greek healing pantheon find their historical parallel, for instance, in the witch-healers. The latter were, in the Middle Ages, "often the only general medical practitioners for a people who were bitterly afflicted with poverty and disease."[15] These wise women worked within the community as practical midwives and herbalists. Many of their herbal remedies have found places in modern pharmacology.

As part of the revival of holistic thinking, the contributions of traditions once neglected because of prejudice are being re-valued. New studies are also reintegrating some of the traditions outlined here with cosmopolitan medicine. Broadening our temporal perspective increases our consciousness of how the progress brought about by scientific and industrial models (outgrowths of Cartesian philosophy) has weakened more holistic, historical attitudes. It also makes possible a strengthening and recovery of those attitudes, which are today gaining new interest and respect.

NOTES

1. Denise Levertov, "The Cold Spring," in *Relearning the Alphabet*. New Directions, 1970.
2. Charles Leslie, ed., *Asian Medical Systems: A Comparative Study*. University of California Press, 1976.
3. Walt Whitman, "Song of Myself," in *Whitman Selected by Robert Creeley*. Penguin, 1973.
4. Laura Riding, "The Wind Suffers," in *Selected Poems: in Five Sets*. Norton, 1970.
5. See Rick J. Carlson, *The End of Medicine*. Wiley, 1975.
6. *Ibid.*
7. Leslie, *Asian Medical Systems*. University of California Press, 1976.
8. Gabriel Garcia Marquez, *One Hundred Years of Solitude*, translated by Gregory Rabassa. Avon, 1970.
9. Walt Whitman, "Starting from Paumanok," in *Whitman Selected by Robert Creeley*. Penguin, 1973.
10. See Allen G. Debus, *The Chemical Philosophy: Paracelsian Science and Medicine in the Sixteenth and Seventeenth Centuries*. Science History Publications, 1977.
11. Stephan Palos, *The Chinese Art of Healing*, translated by Translagency, Ltd. Herder and Herder, 1971.
12. Rene Dubos, *Man Adapting*. Yale University Press, 1965.
13. Michel Foucault, *The Birth of the Clinic: An Archaeology of Medical Perception*. Pantheon, 1973.
14. As quoted in *ibid.*
15. Barbara Ehrenreich and Deirdre English, *Witches, Midwives, and Nurses: A History of Women Healers*. Glass Mountain, 1973.

SUGGESTIONS FOR FURTHER READING

Charles Singer, *Science, Medicine, and History*. Arno Press, 1975.

Arthur Edward Waite, *The Hermetic and Alchemical Writings of Paracelsus*. Shambhala, 1976.

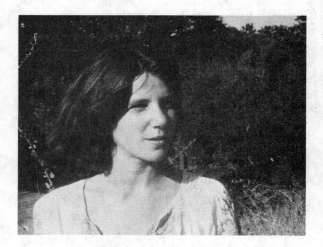

Barbara Einzig has worked as a manuscript editor for the University of California Press, Panjandrum Press, and TRATEC of Los Angeles; she has worked on narration for Umbrella, *a PBS documentary, and collaborated on a study of medical training in the United States at the UCLA Medical Center. Her translations of Russian literature have appeared in many journals. Two books of hers have been published to date:* Color *(Membrane Press, 1976), and* Disappearing Work *(The Figures, 1979).*

The American Popular Health Movement
Alex Binik

This article discusses the rise and fall of the mass-based health movement during the nineteenth century in the United States. The issues debated and struggled with during that era, especially the questions of licensing and the free choice of health-care delivery systems, persist in large measure today.

The rivalry between popular medicine, with its grass-roots supporters, and the emerging American Medical Association, with business and governmental backing, is an instructive historical footnote to our contemporary advocacy of an integrated approach to health and medicine.

ew ideas seldom arise out of a total void. Indeed, the holistic health movement is based largely on principles that underlie the healing arts of more than 2,000 years, both in the Western world and in the Orient. Sociologically, holistic health has a more recent predecessor: a nineteenth-century, mass-based health movement in the United States. The issues debated and struggled over during that period—especially questions of licensing and of the right of individuals to choose their form of health care—persist today. Perhaps an examination of this movement—its rise and ebb—will be useful in addressing current health-care issues.

Among the white settlers in North America, before and shortly after the Revolutionary War, healing work was primarily an informal, nonprofessional activity. As in England, only enough university-trained doctors were available to treat the upper classes; the rest of the population relied upon self-treatment or assistance from lay healers with local reputations, often women (e.g., herbalists, apothecaries, midwives, etc.). These non-physicians, who came to be known as "irregulars" or "botanic doctors," were almost always trained by means of apprenticeships. They lived and worked for the most part in the countryside or in small towns, and often did other kinds of work in addition to practicing the healing arts. And payment for their services, often as not, was in the form of goods or services rather than cash. The techniques of the "irregulars" were primarily those of "nature cure": diet, sweating, and herbs (including Native American remedies).

The so-called "regular doctors," on the other hand, were typically graduates of British medical colleges with no clinical facilities; by 1780 there were enough of them practicing in the cities and larger towns to form a small medical elite that relied on the money economy. They based their "heroic medicine," as it was called, nearly exclusively on massive amounts of calomel (a drug based on mercury), opium, and bloodletting. The term "heroic" was perhaps most appropriate in referring to their patients, for whom extensive trauma was common, and recovery unlikely.

By the early nineteenth century, the "regulars" began to feel the pinch of competition for sufficiently well-heeled patients, both from their own increasing numbers and, to a great degree, from the lay healers (who also tended to charge lower fees). In most states the physicians managed to achieve sufficient influence to gain enactment of licensing laws (the same was true for lawyers). By 1825 the majority of states had passed statutes making medicine a legal practice only when licensed or with permission from a medical society. Typical laws banned practice by herbalists; violators were fined and imprisoned. A New York law of 1818 required one year of training under an *approved* doctor; by 1919 the law was amended to require *four* years of training. According to one medical historian, "Laws were passed in the different states clearly resembling in spirit, as well as in form, those providing for the discovery and punishment of witches." To protect their economic interests, the regulars allied themselves with their legislators, with whom they typically shared social circles.

The new licensing laws threatened not only the botanic healers themselves, but also their patients. The majority of Americans could not afford the services of an "approved" physician, and were in many cases opposed to the officially sanctioned treatments. Further, in the rural areas of the country (by far the largest regions) legal treatment was virtually non-existent; most of the "regulars" had chosen to remain in the cities and larger towns. Rural women, traditionally responsible for the health of their families, found even their access to relevant information cut off. Women also suffered from being suddenly denied legal right to practice midwifery or other forms of healing arts. The officially sanctioned medical schools did not admit women.

Out of this rampant popular dissatisfaction there emerged what soon assumed the proportions of a social movement. This social and political revolt mobilized a broad spectrum of Americans to challenge the official health-care system—at first informally (by their own health practices), and later by direct pressure on their state governments. Today it is generally referred to as the Popular Health Movement (PHM).

The largest and most organized group within the PHM was known as the Thomsonians. Their leader, Samuel Thomson, was born into a poor farming family in New Hampshire in 1769. His introduction to the study of healing occurred as a young boy, by way of a local woman herbalist. He later began his medical practice, not as a conscious profession, but gradually and in response to need. In this respect he was similar to many or most of his followers. He had watched his mother die after treatment by "regular doctors," who, he said:

> "gave her over and gave her disease the name of galloping consumption, which I thought was a very appropriate name; for they are the riders, and their whip is mercury, opium, and Vitriol, and they galloped her out of the world in about nine weeks."

After seeing regular physicians unable to treat his wife and children adequately for a number of serious illnesses, he increasingly began serving as their family doctor. Neighbors began to turn to him for assistance, and his treatments were so successful that his reputation quickly spread over a wide area. (By 1814 he was practicing and lecturing as far away as Philadelphia.) He believed that the body would heal itself, once free of toxic accumulations; to this end he used sweating, vomiting, and enemas, as well as restorative herbal teas.

Thomson was committed to teaching people the fundamentals of preventive medicine and self-treatment; to this end, in 1811, while in Maine, he founded the first Friendly Botanic Society (FBS). Members were taught the nature of his theories and practice, and were provided with a stock of his medicines to use. Similar organizations soon sprang up throughout New England and then throughout the country. Within each FBS, people gathered to exchange cures and herbs and to obtain treatment advice for particular illnesses. Occasionally, guest speakers were invited to talk on some pertinent medical issue. Simple language was emphasized both in such lectures and in the FBS journals. And each member assumed the responsibility to treat and educate any other member in need.

By 1832 the Friendly Botanic Societies were linked in a nationwide FBS organization that was to assume pivotal importance in the political struggles to come. In that year they held a convention to compare experiences and treatments of the massive cholera epidemic that was sweeping the country. Their treatments proved to be tremendously more effective than those of the regular doctors, and millions of Americans joined the burgeoning movement. Other forms of the Popular Health Movement were also in the upswing, sharing a common rejection of the calomel and bleeding treatments. Notably, in many cities, self-help clinics known as Ladies' Physiological Societies came into being, and served much of the public. The Thomsonians, though, appear to have been the most organized, the most outspokenly anti-elitest, and the largest group. (Of a total U.S. population of about 17 million, they claimed four million adherents.) Meanwhile, countless regular physicians began adopting some Thomsonian principles and techniques.

The larger the Popular Health Movement became, the more pronounced became the efforts of the regulars to limit competition. For example, in 1827 a law was passed in New York State preventing unlicensed practitioners from practicing; as a result, many irregulars were jailed. The following year, Thomson's son, John, set out to have the measure repealed by forming an alliance with the radical Jacksonian "Workingman's Party" and the "eclectic"[1] movement. Despite the tremendous mass pressure that was created, the repeal was repeatedly stalled in the New York Assembly, where the regular physicians were strongly entrenched. Finally, after 16 years of struggle, Thomson was able in 1844 to present the legislature with a mass of repeal petitions signed by the majority of the state's voters, and victory was achieved. Similar fights were concurrently waged successfully in many other states, and by 1844, their organization and hard work had paid off: most states had repealed all their restrictive medical legislation.

Already, though, other forces were at work which would eventually lead to the reinstatement of these laws. A major divisive element arose *within* the ranks of the Popular Health Movement and was instrumental in its demise. This was the increasing number of "professional" irregular healers who were concerned about gaining official "respectability" for themselves and their work. In seeking legitimization by the wealthy elite, they chose to achieve a more polished and learned image. Splits occurred within the Thomsonian movement; rival Botanic Societies and schools of higher education were formed, and "accreditation" was demanded. Samuel Thomson was outraged, expressing the fear that, because of this tendency, "the benefit of my discoveries will be taken from the people generally, and like all other crafts monopolized by a few learned individuals." However, the move away from the "every man his own doctor" approach was gaining adherents everywhere, many opportunistically seeking status and economic power. In fact, John Thomson himself, in the aforementioned licensing struggle, had at times sought *not* repeal of the laws entirely, but rather inclusion of professional Thomsonians.[2] And with the abandonment of emphasis on layperson education, the movement began to lose much of its mass political strength.

This move toward "professional" respectability and status was echoed by the eclectic physicians and the homeopaths. Each group founded its own medical societies and schools, and sought to increase its influence on the well-to-do. By the second half of the nineteenth century, the homeopaths and eclectics in New York and Boston were among the most cultured, wealthy, and well-educated physicians, serving a clientele much like themselves.

Meanwhile, another group of physicians with similar class interests was gaining prominence. These were the European-trained "scientific physicians," who were greatly influenced by the "germ theory" of specific, single-factor disease etiology. These doctors also came to represent the increased use of surgery and the focus on specialized parts of the body for their research and practice.

The regulars had formed the American Medical Association in 1848, to fight not only the botanic healers but also the "sectarians" (i.e., eclectics and homeopaths). Now, however, they were being opposed by their own "scientific elite," who saw a coalition with these influential groups as the sure way to reinstate the licensing laws. When the scientific physicians threatened to pull out of the AMA and form their own organizations, the regulars gave in. The coalition that resulted had sufficient political power to get new laws passed in most states (between 1880 and 1900) regulating the practice of medicine. State licensing boards were set up, consisting of regulars, homeopaths, and eclectics.

By 1901 the scientific elite was firmly established as the reigning power group within the AMA. A Council on Medical Education was formed in 1904 to "elevate standards." And in 1910 the Carnegie Foundation issued its Flexner Report, which concluded that most U.S. medical schools were grossly inadequate. Johns Hopkins, a bastion of the new scientific approaches, was to be the model for future medical education. And only those schools which followed that model (necessarily raising dramatically the cost of medical education) could receive foundation support.

A major effect of this report was the subsequent closing of nearly all the numerous homeopathic, eclectic, botanic, women's, and Black medical schools throughout the country. These schools had typically been operating on a slim financial margin already, and could not survive the cutoff of outside funds. Thereupon, the opportunity to be trained for and practice a medical career could be directly restricted by admissions standards and quotas. And, for at least the next 50 years, such opportunities were effectively closed to nearly all but the middle- or upper-class white male. With the uniformity of standards and selection, a further control was also achieved: only one set of basic philosophical attitudes toward healing was presented. Moreover, these did not even need to be stated explicitly, but, rather, could be treated as *the* underlying reality; scientific method, technology, and *truth* were to be presented as facets of one unity. The physician was trained to believe that all truth emanated from medical laboratories and was thereupon passed on via medical training. Thus, for example, if doctors were not trained in nutrition, then —a priori—nutrition could not be a major factor in health or illness.

Happily, this situation is undergoing change today. Medical schools are beginning to emphasize a return to family practice, and some are including courses in nutrition, "bedside manner," and holistic philosophy. However, other modalities remain beyond the pale of medical education—particularly those such as acupuncture and homeopathy, for which medical science cannot yet conceive any sort of biochemical explanation.

This history raises several major questions about our current experience:

1. To what degree do current licensing laws *actually* protect the public? To what degree do these

laws serve to buttress entrenched interests and stall positive change?

2. Can we find methods to unmonopolize the provision of health care and education—to provide the public with freedom of choice and opportunity for self-responsibility, while still offering some level of protection?

3. Will the increased professional recognition of holistically oriented practitioners serve to absorb dissent into a multi-billion-dollar industry, or will the movement continue to focus on the empowerment of the public?

I believe the kinds of decisions our society ultimately makes about these and similar questions will help shape the direction of future health care.

NOTES

1. These were medical reformers who believed in combining botanic and regular medicine on pragmatic grounds.
2. He, however, was forced by Workingman's Party pressure to move for complete repeal.

SUGGESTIONS FOR FURTHER READING

In compiling this history, I found an especially valuable resource in an unpublished book by Altman, Kuhin, Kwasnik, and Logan, *The People's Healers.* Other useful references were the following.

Harris Coulter, *Divided Legacy—A History of the Schism in Medical Thought.* Wehawken Books, 3 vols., 1973-77.

Barbara Ehrenreich and Deirdre English, *Witches, Midwives, and Nurses.* Feminist Press, 1973.

William Rothstein, *American Physicians in the 19th Century: From Sects to Science.* Johns Hopkins University Press, 1972.

Richard Shryock, *Medical Licensing in America, 1650-1965.* Johns Hopkins University Press, 1967.

———, *Development of Modern Medicine.* Knopf, 1947.

———, *Medicine and Society in America, 1660-1860.* New York University Press, 1960.

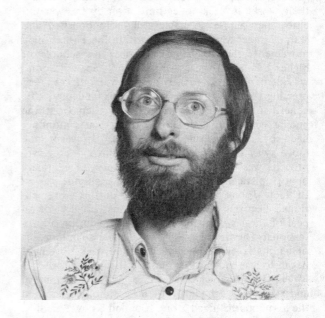

Alex Binik is a practitioner of stress reduction and bodywork, health and lifestyle counseling, and emotional-process work. He has a special interest in the role that myth and meaningful ritual may play in facilitating wholeness in our lives, and is cofounder of PassageWays Center for Myth and Ritual (Berkeley, California), which assists people in ceremonially marking significant life-transitions.

Holistically Oriented Politics
and the Holistic Health Practitioners' Association:
A Model for Personal and Social Health
Steven Jay Markell

The term "self-responsibility" expresses a fundamental axiom of holistic health. It pervades other aspects of New Age thought and action, including lifestyle, health hygiene and habits, mental growth, emotional expression, and political action. Furthermore, the business community, the health and medical industries, and the government are all examining the concepts of self-responsibility and self-care as possible remedies to such problems as the question of blame in medical malpractice, workplace hazards, and environmental pollution and destruction.

This article clarifies the view of the holistic community toward self-responsibility and social health, and includes a recent history and analysis of trends emerging and likely to emerge in the future.

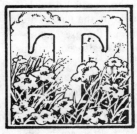

he last few years have seen an explosion in and around the health field. The proliferation of practitioners offering a cornucopia of alternative, nontraditional, and nonmedical healing arts and health education has been massive. Pressure has increased from clients, patients, consumers, and government who want the health and medical industries to change their style and reduce the high price of health- and disease-care delivery by adding more humanistic, "whole person," and preventive services that pose less risk to their recipients. One need only pick up a newspaper or popular magazine on any day of the year, and the evidence for this demand presents itself loudly and clearly.

At the same time, Americans are asking more questions of their health- and disease-care providers and are becoming increasingly involved in their own care. "Do it to me" is less and less the basis for the provider-patient relationship. In experiencing self-responsibility, people are discovering that by participating in more decision-making, they are helping themselves to get well.

In answer to this rapid expansion of interest and the subsequent lag of available services, a new category of people who are developing professional practices in these alternative healing arts and roles has emerged. They come from diverse backgrounds, including the traditional medical and allied fields, teaching careers, social and human services, as well as directly from high schools, colleges, and graduate and professional schools. People of all ages, political, social, and religious persuasions, in looking for new direction and meaning in their own lives, have discovered the holistic health field as a vehicle for personal and vocational development. People can walk into classes or conferences and learn beneficial and powerful skills to help themselves and others, and pass on these tools and knowledge, in turn, to clients and students. All of this has offered a boost to the health-care community, *until recently*.

Competition is one of the basic principles of a healthy free-market system. However, this ballooning effect has led to some major problems:

1. Many people are calling themselves holistic practitioners. Some may actually *be* holistic in their work; most are not.

2. Unreliable or poorly skilled people are misleading consumers in their search for better health and disease care.

3. Consumers are patronizing anyone who uses the term holistic, hoping these practitioners will not treat them in the same ways that their regular physicians do.

4. False hopes are raised by poorly developed or scientifically untested techniques;

5. Within the provider community the gap is widening between lay and licensed practitioners, creating tensions and increased lack of communication between the two.

The influx of unconventionally trained "health professionals" has also directed new attention to the quality of care being offered by them and by the orthodox medical system. Do these lay providers have adequate skills and insights to perceive the limits of their own abilities? For that matter, are nontraditional approaches any safer when applied by licensed professionals? Can the public be assured of quality care and assistance from both lay and licensed practitioners in a manner more equitable than the current system used by the State Boards of Medical Examiners and Quality Assurance to police the traditional ranks against malpractice and medical quackery?[1]

Benefits gained by posing these questions include the following:

1. Previously unscrutinized values are now receiving attention in both business and government policy-making circles.

2. Crucial research fields are expanding to explore the definition of optimal health, rather than limiting study to the nature and control of disease.[2]

3. The prevention, rather than merely treatment, of chronic degenerative disease is becoming a focus of research.

4. Methodical study is underway to discover and explore less toxic or nontoxic alternatives to conventional treatment of illness.

5. The tendency to relegate decision-making to experts and the courts is gradually reversing.

More people are acknowledging the dis-ease within the health and medical (disease-care) community and the limits of "objective analysis." These people are seeking to develop *political* strategies for cleansing, rebalancing, and rebuilding our health-care system, knowing that true dysfunction can only be effectively addressed at its root, not just at the level of symptom.

A MULTI-DIMENSIONAL RESPONSE

Response to this concern has been fourfold. First, the medical community has initiated numerous investigations, often employing nonscientific methods to evaluate nonorthodox tools. Lay and nontraditional licensed practitioners have experienced harassment and prosecution by medical societies and licensure boards, who are bent on repressing nontraditional health practices. Charges have included practicing medicine without a license, being a public nuisance, and murder.[3] Second, legislators and regulatory boards at the state level are reviewing and redefining the practice of medicine and the medical licensure system, to see if they can include and control the rapidly growing community of holistically oriented providers, perhaps by creating another licensed niche within the existing system, or an alternative licensure system that would include all practices. Third, lay and nontraditional providers are organizing themselves into professional societies that address these

concerns, and are developing solutions that include *self-responsibly* from *within* their peer group, rather than expecting policies and regulations to come from *without* (as in the two previous responses). In California, for example, acupuncturists, masseuses, and midwives, by forming special-interest pressure groups, have generated legislation that works *against* independent professional recognition. The resultant misdirected judicial decrees (excluding the Doshi case in San Luis Obispo; see *Holistic Health Review,* Spring 1979) have caused loss to these practitioners and their clients. Practitioners continue to cope with the side-effects of these actions. Fourth, the lay-practioner community has been forced deeper "underground" in some areas, and open, honest practice has become more difficult.

IMPACT UNFOLDING

The effects of public and professional interest in holistic health continue to grow. Conferences have been held in Washington, D.C., for the federal government, and in Sacramento and Berkeley, California, and other local communities for the state government. Congressionally chartered offices are holding hearings on "The New Health Technologies." Legislators and regulatory boards throughout the nation are voicing concern for public safety as the use of nonorthodox philosophies and tools in health education and promotion, as well as in disease treatment and prevention, increases. Federally funded research projects are measuring, dissecting, and developing new models of professional training and practice; an example is the National Institute of Mental Health's funding of the Collaborative Health Program in San Francisco, California. National health insurance and health service legislation is boiling on the dockets of both houses of Congress. Professional associations are underway nationwide, including the American Holistic Medical Association, the Association for Holistic Health, the American Holistic Nursing Association, the Alternative Medical Association, the National Council on Wholistic Therapeutics. Holistic health associations have formed in Canada; Washington State; Sacramento, San Diego, and San Francisco, California; Tucson, Arizona; Austin, Texas; New England; New York; the Princeton area of New Jersey; and Colorado. Hundreds of schools in every corner of the United States offer training, certification, or degrees through residential and correspondence courses in many of the holistic principles and practices.

Although limelighting the need for medical diversity, this fascination with holistic health has also revealed the lack of cohesion within the newly forming field. There is a scarcity of the generally acknowledged definitions, axioms, standards, and checks and balances that are usually found within traditional medical schools of thought and professions. There is a growing demand for quality assurance, greater accountability, and public access to these providers. When there is enough public demand to meet these conditions, the government will attempt to answer the outcry. Officials will ask the "experts" what to do. Will the holistic health field have its own team of experts primed and ready, with refined strategies backed by an organized constituency? Or will the prevailing economic and political influences and special-interest groups dictate policy for governing the holistic field?

ADDRESSING THESE ISSUES

The active and vocal practitioner constituency in the San Francisco Bay Area is preparing to play an influencial role in the formation of government policy. They have formed the Holistic Health Practitioner's Association (HHPA) to address these very issues.

Members of the HHPA are discussing the concept that their own professional well-being depends on guaranteed freedom of choice for themselves and for their clients. Hence, they are taking steps now in an effort to prevent later legal and health policy disputes. Members are taking an active, self-responsible role in public protection, in order to assure that the State of California takes a truly responsible and balanced position. In the past, the state legislative bodies have been greatly influenced by the state's largest lobbying body, the California Medical Association. The HHPA can provide strong leadership by offering a methodical and scientific framework in which to examine the myriad approaches and techniques in the holistic collection.

LIVING HOLISTICALLY

The holistic perspective on dealing with and solving problems considers the impact of their physical, emotional, mental, spiritual, and environmental (including ecological, political, and cultural) aspects. Members of HHPA are applying this model to health, the practice of health education and care, and their own lives. To be fully consistent with the advice and counsel offered to clients, holistically oriented health-care practitioners pursue physical, emotional, mental, and spiritual health, and are actively involved in healing the environment. Ecologically, their awareness tends to be more developed than that of traditional health providers. They frequent recycling centers, minimize their contribution to pollution, and support related economic concerns. Culturally, they participate in community/ethnic/religious activities. Politically, they support the causes of choice, participate in discussion groups, lobby their governmental representatives, vote, attend rallies, etc.

The HHPA is also addressing the need to integrate the recognition, legitimization, and utilization of alternative therapies and approaches into available health care. This your.g organization is concerned with access to holistic practices in the Third World, as well as for youngsters and elders; reimbursement for holistic therapies by third-party payment systems; arbitration of disputes between providers and consumers; and coordination of resources, such as in the areas of funding, research, and networking.

HHPA committees meet monthly to develop position statements on ethics, standards of practice and training, and definitions of holistic health and practice. Additional committees convene to discuss primary and continuing education for practitioners, communication and public outreach, organizational development, legality of holistic practice, contracts in practice, and facility collaboration.

Underpinning the HHPA structure is its members' insistence that the association reflect in its framework and process the values expressed within the holistic perspective. Meetings and activities are personally and socially rewarding and healing. The HHPA deals with key issues such as: how to have an inclusive membership policy rather than an elitist one; how to encourage member practitioners to "practice what they preach"; how to make decisions that incorporate and balance each member's view; how to have freedom of choice in offering and seeking care while maintaining quality; how to decide who may be called (or call themselves) a holistic health practitioner.[4]

The HHPA was initiated in the San Francisco Bay Area and is currently concentrating on local, grassroots organization. However, once the financial and organizational foundation is laid, membership will be expanded throughout California. Concern for the thoroughness and professionalism of its actions and image has judiciously guided HHPA's growth. Each county and state has its own individual characteristics and needs for the formation of a professional organi-

Implications of Holistic Health
George Leonard

We have a situation in which almost every new triumph in surgery and life-support brings the system nearer to bankruptcy without adding very much at all to general life expectancy or well-being.

Let's face it, powerful new drugs won't solve the problem; they may make it worse. Miraculous new surgical and life-support techniques won't solve the problem and may make it worse. National health insurance, though perhaps humane and needed, won't solve the problem, but may make it worse by strengthening

Reprinted from *The Journal of Holistic Health,* Vol. 3. By permission of The Mandala Society and The Association for Holistic Health, P.O. Box 1233, Del Mar, CA 92014.

the dead bureaucratic hands of the third party involved in medical payment; nor will new sophistication or computerization in health-care delivery systems, nor will even iridology, homeopathy, acupuncture, Rolfing, reflexology, biofeedback or fasting: none of these in themselves will do it.

What, then, will solve the problem? Something very, very simple: a change in our national lifestyle, along with a more dignified, realistic approach to the process of dying. These simple, sweeping measures would have a drastic effect on national health and would certainly reverse the oncoming tide of health-care bankruptcy. And nothing drastic at the outset would be needed to demonstrate the efficacy of this approach. A small change in lifestyle would probably create a small change in national health, moderate change would show commensurate effect, and so on.

You're probably familiar with Dr. Arthur Breslow's survey of 7,000 Californian adults, in which he rated life expectancy in terms of

---

zation. Local groups in other areas are also banding together for their own mutual benefit and later representation in a state-wide organization.

At this writing, HHPA membership is expanding rapidly, and the group has a very positive prognosis. Members are excited about the group support they have created within HHPA, and they are encouraging other practitioners throughout the nation to follow suit.

The holistic health field, born of the social, political and individual issues of the 1960s, has a long and challenging road ahead. The momentum generated toward social evolution in the Sixties can be sustained, and the solutions to our current social dilemmas can emerge during the Eighties only by means of internal personal and external political involvement.[5]

NOTES

1. It is not within the scope of this article to criticize the safety assurances offered by the medical examiner/licensure system. Both benefits and faults have been illustrated. For a critique of licensure and proposed alternatives, see the articles by Dana Ullman and Stanley Gross in the list of suggested readings.

2. See the article by Brendan O'Regan and Rick Carlson in the list of suggested readings.
3. Acupuncturists have subsequently won the right to see clients without the need for physician prescription, but still have great difficulty in gaining access to the examination and certification process.
4. Is a holistic health practitioner one who earns a living providing holistically oriented health service? Is a person living holistically a self-practitioner? Is a person working as a lawyer, author, or administrator to influence society with holistic perspectives also a holistic health practitioner?
5. For more information about the Holistic Health Practitioner's Association, send a self-addressed stamped envelope to: HHPA, 396 Euclid Avenue, Oakland, CA 94610. For information about the *Holistic Health Review,* write to Human Sciences Press, 72 Fifth Avenue, New York, NY 10011.

SUGGESTIONS FOR FURTHER READING

Marilyn Ferguson, *The Aquarian Conspiracy: Personal and Social Transformation in the 1980's.* J. P. Tarcher, 1980.

Friendly Shared Powers: Practicing Self-Mastery and Creative Teamwork for Earth's Community. Clear Marks, 1979.

Stanley Gross, Ed.D., "Professional Disclosure: An Alternative to Licensing," *Personnel and Guidance*

what might be called "Grandma's seven old-fashioned health hints." They go like this: no smoking; moderate drinking; seven or eight hours of sleep at night; regular meals with no snacks in between; breakfast every day; normal weight; and regular moderate exercise. The positive correlation between these elements of lifestyle and health are truly amazing.

For something more dramatic, but still incomplete, because there's even more to it than this, we could ponder a thought experiment given to me by Dr. Phil Lee, one of our most distinguished preventive-medicine experts: if by the snap of a finger, we could magically end all abuse of tobacco, alcohol, and automobiles, suddenly one-half of all our hospital beds would be empty—and he says that's a conservative figure. He says that probably more than 50 percent of those in hospitals today are there for something related to the abuse of tobacco, alcohol, or automobiles: these are the dreadful environmental effects that go along with our present lifestyle, a mad, pell-mell, frantic drive

for exponential growth. Here in the U.S. we've increased the amount of toxic substances spewed into the biosphere fifteen-fold since World War II. And now 60 to 90 percent of cancer is triggered by environmental irritants. A recent report to the U.S. Senate subcommittee on health and science warned that most mother's milk today in the United States is dangerously contaminated with pesticide residues and other toxic chemicals, and they warned little infants against drinking it.

George Leonard has been associated with the human potential move.nent for many years. Former vice-president of the Esalen Institute of San Francisco, and former senior editor of Look Magazine for seventeen years, he is author of the best-seller, Education and Ecstasy, *and more recently* The Transformation. *He holds a black belt in Aikido, and is currently on the board of advisors for the Association for Holistic Health.*

Journal, 55, no. 10 (1977), 586-588. Reprinted in *Holistic Health Review,* Fall 1978 and Spring 1979.

Melvin Gurtov, *Making Changes: The Politics of Self-Liberation.* Harvest Moon Books, 1979.

Brendan O'Regan and Rick J. Carlson, "Defining Health: The State of the Art," *Holistic Health Review, 3,* 2, 86-102.

Michael Rossman, *New Age Blues: On the Politics of Consciousness.* Dutton, 1979.

Mark Satin, *New Age Politics.* Delta Publishing, 1978.

Dana Ullman, "Regulated Freedom of Choice: An Alternative to Licensure." *Holistic Health Review, 4,* 1, 1980.

Steven Markell, co-editor of the Holistic Health Review, *has been expressing his own brand of self-responsible social health action through a variety of projects and organizations during the past five years. He is one of the founding members of the Holistic Health Organizing Committee and the Holistic Health Practitioners' Association. He is in private practice in Berkeley, California, as a Life Choice Awareness Consultant, incorporating Casetaking in the Empirical Tradition, iridology, nutrition/biochemistry, career and lifestyle counseling, and an eclectic synthesis of biomedical and spiritual perspectives in his work with individuals and organizations.*

Health: As If We All Mattered
James T. Carter, O.D.

We are witnessing the beginning of a shift from fragmented, depersonalized, expensive, illness-oriented health care, to a system of health development and promotion in which the individual is in a position to act as his or her own health provider.

All factors, great and small, personal, social, and environmental, affect the quality of our health. Dr. Carter underscores the importance of lifestyle decisions for restoring health. Consumers, health providers, educators, policy makers, and researchers are recognizing the benefits of holistic health. Data from a recent Canadian Health study substantiate the claims that health education and preventive measures are making a positive impression on national health and economic priorities. We can no longer take a small view of our own problems, or their solutions.

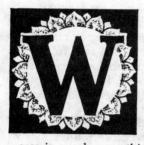 e all know what a blessing it is to be in a state of glowing, radiant, vibrant health. Yet, somehow, few of us have been able to experience this, or if we have, it seems to pass quickly. Too many of us have been taught to think that disease is merely something we "get"—or illness is something we catch. And, once we've caught an illness, we go to a health practitioner to have him "take away" the problem.

It is time to challenge this concept of illness and to acknowledge that the passive acquiescence to disease is a comfortable cultural myth, oftentimes a product of the ignorance of the personal and social realities around us. New health practitioners tend to see both health and disease as something people "do" and not just something people "get." With this definition, disease and health come from inside as well as from outside the individual.

Reprinted by permission from *Holistic Health Review*, 2, no. 2 (Spring 1979), 6-9.

In the 1950s and 60s doctors stressed technology, medical intervention, and the need to isolate and study disease. By contrast, in the 70s the new practitioners of holistic health emphasize preventive care, personal responsibility, and the need to view any illness in the essential context, that of the experience of the true inner self and its expression in the world.

An important principle of holistic health today is that we should not look at any effect in isolation; the illness is not separate from the rest of the person, and sick individuals cannot be isolated from the social and cultural environment which surrounds them. As an ancient Tibetan Buddhist sutra points out,

> "If a leg is cut, is it true that the hand does not need to tend the wound because the leg only has sustained the injury? Since the person as a whole experiences the suffering, it is natural for the hand, although not affected, to take action. In the same way we should be responsible for helping others."

ACTIVATED PATIENT

The new practitioner stresses both self-reliance and social responsibility. To be self-reliant and socially responsible we need to be not only well-informed but encouraged to creatively solve our health problems. This means an *active* posture, not just for practitioners, but also for patients, because sickness is essentially the most powerful opportunity for self-renewal and the most potent time for responsible personal and, oftentimes, social transformation.

Sickness also presents to individuals a time for careful reexamination of ourselves and our environment. We have to understand the pressures generated by new urban lifestyles, the health impacts of the environment and the changing roles of the individual in society. For many years we have virtually ignored the behavioral, social, and environmental factors contributing to health and well-being. Without a better understanding of the impact of these factors, we cannot even begin the task of educating the individual patient to make consistently responsible choices concerning his own health care.

We are beginning to get some research results which will help improve our information about health-care priorities.

THE CANADIAN PERSPECTIVE

One of the best frameworks for assessing these priorities was provided by the landmark study by Canadian Minister of Health and Welfare, Marc Lalonde, called *A New Perspective on the Health of Canadians.*

The Lalonde study concentrated on the major diseases which parallel the best-known cripplers and killers in the United States: cancer, heart disease, suicide, alcoholism, etc. The study set out to discover the most important factors in the crippling and killing powers of disease.

Four interdependent factors stood out:

(1) the amount of *medical research* being done on the disease;

(2) the availability of *health services* for those afflicted;

(3) the *environment* of the disease;

(4) the *lifestyle* or set of personal choices associated with the disease.

The report's most provocative conclusion was that lifestyle changes had the greatest effect on reducing a disease for all major age groups and in all major diseases studied. The second largest effect was in the area of environment. Less importance was placed on health services, and the least return (from an economic perspective) on reducing disease was from medical research.

The research concludes that we need to shift from our fragmented, depersonalized, costly, illness-oriented system to a system of health development and health promotion with the individual in a position to act as his or her own provider.

In the U.S. we still have our economic priorities reversed; most of our health-care dollars are going to support the out-moded social definition of health and disease. Identifying the economic problems in such a transition in a major address before the American Public Health Association, APHA president George Pickett, M.D., recognizes the present revenue-seeking position: "In no other system does rising demand produce price increases and supply decreases simultaneously. In no other economic system does the boss make all the decisions while everyone else takes all the risks."

An annual price tag of half a trillion dollars for health is projected within ten years if we try to hang onto the old perspectives. It is thus obvious that economic pressures will be instrumental in reforming the health-care delivery system.

The Canadian report establishes some clear-cut economic priorities: lifestyle and environmental factors are the most cost-effective concerns to pursue. Improving health status by changes in lifestyles requires a reconciliation of personal and social values with new living patterns.

Coming to know ourselves better is one of the challenges implied in changing our lifestyle patterns. Our lifestyle can be devastating to our health. Recognizing that our attitudes and emotions have dramatic, direct impact on our bodies is a first step in this process.

A subtle cultural value which affects lifestyle is the aggressive competitive behavior socially accepted in the American culture. This "survival of the fittest" attitude can initiate internal organ malfunction in the body as well as communicable stress in the social environment of the distressed individual. Other health impacts of cultural values can be found by studying the way we drive a car (58,000 deaths, two million injuries per year), the choices we make to solve our crises in personal growth (aggression, suicide, rape, etc.), the ways we choose to eat and distribute food (obesity, ulcers, starvation, hunger, vascular disease, etc.), and the ways we choose to express our bodies (over half the population is essentially sedentary).

EMERGING HEALTH TRENDS

Today there are many positive lifestyle trends which are supported by newly emerging cultural values. Health is becoming a status symbol. Women who are athletic are no longer viewed as unfeminine. Even *Vogue* magazine has declared that it is "OK to Sweat" and has devoted editorial space to fitness routines as well as beauty. There is wider recognition and encouragement for utilizing personal resources (meditation, inner healing, physical activity, etc.). There has been an explosion of self-help books and how-to-run, dream, and control-your-diet manuals. And the traditional value—*physician, heal thyself*—has emerged again among the holistic health practitioners.

Another powerful trend in the area of "social lifestyle" is growing willingness to live peacefully with all beings on our planet. Increased understanding of the community of life and the oneness of the human race, coupled with the growing personal participation in the processes of individuation, ultimately make up the most powerful health trends operating in our present culture.

Our second most important way to affect health is in the environment. The effects of home and working environments on personal, family, and community health are being studied. The impact of toxic industrial wastes, atmospheric pollutants, and noise has been documented. Carcinogens in the environment, foods, and other personal items are also being recognized. Even geothermal power once thought "clean" is found to bring "acid rain" for miles from its source. Many are recognizing that how we live in

the world around us (lifestyle/environment) has more influence on our health than the medical care we use.

The publicity about the effects of radiation in the environment is causing alarm. One medical example is doctor-administered radiopharmaceuticals (10 million patient doses per year). Jacobson, Plato, and Toeroek at the University of Michigan found that treated patients emit so much radiation that they would be refused passage as cargo in a jet plane; yet they can sit next to an unsuspecting person and irradiate their neighbors with up to half the radiation they received from the doctor. Indeed, it has been said that discharged radiation from a medical center

U.S. Health-Care Cost-Effectiveness
William Stanniger

Individual health-care costs in our country have increased nearly tenfold since 1950, from an average of $87 to $830 per person annually. Costs have been projected to reach $1,000 per

person by next year. Despite this alarming acceleration in costs, chronic diseases such as heart disease, cancer, and diabetes are increasing, even amongst teenagers and children. We must ask the questions, "Why?" and "What can be done to change this trend?"

Although our medical system is estimated to affect only 10 percent of the factors influencing health, it receives about 96 percent of our annual health-care expenditures. We know

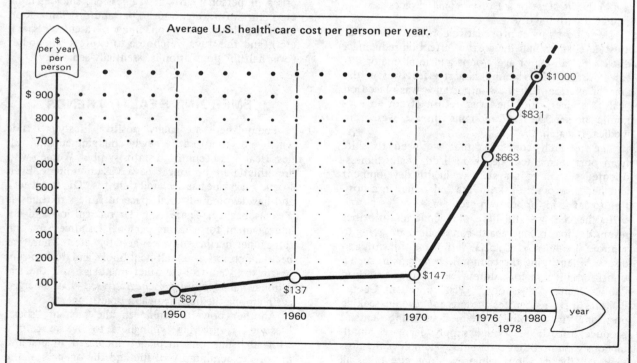

Average U.S. health-care cost per person per year.

can far surpass that released from a nuclear plant.

Perhaps the most powerful emerging trends in environment are the philosophy that we are inextricably interwoven with the world around us and the realization that there is an abundance, not a scarcity, of appropriate resources (food, energy, space, grains, solar energy, new types of structures). This ecological perspective has given rise to a spiritual view: we must come to terms with our interdependence.

Health services and medical research should be thought of as secondary influences on health and well being. These influences come into play when the two primary issues of lifestyle and environment are in irreconcilable disorder. In the mainstream medical approach, these secondary factors are treated as primary, and holistic health practitioners see them as relevant only when we have exhausted our personal and social resources.

Aside from the basic neglect of the effects of lifestyle and environment, the negative trends appear to arise from five problems inherent in the present system: uneven distribution of professionals and services; unwieldy fees and accelerating costs; inadequate accessibility of services; excessive use of hospital and institutional care; and the absence of basic principles and practices of care.

---

that "an ounce of prevention is worth a pound of cure," yet only 4 percent of our health-care dollars go toward preventive health-care programs.

In order to reverse the trend of spiralling costs and poorer health, we must put more energy toward prevention, and toward the promotion of health. We must provide more effective alternatives to augment our often dehumanized, technological, sick-care system. We need education that fosters increased individual- and family-centered responsibility for all levels of health—from birth to death, and in body, mind, and spirit. And we need to reinvest in human warmth, the dynamic of the healing relationship, and the support of each individual to be self-determining.

Reprinted by permission from *Holistic Health Review*, 1979.

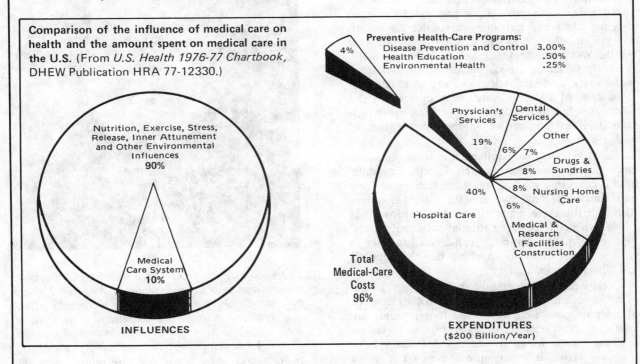

Comparison of the influence of medical care on health and the amount spent on medical care in the U.S. (From *U.S. Health 1976-77 Chartbook,* DHEW Publication HRA 77-12330.)

Nutrition, Exercise, Stress, Release, Inner Attunement and Other Environmental Influences 90%

Medical Care System 10%

INFLUENCES

Preventive Health-Care Programs:
Disease Prevention and Control   3.00%
Health Education   .50%
Environmental Health   .25%

4%

Physician's Services 19%

Dental Services 6%

Other 7%

Drugs & Sundries 8%

Nursing Home Care 8%

Medical & Research Facilities Construction 6%

Hospital Care 40%

Total Medical-Care Costs 96%

EXPENDITURES
($200 Billion/Year)

The above result in symptom-related services that often necessitate the excessive use of drugs, surgery, and high-level technology. Even the United States Public Health Service recently acknowledged in its annual report on the health of the Nation:

> "There is a lack of valid clinical information regarding the efficacy and effectiveness of current medical practice. Despite substantial Federal effort in this area of biomedical research there is still great uncertainty about what constitutes the most effective diagnostic and therapeutic procedures."

There are, however, many positive trends emerging in the health service area. Many new professionals are willing to reconsider the principles and practices in which they were trained, and are expanding to a holistic model similar to Lalonde's example. Additionally, increased consumer involvement at all levels of health care, from planning and quality assurance to budget management, is producing constructive change.

Indeed, a growing public mandate for improvement in health services is becoming a potent tool for change. There is a trend toward new classifications of health providers, some professional and some lay, to expand care, extend availability, and reduce patient dependency on physicians and hospitals. This trend is linked to expanded preventive and predictive care, stressing education, nutrition, personal involvement, and community action. In addition, there are new (to the West) practices such as acupuncture, iridology, body therapies, clinical nutrition, inner healing, biofeedback, and meditation, and new products such as educational materials, nutritional supplements and substitutes, health retreats, and sports facilities which serve the development of an expanded notion of health services.

The other secondary influence is from the sacrosanct ground of medical research. Except for public-health concerns, medical research techniques have been limited to looking at diseases in total isolation. Although this molecular and biological approach has yielded tremendous information about structure and function of the human body, it has failed to make as great a contribution to knocking out the cripplers and killers in contemporary society.

Overspecialized reductionist research is now broadening to include the biological (and social) concept of multiple causation. We can no longer simply say cigarettes cause cancer, or even that a bacterium causes a disease. We are beginning to see that one disease may have a different cause or even set of causes in different settings with different people. In addi-

tion, we are beginning to see that only when we combine the rational/technical mode of examination with the subjective/intuitive process of exploration will we have true scientific inquiry which is ethically balanced and socially responsive.

We have briefly examined those major areas influencing health and disease. We must master the way we live our life (lifestyle), where we live our lives (environment), and with what help (social health services, educational/industrial/political institutions) we live our lives if we are to enjoy better health and see the seeds of a new image of humankind mature.

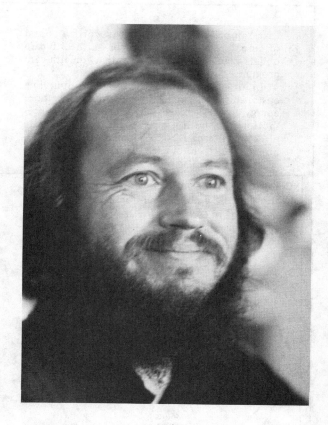

James T. Carter, O.D., is a natural-health practitioner, optometrist, and research scientist. He has successfully developed iridology as a clinically effective evaluation tool. His practice unifies Chinese medical philosophies with Western biological sciences. His work has helped to initiate and clarify new health policies and provide for the integration of public health strategies and emerging health practices.

Section II:
Body/Mind
Body Awareness, Nutrition, Exercise, Relaxation

"Leave thy drugs in the chemist's pot if thou can't heal the patient with food."

Hippocrates

"I discovered the middle path of stillness within speed, calmness within fear, and I held it longer and quieter than ever before."

Steve McKinney
(recalling how he felt
when he broke the world downhill ski record)

"Simplify, simplify, simplify. Live unknown, make your wants few.
Shed this externalized clutter, these needless needs; they are merely a form of bondage and hinder man's journey."

Robert S. de Ropp

"Mind and body are different expresssions of the same thing; the unique part of the universe that is you."

Jack Schwarz

"Don't you know that four-fifths of all our troubles in this life would disappear if we would just sit down and keep still?"

Calvin Coolidge

"Health is a consummation of a love affair of the organs of the body."

Plato

Introduction
BODY/MIND: Body Awareness, Nutrition, Exercise, Relaxation

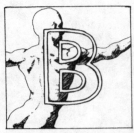

y calling this section Body/ Mind, we represent the concept that the body and mind are not two separate entities, but are one and the same. Our body sensations are experienced by the mind; our mental process is experienced by the body. Our thoughts and feelings affect the way we breathe, hold ourselves, and move. Whatever we do that affects the body affects the mind, and what affects the mind likewise affects the body.

Our Body/Mind section is the largest in the book. In this section we have articles representing four major subjects: body awareness, nutrition, exercise, and relaxation.

The body is a great teacher. It manifests both our inner harmonies and our imbalances for all to see. It has been said that the mind can tell a lie, but not the body. In order that we may know how to listen to our bodies tell us the truth, we are presenting articles that will help you to see, experience, feel, and listen to your bodies in order to reach a greater state of harmony.

Attunement with our bodies' individual needs is our best source of nutritional guidance. There is no one diet that will work for everybody. We need to experiment carefully and see what works for our-selves. Our articles on nutrition offer practical advice, address the subjects of vitamin, food, and mineral supplements, and introduce different approaches to nutrition.

It seems that people are exercising, taking care of their bodies, and enjoying the results like never before. To care for oneself by regular exercise provides physical well-being and a sense of being vitally alive. The various approaches to exercise offer everybody an opportunity to find an individual approach. In our articles representing some of these approaches, you'll find practical information that will help you to enrich an already existing exercise program, or inspire you to begin a new one.

A relaxed body/mind is better able to deal with life situations than a stressed one. Learning to control and balance stress with relaxation is an essential part of Holistic Health. The articles about relaxation offer some new variations on old themes, such as the use of water, sound, and breathing techniques, and there is an excellent article on stress management.

The care of our body/mind need no longer be thought of as dutiful and boring calisthenics, a vegetable diet, or eight hours of sleep. Rather, it can be seen and experienced as a process of enriching our lives by the choice of what brings us satisfaction and a sense of well-being.

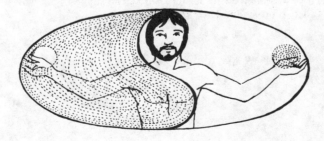

Body/Mind Survey

How well does each statement describe your patterns
of thought and action?

1. I actively view my body as a whole, composed of interrelated parts.
2. My mind exerts a direct influence on my body.
3. I enjoy my body.
4. I have plenty of energy.
5. I am aware of the effects of social and environmental influences on the health of my organism.
6. I eat nourishing, well-balanced meals.
7. I follow regular eating habits.
8. Mealtimes are free from tension and disagreement.
9. I enjoy cooking for myself and others.
10. I am aware of how my diet effects my mood.
11. I read labels on canned or packaged foods.
12. I eat plenty of fresh seasonal vegetables and fruits.
13. I drink chemical-free, pure water.
14. I take vitamin and mineral supplements.
15. I buy the highest-quality food I can find.
16. I feel physically fit, optimally alive.
17. I do regular vigorous exercise that is good for the circulation.
18. I like to dance.
19. I do not feel "out of shape."
20. I participate in some creative movement, such as dance, sports, etc.
21. I want to incorporate an exercise program into my daily routine.
22. I feel relaxed.
23. I do not have difficulty relaxing.
24. I balance work with pleasure.
25. My lifestyle provides periodic times for rest and meditation.
26. I feel capable of making changes in my life to alleviate stress.
27. I do not use tranquilizers.
28. I have personally used:
    a. autosuggestion (self-hypnosis)
    b. progressive relaxation exercises
    c. diaphragmatic breathing
    d. guided visualizations
    e. affirmations
    f. meditation

The High Priest
Richard Selzer, M.D.

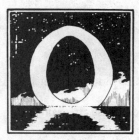

On the bulletin board in the front hall of the hospital where I work, there appeared an announcement. "Yeshi Dhonden," it read, "will make rounds at six o'clock on the morning of June 10." The particularities of the meeting were then given, followed by a notation: "Yeshi Dhonden is Personal Physician to the Dalai Lama." I am not so leathery a skeptic that I would knowingly ignore an emissary from the gods. Not only might such sangroid be inimical to one's earthly well-being, it could take care of eternity as well. Thus, on the morning of June 10, I joined the clutch of whitecoats waiting in the small conference room adjacent to the ward selected for the rounds. The air in the room is heavy with ill-concealed dubiety and suspicion of bamboozlement. At precisely six o'clock, he materializes, a short, golden, barrelly man dressed in a sleeveless robe of saffron and maroon. His scalp is shaven, and the only visible hair is a scanty black line above each hooded eye.

He bows in greeting while his young interpreter makes the introduction. Yeshi Dhonden, we are told, will examine a patient selected by a member of the staff. The diagnosis is as unknown to Yeshi Dhonden as it is to us. The examination of the patient will take place in our presence, after which we will reconvene in the conference room where Yeshi Dhonden will discuss the case. We are further informed that for the past two hours Yeshi Dhonden has purified himself by bathing, fasting, and prayer. I, having breakfasted well, performed only the most desultory of ablutions, and given no thought at all to my soul, glance furtively at my fellows. Suddenly, we seem a soiled, uncouth lot.

The patient had been awakened early, told that she was to be examined by a foreign doctor, and requested to produce a fresh specimen of urine; so

when we enter her room, the woman shows no surprise. She has long ago taken on that mixture of compliance and resignation that is the facies of chronic illness. This was to be but another in an endless series of tests and examinations. Yeshi Dhonden steps to the bedside while the rest stand apart, watching. For a long time he gazes at the woman, favoring no part of the body with his eyes, but seeming to fix his glance at a place just above her supine form. I, too, study her. No physical sign nor obvious symptom gives a clue of the nature of her disease.

At last he takes her hand, raising it in both of his own. Now he bends over the bed in a kind of crouching stance, his head drawn down into the collar of his robe. His eyes are closed as he feels for her pulse. In a moment he has found the spot, and for the next half hour he remains thus, suspended above the patient like some exotic golden bird with folded wings, holding the pulse of the woman beneath his fingers, cradling her hand in his. All the power of the man seems to have been drawn down into this one purpose. It is palpation of the pulse raised to the state of ritual. From the foot of the bed, where I stand, it is as though he and the patient have entered a special place of isolation, of apartness, about which a vacancy hovers, and across which no violation is possible. After a moment the woman rests back upon her pillow. From time to time, she raises her head to look at the strange figure above her, then sinks back once more. I cannot see their hands joined in a correspondence that is exclusive, intimate, his fingertips receiving the voice of her sick body through the rhythm and throb she offers at her wrist. All at once I am envious—not of him, not of Yeshi Dhonden for his gift of beauty and holiness, but of her. I want to be held like that, touched so, received. And I know that I, who have palpated a hundred thousand pulses, have not felt a single one.

At last Yeshi Dhonden straightens, gently places the woman's hand upon the bed, and steps back. The interpreter produces a small wooden bowl and two sticks. Yeshi Dhonden pours a portion of the urine specimen into the bowl, and proceeds to whip the

This article originally appeared in *Mortal Lessons,* by Richard Selzer, M.D. It is reprinted here by permission of the author.

liquid with the two sticks. This he does for several minutes until a foam is raised. Then, bowing above the bowl, he inhales the odor three times. He sets down the bowl and turns to leave. All this while, he has not uttered a single word. As he nears the door, the woman raises her head and calls out to him in a voice at once urgent and serene. "Thank you, doctor," she says, and touches with her other hand the place he had held on her wrist, as though to recapture something that had visited there. Yeshi Dhonden turns back for a moment to gaze at her, then steps into the corridor. Rounds are at an end.

We are seated once more in the conference room. Yeshi Dhonden speaks now for the first time, in soft Tibetan sounds that I have never heard before. He has barely begun when the young interpreter begins to translate, the two voices continuing in tandem—a bilingual fugue, the one chasing the other. It is like the chanting of monks. He speaks of winds coursing through the body of the woman, currents that break against barriers, eddying. These vortices are in her blood, he says. The last spendings of an imperfect heart. Between the chambers of her heart, long, long before she was born, a wind had come and blown open a deep gate that must never be opened. Through it charge the full waters of her river, as the mountain stream cascades in the springtime, battering, knocking loose the land, and flooding her breath. Thus he speaks, and is silent.

"May we now have the diagnosis?" a professor asks.

The host of these rounds, the man who knows, answers.

"Congenital heart disease," he says. "Interventricular septal defect, with resultant heart failure."

A gateway in the heart, I think. That must not be opened. Through it charge the full waters that flood her breath. So! Here then is the doctor listening to the sounds of the body to which the rest of us are deaf. He is more than doctor. He is priest.

Now and then it happens as I make my own rounds, that I hear the sounds of his voice, like an ancient Buddhist prayer, its meaning long since forgotten, only the music remaining. Then a jubilation possesses me, and I feel my self touched by something divine.

Richard Selzer, M.D., teaches surgery at Yale, and is the author of several books of essays, memoirs, and short stories.

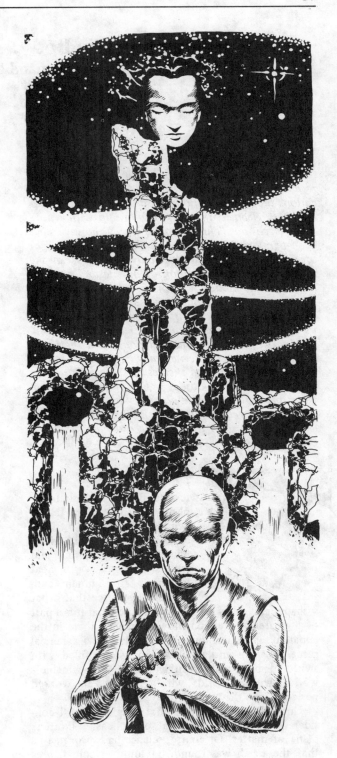

The Microcosmic Body: Discovering the Implicit
Armand Ian Brint

Part of the movement to holism is an attempt to recapture the wisdom of the past. Many ancient civilizations provided traditional wisdom from which their members gleaned a proper relationship with nature and the cosmos. This profound legacy, however, has been temporarily buried in the West under the weight of a mechanistic reality. It is only now, as we awake to the senseless destruction of our natural environment and the modern epidemics that ravage our bodies, that we begin to question the indoctrination that spawned this estrangement. As something deep within us begins to stir and reach out for a purposeful connection with life, the old "religions" and their contemporary counterparts magically emerge.

One of the common themes of these philosophies is the view of the body as a tiny reflection of universal principles. By studying the natural inclinations and subtle forces active in the body, one is led into a realignment with the intrinsic order and meaning of life.

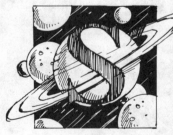

Stewart Brand said that the photograph of the Earth (taken from outer space by a satellite) that shows the whole blue orb with spirals and whorls of cloud was a great landmark for human consciousness. We see that it has a shape, and it has limits.[1] We also see that it is a part of a greater whole: somehow suspended there in the apparent emptiness of space, it fits like a spherical piece in a gargantuan puzzle, a whole, filled with swirls of blue and green and hues unimaginable—worlds within worlds within worlds, all worked perfectly into the pattern.

Until the time of this photograph, we still considered the Earth to be flat or at least a limitless plane of matter. Of course, science had informed us that the Earth was round, but only in cold figures and schematic representations. We had not tasted its roundness, and therefore clung desperately to our old two-dimensional sense of sovereignty.

The pre-Columbus Earth was insured of its isolation by monsters threatening at its edge. With the rise of "manifest destiny" these mythical beasts were neatly severed from our consciousness by "scientific crusaders," and in their stead we were left to ponder the vastness of unfriendly space, our isolation completely intact. We merely replaced the frightful imaginings of the Middle Ages with the existential imaginings of our own "age of reason."

Now what does all this talk of fantastic creatures at the fringe of the world and snapshots of planet Earth have to do with the body? A great deal, I submit. The same beliefs that precipitate the way we view the cosmos out there apply to the way we view our bodies in here. No matter how much we fragment our thinking or display apparent contradictions in our actions, there is a thread of consistency that maintains a unified point of view, in spite of ourselves. If we are fearful of space and attempt to conquer it, then chances are we are just as fearful of the immediate space of the body and will attempt to conquer it. The familiar cinematographic scenerio of the gallant space-fleet commander who subjugates alien planets with his laser beams is not unlike the doctor who, by "heroic intervention," claims dominion over the alien body, with the assistance of what Rene Dubos calls the "magic bullets" of the medical arsenal. It is Hollywood and science all rolled up into one magnificent ideology. There is only one problem—it doesn't work. Jacob Needleman puts it this way:

> "The whole vision of the technological conquest of nature has proved to be a mirage. Both the harmony of the body and the harmony of the environment seem to be far subtler and more powerful than we have realized."[2]

We are slowly, as a people, coming to this inevitable understanding. Along with this disturbing realization, we in the West have begun to witness the breakdown of the heretofore prevailing Cartesian world view, that which designates "them" and "us," the dichotomy between the tangible and the intangible, the compulsion to maintain a separation from nature, etc. The last two decades have heralded the rediscovery of the implicit—the wholeness and integrity of life. This wholeness pertains not only to discrete organisms (body, mind, and spirit), but to life-forms and their environment, as spheres of interlocking energy.

The picture sent from outer space is one reminder of a world organism, a great body composed of smaller bodies—land masses, oceans, mountains, rivers. Even the smallest subatomic "body" is integral to the whole. It is as if you could step outside of your own body and take an objective look at the form before you. All illusion would quickly vanish, all ego-inspired fantasies of limitless isolation gone. Only the bare-boned truth of the organism would remain. And what you would see, like the photo of the Earth, would be one body, composed of many cells, tissues, and organs, all interdependent and intimately connected with the environment, just as the Earth is sustained by the envelope of space.

Long before the advent of the scientific/mechanistic view of nature vis-a-vis the body, our physical nature was considered a tiny reflection of those principles ordering the whole of the cosmos—a microcosm(os). The Islamic philosopher Al-Ghazzali articulated what countless other thinkers had realized through the ages: "Man has been truly termed a 'microcosm,' or little world in himself, and the structure of his body should be studied not only by those who wish to become doctors, but by those who wish to attain to a more intimate knowledge of God."[3]

Jacob Needleman suggests that it was only gradually, as humanity began to place the fear of illness and death before its search for self-knowledge, that its natural position in the universe became obscured and finally lost to many. The movement of holism is largely an attempt to reinstate this primordial fact in our stubborn consciousness.

SYMBOLS OF HOLISM

The notion that the body is an aspect of a larger whole which is, in some mysterious fashion, also simultaneously reflected in the body, has been symbolized from time immemorial by the circle, a form without beginning and without end. Dr. M.-L. von Franz explains:

"Whether the symbol of the circle appears in primitive sun worship or modern religion, in

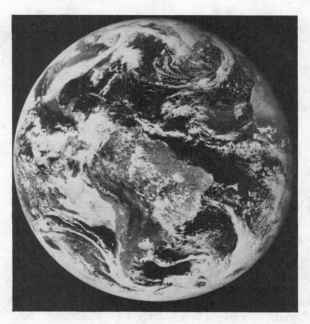

The same beliefs that precipitate the way we view the earth and the cosmos apply to the way we view our bodies.

myths or dreams, in the mandalas drawn by Tibetan monks, in the ground plans of cities, or in the spherical concepts of early astronomers, it always points to the single most vital aspect of life—its ultimate wholeness."

We may be able to dismiss the idea of wholeness from our cognitive mind, but the deeper urges of the psyche will not be denied. This archetypal form, ubiquitous in the revolving wheels of our technology, in the face of the sun, and in the shape of our own eyes, is etched in the depths of our awareness, and its symbolic meaning is projected onto the outer world. It is the truth of our being and we hunger for its recognition by the conscious mind. But until that time comes, we suffer the self-imposed chains of the body. We are at odds with the body because, as I said, we are at odds with nature and the universe at large. On the other hand, an enlightened exploration of the body may provide us with our best opportunity to understand our environment, and with it a rediscovered "passage to the stars."

If we look at the very seed of our bodies, the DNA code, we observe an intriguing phenomenon. The structure of this double-helix bonded chain readily suggests the formation of a spiral. This configuration is not accidental or arbitrary. Rather, it embodies the symbolic circular movement of energy as expressed by the ancients on cave walls, pottery, and sculpture long before the birth of so-called modern civilization. A more recognizable representation has survived to the present day in the form of the caduceus. "Like the spiral, energy is labyrinthine in its forms of being and in the passageways between these forms." The spiral, a variant of the circle, suggests the movement of invisible forces, from subtle to gross, which constitutes our universe. Our bodies merely occupy a particularly dense space along this continuum, and as such are an example of a continuous process in its manifest form. Seeing that the rugged stuff of our bodies is formed out of the chemical information stored in the chromosomes of the nuclei of cells, we are led to consider the words of the philosopher/poet Lao Tzu, "The wise man looks into space and does not regard the small as too little or the great as too big; for he knows that there is no limit to dimensions."

The study of DNA has unwittingly unveiled a profound metaphysical truth: each part of the whole contains a blueprint of the whole, just as each cell contains a tiny DNA blueprint for the entire body. This fundamental understanding of "reality" is also reflected in the revolutionary "holographic theory" put forth by Dr. Carl Pribram, physicist David Bohm, and others.[4]

THE ENERGETIC BODY

The secrets of DNA and the mathematical formulae of the holographic paradigm are perhaps more accessible in the "reflexive" body therapies. This group of techniques commonly embraces the concept that the body is an integral whole and that parts of the body, if observed properly, yield a picture of the whole. The word "reflexive" is in this case meant to describe processes which reflect the total organism. The idea is not very different from "Sherlock Holmesian" inductive reasoning, where, for example, the physical constitution of an assailant is calculated from the size of the suspect's footprints and the distance measured between them. Practices such as iridology, hand and foot reflexology, physiognomy (facial analysis—see Figure 1), even the systems of chiropractic and acupuncture, fall under this category. Such systems continue to be part of the sacred healing heritage of civilizations that did not adhere to a mechanistic reality. Ironically, in light of recent discoveries, they offer our technological sensibilities a holographic image of the body which unequivocally unites the realms of science and metaphysics.

When we employ a system such as physiognomy, we are embarking on a new way of perceiving the body. We have left the reductionist coordinates behind and are directly observing the energetic makeup of the body. We must shake loose the fetters of linear rationality, and consider ourselves on the brink of a new world, as the insight of Shakespeare directs: "And therefore as a stranger give it welcome. There are more things in heaven and earth, Horatio, than are dreamt of in your philosophy."

"Energy" is not just an appellation for a subtlety that science has yet to explain, but a genuine quality that defies analytic explanation. It is as difficult a problem for the intellect to subdue as the reason birds sing in the early morning, or seasons change—they just do. When we have come to understand the mysteries of nature, then we will have arrived at the threshold of our cosmic self.

It is by learning to understand the movement and cycles of energy through tangible forms—changing seasons, flow of rivers, our own thirsts and hungers—that we are taught to order our lives, and can reach a deep spiritual attunement. Paradoxically, by contemplating the true nature of the physical plane, we are led to the spiritual, which is its initiator. As expressed in "The Cauldron" from the *I Ching,* "All that is visible must grow beyond itself, extended into the realm of the invisible. Thereby it receives its true consecration and clarity, and takes firm root in the cosmic order."

In attempts to understand the invisible laws of nature, many creation myths speak to a single source-energy that is the Mother of all things. Consequently, many ancient systems of healing assert that there is one fundamental energy which gives life to the organisms and from which all other bodily functions are born. This energy has been christened variously according to the culture. In Chinese medicine it is *chi,* Ayurvedic philosophy calls it *prana* (life-breath); in the West this idea was associated with the school of Vitalism.

It generally follows that this source energy is, by the machinations of nature, subdivided into two poles of energy and then into a small number of primary energetic qualities. The host of manifest forms, of which we are but a part, is the result of subsequent diversification, and subtlety arises from the permutations of these "primary" energies.

In the Chinese system of medicine we find a clear example of this process. The original *chi* energy gave rise to polarity, *yin* water and *yang* fire. The interaction of these two forces created the qualities of earth, air, and wood. (As you can see, the language used to describe these archetypal energies is highly poetic. This feature, characteristic of ancient medicine, will

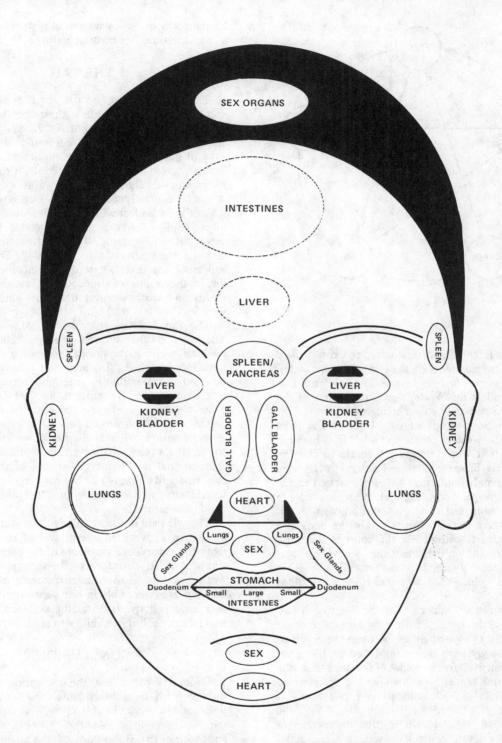

Figure 1: Systems such as physiognomy embrace the concept that the body is an integral whole and that a part of the whole reflects a picture of the whole.

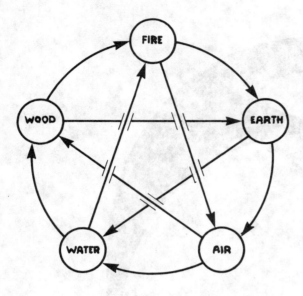

Figure 2.

be discussed later.) The diagram used to express these forces is a circle connecting the fire, earth, air, water, and wood elements (see Figure 2). This structure roughly parallels the Western esoteric notion of the pentagram: man plus the four elements of nature.

The Chinese concept of causal forces has been translated in Western texts as the "Five-Element Theory," but it would be more accurate to describe it as the "Five-Element Change Theory." It has been said that the only thing that remains constant in the universe is change. Accordingly, the Chinese attribute all phenomenological events to the constant interactions of these primary forces within the body and their counterparts without. In this context, the traditional teacher admonishes his students never to treat the same disease twice, because even if there is no symptomatic change in a patient, all conditions *are* dynamic.

The question of balance is integral to any discussion of energetic forces. Health may be said to occur when there is a proper balance between these forces. By definition, systems of healing based on the interplay of elemental forces include the idea that the body's natural tendency is to maintain its state of equilibrium. As such, it is understood that disease is not arbitrarily inflicted on us, but invited into the organism when, by our own volition or by circumstances beyond our control (genetic factors, pollution, etc.), we stray from our natural disposition and relationship with nature. This thought may be found

in the roots of our own medical system in the Hippocratic doctrine, "vis medicae naturae."

THE TAO

The Chinese addressed the question of balance in many texts, but perhaps its highest expression is to be found in the 81 chapters of the *Tao Te Ching*. This timeless work, simple yet profound, describes the flow of natural forces in man and nature. For the last 2,500 years it has guided the conduct of its readers by means of adherence to the natural order of life. As we have already seen, such obedience to the "real" laws of the manifest world ultimately lead to a deeper understanding of the spiritual world. Chapter 43 serves as an example: "The softest thing in the universe overcomes the hardest thing. That without substance can enter where there is no room. Hence I know the value of nonaction. Teaching without words and work without doing are understood by very few."

The *Tao Te Ching,* like the "Five-Element Change Theory" and other naturalistic cosmologies, is a metaphorical work, metaphorical perhaps in the original sense of the word, "to carry over." An ancient Chinese axiom states that if something is true, it must be true on all levels. Therefore in the *Tao Te Ching,* because we live in a reflexive universe, the conduct of a person or a nation should follow the observable patterns of nature. When in chapter 28 we are instructed to "Be the stream of the universe!" it means exactly that; so that by "Being the stream of the universe, ever true and unswerving," we may regain our natural spontaneity and innocence or, "Become as a little child once more."

The elemental forces alluded to in the *Tao Te Ching* are at work in every level of our evolution, from the embryonic unfolding of the organism to the ways in which we interact with society. They are at work not only as the unseen forces ordering visible life, but are discernible in our very structure, appearance, and activity. It is not the evidence of this fact that is lacking, but our ability to see it.

CONCLUSION

Buddhists often use the metaphor of the sun shining forth from behind the clouds to indicate a sense of discovery. In this essay, the discovery pertains to the implicit order and unity operating behind and within the framework of the manifest world, specifically the body. It is a curious thing that we use our bodies more like mundane tools than the architecture of the heavens. But then the clouds can get awfully thick. Since we lack a sense of the universe, our bodies become the oxen that bear the yoke of our daily fears and desires. Each time we inflict needless harm on our body or that of another, a ripple is sent throughout the vast circle of the cosmos, the stars in their celestial niche are shaken slightly, and the Earth lets loose a muffled groan. What we fail to consider is that the cloth of flesh we wear so carelessly is the material of the spirit, a direct descendent of the universe, and therefore precious.

> "As above, so below.... For the fundamental laws... penetrate everything and should be studied simultaneously both in the world and in man."

NOTES

1. Gary Snyder, "Re-inhabitation," in *The Old Ways* (City Lights Books, 1977), p. 62.
2. Jacob Needleman, *A Sense of the Cosmos*, p. 41.
3. P. D. Ouspensky, *In Search of the Miraculous*, p. 280.
4. For more information, see the article here by Marilyn Ferguson.

SUGGESTIONS FOR FURTHER READING

Jose and Miriam Arguelles, *Mandala*. Shambhala, 1972.

Rene Dubos, *Mirage of Health*. Harper, 1979.

Gia-Fu Feng and Jane English (trans.), *Tao Te Ching*. Vintage, 1972.

Carl G. Jung, *Man and His Symbols*. Dell, 1977.

Jacob Needleman, *A Sense of the Cosmos*. Dutton, 1976.

P. D. Ouspensky, *In Search of the Miraculous*. Harcourt, Brace, 1949.

Armand Ian Brint has, for the last six years, been an active contributor to the field of holistic health. He is the founder of the Berkeley Holistic Health Center, and co-editor of the Holistic Health Handbook *and of this volume. Armand also teaches courses on iridology and the Chinese Five Element Theory, and writes and lectures on the subject of holistic living.*

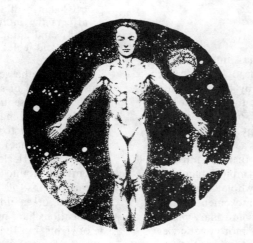

Touch for Health
Susan Koenig

Touch for health. This simple directive sets the tone for an extraordinary new self-help system. It is an active method, for it must be experienced to be fully appreciated. It is active, moreover, in the sense that you become a participant in your own healing. With these thoughts in mind, Ms. Koenig intends to help you put the system of Touch for Health to a practical test in your own life. Because Touch for Health is arranged as a simple and methodical series of techniques, it is accessible as an educational tool to both lay and professional health providers. It is truly people's health care.

Touch for Health is another example of the marvelous subtlety of the body. It enables us to reach into a realm which, to the unenlightened intellect, appears as nothing short of magic, but in reality stands as a true representation of the operation of our bodies.

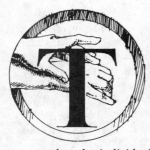
he body has more than 100 distinct sets of muscles, each nourished by the same blood and energy that animate your organs and other body parts. If we accept the premise that the body is a unified ecological system, then we must reason that the individual parts are symbiotic and function for the preservation of the whole. Organs give the being life, and muscles allow movement through space. Together they fulfill the evolutionary plan of the organism. If we take a slightly more poetic view, the muscles may be seen as an extension of the internal physiological processes that sustain life. If there is a drought on the land, the crops will fail; so, too, if the organs are deficient, their structural counterpart will similarly fail. This simple analogy illustrates the working hypothesis behind Touch for Health.

Headaches, backaches, hypoglycemia—whatever your complaint, the effect on the body is felt through the musculature. This is the key to Touch for Health, which views muscle function as an indication of internal homeostasis (balance). For example, your problem may involve a tight muscle. An analysis of that constricted muscle reveals the larger process of which it is a part.

"If there is a tight muscle in the hip, for instance, [resulting] from a corresponding weakness on the opposite side, then that hip is favored because of the tension restricting its motion. That puts a different strain on the foot, and with the foot in a different position, there will be a strain on other sets of muscles. This is going to change the body's general posture, affecting the positions of the internal organs. That, in turn, restricts the nutrition to the organs and changes the excretions and hormonal functions. The chemical/psychological balance of the person is changed, and this affects the individual cells in the body. As the body and mind are affected, the person will think and feel differently."[1]

Although the actual chain of events is never quite this sequential or simplistic, the outcome is often the same. The consequences to the body are determined, among other things, by the person's general health, age, and ability to check a further erosion of normal function (balance).

Touch for Health represents a body of knowledge assembled around the central principle that the relative strengths of isolated muscles indicate specific meridian organ imbalances. The exact muscle/organ connections have not been traced in the most scientific of terms, but these "reflex" relationships have been proven by years of empirical study. By applying various systems of correction, including acupressure and massage, one teaches the body to regain and regenerate its own natural vitality. Touch for Health is therefore a powerful self-healing tool.

The creator and spirit behind Touch for Health is Dr. John Thie, a dynamic teacher and practicing chiropractor, chairman of the International College of Applied Kinesiology, and professor of Kinesiology in sports medicine at Pepperdine University, Malibu, California. When Dr. Thie graduated from chiropractic school, he did not feel he was the qualified "expert" his degree and license declared him to be. His search for knowledge led him in the mid-60s to a lecture demonstration by the chiropractor Dr. George Goodheart. There he had the profound experience of seeing and feeling muscle testing for the first time. Dr. Goodheart had realized that, as indicators of internal body function, muscles were an important analytical tool. This understanding, coupled with his eclectic studies in physiological research and Chinese medicine, eventually produced the unified practice of applied kinesiology.[2]

After years of daily application in his own practice, John Thie became convinced of the validity and importance of Dr. Goodheart's work. In fact, he began teaching his patients how to take care of themselves using these techniques. Urged by friends and clients, he undertook the immense task of compiling, organizing, and editing more than a decade's worth of related notes and documentation. Undaunted by the criticism of his professional colleagues, who were wary of teaching lay people professional secrets, he finally published, with the assistance of his associate, Mary Marks, the *Touch For Health* book in 1973.

MUSCLE TESTING

Muscle testing is our biofeedback tool. The actual technique is quite simple, and must be done with a partner. You position a part of your partner's body, for example, the arm, so that only a certain muscle will be involved in a particular movement, or "range of motion" (see *Touch For Health* manual for specific muscle tests). Take the person through the range of motion before actually doing the test so that the specific movement is made perfectly clear to the brain. Tell the person to "resist," meaning to hold that position while you pull or push. All muscle tests are done first on one side, then on the other (bilaterally). We push or pull muscles according to a person's relative strength. Therefore, a strong, muscular individual will require more pressure than one of less muscle tone. Muscle strengths from both sides of the body are compared in all the tests, so that we have a total picture of the person's strong and weak muscles.

Muscle testing is also used to measure the effectiveness of the corrections one has made. Any muscles that were originally weak are retested after each correction to see if the strength and range of motion of the muscle has been affected. By achieving muscle balance, we are promoting total body balance, a condition wherein all body parts are working properly in relationship to one another.

All muscles used in Touch for Health relate to one of the 14 major acupuncture meridians, or energy pathways, in the body as defined and "mapped" by the Chinese more than 3,000 years ago. Each muscle also relates to an organ, gland, function, or body part such as the ears and eyes. Certain muscles are directly related to a specific organ because they may share, for example, a lymph vessel or an acupuncture meridian. Restoring the energy flow to that muscle will also give relief to the shared organ and meridian. Energy blockages in the meridian are diagnosed by means of the muscle tests. Once a blockage is located, the methodical use of one or several of the systems of correction will restore balance.

WHAT ARE ENERGY BLOCKAGES?

Many basic assumptions of holistic philosophy originate in the East. The term *chi,* meaning vital force or life energy, may be familiar to some of you. This life energy activates, animates, and maintains the very life process, and is derived from our environment by such processes as respiration and nutrition.[3] It permeates every living cell and tissue, and circulates through the body by way of the meridian pathways. When vital energy is impaired or blocked, less energy is able to move through us. We call this an energy blockage. Sometimes vital energy is referred to as our body's "innate intelligence," because it inherently seeks to maintain balance; thus the tendency of the body to heal itself. Any disturbance of natural or proper balance which continues to prevent the free flow of energy will eventually manifest in some form of malfunction. The body often tells us when the natural flow of energy has been blocked by producing pain (although pain is not always the result of an energy blockage). The goal of balancing the body's energy is to allow the life force to flow uninterrupted throughout the body, so that the organism can heal itself and experience optimal health and well-being.

MERIDIANS

Meridians are currently under medical research, and have thus far been described as acupressure vessels,

> "... located throughout the body. They contain a free-flowing, colorless, noncellular liquid which may be partly actuated by the heart.

These meridians have been measured and mapped by modern technological methods, electronically, thermatically, and radioactively. There are specific acupuncture points along the meridians. These points are electromagnetic in character and consist of small, oval cells called bonham corpuscles which surround the capillaries in the skin, the blood vessels, and the organs throughout the body."[4]

Each meridian takes the name of the organ, function, process, or system it governs (i.e., kidney meridian). There are twelve "organ meridians" that have symmetrical pathways, one on each side of the body. Two meridians, the central and governing, run up the front and back midline of the body respectively. Since proper body functioning is largely dependent on the free flow of *chi*, any energy blockage in a meridian may also result in an energy blockage in its related organ, with disease as a possible result. Drugs, tension and stress, illness, faulty digestion, even lack of sleep can impair or reverse meridian energy flow.

The muscles can be strengthened by tracing or running the meridians on or close to the surface of the body with the fingers, in the direction the energy currents naturally flow.

NEURO-LYMPHATIC MASSAGE POINTS

The lymphatic system is often referred to as the "garbage disposal system" of the body. It's not only important for detoxification and fluid drainage, but also transports proteins, hormones, and fats to the cells. There are twice as many lymph vessels and lymph as there are blood vessels and blood in the body. Lymph also constitutes one quarter of the white blood cells and aids in the production of antibodies.

The nero-lymphatic massage points are located mainly on the chest, head, and back. They are massaged for 10-30 seconds with fairly deep pressure. They may be tender or ticklish when touched, and the sorest points are probably the ones that are most in need of massage. Massage increases the flow of lymph and other body fluids that have been sluggish or blocked. When the energy of the lymph can again flow to the muscle and its related organ, the muscle will respond more efficiently to retesting.

NEURO-VASCULAR HOLDING POINTS

These points are located mainly on the head and are "believed to be the primitive pulsation of the microscopic capillary bed in the skin."[5] They are held lightly with the pads of the fingers for 20 seconds to 10 minutes, depending on the severity of the problem. A few seconds after contact a pulse is felt. When we hold these points lightly until the pulses synchronize, muscles are strengthened, blood circulation to both the muscle and the related organ seems to improve.

ACUPRESSURE HOLDING POINTS

These are traditional acupuncture points that are held with finger pressure for 15 seconds up to a few minutes. Two points are held at the same time on the same side of the body, with one hand holding an arm point and the other holding a leg point. In order to strengthen the muscle(s) involved, both sets of designated points are held, and, of course, the muscle(s) are retested.

THE TOUCH FOR HEALTH BALANCING SYSTEM

Touch for Health is a unified system of techniques and concepts, arranged in orderly procedures. Absolutely essential for understanding this system is the *Touch for Health* book (see bibliography), a "how to" manual for each muscle test and all corrective reflex point locations. Since the book's publication, the system has undergone considerable refinement, and much of the following information is not found in the *Touch for Health* book. This article is designed to introduce the subject and, along with the *Touch for Health* book, put it into practice.

"The Wheel" (see Figure 1) is a visual aid for understanding the organizational principles of Touch for Health. Starting at the stomach meridian, read around the wheel clockwise, proceeding to the inner circle. Each section from top to bottom contains: (1) the name of the meridian; (2) the indicator muscle for that meridian, and (3) the names of other muscles associated with the meridian (and in parentheses the names of the related organ, gland, function, or system).

The analogy of a beaver building a dam in an irrigation ditch can help us understand the wheel. The meridian pathways represent an irrigation ditch with 14 major junctions. The dam represents an energy blockage somewhere in the system, let's say, at the heart junction. Since little or no water can pass beyond the dam, several important junctions may not be getting any water flow. The root of the problem is at the heart junction, not at the others. Once the heart channel can be cleared, "water energy" again

(Text continued on p. 50)

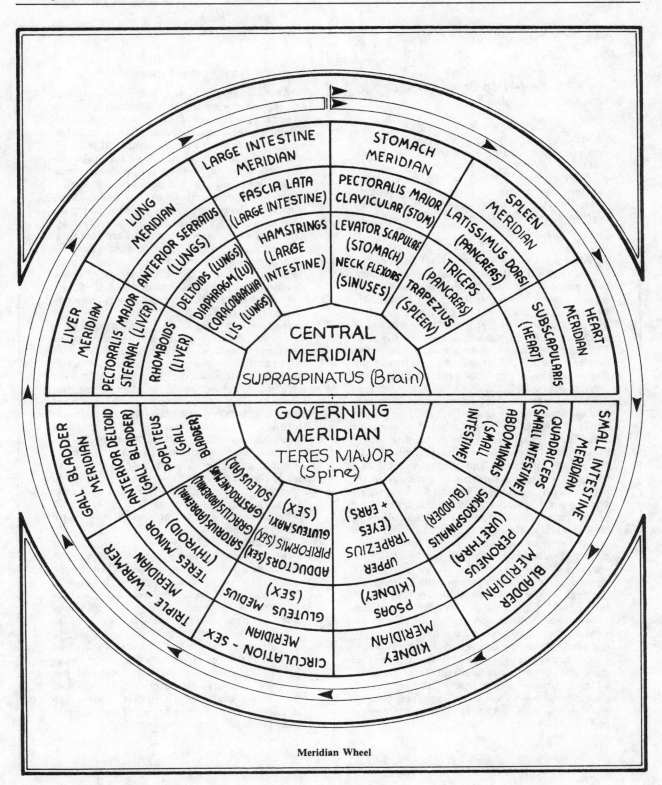

Meridian Wheel

Self-Help Program
Susan Koenig

Although Touch for Health is primarily designed as a two-person process, all reflex correction points and meridian tracing can be done by oneself. Only muscle testing itself demands a partner. Cross-crawl exercises and self-massage are two highly recommended health-maintenance practices.

SELF-MASSAGE

Touching our body helps us get to know it. In Touch for Health, we suggest you massage the easy-to-reach, major reflex points, located mainly on the chest, belly, thighs, shoulders, and neck (see Figure 2). Begin under the clavical (collarbone) and proceed down each side of the sternum (breast bone) between the ribs. Think of the ribs as mountains and the spaces between them the valleys. As you run your fingers down the ribs beside the sternum, your fingers naturally sink down into the valleys. That's where you want to massage. Then follow the longer valley under both breasts. Linger where the spots are more tender. Use as much pressure as you can without tensing other muscles, and remember to breathe. Spend 10-20 seconds on an area and then move on. I like to massage using a rotating or back-and-forth motion with my fingers. The idea is to systematically cover the areas indicated. Massage your navel, the area on either side of it, and above it on both sides. Massage on and just inside the hip bones. Now massage up and down the insides and outsides of your thighs. Again, linger where it is especially tender. If you're not finding tender spots, use more pressure. Finish on the back of the neck and shoulders, and under the ocipital ridge. To find this ridge, bend your head forward a little and bring your fingers up your neck until you feel a ridge near the base of the skull. Massaging this area is especially helpful for headaches. Now massage the nape of the neck and on either side of the large vertebra which protrudes at the base of the neck. End your session with some cross crawls (see below) and feel renewed and ready to start the day or to pick up after a work break.

THE CROSS-CRAWL

Any movement in which the opposite arm and leg are moving together is a contralateral or cross-crawl exercise. Walking with your arms swinging freely and opposite arms and legs working together is a good example. It is a well-known fact that the right side of the brain controls the left side of the body, and vice versa. Cross-crawls aid in maintaining the normal neurological organization of the brain. Cross-crawls can be done by crawling around on the floor, marching in place, or lying down face up. Although all cross-crawl exercises are beneficial and energizing to the body, applied kinesiologists consider the latter position the most therapeutic. When the body is lying down, gravity forces the muscles to do more work.

Do at least 25 sets of cross-crawls every day as part of your exercise program (one client does them first thing in the morning while she's still in bed). As a school teacher, I used cross-crawl exersises one to four times a day with children that were hyperactive and had learning and coordination problems. Not only did I see it do miracles for some of the children, but I began feeling more energetic and able to cope with the stress of teaching. Many Touch for Health instructors are out in the field doing cross-crawl exercises with all kinds of people, including senior citizens, Down's Syndrome children, and athletic teams, with very exciting and healing results. Perhaps the most publicized achievements are those of Dr. LeRoy Perry, D.C., who successfully uses Touch for Health techniques, including the cross-crawl, with Olympic champions.

Homolateral exercises, such as jumping jacks or the swimmer's breast stroke, actually have a weakening effect on most people. Even though balance is restored quickly in healthy people, it's a good idea to intersperse and conclude your exercise program with the strengthening effect of cross-crawls. If you are not used to exercising, a moderate walk is a good way to start. Cross-crawls are fun and easy to do, and you can make up many variations. For example, do the regular cross-crawl movement but reach way out with your arms and legs and give your belly a stretch too. Or do the twist, with the right elbow touching the left knee, and vice versa. Try cross-crawling to music!

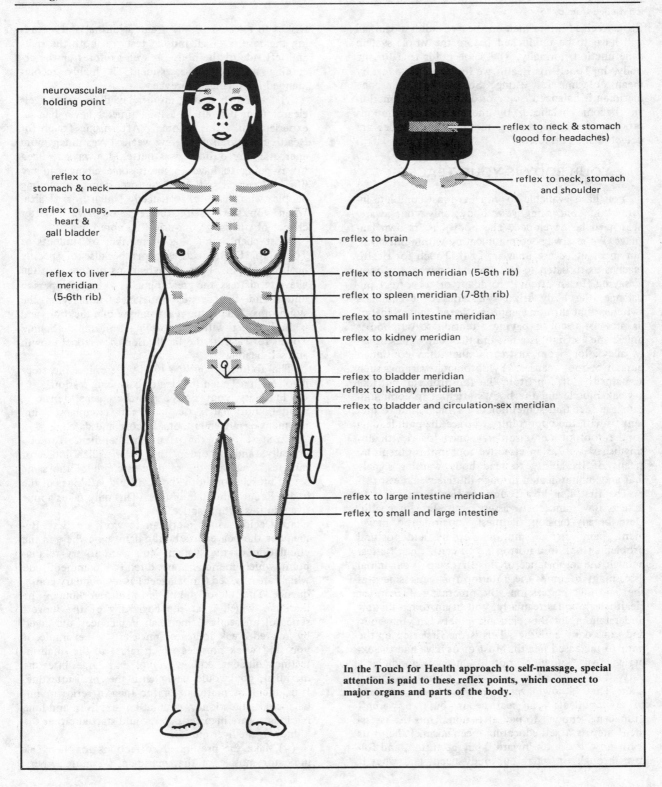

neurovascular holding point

reflex to stomach & neck

reflex to lungs, heart & gall bladder

reflex to liver meridian (5-6th rib)

reflex to neck & stomach (good for headaches)

reflex to neck, stomach and shoulder

reflex to brain

reflex to stomach meridian (5-6th rib)

reflex to spleen meridian (7-8th rib)

reflex to small intestine meridian

reflex to kidney meridian

reflex to bladder meridian

reflex to kidney meridian

reflex to bladder and circulation-sex meridian

reflex to large intestine meridian

reflex to small and large intestine

In the Touch for Health approach to self-massage, special attention is paid to these reflex points, which connect to major organs and parts of the body.

(continued from p. 46)

flows freely. If more than one beaver builds a dam, all will have to be unblocked before the whole system can function normally. The same holds true for the body. In Touch for Health we look for the dams by means of muscle testing. Sometimes when one meridian is balanced, some or all of the other meridians become balanced. By means of a continuous process of muscle testing, meridian imbalances are detected and corrected.

YOUR BODY IS YOUR TEACHER

You have available to you the most complete information concerning *your* body; only your awareness need be developed. The body has its own language. We're always communicating within ourselves, but most of us are unaware of it. Touch for Health teaches us to listen to and understand what the body is saying. In an attempt to adapt or to correct imbalance, the body triggers a series of events like switches that turn on symptomatic red lights. Most of us are not used to paying attention to our bodies unless the "signal" is pain, and then our goal is usually alleviation from distress, rather than continued pursuit of root "causes." Symptomatic warnings such as pain do not constitute the full problem, but like a weak muscle are the body's attempt to communicate the fact that something is "wrong," and to present us with the opportunity to trace the path leading to the root of our disorder. Touch for Health distinguishes itself as an effective tool in this pursuit by means of its ability to read body warning signals that are communicated through muscle weaknesses.

The first step in a Touch for Health session is to take a few minutes to assess your state of health. Describe any tension, tightness, impairment of movement, pain, mental/emotional upsets, and postural problems (look in a mirror if you can). I can't stress enough the importance of this first step. Your initial assessment becomes the criterion for reassessment at the end of the session. By practicing Touch for Health techniques regularly, you begin to have a new understanding of the relationship between your body and your daily activities. This is the first step on the path to increased health. Most of us have had the experience of "knowing" not to eat some goodie at a party, but indulging anyway, and "paying the Piper" later. That "knowingness" was our body's attempt to communicate our real needs, but we weren't "tuned in" enough to pay attention. Thus the assessment step is a self-educating mechanism. It helps us learn how to "look inward," pay attention, and follow through on what our body needs and what it

wishes to reject. Keeping a dated journal and recording the results of all muscle tests on both the right and left side of the body, as well as notes on the beginning and ending assessment, is highly recommended for further reference.

"I feel much better, more relaxed, my head feels clearer than it's felt in a long time. I never had an experience like this before." "After using Touch for Health on myself for a few weeks I was much more energetic, my outlook was better. I always realized I was going to have to make some changes in my life." Comments like these are common among people who have experienced Touch for Health. When you start feeling better, you have a better chance of changing your priorities about health.

Most clients and a good number of students of Touch for Health classes come because of specific health problems. Even though an instructor can often alleviate distress, the greater goal is to help the person understand the deeper imbalances underlying the symptoms. This is the real meaning of education, and is in keeping with the guiding philosophy behind Touch for Health: the facilitation of personal growth and self-healing.

The following outline briefly describes the steps involved in a Touch for Health balancing session.

(1) Assess your body: posture, pains, tensions, mental/emotional state, common complaints, impairment of movement, etc. Record and date.

(2) Start with the stomach meridian. Test bilaterally, and in order, the 14 meridian indicator muscles. Compare the relative strength of the same set of muscles on both the right and left sides of the body. Record and date results. (This only takes about five minutes with practice.)

(3) Decide which meridian to work on first. Remember the beaver has built a dam somewhere in the circulation of the system. You want to try to pinpoint which meridians are directly "dammed" and which are blocked (imbalanced) as a secondary consequence. The rule of thumb is to start working on the meridian which is at the beginning of the longest series of consecutive meridian imbalances, displayed by related weak indicator muscles. For example, if you find weak muscles which relate to the small intestine, bladder, kidney, lung, and large intestine meridian, you would begin with the small intestine. It is the first meridian of the longest series of imbalances. If the kidney, circulation-sex, liver, and lung meridians were involved, you would start at either the kidney or the liver meridian.

(4) Make the prescribed corrections for the weak indicator muscle of that meridian. (A more experi-

enced "Touch for Healther" would test and correct if necessary, all muscles related to that meridian.) Any system of correction can be used in any order. I prefer: (a) neuro-lymphatic massage points; (b) neuro-vascular holding points; (c) meridian; (d) acupressure holding points.

(5) Retest the weak muscle(s) from #4. If weak, repeat #4.[6] When previously weak muscles for that meridian test strong, you are ready for the next step. Continue to record pertinent data.

(6) Retest all previously weak meridian indicator muscles. Some or all may now test strong. (Particularly if the first meridian corrected contained a "major" dam).

(7) Reassess the picture of the remaining weak indicator muscles. As in #3, choose the next meridian to work on, which is the first of the longest series of consecutive meridians displaying related weak indicator muscles.

(8) Repeat #4, #5, #6, and #7 until all previously weak muscles test strong.

(9) Reassess your body based on the criteria of #1. Date and record as relevant.

(10) A Touch for Health session may take from 15 minutes to one hour. I try to accomplish a complete balancing within an hour. Beginners, however, should not feel they must achieve this goal. The important point is to work only as long as the quality of your energy and attention remains high. Even a partial balancing can bring positive results.

(11) Start a daily program using (and expanding over time) Touch for Health techniques. These can easily be combined with other healthful practices, such as exercise and a good diet.

CONCLUSION

Touch for Health is a holistic discipline intended to help the general public better understand the healing process. We are individuals, not a "runny nose" or an "arthritic," and our whole being must be taken into account. Touch for Health is not a panacea for all health problems, but it does offer guidelines for health maintenance and revitalization with safe, simple, and easy-to-use techniques. One of the basic goals of the holistic health movement is to make practical self-help skills like Touch for Health available to the public. Touch for Health also offers career training and adds to the repertoire of the health professional. It provides techniques which may be used adjunctly, or easily integrated into existing therapies.

Touch helps foster communication between people, and develops a greater trust between family members and friends. We are social beings; touch helps us express our caring nature, and is perhaps the most direct form of healing we can share. Therefore, we should take to heart the advice of this system, and sincerely set about learning how to "Touch for Health."

NOTES

1. John F. Thie, *Touch for Health*, p. 7.
2. Salient aspects of applied kinesiology are drawn from: (1) the technique of muscle testing demonstrated by Kendall and Kendall, two physiotherapists who first used it to evaluate the function and effectiveness of muscles; (2) the research of Bennett and DeJarnette, two pioneers in the study of reflexes who revealed how muscles could move bones by the activation of skin areas with deep massage and light touch; and (3) Dr. Frank Chapman, an osteopath who demonstrated the healing benefit to various organs and body functions through the massage of tender lymphatic areas. The results of Dr. Goodheart's research are recorded and available in his numerous "Research Manuals."
3. Mary Austin, *Acupuncture Therapy*, p. 1.
4. *Touch for Health*, p. 16.
5. *Touch for Health*, p. 15.
6. Here the system employs a technique called "challenging," which enables the tester to check which system(s) of correction are the most effective in restoring muscle balance.

SUGGESTIONS FOR FURTHER READING

Mary Austin, *Acupuncture Therapy*. Turnstone Books, 1972.

Carl H. Delacato, *The Diagnosis and Treatment of Speech and Reading Problems*. Charles C. Thomas, 1963.

George J. Goodheart, *Applied Kinesiology Research Manuals*. 1964-71.

Shafica Karagulla, *Breakthrough to Creativity*. DeVorss, 1919.

Henry O. Kendall *et al.*, *Muscles: Testing and Function*. Williams and Wilkins, 2d ed., 1971.

Stephen Rogers Peck, *Atlas of Human Anatomy for the Artist*. Oxford University Press, 1951.

John F. Thie, with Mary Marks, *Touch for Health*. DeVorss, 1973.

Susan Koenig is an administrator of the Berkeley Holistic Health Center and coordinator of the Continuing Education (CE) program for nurses. She is a certified Touch for Health instructor and a California State Certified Masseuse. Susan is on the teaching staff of the Berkeley Holistic Health Center and is in private practice in the Bay Area.

The Teachings of Moshe Feldenkrais:
Seeing Movement as the Embodiment of Intention
Layna Verin

The teachings of Moshe Feldenkrais are not a routinized set of exercises, but rather a process as alive and animated as the teacher himself. The basic idea is to reeducate the movements of the body in order to eliminate habitual responses in the brain— responses that hamper our movement, and therefore our total energy and creativity.

According to Feldenkrais, the key to a natural expression of movement, "as the embodiment of the organism's intention," is to affect the cortex of the brain via the motor system. In his own words, "what I'm after isn't flexible bodies, but flexible brains."

In this beautiful article which Moshe Feldenkrais calls "perhaps the fullest and best description of what goes on in my workshops," Ms. Verin captures the joy of Feldenkrais, the man and his teachings.

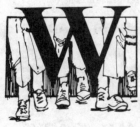isdom is always the same. Its application varies, but its use is invariable—to free the human spirit.

Among the wiser men in this world is one Moshe Feldenkrais, originator of a unique kind of body reeducation which, I believe, is to have exceedingly far-reaching application and influence.

Like other great innovators of our time, Feldenkrais bases his method on the importance of awareness in human functioning. What makes his work unique is the fact that he has discovered something fundamental about learning and change that no one before him, in either the Eastern or the Western world, has scientifically understood, though they may have sensed it intuitively. Because of this understanding, he has devised a way of learning so deeply rooted in common sense and so profoundly simple that it is within the capacity of anyone, from the most supple athletes to those crippled by deformations.

This article first appeared in *The Graduate Review*, June 1978.

Awareness, to Feldenkrais, has a very special meaning. To him, we live in four possible states: asleep, awake, conscious, and aware. Consciousness is a higher aspect of being awake, but awareness has to be cultivated.

Awareness is consciousness allied with knowledge. It includes being attentive to what goes on both inside yourself and in the external world. For the external world, the surrounding environment of space and society is as intrinsic a part of us as the nervous system and its body envelope.

Awareness cannot be taught; it has to be experienced. And in order that it may be experienced, a particular learning situation has to be created. This situation must both stimulate awareness and pose problems that only heightened awareness can solve.

By creating this kind of learning situation, Feldenkrais has also created a new kind of learning—a learning that is non-cerebral and non-coercive, in which there is no "correct" way of doing things, no competitive striving, no "perfect" or "imperfect." A learning that is as much play as it is work. A process, in fact, in which the mind/body plays/works.

This learning, like that of the infant, is self-directed. It is the antithesis of the authoritarian learning by rote to which we are accustomed. It circumvents the twin demons of anxiety and habit, replacing willpower and compulsive effort with curiosity and pleasure.

The changes it produces are immediately and dramatically visible, affecting body, mind, and feeling simultaneously, and resulting in a new and heightened sense of self—a new self-image.

Feldenkrais is a great teacher who insists that he teaches nothing. What he teaches is learning to learn. What he does is make it possible for you to experience your body and to replace habitual ineffective movements, which he calls "parasitic" movements, with free, unhampered movements that do what they are intended to do with the least expenditure of energy.

Nevertheless, he says, "The movements are nothing. They're an idiotic thing. What I'm after isn't flexible bodies, but flexible brains. What I'm after is to restore each person to their human dignity."

What is astonishing is the simple and direct means he has devised to accomplish this.

Feldenkrais works through the motor system. He sees the motor system not as related to the mind, but as inseparable from it. Thus, any change in the motor system will alter the patterns in the motor cortex of the brain, with results that diffuse throughout the nervous system.

"Without motor functions," he says, "the brain wouldn't think, or at least the continuity of mental functions is assured by corresponding motor functions."

Movement is the essence of life. It is also the embodiment of intention—the intention of the organism. Every thought and emotion finds its expression in movement, whether the movement consists of the gross muscular transformations of rage and fear, or the infinitesimal change in the eye's pupil caused by a fleeting thought.

Movements are concrete and simple. They are easy to differentiate. And learning depends on the ability to distinguish and differentiate.

When we move, an image of the movement is transmitted to the brain. If our image self is distorted, that distortion is incorporated in the message. Each time the movement is repeated, the distortion is repeated, and its repercussions in the body become more and more destructive.

If a new message can be transmitted to the brain, a change takes place in the cortex, freeing it from the old patterns, and the brain will transmit new messages to the body. This reversibility in the nervous system is distinctively human, and is what makes relearning possible.

"That being so," Moshe would say if he were talking to a class (all his students call him Moshe—pronounced Mo-shay')—"that being so, lie down on your backs on the floor."

His lessons usually begin with a simple movement, such as flexing and extending one foot, or placing the feet near the body so that the knees are bent, and lowering the legs first to one side, then the other.

Such movements may feel totally unfamiliar, even though you may have done them when you were a baby. Babies haven't yet lost their native intelligence, and they intuitively exercise every muscle and every sense with no direction or compulsion from anyone, without even a guru.

Nonhabitual movements are added to the habitual ones—turning the head in opposition to the shoulders, or the eyes in opposition to the head. They form

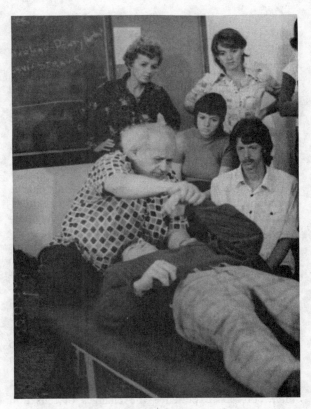

Feldenkrais bases his teaching on the importance of awareness in human functioning.

combinations and variations of combinations, culminating in a reorganization of the whole body. At that point, what Moshe would call "a funny thing" happens, the "funny thing" he has been leading up to all along.

He asks the class to do one more movement. This last movement isn't simple at all. It is quite complicated. It demands flexibility, coordination, balance, a fine adjustment of intent and impulse, none of which you had to the necessary degree when the lesson began. Yet, to your delight, you do it. Effortlessly.

You may be arching your body in a way that is usually achieved only after weeks or even months of arduous hatha yoga stretches. Or find yourself swinging your body around in a full circle on your pelvis, like a child. Or, with utmost ease, touching your knee to the opposite elbow. The details are unimportant. What is important is that in a ridiculously short time you have accomplished something that you were certain you couldn't do, and accomplished it with ease, enjoyment, and zest.

"Stand up," he says. "Walk around. How do you feel? Do you walk differently? Look at the people around you. Look at their faces. Do they look different? Have their eyes changed? Their shoulders?"

Indeed they have. The eyes are brighter, more open. In some people, they appear to have changed position slightly. The shoulders are looser, the expressions more intelligent, more alive. And indeed you walk differently. Your feet feel more balanced. They get the same stimulus from the floor that they did earlier, but they respond differently.

You have demonstrated to yourself the apparently changeless rule of change: when you can't change the stimulus, change the response. You feel exhilarated. Centered. Receptive. Even kind of loving, maybe. What has happened? How did he do it?

He did it in the most delicate, the most ingenious way. By enabling you to become more sensitive to differences. By devising a configuration of movements that cannot be performed without this refinement. By making you aware of the minute interval between the time your body mobilizes itself for a movement and the time when you actually do that movement—the minute interval that allows you to exercise that capacity for differentiation, and to change.

Periodically he stops and asks the students to scan their bodies. "Experience the changes of sensation in the side of the body that is being worked on," he says. "Feel the difference in the way the spine lies on the floor, the difference in the way the limbs are lying. Notice whether the backs of the knees touch the floor." Amazingly, one side of the body seems to shrink, the other to expand and swell. It seems to grow warmer, more alive, more expressive.

He may ask for a large movement, then reduce it to a smaller and smaller one. He may ask for a slow movement, then quicken it so that there is less willful control. Or retard it even more, so that the experience of sensation is stronger.

If the work begins on the right side, the movements may be repeated on the left side in exactly the same way. Or he may ask the class to imagine doing the movement on the left side several times before actually doing it. You discover that when you image the movement, the body mobilizes the muscles for action. Then, when you do the movement, it not only feels as if you had already worked on it, but it is more fluid than it was on the right side because you have discarded your previous mistakes.

Sometimes he has the class imagine the movements on the unworked side and never do them at all. And, occasionally, the work is done only on one side, so

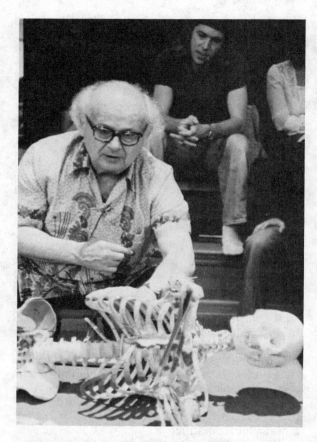

There must be an awareness of the skeleton itself, of its orientation and movement in space.

that you can experience how the learning diffuses through the nervous system into the muscles on the unworked side.

What is most extraordinary about all this is not the magnitude of the change, or the ease and swiftness with which it is effected, but that it is a complete reversal of ordinary learning. It is discovery. Discovery not about things, but about processes and change. The whole self is involved—mind, body, and feeling. The obvious difference in posture and movement is the outer sign of an inner change. There is a new attitude to both the inner and the outer environment, the beginning of a new facility in dealing with both.

"Learning that is not conducted through a new way of action is not learning," says Feldenkrais. "You only learn what you already know, what you have experienced. Learning is the crystallization of the experience." The experience isn't verbalized. Nevertheless, it isn't complete until it becomes verbalized, so that the differences between the old and the new way are understood. It must also become so familiar that it is automatic, or even unconscious.

In ordinary learning, a habit confronted with a situation in which it is useless is resistant to change. Confronted with a similar situation, a movement or attitude that is learned with awareness can be modified or changed by virtue of that awareness.

Feldenkrais never presents a lesson twice in exactly the same way. There is always a new variation, a new realization to be shared. "He has the ability to see new things every single day," says one of the students he is training to carry on his work. "He uses no notes, and every day he comes up with something new—not just a new movement, but a new perspective, a new way of looking at things. A most incredible teacher."

While the class is learning, he pleads, groans, cajoles, reminisces, lives every moment of comprehension or incomprehension. He never minces words. Says exactly what he means, with jokes, laughter, exasperation, and wisdom. His vulgarity is hilarious. Even his irascibility is tinged with humor. "As I've said a thousand times," he says for the thousandth time, "when people are in a mood where they're ready to smile, their minds are working. You tell everybody to be serious, they're unable to think anything for themselves."

"Stop, everybody!" he said suddenly in the midst of a workshop, just as we had begun a movement of bringing the head toward the left knee. "Watch her!" He pointed to a woman off near the corner in the front row. (Of the hundred or more people in the hall, she was perhaps the furthest from bringing knee and head together.) "You see the tiny movement she is making? She has self-esteem. She doesn't try. She does what she can. She doesn't have to prove anything to herself. And she will be one of the first to touch her head. You'll see."

He turned to the woman. "Here and now I say that you will touch better than all the others, because you have respect for yourself."

The class resumed. "Aha! Did I tell you she would get there first?" Everyone sat up. The woman was doing with ease what others who were able to "almost" do from the beginning and who were working with effort were still unable to do.

"Well," he asked, "did she grow stronger in this time or did she use her brain better? I say anybody can do it provided you correct your self-esteem. Only you can say if you are good. Nobody else. And you can learn now in an hour what, otherwise, people can't learn in years."

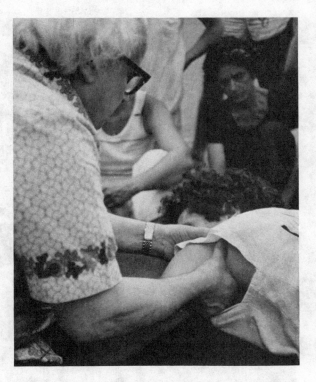

If a new message can be transmitted to the brain, a change takes place in the cortex, freeing it from the old patterns.

"You don't have to break your neck to show me how clever you are," he continued. "I know you're clever. More than you believe you are. Don't strain. It's a sign of internal impotence. And impotence is not a thing to be cultivated." Adding, "By the way, that's the way to cure real impotence—to learn to do it, not by 'curing' it."

There are many "first time in my life" experiences in the Feldenkrais classes. A young woman lying next to me in one of the first sessions I attended told me, "All my adult life I've felt awkward and ungainly. This is the first time I've ever done a movement and felt graceful."

A woman violinist who for seven years had been vainly trying to achieve a vibrato effect, and who, in desperation, was about to relinquish her hopes of becoming a concert violinist, came home after the third lesson and played vibrato without knowing how or why. The old, ineffectual impulse—the "parasitic" one—had been inhibited and superseded by a new, organic one.

As for me, I experienced my skeleton for the first time in one of the classes. Became aware of my bones. Felt myself as a structure of bones and joints

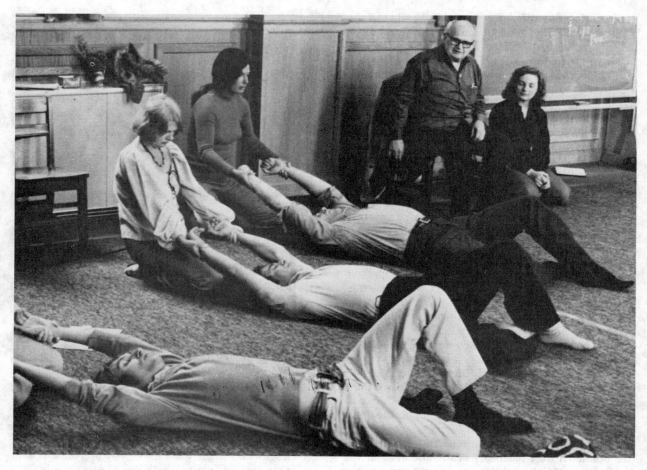

"People are not a bunch of properties," Feldenkrais says, "They are a process. All life is a process. Improve the quality of the process and the rest will take care of itself."

—a "skellington," as a child described by Sylvia Ashton Warner wrote in his composition. Feldenkrais teaches that to become aware of what is happening in the muscles is basic, but it isn't enough. There must be an awareness of the skeleton itself, of its orientation and movement in space.

What I have been describing is only one aspect of the Feldenkrais work, the group aspect, known as Awareness Through Movement. The other aspect, an outgrowth of this original work, consists of manipulation, and is called Functional Integration.

In this work with individuals, Feldenkrais treats the nervous system primarily through the skeletal structure. He gives physical support to the body members to offset the influence of gravity, thus returning the body to an early childhood state. Then he gently manipulates them, using the same configurations as in the Awareness Through Movement group sessions.

People come to him for treatment of deformations, injuries, congenital illnesses, and a multitude of physical problems with an emotional source. His reputation in restoring physical function, or as a student put it, "re-able-ization," is worldwide. "There is no limit," he says, "to possible improvement in functioning, and no limit to human potential."

I discontinued sessions with a chiropractor when I began the classes with Feldenkrais. I have a bad back —bone spurs, damaged disks, a severe curvature, a rotation in the upper spine. One manipulative session with Moshe accomplished what years of osteopathy and chiropractic had failed to achieve. The session lasted less than 15 minutes. I was stunned. "Can this be all?" I wanted to say.

I asked Moshe if the results would last, not believing that they could. He said that they would if I could manage to retain the sensation I was experiencing. I did, for more than three months, and would have done so longer had I not interrupted the awareness exercises.

To startle my chiropractor, I visited him again and asked him to examine my back. He did and gasped. "It can't be," he exclaimed. "Your back is entirely different."

Feldenkrais never speaks of his work as therapy. He never uses terms like "emotional disease" or "character disorders." He speaks only of faulty learning. Malfunctioning bodies are not diseased. The distressed psyche, unable to cope with the stresses of continuous coercion and repression, is not diseased. Both are simply poorly taught.

A person who realizes that his education has been faulty does not regard himself in the same way, nor is he regarded in the same way, as a person who is "sick," regardless of what euphemistic jargon disguises the "sickness." If we feel awkward, dull, somehow shameful, we will behave in an awkward, dull and shamed manner. Feeling free and uninhibited, we will behave spontaneously.

A physical distortion exists in the brain as literally as in the vertebrae. The corrective lies in releasing an inhibition in the brain cortex, so that the old pattern of response is broken and can be replaced with a useful response. Once that is done, the change in behavior is already begun.

We live in a civilization that demands finer and finer adjustments in order to function in a human way. Yet, from our birth, that civilization represses in us the qualities we most need to develop. Feldenkrais seeks to undo the emotional and physical havoc caused by this suppression of our most vital impulses. He says that he has barely scratched the surface of the study of the human nervous system and the ways of bettering its function. He has taken only one aspect and worked on it, but the possibilities are immense.

"People are not a bunch of properties," he says. "They are a process. All life is process. Improve the quality of the process and the rest will take care of itself."

SUGGESTIONS FOR FURTHER READING

Moshe Feldenkrais, *Awareness Through Movement.* Harper and Row, 1972.

———, *Body and Mature Behavior.* International Universities Press, 1975.

———, *The Case of Nora: Body Awareness as Healing Therapy.* Harper and Row, 1977.

Layna Verin is a writer, poet, and lecturer. She is also a psychic counselor and holistic health practitioner, conducting workshops in Hatha Yoga, sexuality, and preparation for natural childbirth. Her articles on aspects of holistic health have appeared in a variety of publications, including Energy and Character, Humanizing City Life, The Berkeley Monthly, *and* The Graduate Review.

Bodymind

Ken Dychtwald, Ph.D.

The Western world has inherited the notion that the body and the mind are two separate entities, almost coincidentally sharing the same space. Even the word "psychosomatic," one of our culture's few allusions to a body/mind interaction, merely conjures up images of an overactive imagination, rather than any meaningful understanding of body/mind intercommunications.

Fortunately, many have come to the realization that the body and mind not only are intimately related, but may be indivisible. In this provocative article, Dr. Dychtwald suggests that the disposition of the body is largely an extension of the mind. The implication is clear: as long as we can maintain a graceful, balanced state of mind, we will naturally inherit a graceful, balanced body.

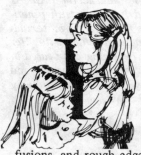 f you were a physician you would no doubt say that I am in good health and that I am lucky to have such a vital, well-toned body. When I examine myself closely, however, I notice that there are all sorts of imbalances, confusions, and rough edges within my tissues, as surely as there are within my soul; conflicts that have come to form my physical body as definitely and as distinctly as they have also molded my character and life.

In fact, my body is incredibly lopsided. My right leg is longer than my left; my left hand is smaller than my right; my right shoulder is lower than my left; the top half of my body is more muscular than the bottom half; my pelvis is rotated a bit in a clockwise fashion; my neck is angled slightly to the right; my spine is not as straight as it is supposed to be; my feet are somewnat archless; my right hand is more coordinated than my left hand; my left leg is tighter than

---

Sections of this article have been excerpted from *Bodymind* by Ken Dychtwald (Jove Publications), and are reprinted here by permission of the author.

my right leg . . . and on and on. There are an infinite number of asymmetries and imbalances within my body.

I am not smooth, for my life has not always been smooth. I am not perfectly balanced, for my feelings are not always balanced. My muscular strength is not equally proportioned throughout my body, just as my interests are not equally distributed throughout my life. In a way, my body is like the Earth, whose mountains, valleys, river beds, and uneven topography tell the story of its history and creation as surely as my body expresses the trials and creative changes that I have experienced throughout my lifetime.

In my attempt to explore the terrain of my own life and being, I have discovered that my body and my mind are reflections of each other, and that the emotions and experiences which have formed my personality have affected the formation and structure of my muscles and tissue. As I have become more aware of my own history and the realm of possibilities that it reveals, I have also come to appreciate some of the ways that these body/mind relationships can be discovered, examined, and improved upon.

In my own life, I have given up on the notion of the "perfect" bodymind or the "ideal" life, for there are no such things. Rather, I have allowed myself to become more aware and enlightened about my own potential, and by so doing have begun to discover the unique life and bodymind that is "ideal" for my specific needs and dreams. I notice that when I approach my growth and self-exploration from this perspective, they become pleasurable adventures rather than tedious chores.

FORMATION OF THE BODYMIND

Traditionally, five components have been identified as influential, in the formation of the human bodymind: (1) heredity; (2) physical activity and exposure; (3) nutrition; (4) environment; and (5) emotional and psychological activity and exposure.

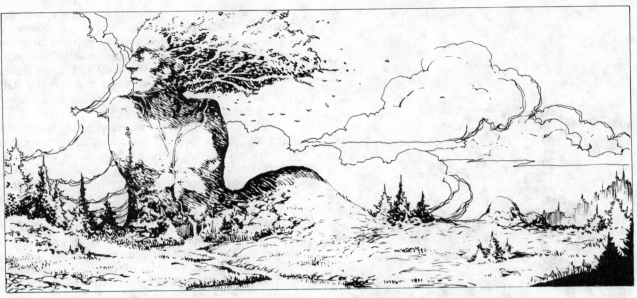

My body is like the earth, whose mountains, valleys, river beds and uneven topography tell the story of its history and creation as surely as my body expresses the trials and creative changes that I have experienced.

Heredity includes all factors that are with us at birth. This information and structure is passed on from our parents to us, and is, no doubt, a critical factor in the formation of our own unique bodyminds. For obvious reasons, it is very difficult to isolate those aspects of the physical and psychological self for which heredity is entirely responsible.

The second influential component, *physical activity,* includes all the physical actions, activities, and encounters that we experience throughout our lives. Walking, sleeping, bicycle riding, pounding nails, sitting, giving birth, and playing the piano are all activities that, regardless of their hereditary and psychoemotional components, mold and shape our bodyminds. What we have done with ourselves, how we have done it, how frequently we have done it, and how it felt to be doing it are all reflected in the way we have developed our muscles, bones, and neuromuscular coordination.

The third major component in the creation of the bodymind is *nutrition.* By nutrition, I mean all the fuel, psychological as well as physical, that the bodymind takes in and digests in order to supply itself with the necessary elements for regeneration and continued growth. Although there is controversy about what fuels are most healthful or appropriate, there is definite agreement about the important role that nutrition plays in the creation and maintenance of the bodymind.

Environment is the fourth major component that influences the formation of the human bodymind. By environment, I mean all the physical, social, and psychological structures within which we live our lives. Like heredity, environmental factors are "givens" that we receive as we enter life at a particular time and in a particular location. They differ from heredity, however, in that we have the ability to change them—and, therefore, their influence on our personal development—by taking steps to alter them, or by simply changing locations. As a result, our relationship to our environment is a dynamic process that is continually open to change, rearrangement, and re-creation. It is extremely difficult to separate ourselves from our environment, for, in a sense, it is as much within us as it is outside us.

The fifth component, *emotional and psychological activity and experience,* is the one that fascinates me the most. Although most people will agree that feelings, attitudes, and experiences have an effect on the conditions of their bodyminds, there is very little agreement about *how much* effect they have. For example, if I am nervous and I feel butterflies in my stomach, I naturally associate my physical symptoms with the emotional stress. Or, if I have just had a fight with my girlfriend and I notice that my neck is stiff and I've got a headache coming on, I'll probably admit to myself that the argument caused the tension.

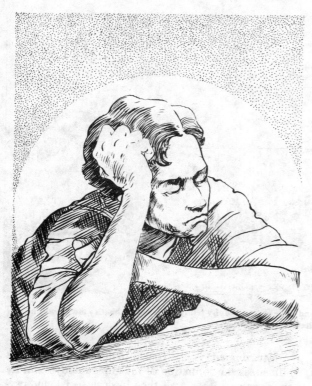

The body forms around the feelings that animate it; those feelings become habituated and trapped within the body tissue.

Yet, how far will I carry these psychosomatic associations? When I have a sore throat, do I associate it with restrained anger? If I sprain my ankle, did I do so at a time when I was feeling emotionally ungrounded? If I am asthmatic, am I this way because it is hard for me to take responsibility for the rage that is trapped in my chest? If I have hemorrhoids, is it because I have been holding on to all my feelings too tightly? If I am blissfully happy, is it because my bodymind is healthfully relaxed and integrated?

Chances are that most of us do not relate every one of our emotional attitudes and experiences to specific physical symptoms and conditions. Conversely, how many of us associate our body structures with personality preferences and emotional histories? Yet, there is increasing evidence that our feelings and attitudes very directly affect the way we hold ourselves, move, breathe, and grow, and that just as we partly form ourselves with physical activity, so do we mold ourselves with selective emotional activity and experience.

For example, imagine that you are extremely nervous and upset. With this feeling, allow the accompanying physical sensations in your belly, and perhaps, a shortening of breath. What would happen if you practiced this psychosomatic pattern for a few minutes each day? Surely after months and years of exercising yourself in this fashion, the muscles of your belly and chest would begin to reflect this state of nervousness, with its accompanying tensions and blockages.

Or imagine that you are very unhappy and depressed. Allow yourself to assume the posture that would reflect these feelings. Chances are, your shoulders would slump, your chest would become sunken, and you would project an over-all feeling of heaviness.

Emotional stimulation of muscles can have the same effect on the body as purely physical activity, except that it is usually more difficult to detect the source of stimulation and the way in which it has been selectively, and often unconsciously, exercised. The body begins to form around the feelings that animate it, and the feelings, in turn, become habituated and trapped within the body tissue. The bodymind then, when seen from this perspective, is to some extent the continually regenerating product of a lifetime of emotional encounters, psychological activities, and psychosomatic preferences.

I have isolated these five approaches for academic purposes, but in reality they are inseparable. In this article, I will focus primarily on several aspects of the fifth component of bodymind formation, that of emotional activity and psychological preference. Although this path is intimately connected to all the others, I feel that it is the most important because of its effect on the creation of the human bodymind. A growing body of evidence suggests that emotional experiences, psychological choices, and personal attitudes and images not only affect the functioning of the human organism, but also strongly influence the ways in which it is shaped and structured. This is not to say that heredity, physical activity, nutrition, and environment do not influence the bodymind; they unquestionably do. Rather, I am suggesting that when all these forces are merged in the creation of a human being, the force of the aware human psyche seems to be the most powerfully formative.

The study of the relationships that exist between the mind and the body is not new. As long as human beings have reflected on their health, survival, passions, thoughts, dreams, lives, and selfhood, there have been questions about the nature of this most precious and elusive of all unknown territories. In the East, as exemplified in the Oriental and Indian cultures, the body and the mind have traditionally been viewed as inseparable aspects of the same human essence. The health practices, educational forms, religious insititutions, and psychoemotional disciplines of that part of the planet all suggest a holistic approach to life and life-development.

Here in the West, we have chosen to make a duality of the bodymind, separating it into two parts: the psyche, which is considered to dwell somewhere in the skull between the eyes; and the body, which lives and moves beneath it. This mind/body dualism is reflected in all our institutions and cultural processes. By intellectually dividing ourselves into unrelated parts, we encourage intensive specialization and differentiation in all our activities, thereby further encouraging mind/body separatism, rather than holism. Because of this split, it is not surprising to find that our minds and bodies often compete and argue, for they lack communication.

In reality, every cell in your body is both structurally and functionally related to every other cell in your body. Similarly, all your thoughts, beliefs, fears, and dreams are dynamically connected within the structure and function of your psyche. I would also like to suggest that your cells and your thoughts are more directly interconnected than you probably believe at present. In this article, I present two major splits that can be observed in the bodymind. These descriptions are not intended as definitive studies, but should allow you to begin to see some of the ways in which the shape of the physical body is reflective of the psychological body that is housed within it.[1]

First, it might be helpful for you to take a few minutes to explore the over-all form of your own bodymind. This is best done in the nude, and it is helpful to stand in front of a full-length mirror in order to get a total view of the way your body is shaped.

As you look at yourself, try to be nonjudgmental, and avoid commenting to yourself about things you need to be doing for yourself (like dieting or exercising), or changes that have affected your posture (like aging or illness). Simply view yourself and allow yourself to get a sense of the way you are shaped and molded in every part of your body. Pay particular attention to the relationship between the left and right side of your body. Does one side appear to be larger or more powerful than the other? Is one side more healthy looking than the other? How about the top and bottom halves of your body? Do they seem to be proportionately related, or is one of the halves larger and heavier than the other? Take a few moments to explore your body with respect to areas of strength or weakness. As you look at yourself, see if you can make a mental map of your body, charting points of vitality and health, as well as points of disease and illness.

Sometimes, it's helpful to make a sketch of your body, front and back, and then color in the various experiences, incidents, and traumas that have contributed to your physical structure. To do this, take a large sheet of paper (perhaps butcher paper) and first outline your body. Then with different colored crayons or pencils draw in all the locations on your body where you have experienced either pain, stress, accident, or illness. Be sure to include all the little injuries and strains as well as the larger dis-eases and problems. Then, with other colors, highlight all the parts of your body that give you, or have given you, great joy or pleasure. Be sure to include all those parts that you consider vital and healthy. You might even discover that some of these locations coincide with the unhealthy zones. When you have completed this part of the drawing, look at yourself and try to get a sense of what parts of your body seem to project a glow of vitality. For example, you might feel that your face gives off a pleasant shine, or perhaps your hands generate a great deal of love or energy. In any case, once you have decided what part or parts of you are exceptionally vital and outpouring, color them as auras that project outward from the surface of your body.

While you are creating this body map, it is important that you take the time to sense how you feel about the different aspects of your body. See if you feel intimate with certain parts of yourself, and more of a stranger to other parts. Make notes to yourself about your discoveries, and save your drawings (front and back), for these will be helpful references as we discuss the following bodymind functions and qualities.

RIGHT/LEFT SPLIT

The first separation that I will discuss is the one between the right and left sides of the bodymind. Although these sides seem extremely similar to one another, they often house and animate different aspects of character and personality. It may be helpful to remember that the left cerebral hemisphere controls most of the right side's motor and neuromuscular functioning, and that the right cerebral hemisphere controls the left side of the body.

In recent years, several fascinating studies have explored right/left brain activity, and these have indicated strong differentiations between the character and quality of right- and left-hemisphere activity. According to Dr. Robert Ornstein, a pioneer in this

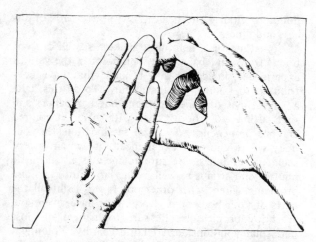

The right/left split is seen in how we shape our muscles and tissue, in the way we move and use our body parts.

field, the left hemisphere "is predominantly involved with analytic, logical thinking, especially in verbal and mathematical functions." The right hemisphere, on the other hand, "is primarily responsible for orientation in space, artistic endeavors, crafts, body images, recognition of faces."[2]

Correspondingly, the right side of the bodymind is usually considered the "masculine" side, having to do with logic and rational thought, and with such aspects of personality as assertiveness, aggressiveness, and authoritarianism—in the Chinese cosmology, the *yang,* or creative forces. The left side of the bodymind is considered to be related to the feminine aspects of the character. Personality constructs such as emotionality, passivity, creative thought, holistic expression, and the *yin,* or receptive forces, are said to inhabit and animate this side of the bodymind.

The easiest way to detect the right/left differences is simply to observe people while they are expressing themselves. The most obvious displays of right/left preferences occur when emotions are being released and acted out. I have found that encounter groups, sensitivity workshops, and group-therapy sessions have proved to be the most rewarding of all laboratories within which to explore these psychosomatic relationships.

The right/left split can be seen in the way we shape our muscles and tissue, in the way we move and use our body parts, and in the way we nonverbally express and communicate our attitudes and emotions. It is important to keep this particular separation in mind, for as we crisscross the bodymind and isolate specific regions and limbs, this particular duality will help to pinpoint more specifically the blocks and

character traits that animate our bodyminds. For example, in the case of one's hands, which have to do with reaching out and making contact, the left hand is associated with reaching out in a passive, receptive way, and the right hand corresponds to reaching out in an active, aggressive fashion.

TOP/BOTTOM SPLIT

Another major psychosomatic separation in the bodymind is that which is reflected in the top and bottom halves of the body. In many people this split tends to be more dramatic and obvious than the right/left split.

The bottom half of the bodymind, functionally considered, is the part of the organism that makes contact with the Earth. It is concerned with stabilizing, moving, balancing, supporting, and establishing a comfortable condition of groundedness. The top half of the bodymind, on the other hand, has to do with seeing, hearing, speaking, thinking, expressing, stroking, hitting, holding, communicating, and breathing.

Psychosocially, the bottom half is oriented toward privacy, support, introspection, homeyness, emotional stability, dependency, and motion/stasis. The top half is concerned with socializing, outward expression, interpersonal communications and manipulation, self-assertion, aspirations, and action.

One of the easiest ways to tell how a person relates to these aspects of his life is to observe the way his weight is distributed throughout his body. When diagnosing the bodymind in this fashion, remember that an individual must be viewed in terms of himself and the way he is proportionately structured, and not by comparing his top half with another individual's top half. Each person must be explored in his "wholeness," for it is from this wholeness that the unique personality emerges.

There are a number of ways in which people construct the proportions of their tops and bottoms. The easiest cases to observe are the ones that show extreme differences in structure from top to bottom, and there are a great many people who are shaped in these ways. The extreme examples of this duality are people who are very large and heavy from the hips down, and narrow from the waist up, or people who are large and overdeveloped from the waist up, and narrow and contracted from the hips down.

When the lower body half is proportionately larger than the upper half, it suggests that the individual has great comfort and facility in dealing with the stabilizing, homey, grounded, and private aspects of his life. In a sense, he has "filled out" these forces for support and identification, but will also usually tend to develop a lifestyle that insures the continuance of these relationships and contacts. The top half of the bodymind, which has to do with assertion and communication, is underdeveloped and contracted. With this bodymind split, weight distribution can be roughly correlated to attention distribution.

Since this person has overdeveloped the private aspects of himself to the exclusion of the expressive parts, he might tend to feel more comfortable expressing himself inwardly than outwardly. Emotions that can't find release through the natural channels of the hands, chest, heart, mouth, jaw, and eyes will bounce around inside until they are translated into a comfortable and appropriate means of self-expression. This person may often tend to be what is called a "feeling" or "being" person, rather than an "action" or "doing" person.

What if the top half is large and the bottom half is small? We all know people like this, who have large barrel chests, skinny legs, and contracted backsides. This person will be overdeveloped in his ability to be expressive, social, assertive, and outgoing, but his thin legs and hips will reflect a lack of emotional stability and self-support. As a result, he will have to "stand his ground" with his back, chest, and head (which are his active, assertive aspects) to compensate for the weakness in his legs and emotional roots. This person will probably be more of a mover than a homebody, more prone to action than to stasis.

These two bodymind extremes are located on opposite sides of a long continuum that includes the whole spectrum of top/bottom possibilities. Although very few people fit these descriptive extremes, most of us do lean in one of the two directions. The degree to which we prefer one style of being over the other is reflected in the amount of top/bottom balance in our bodyminds.

It is important to remember that there is no bodymind structure that is the "right" one. Some people have large tops and small bottoms, others have small tops and large bottoms, others have equally balanced tops and bottoms. Some people injure themselves frequently; others remain healthy and unblemished throughout their lives. Each body is reflective of a unique person, with his own unique style of being. Therefore, what is most important about this information, no matter what your particular shape happens to be, is that you realize that your bodymind is made up of many different components, and that some of these different preferences and qualities will be reflected in the structure and functions of the top

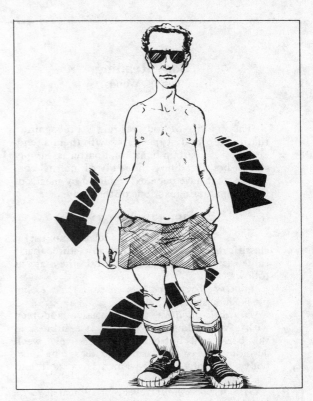

Emotions that aren't released bounce around inside until they are translated into a comfortable and appropriate physical means of self-expression.

and bottom halves, as well as the right and left halves, of your bodymind.

Now, I'd like to ask you to observe yourself once again in a full-length mirror. As you look at yourself this time, pay attention to the various bodymind splits that I have just described. See if you can be more aware of any imbalances that exist in your bodymind, and allow yourself to relate these imbalances to the corresponding preferences and habits that highlight your character and lifestyle. As you view yourself in this fashion, try to see the parts of your bodymind that are undeveloped not as points of weakness, but rather as untapped regions of yourself that are to be further explored and developed.

As you listen to the messages of your own bodymind, enjoy the way your muscles and limbs have come to tell the stories that are alive within you, stories that tell of experiences past, passions present, and dreams future; for when we realize the degree to which we have actually influenced and shaped our own bodyminds, we find ourselves in a position of increased self-awareness and greater self-responsibility.

(Text continued on p. 66)

Body Reading
Patrick Woods

The practice of body reading is a recognition that certain body types carry with them a tendency toward certain behavioral patterns. Simply stated, body reading is the study of internal conditions that have been externalized by means of the sympathetic reactions of the body.

A BRIEF LOOK AT TYPES

W.A. Sheldon presents a clear and useful classification of body types into three basic categories.[1] Loosely paraphrased, they are as follows.

(1) *Gut dominance* (viscerotonia). An example is Shakespeare's Falstaff.

Physical qualities are a massive abdomen with a protruding belly. There is a fullness in the belly and buttocks, but relatively weak development of the arms and legs. The face, body, and physical movements are soft and relaxed.

The temperament reveals a typical love of physical comfort, indulgence in overeating, oversleeping, and excessive amiability. Viscerotonians show a pronounced tendency to inertia.

(2) *Muscle dominance* (somatotonia). An example is the Tarzan type.

Physical qualities are a firm body with a typically large chest and narrow hips.

The temperament is characterized by a vigorous propensity for action. Somatotonians tend to hurl themselves head-on at the task at hand, often losing sensitivity both to themselves and to others. People of this type need to learn to relax and to become more receptive, so that they can achieve balance in their lives.

(3) *Nervous-system dominance* (cerebrotonia). An example is the Ichabod Crane character type.

Physical qualities include a fragile body that is delicate and linear. Cerebrotonians have slender limbs with poorly developed muscles. They lack padding, and their nervous systems are "overexposed."

The temperament is characterized by introversion and a tendency toward dreaminess. They typically overreact to practically everything, and are generally tense, repressed, and anxious. Their greatest need is to learn how to slow down and relax.

Using the preceding types as an overview, let us now look at another area of body reading that can give us added insight into peoples' dispositions and self-concepts.

BODY READING BY POSTURAL STRUCTURAL ANALYSIS

Our bodies can be seen as indicators of our relationships with the world. Our muscles contract under stress and relax to experience pleasure. The body is the lens through which we experience the world around us. It receives external stimulation and expresses or suppresses internal impulses. The body responds in basically the same way to any tension, whether it be physical or emotional, so that the body actually bends and is beaten down under an emotional weight as if the weight were a physical object. As we react to various recurring situations, certain habitual patterns begin to form, both in our inner (emotional) responses, and in our outer (bodily) responses.

A WORKING MODEL

The legs can be compared to a tree trunk, which supports the tree and gives it a solid foundation. In the same manner, we depend on our legs to give us a sense of stability. Underdeveloped, weak, or chronically tense legs fail to provide this feeling of support and confidence that is necessary for us to "stand up for ourselves."

The knees, if weak or rigid, may be a key cause of unstable or stilt-like legs. We have probably all heard the expression "weak-kneed," which is used to describe a condition of fear. Shaky knees and legs may transmit feelings of uneasiness and a sense of possible collapse.

The feet can be thought of as our "roots." They are the part of us that makes contact with the ground we stand on. Feet that do not grip the earth easily and securely may cause feelings of uncertainty and imbalance throughout the entire body and psyche.

The buttocks/pelvic area houses the fundamental life processes (i.e., elimination and reproduction), and it is the center for our basic survival instincts. Frequently ideas of survival or sexuality are in conflict with current social values, thereby creating basic survival fears and a corresponding lack of movement and awareness.

The abdomen/belly area contains the forces that generate our active life power through the process of digestion. Likewise, the belly is viewed as the place where we generate our power to assert ourselves in the world. The inhibition of this assertive power will be manifested in the belly, and the conscious experience will be that of fear. Stomach ulcers, constipation, rigid abdominal muscles, and other similar abdominal problems may indicate a withholding of one's own power, or perhaps a condition of being overpowered by others.

The chest/heart area houses feelings such as love, compassion, and receptivity. From here we experience our "heartfelt" emotional connections to the world. Chests that are collapsed —perhaps protected by slumping shoulders— indicate a probable attempt to withdraw from the real or imaginary hostile feelings of others. Heavily muscular, rigid, or "puffed-out" chests transmit feelings of protectiveness and overcompensation that are a response to a world that the individual doesn't feel able to deal with in a sensitive manner. All the above indicate protective responses caused by feelings of vulnerability.

The shoulders and arms are instruments of expression and action. Slumped shoulders may indicate feelings of heavy burden, i.e., "carrying the weight of the world." Raised shoulders may indicate an attitude of fear or anticipation. Shoulders pulled back in an exaggerated position usually accompany the puffed-out chest in an expression of false bravado. Tense forearms indicate frustration or a suppression of anger, for the expressive energy is never fully released through the arms and hands.

The neck and throat are the channels for vocal expression. Tension in this area indicates a "choking off" of the natural tendencies to express or respond. Perhaps there is the sensation of being forced to swallow something distasteful (either physically or emotionally). Tension here is readily observable, both to the eye and to the touch.

The jaw, likewise, deals with expression. A strongly held jaw indicates a tendency to repress feelings in a strong way. This can be seen as a literal sort of "biting the bullet."

The chin is an indicator of how we endure under stress. A soft weakly held chin usually indicates a weak personality in this respect; a square or solidly held chin suggests a person who is ready to meet the forces of the world "head-on."

The face often shows what the person (consciously or unconsciously) thinks the world wants to see. Sometimes this is not compatible with what the person actually feels. Frequently there is the complaint of feeling trapped behind a rigid "mask" of tension.

The compulsive smile generally indicates a compulsive need to be liked. Usually these people have strong muscular development in the face, especially around the cheekbones.

The eyes have been said to be the mirrors of the soul. Certainly they give us a direct look into a person's inner emotional nature, showing feelings of anger, sadness, joy receptivity,

(continued on p. 66)

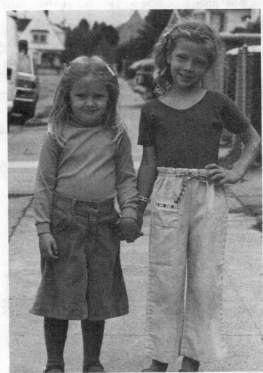

The body types of these two young ladies will influence their disposition throughout their lives.

(continued from p. 65)

hostility, wonder, and surprise. The more re-laxed the person's eyes, the more relaxed is that person's vision in terms of his or her ability to see things, including conceptual things, clearly. Tension around the eyes is often mani-fested in the eyebrows.

Tense, knotted eyebrows generally shows a straining to see things—a straining to figure things out mentally. This straining blocks the ability to see beyond personal concepts, and it hinders clear understanding and receptivity. Receptivity comes best in a relaxed state.

These above descriptions constitute only a rudimentary study of body reading. Readings who are interested in the concept of "body-mind" are encouraged to explore this develop-ing field further.

Patrick Woods is a bodywork therapist and personal growth counselor in Berkeley, Califor-nia. He teaches classes in deep-tissue bodywork therapy, and is a health educator at the Berke-ley Holistic Health Center.

NOTES

1. Robert De Ropp, *The Master Game* (Dell, 1968), pp. 106-126.

(continued from p. 63)

NOTES

1. Other major splits include front/back, head/body, torso/limbs, and are described in the expanded version of this arti-cle, "Major Splits in the Bodymind," *Alternatives Magazine* (October 1978).
2. Robert Ornstein, *The Psychology of Consciousness* (Vi-king, 1973), p. 52.

SUGGESTIONS FOR FURTHER READING

Frederick M. Alexander, *The Resurrection of the Body*. Dell, 1974.
Ken Dychtwald, *Bodymind*. Jove Books, 1978.
Ron Kurtz and Hector Prestera, *The Body Reveals*. Bantam, 1977.
Alexander Lowen, *The Language of the Body*. Col-lier Books, 1971.
Robert De Ropp, *The Master Game*. Dell, 1968.

Ken Dychtwald, Ph.D., psychologist, is a well-known pioneer in the holistic-health and human-development fields. He is president of Ken Dycht-wald, Ph.D., and Associates, was founding president of the Association for Humanistic Gerontology (A.H.G.), and was formerly a director of The SAGE Project, the highly acclaimed holistic-health center for elders in the San Francisco Bay Area.

In addition to lecturing and conducting seminars nationwide on bodymind development, holistic health, life-design, and aging/longevity, he serves as a consultant to government, industry, and media, and is an adjunct instructor in psychology, gerontology,

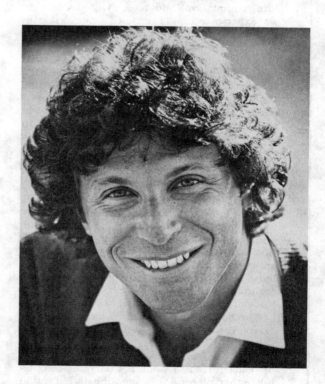

and health-related sciences at several colleges and universities.

His publications include: Bodymind *(Jove, 1978);* Millenium: Glimpses Into the 21st Century, *with Dr. A. Villoldo (J.P. Tarcher/Houghton Mifflin, Winter 1980);* The Aging of America *(J.P. Tarcher/ Bantam, 1981); and numerous articles in professional journals and popular magazines.*

Evolution and Biopsychology
Frank Wildman

In the world of body/mind therapies there is not yet a unifying framework that encompasses the therapies as a whole. Individual methodologies tend to be viewed as autonomous systems, with little communication or understanding between them. The resulting confusion diminishes the efficacy and credibility of the entire spectrum of body/mind disciplines.

In his rigorous article, Mr. Wildman suggests that there is a theory capable of providing this much-needed paradigm. He postulates that Darwin's theory of evolution is dynamic enough to account for the constantly changing qualities of the body/mind, and the therapies that are applied to "it."

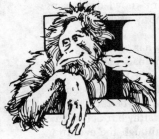

In surveying current discussions of the various body-oriented therapies, I am reminded of the situation of the preevolutionists who began investigating biology, geology, palaeontology, and other natural sciences. In attempting to make sense out of the profusion of newly observed phenomena, these investigators proposed many theories that now seem strange indeed. There was the theory of the spontaneous generation of life; the theory of acquired characteristics; the theory of the diluvianists, who believed the world had been destroyed in periodic great floods; the theory of the vulcanists, who believed the world had been repeatedly inundated with lava. That there was a progression and a hierarchy of life forms was observed time and again, but no one could propose a theory that could account for all the data, and explain how life began or how and why life moved in time toward ever-greater complexity.

This impasse was dissolved during the last third of the nineteenth century by Darwin's theory of the evolution of life by natural selection. It was the most creative, important, and far-reaching perception of life that Western civilization had developed for millennia. Darwin's theory quickened the thought of the world, tied together many confusing and fragmentary loose ends in all fields of science, and changed our view of life and our place in it forever.

Today, faced with all the confusing and sometimes contradictory methods that are included under the terms "body therapies" or "bodywork," therapists have at best only fragmentary approaches to understanding the complexities of the human bodymind. In talking with and experiencing therapists of differing approaches, I am reminded of the starfish, which, when overly excited, can actually tear itself in two merely by the antagonistic activity of its own feet. Many techniques have little or no common ground, either theoretical or practical, with other techniques that may approach the same body. These antagonisms and contradictions are not always apparent, since they are frequently glossed over or ignored for the sake of "solidarity" and social peace.

Some practitioners of body therapies believe their own particular approach to be the most comprehensive, accurate, and effective in dealing with their client's problems; others place their faith in vague syncretic gestures. (Some currently popular examples of the latter are Neo-Reichian Polarity therapy, Reichian Rolfing, Bioenergetic-Gestalt therapy, Feldenkrais and Gestalt.) I believe that any such conviction is premature and fundamentally ill-founded. No theory yet advanced has rigorously integrated, explained, or even classified the data and insights of all the various methods. There are many scattered therapeutic techniques, explorations, and explanations, but no true science of biopsychology has yet emerged.

This situation is understandable in view of the fact that psychology (especially as applied to the body therapies) has been going through a natural-history stage of development, similar to that of biology in the early nineteenth century. Some attempts have been made at system building, but what currently passes as theory is really a labeling of phenomena and concepts, as in natural history, and efforts at synthesis commonly consist of cross-referencing different sets of definitions and metaphors erected by the more imaginative thinkers, such as Reich, Lowen, and Feldenkrais, also as in natural history. I believe that, today, given the increasing richness of experimental and descriptive data at all levels of science and in the many bodywork and therapeutic methods, psychology, biology, and ethology can merge to yield the first phenomenological laws that pertain to the human bodymind.

What is both needed and possible today is a truly synthetic and coherent theoretical framework—a *paradigm*—for a "Biopsychology." A paradigm constitutes a basic interpretive framework in which we can organize our inputs from the natural world. A paradigm is also a way of thinking about and connecting our observations and experiences of the world, leading eventually to a set of mutually shared assumptions upon which further experience and knowledge may rest. The matrix of the paradigm is the unifier of our experience. A paradigm also functions as a perceptual filter; it permits the reception of certain information and screens out data that do not fit the matrix. Thus it also restricts our worldview and sets limits on the phenomena of which we are aware, often without our consciously realizing it.

But this apparently restrictive process is also intensely creative. It is the movement from emptiness to form. It patterns our collective perceptions and our social order, and establishes the boundaries of research. Thus, a good paradigm accounts for what is known and suggests what will probably be the most fruitful directions for future research, but does not attempt to rigidly explain everything. It should be useful, adjustable, and susceptible to refutation—flexible but clearly formed, like a healthy animal.

Without an adequate paradigm, students of therapy and bodywork resemble a gaggle of spiritual neophytes, rushing to sit at the feet of one guru after another, eagerly seeking some form of generalized enlightenment. The time has come for the body therapies to have a paradigm of their own, within which they can organize their many disparate and sometimes antagonistic elements into a deeper understanding of what happens when clients alter their breathing and their movements, what happens when you lay your hands on them, manipulate their tissue, talk to them, or interact with them in any way for the purpose of increasing their awareness, health, or growth.

In order for a theory to be useful to an emerging biopsychology, it must meet certain requirements. First, it must be nonobvious. A "theory" that can be arrived at by observation only, without reasoning, is not scientifically acceptable. Second, it must go be-

yond what could be grasped from unaided intuition or scattered concepts. And third, it should be *testable* in natural systems. A useful theoretical framework must expand and improve our working perceptions.

I propose that evolutionary theory may constitute the much needed theoretical framework upon which to build a science of biopsychology. Evolutionary theory is a broad and flexible paradigm that is well-integrated and can include highly diverse forms of information. It fulfills the requirements of a useful theory for a true biopsychology, and it is already the great ordering principle in biology. The diversity of life forms, patterns of animal distribution, the massive accumulation of observations of animal behavior, adaptation, and social interaction—all this was merely a bewildering chaos of facts until it was given meaning by the evolutionary theory.

There is no area of the life sciences in which evolutionary theory has not served as an ordering principle. From genetics to primate ethology, from zoological classification to palaeontology, from anthropology to geology, evolution is the underlying principle that gives meaning and order. The study of the origin of the universe, of our planet, and of life itself are all unified as part of a great body of knowledge because of the often disregarded and poorly understood paradigm of evolution.

To the lay person, evolution has something to do with dinosaurs, or with how human beings evolved from apes by survival of the fittest. Even to most biologists, it has been merely a historical document, an explanation of how things got to be the way they are. Most scientists profess the faith, but act in their daily teaching and research as though the evolutionary paradigm that organizes their discipline were somehow irrelevant, or as if, somewhat as in the "God is dead" movement, evolution may have originated things, but isn't relevant to the actual, present-day workings of the world. But evolution *is* relevant to living things today. It is not only an explanation of how life came to be and of the mechanisms that are responsible for changes in the future; it is also the guiding principle that makes sense out of why living things are as they are.

As I define it, evolution is an account of the ongoing, mysterious forces that have swept the energy of the cosmos into material form and shaped those energy forms into living tissue that grew in complexity until they became aware and eventually able to conceive of the process of their own formation.

Evolution offers a biospiritual attitude toward life. The similarities in chemical composition between the distant stars and all life on Earth, the recapitulation

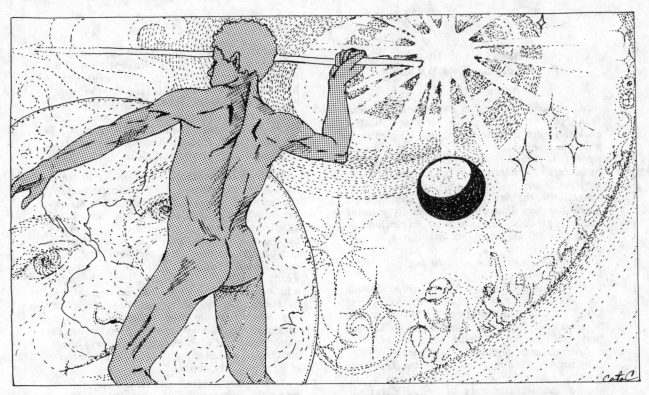

Evolution is not only an explanation of how life came to be and of its mechanisms for change; it is also the guiding principle that makes sense out of why living things are as they are.

of the stages of phylogenetic development that all our bodies must pass through as embryos—such facts link us to the cosmos and to all life. Human evolution is both a result and a continuation of the complex bio-social interactions, adaptations, and perceptual developments of our primate ancestors that led to behaviors of increasing complexity that required higher and higher levels of neural integration. Human evolution is thus part of a tendency toward a more refined and complicated organization of matter in the on-going evolution of the cosmos. The evolution of biological structure and the evolution of consciousness are inseparable. It is because of this coevolution of structure and consciousness that biopsychology can exist.

Evolution is also a grand, explosive cosmic myth, full of fire and blood and extinct monsters. It is both a myth supported by rigorously interpreted data and a myth that necessitates speculation and imagination. It is an open-ended interpretation of the story of creation. It is a wonderfully unfinished and yet well-defined story, a story we all participate in and unwittingly help direct in the course of our lives.

Few understand that evolutionary theory laid a groundwork which began to undermine Western civilization's predilection for mechanical, static, and reductionist views of life. Evolutionary theory differs radically from traditional Western paradigms, in that it involves process or dynamic thinking. Western science has so far been involved primarily with structure. Our bodies, our social institutions, and our ideas are mainly described in structural terms, that is, in terms of relations between solid objects or discrete ideas. Hence, therapists speak of "dissolving body armor," and clients bring us problems to be "solved," just as something solid may be dissolved in a liquid. This language parallels that of mechanistic engineering systems. No wonder, then, that in such mechanistic views, the preservation of structure is of foremost concern.

In a structural view, dynamic phenomena are described as processes determined by structure, much like a liquid flowing in a pipe or the combustion process in an engine. In application, this view of the body causes one to focus either on how to preserve a given structural state by creating or maintaining static

What Is Evolution?
Ron Fielder and Frank Wildman

Evolution is defined as a process of development, formation, or growth. More specifically, evolution refers to the theory that all species of plants and animals developed from earlier forms by hereditary transmission of slight variations to successive generations. Though this theory is a virtually unquestioned part of our modern scientific world view, the notion that all life on Earth developed as part of a wholly natural organic process represents a revolution in human belief. In prescientific cultures, for example, supernatural agencies of various kinds were almost invariably held to be responsible for the development of life.

For Christian Europe, the accepted dogma was the doctrine of Special Creation, which held that God had performed an individual act of creation for each of the millions of species that exist or have existed on Earth. In the eighteenth and nineteenth centuries this doctrine was disputed by a few daring thinkers who saw that the evidence of fossils in rock strata argued against the theory of Special Creation. The geological record strongly indicated that species underwent gradual modification during the course of generations. However, the mechanism by which these modifications occurred and led to the adaptation of species to their environments remained an unsolved mystery to the early evolutionists. Evolutionary theory could not prevail against Christian dogma until this critical conceptual lacuna had been filled.

The question of precisely how evolution worked was persuasively answered by Charles Darwin in his book *On the Origin of Species by Natural Selection,* published in 1859. Darwin observed that there is considerable variation in specific characteristics within species. His great and original contribution was the identification of the mechanism by which these naturally occurring variations were turned to adaptive ends: the principle of natural selection. A passage from the introduction to his book summarizes his view of this mechanism.

"The struggle for existence amongst all organic beings throughout the world, which inevitably follows from the high geometrical ratio of their increase, will be considered . . . . As many more individuals of each species are born than can possibly survive; and as, consequently, there is a frequently recurring struggle for existence, it follows that any being, if it vary however slightly in any manner profitable to itself . . . will have a better chance of surviving, and thus be *naturally selected.* From the strong principle of inheritance any selected variety will tend to propagate its new and modified form."

Darwin saw natural selection as a consequence of the competition for life itself among the supernumerary young of each species. Those whose modifications made them better adapted to their species' ecological niche would, he concluded, survive to reproduce in greater numbers than those less well-endowed. Conversely, individuals with unsuitable variations would tend to be eliminated from the reproductive pool by the same struggle for existence. In short, because of intense and unrelenting population pressure, the conditions of specific environments become screening factors in the reproduction of each generation, always orienting change within a population in the direction of improved adaptation.

Today the principle of natural selection remains the cornerstone of evolutionary theory, although Darwin's ideas about its actual operation have been modified somewhat. In particular, his emphasis on the struggle for life and the physical failure of less competitive forms has itself been eliminated. Natural selection is now seen to result from the simple fact that in any population some individuals produce more offspring than others. Under natural conditions, these more prolific breeders tend to be the ones who can best exploit the niche already occupied by their species, or another accessible niche. (However, this correlation is not automatic; it is only the general rule.) Thus, natural selection is seen to favor improved adaptation to existing or new conditions, rather than the development of populations that are ever more "fit" to prevail in a life-and-death struggle.

Modern evolutionary theory incorporates other important advances over Darwin's understanding of the process, most significantly in the area of hereditary laws and mechanisms. The science of genetics has revealed that heredity is transmitted from generation to generation by genes, minute but extremely complex chemical structures that exist in paired sets in the nuclei of most body cells. In sexual reproduction, the genes of the parents are mixed to produce the genetic blueprint for the development of the new individual. This constant reshuffling of genes produces much of the variation in characteristics whose source remained a mystery to Darwin. The other source of genetic variation is the mutation of genes in the production of reproductive cells. Together these two mechanisms produce the raw material of random hereditary variation upon which natural selection acts to further adaptation.

Such is our contemporary understanding of the evolutionary mechanisms that have produced the myriad forms of life on Earth. The evolution of the organic world continues today, of course, but mankind's impact on the environment has radically altered the process. Whole species have been exterminated, and the natural ecosystems of vast areas disrupted, by the direct or indirect effects of man's activities. In less obvious ways, too, man's activities have created selective pressures that could only be called "natural" by the most liberal extension of the meaning of the word.

Man's profound impact on the environment and all its processes, including evolution, is an outgrowth of his awesome adaptability. The evolutionary consequences of this adaptive success are most profound for *Homo sapiens* himself. By transforming the pattern of natural processes so radically, he has largely unhooked his own evolution from the mechanism of natural selection. For humans the predominant source of adaptive challenges and selective pressures is the social environment, rather than the physical or the biological. In the other primate families, social behavior is directed by unyielding group pressures. Until recently, human society has evolved primarily because of political, religious, and educational pressures which have also imposed narrow views and limited behavioral alternatives.

Today, the therapeutic and healing professions offer another alternative to the traditional institutional molders of human consciousness. A more individualized, self-directed consciousness may be evolving on the planet, with more freedom of choice than ever before. The issues of choice and responsibility are of importance to anyone involved in the healing and therapeutic professions. In these circumstances, it becomes increasingly clear that the course of man's future evolution will be determined by his own acts, however they are determined. The great issue before humanity today is whether and how we will employ the rapidly developing means, both social and biochemical, of directing our evolution more consciously.

boundaries, or on how to engineer a transition to a new structural state by using manipulative and therapeutic "technologies." A structure-oriented approach deals with a body as if it were a machine to be engineered and controlled from the outside; it takes an inherently elitist attitude. This attitude is endemic to most therapeutic schools in existence, be they traditional or nontraditional. The structural view is an unhealthy attitude for the body therapies, and creates only a "New Age staticism."

Some of humankind's oldest religious systems and paradigms, such as Buddhism, Taoism, and Hermetic philosophies, were cast in process terms. In their pure forms they did not incorporate ideal notions of structure, such as God, or essence, or a static self. A deeper understanding of natural (as contrasted to engineering) processes likewise reveals a world in a state of constant dynamic fluctuation. Evolution concerns changes in organization rather than in substance. In an open-ended biosphere, where "order through fluctuation" is the rule, process and structure become complementary aspects of the over-all changes—the evolution—in the organization of matter.

The basic complementarity of process and structure has never been grasped as precisely as it can be today in the dynamic vision of evolutionary theory. Evolution provides a paradigm in which the East's profound grasp of process in nature is wedded to the rigorous empiricism of Western science. In this synthesis, knowledge of the human bodymind gleaned from both cultures can be synergistically exploited. With evolutionary theory to guide the tremendous body of knowledge we have discovered about the operations of the natural world, we can begin to understand the purposefulness of living things. Within the framework of evolution, "Why?" and "What for?" and even "So what?" become interesting and meaningful questions. The dynamic relationship between structure, function, and behavior, which cannot logically be studied or understood apart from one

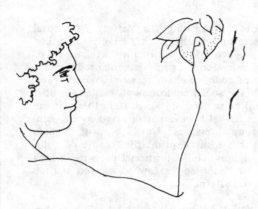

If we consider the hand and arm, we can see how their structures and functions established a new relation between the human animal and its environment.

another, becomes illuminated in a meaningful and revealing fashion.

Studies of the human body such as anatomy, physiology, and embryology become interrelated, become truly "life sciences" within the dynamic view of the body that evolution posits. We cannot know what a biological structure "means" unless we know why it is as it is and what it is for, unless we know the entire physical, social, or cultural environment that has shaped it. For example, in the human animal, the shape and function of the body is determined in every detail by the upright psoture. If we consider the hand and arm within the framework of an upright posture, we can see that the peculiar structure and function of arm and hand have established a new relation between the human animal and the world. We become creatures that reach out into the world and bring it to us. We become a touching, grasping animal. The anatomical description that deals only with the structure of the hand is an analysis of a dead body.

Psychotherapy and psychology have largely ignored evolution, as though structure, function, behavior, and feelings were not integrated factors in the process of living. Experimental and behavioral psychology and learning theory are useful for manipulating behavior, toilet training a child, or designing teaching machines, but they are not very useful for explaining the complex patterns of human behavior. Behavioral psychologists recognize that the behavior of other species can shed light on certain aspects of human behavior, but have not incorporated evolutionary thinking into their work. As a result, comparative psychology has become characterized by studies of bar pressing and maze running, which provide little insight into the natural behavior of free-living animals. They do not help us to understand why robins sing in the spring, why wolves live in packs, why the social structure of a primate community is designed as it is, or why human animals seek love and are so curious about the future.

Most body therapies recognize the integration of the physical body and the feeling body, at least to some degree. This recognition is the source of their efficacy. But, as I pointed out earlier, the numerous descriptions of how body and mind relate are diverse and often contradictory. With evolutionary theory as a guide, psychology can blend with biology, and perhaps Freud's dream of a scientific but humane psychology can be realized.

To help create this union, we must expand our interpretation of evolutionary theory into the sphere of biosocial interaction. Human behavior in the physical environment is only one aspect of human existence. The biosocial, the biocultural, and the biospiritual are all two-way interactions in dynamic environments which, in their totality, link human consciousness with evolution. Experience, then, is no longer to be interpreted as an accumulation of things (sensations, perceptions, thoughts, and feelings) in places (the soul, the mind, the consciousness, or the unconscious). In the process-thinking of evolution, man is always changing his organization, is always in flux, and experience is always a relationship with other dynamic structures and processes.

A new vision of consciousness, with its own set of problems and questions, must emerge as part of a new science of biopsychology, which will link fringe elements of therapy and obscure techniques with great and established bodies of knowledge. Much research has been done tracing the structural evolution of living matter. No one has yet traced an evolution of consciousness and tied it to that of structure and function.

As biological systems grow in size and complexity, they reach a limit where a new level of hierarchical control is necessary if the system is to function properly. What were the factors in the social adaptations of man and the primates that led to the conditions of awareness? What conditions relate the growth of awareness to present or past survival functions for the species? What is the evolutionary biology of an animal that perceives both its interior and its exterior environment?

On a more pragmatic and clinical level, some questions are: What is involved in the process of evaluating someone's body? What are we seeing? How does the therapeutic interaction appear if viewed from the standpoint of animal behavior and primate ethology? What is pathological behavior? Before we can assess biological norms of behavior, we will have to realize that behavior which seems abnormal is usually a product of processes which, in other surroundings, would have led to normal adaptation. Even the severe repression of the "instincts" which Freud considered the dynamic basis and inevitable cost of civilization is not by itself an indicator of pathology—some non-human primate troops are also regulated by internalized repression. The vision of a nonrepressive society, wherein the instincts regain their precivilized status or the bioplasma flows with perfect freedom, is based on a misapprehension. It is another form of New Age staticism.

Among the higher mammals whose social-group life dominates adaptive behavior strategy, evolution by natural selection adapts the individual to the social norms of the group more than to the physical environment or to individual survival. The social Darwinists helped foster the popular image of evolution as a series of epic adventures, but survival of the fittest individuals has been replaced by the survival of the fittest populations. Love, joy, hate, aggression, fear, expansiveness, and withdrawal are all orchestrated in blends that promote not the happiness or even survival of the individual, but maximum survival of the species. In humans, some measure of inhibition, fragmentation, introversion, and vicarious fulfillment—all of which can be symptoms of pathology—may also be part of the legacies of consciousness inherited from the archaic patterns of biosocial organization among our ancestors. If expansiveness and love, perceptual and behavioral plasticity, and higher neural organization (or higher consciousness) have been bequeathed to us by our ancestors because they were essential for group survival, frustration and dissatisfaction were and are survival devices in precisely the same way.

It is obviously beyond the scope of this essay to draw specific conclusions or outline a complete biopsychology. I hope to do so in a book I am currently planning. Meanwhile, I hope this essay will stimulate thinking and affect attitudes about the direction the body therapies are taking today. I would like to see people who work with the body appreciate the vast fund of knowledge and the enlightened viewpoint about the human bodymind that evolutionary thought offers. Such an expansion of our horizons might enable us all to begin asking better questions. For instance, the age-old enigma of how the mind and body are unified has plagued many theorists. Most schools of psychological thought make some attempt to unravel that question. However, the better question may not be "How are we embodied?" or "How is the bodymind unified?" but rather "How did living matter shape itself and change its organization (evolve) until it became aware of itself?" and "What forces direct this process?" and "How do we experience this process in our lives and our bodies?"

SUGGESTIONS FOR FURTHER READING

Edward O. Wilson, *Sociobiology: The New Synthesis.* Harvard University Press, 1975.

Gaylord G. Simpson, *The Meaning of Evolution.* Harcourt Brace and World, 1949.

————, *Biology and Man.* Yale University Press, 1953.

Erich Jantsch and Conrad Waddington, *Evolution and Consciousness.* Addison-Wesley, 1976.

E. A. and N. Tinbergen, *Early Childhood Autism: An Ethological Approach.* Paul Parey, 1972.

N. Tinbergen, *Social Behavior in Animals.* Science Paperbacks, 1968.

J. N. Spuhler, ed., *The Evolution of Man's Capacity for Culture.* Wayne State University Press, 1959.

Frank Wildman, a former professional dancer and an innovative teacher of the sciences of the body, directs the Somataxis Institute for Movement Education and Research. He conducts classes and workshops for therapists, movement teachers, and health practitioners, and trains people who use movement in working with older people. He maintains a private practice in movement therapy in Berkeley, California, and is a movement specialist for the University of California Extension.

Frank is presently writing a book on biopsychology stemming from his Bay Area course in "Anatomy Thru Evolution."

Taking Nutritional Responsibility
Edward Bauman, M.Ed.

To eat is human; to digest and enjoy, divine. Instead of Alka Seltzer or Tums for the tummy, how about using nutritional responsibility as a remedy for your dietary errors and excesses?

Mr. Bauman, a health educator from the Berkeley Holistic Health Center, offers a generous feast of practical dietary and lifestyle suggestions. He provides special support and instruction for those of us who wish to change from the commercial fare to a more healthful, vegetarian-based diet.

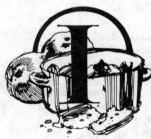

Isn't it astounding that most of us are unconscious of how our bodies operate, and what makes for optimal nutrition? Neither our parents, teachers, nor physicians taught us how to identify nutritional needs and satisfy them. It's time we found out for ourselves, by study and experience, what is fit to eat and what is not.

Can you remember a fresh, nutritionally rich meal, prepared with love and graciously served? The satisfaction of communing with family, friends, and food is immensely rewarding. Eating has a spiritual function, for it fills us with nature's life force. As we digest and assimilate its contents, the essence of our food becomes a part of us.

This leads us to scrutinize the effects of the "Pepsi generation." None of us in the modern world has escaped the impressions that commercialism has made on our psyche and in our bodies. How quickly convenience foods and instant sensory gratification corrode our nutritional morals! Denatured food breeds weak, insensitive, dependent organisms. A 1974 *Wall Street Journal* headline surmised, "Most people have no taste; it's been lost in the process."

Until you are thoroughly sick of self-abuse, you won't make the commitment to be maximally healthy. Nutritional responsibility begins with learning to exercise judgment in matters of diet. For some, it means learning for the first time how to gather, prepare, digest and assimilate food efficiently. Nearly all bad food habits are actually responses to other symptoms, such as depression and fatigue. Moreover, commercial convenience foods merely cover your hunger, without delivering essential nutrients. As hunger becomes craving, need translates into desire, seldom satiated. Dr. Jean Mayer of Harvard University warns, "Enriched junk food is still junk." *Caveat emptor* (Buyer beware)!

This article addresses those people who wish to use sound nutritional principles as a basis for personal healing work. All material is presented as suggestion, not prescription. Use whatever is appropriate for your needs at this time. I emphasize natural foods and nutritional teachings that you can apply on your own, without great expense or risk.

Nutrition is the art and science of *nourishing yourself optimally,* and nutritional responsibility is a process. Three interconnecting phases will be discussed:

(1) Examining the systemic effects of habitual dietary errors and digestive overload.

(2) Preparing to change your diet: general guidelines; personal and environmental considerations.

(3) Adopting the right diet for you: developing a vegetarian basis; suggestions for substituting and combining sensibly.

DIETARY ERRORS AND DIGESTIVE OVERLOAD: CAUSE, CONSEQUENCE, AND REMEDY

Dietary errors inevitably create a digestive overload which denies the body the nutrients it deserves. Before eating a single bite, consider your habitual eating behavior. Are you shortchanging yourself by carelessness and haste? Do you:

(1) eat too fast?

(2) eat too often?

(3) eat poor-quality food?

(4) lack sufficient digestive enzymes?

(5) eat when stressed?

Let's face it, we can all pay more attention to our internal rhythm and pace. The tradition of saying grace before meals is an important and healthy practice. During this brief silence, pressures of the day are released, and gratitude for the gift of food can be expressed. A moment's pause allows blood to drain from your brain and to center in the abdomen, thereby stimulating secretions of digestive enzymes in the stomach, small intestine, and salivary glands. Take time for relaxation after the meal, as well.

According to Dr. Kurt Donsbach, a great way to correct dietary errors is to exercise five minutes before eating. This stimulates the liver and muscle tissues to release glycogen into the blood. This reserve of fuel is oxidized and converted to glucose, a simple sugar, which immediately raises the blood sugar level and allays hunger. After exercise, rest a moment, and then take your meal. You'll be less likely to overeat.

The result of dietary excess is digestive overload. An excess is any amount of food that exceeds the body's ability to handle it efficiently, or any food additive or other substance that is foreign to the human body. Excess compels the digestive organs and glands to work overtime. Their complaints are registered symptomatically. Diseases of overload include diabetes and hypoglycemia (from carbohydrates), hardening of the arteries (from fats), degenerative problems and premature aging (from proteins), and obesity (from all of the above).

When more food is taken into the body than can be completely metabolized, the excess winds up in the intestinal tract. Undigested matter is ripe for bacterial action, virus, and germ infestation. Germs do not cause disease, but are able to multiply in a sick organism because of disturbed function. Undigested fat particles rancidify and collect as cholesterol; carbohydrates ferment, creating gas, and proteins putrify, releasing uric acid. These toxic residues interfere with the formation of the "friendly" bacteria that are necessary for a healthy intestinal ecosystem. The liver filters as much of the impurities as it can, but it, too, becomes fatigued, and polluted blood is relayed to hungry cells. Headaches, skin eruptions, depression, and liver ailments are symptomatic of the need for corrective action.

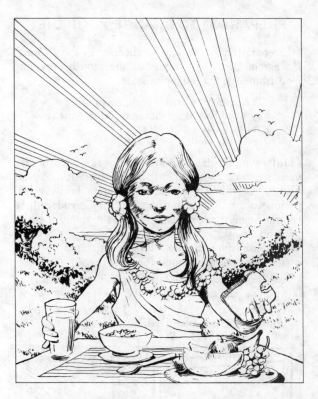

Eating has a spiritual function; it fills us with nature's life force. The essence of our food becomes a part of us.

Natural elements such as whole foods, herbs, and self-control have been proven throughout history to be effective antidotes to the abuses of civilization. Dr. Ann Wigmore of the Hippocrates Health Institute says that in a healthy, relaxed environment, the human body is self-regulating, self-cleansing, and self-healing. She and many others believe that every "incurable" health problem can be treated by cleansing the blood stream, replenishing deficient substances, and stimulating the circulatory system to carry away wastes and toxins.

In order to relieve digestive overload, lighten up on food intake and cleanse the intestinal tract. Increase naturally laxative fresh raw foods and pure fluids—either herb teas, mineral broths, fruit, or vegetable juices. Take an enema or colonic, if desired. Add cultured and fermented foods to your diet. Refined foods, alcohol, drugs, sugars, salt, and chemicals all retard vigorous digestive action. Natural minerals from foods or supplements, plus the vitamin B complex are helpful tonics for weak digestion and assimilation.

PREPARING TO CHANGE YOUR DIET

Preparation is the key to success. In the *I Ching,*
Hexagram 27 (The Corners of the Mouth/Providing
Nourishment), the judgment states:

> "Perserverence brings good fortune.
> Pay heed to the providing of nourishment
> And to what a man seeks
> To fill his mouth with."

Clarify your goals, examine your needs, and solidify
your personal commitment to the restoration of your
health. A gradual reeducation program is always superior to an "all or nothing" plan. Consider these
common-sense guidelines, and begin to apply them in
your own way.

(1) Simplify your diet. Base it on staple foods
that you know are good for you.

(2) Regulate your dietary habits. Train yourself
to chew, sip, and savor. Systematically undereat.

(3) Swear off junk food. Become a health-
conscious shopper and eater.

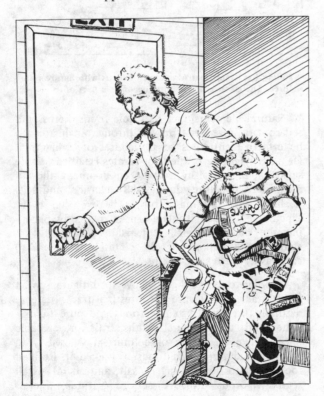

**Mark Twain said that a habit cannot simply be tossed out
the window. Escort it like an old friend, down the stairs, and
out the door.**

(4) Learn how to prepare food that satisfies
your unique taste and temperament.

(5) Select the freshest local food for each
season.

(6) Avoid dogmatism. Let others eat in peace.

(7) Nutritionally attend to your size, age, and
special needs.

(8) Make safe, conscious experiments. Try new
food patterns, and evaluate your responses.

(9) Discuss diet and holistic health with friends
who share similar experiences.

(10) Develop a diet that reflects the best aspects of life—food with strength, wholeness,
and beauty.

Mark Twain said that a habit cannot simply be
tossed out the window. Escort it like an old friend,
down the stairs, one at a time, and out the door. As
old patterns are broken, cravings and feelings of all
varieties will emerge. Be gentle with yourself. Change
of any kind is stressful. As toxins are released, suppressed disease symptoms may reappear for short
intervals. This is known as a "healing crisis." You
must cleanse yourself to make way for new growth.
Relax your expectations and cooperate with Mother
Nature.

Every cell in our bodies has its own life and death.
Cells are constantly wearing out, dying, and being
replaced by new cells. A body's blood cells are completely renewed every 24 to 36 hours, and bone cells
every twelve months. Every seven years you have an
entire renewal of all body tissues. With proper nourishment, we can regenerate organs and tissues.

Once you feel that you have taken charge of examining yourself to the best of your ability, seek
out the advice of one or more health professionals.
Laboratory tests are helpful in revealing dietary
deficiencies. Hair analysis, computerized dietary evaluations, urine and saliva tests, and blood reports give
medical and holistic practitioners data upon which to
base recommendations. Books are valuable resources.
Concentrate on those suggestions that seem to adapt
to your orientation. If you doubt the benefit of a
remedy, it is unlikely to work for you.

Your environment can contribute to your health
and nutritional problem, or to its solution. Consider
these factors:

(1) Keep your house clean, with a good circulation of fresh air. Pollens, molds, dust, and
animal hair put stress on your digestive and
immunological systems.

(2) Inventory your fabrics, toiletries, foods, and utensils. Synthetic fibers and inorganic metals disintegrate and enter your body through the skin, as well as orally. Use natural goods whenever possible.

(3) Drink pure spring water. Tap water contains many chemicals.

(4) Bring green plants into your home. They increase the oxygen indoors, and they neutralize air pollutants.

(5) Screen out harsh noises and unpleasant odors whenever possible.

(6) Learn how to relax. Soothe your mind with recreation and meditation. This will help balance your glands and comfort digestive distress.

(7) Be attentive to personal hygiene. Wash with gentle soap and shampoo.

(8) Follow hot water baths and showers with cold rinses, in order to close the pores and stimulate circulation.

(9) Buy toothpaste, cosmetics, detergents, and household products that are sugar-free and non-toxic.

(10) Examine your work environment and make it as healthful and nurturing as possible.

ADOPTING THE RIGHT DIET FOR YOU

Adopting a new diet can well be compared with buying a new wardrobe. No matter how stylish an outfit might be, if it doesn't fit, you might as well save your money. A sensible diet is well-coordinated and comfortable, accentuating your heritage, background, and true nature. If you are Greek, a traditional Japanese macrobiotic diet will not speak to your food sensibilities. Diets that are foreign to one's natural way simply won't be followed through. After all, your diet is the home base you will return to after an occasional digression into indulgence. Develop your own "nutrition intuition," and let it guide you to the finest diet you can imagine. If your diet is based on nonnutritious staples, begin now to find real alternatives.

A vegetarian-based diet is a good starting point. I suggest vegetarian-based, rather than pure vegetarian, because this allows people who eat meat to significantly upgrade the vegetable portion of their meal, yet minimize their dependence on meat, starch, and sugar.

Why vegetables, and not other food sources, or synthetics? All life is sustained by powers that

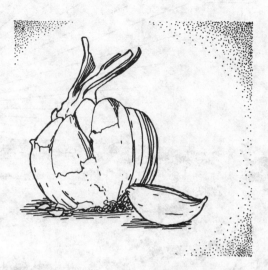

come from the sun. Vegetation covers the earth and absorbs sunlight. By means of the miracle of photosynthesis, green plants transform carbon dioxide and water into new cell formations, which humans and animals eat, and they release oxygen, which we breathe. The chlorophyll molecule is practically identical in composition to the hemoglobin or red blood pigment that transports oxygen to the cells in our body. Rich in enzymes, vitamins, and minerals, chlorophyll is rightly called "liquid sunshine." Abundant in all green vegetables and sprouts, inexpensive, and readily assimilated, it is a necessary healing nutrient. How green is *your* diet?

In their natural state all foods are combinations of protein, carbohydrates, fats, minerals, vitamins, and enzymes. Complete utilization of foods can only take place when all these elements are consumed. Herein lies the dharma (path), the secret benefit of eating whole foods.

Consider grain. Grain is both the seed and the fruit of the grass plant. It contains all essential nutrients for a new cycle of life. To the Native American people, corn (maize) meant "she who sustains us, our mother, our life." Rice, with a 5,000-year-old history as the principal food in the Orient, means (in Sanskrit, *dhanga*) "supporter or nourisher of man." We have lost most of the forty nutrients supplied by the whole wheatberry, with our modern milling and baking processes. By eating whole grain that has been soaked, sprouted, or cooked at a simmer, we can provide ourselves with a staple food that has slow, even digestibility and a balanced mineral content that is ideal for human use. Whole grains and vegetables are stress

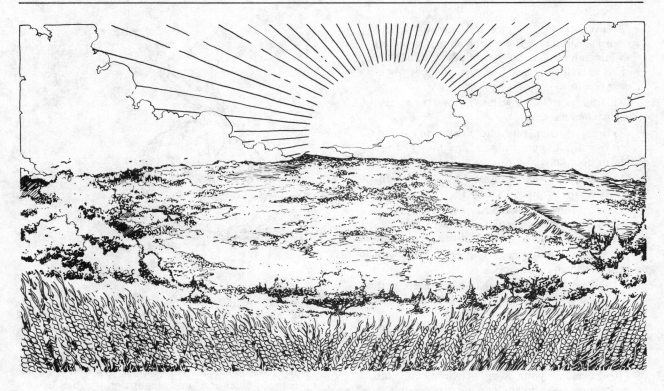

Vegetation covers the earth and absorbs sunlight, transforms carbon dioxide and water, and releases oxygen. Chlorophyll has been called liquid sunshine. How green is *your* diet?

resisters and mood stabilizers, for they help to maintain a constant glucose level in the blood.

When preparing fruits and vegetables, scrub the skins with warm, soapy water or a 1 percent solution of hydrochloric acid to remove chemical residue. The peelings should not be discarded, nor the seeds or structures surrounding them, because they contain some of the most important components. The apple is a good example. The core, including seeds, contains twenty times as much iodine and other minerals as the whole of the rest of the fruit. Beet or turnip greens are likewise far more nutritious than their commonly eaten roots. Egg white and yolk combine to provide an even balance of lecithin and fatty acids.

Chewing is more important when eating vegetables than when eating meat. Starch digestion begins in the mouth, and not the stomach (where protein is broken down). The more you chew grains and vegetables, the more alkaline saliva digests them, and the sweeter they taste.

Try eliminating heavy foods from your diet. You can reintroduce them at a later time when your overall health and digestive vitality is stronger. By diversifying foods you will receive a variety of nutrients.

The most common food allergens are the most over-consumed foods: milk, eggs, cheese, meat, wheat, potatoes, and corn. Like a field that becomes depleted when only one crop is grown on it, our bodies need a rotation of foods to avoid biochemical imbalances. Deficiency symptoms that show up as a lack of brightness, clarity, and *joie de vivre* can be corrected with a stable diet that has been bolstered by vitamin and mineral supplements.

SUBSTITUTION

What a difference it would make if the majority of people began their day with fresh fruit juice and herbal tea instead of coffee. The caffeine rush sets in motion a vicious cycle of stimulation and exhaustion that is cumulatively deteriorating. But how does one break this conditioned stimulus and response, when the aroma and taste of coffee is so tempting and delicious?

One successful approach is to introduce new foods and nutritional supplements in combination, rather than one at a time. In the case of coffee, we seldom drink it alone. We add milk or sugar, or some chemical impersonators. We take it with toast, pastries, or at the conclusion of the meal. What if we chose to substitute herbal tea for coffee? Does bacon and eggs, or steak and potato resonate with camomile tea? Not too well. Coffee seems to be a counterpoint to a diet high in animal products and refined sugars. A breakfast of fresh fruit, granola, and yogurt does not call for coffee to complete the meal. Neither does a dinner of cooked grain such as brown rice, legumes or cheese, and vegetables. Herbal tea (a mild plant beverage) naturally complements a simple, yet completely satisfying, vegetable meal.

An efficient way to reduce meat consumption is to learn to use complementary vegetable protein foods. Many people who stop eating meat rely excessively on dairy products, and they soon find themselves mucous-plagued, allergic, and digestively sluggish. In *The Diet For A Small Planet,* Francis Moore Lappe explains the personal, social, and ecological benefits of switching to vegetable-based protein sources. Simply stated, a vegetable-based diet follows the wisdom of traditional cultures the world over, wherein whole grains such as barley, buckwheat, millet, corn, rice, whole wheat, or cereal grains are combined with 20 to 30 percent nuts, seeds, beans, milk, cheese, or eggs. The limited amino acids of either of these food groups alone is completed when they occur in proper combination. Consult vegetarian cookbooks for recipes and instructions for creating nutritionally balanced, delicious meals.

Several elements of food combining will help you to avoid complication when making dietary changes. They include the following.

(1) Eat foods in their unfired state (raw) if possible. Baking and steaming are preferrable to frying and broiling.

(2) Eat one high-quality protein combination at each meal.

(3) Eat the protein food first, in order to allow gastric juices to act on it.

(4) Eat garlic, ginger, culinary herbs, and fresh vegetables in combination with protein. They add enzymes and stimulate digestion.

(5) Eat only one complex carbohydrate (a grain, potato, or root vegetable) at a meal. Combine it with a vegetable protein companion.

(6) Drink milk alone, or with acid fruits. Cultured milk is predigestible, and is preferred. Sources are yogurt, kefir, and buttermilk.

(7) To avoid washing away digestive enzymes, drink beverages 30 minutes before or after your meal.

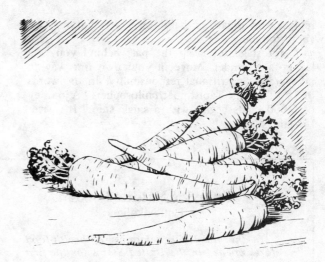

(8) Fruits are best when eaten alone, because they interfere with digestion of concentrated proteins, fats, carbohydrates, and vegetables. Lemons, pineapples, and papayas aid protein digestion when eaten after the meal.

(9) Wait at least one hour after eating before having dessert.

(10) Replace animal fats with unrefined vegetable oils, nuts, seeds, avocados, and olives. Combine with lemons and add to vegetable dishes.

Adherence to these principles promotes efficient digestion and assimilation of foods. If your condition is weak, a mono diet (one food at a sitting) is suggested, or fasting (complete abstinence from solid food), which will enable you to direct more inner attention to elimination, rest, and recuperation. See a responsible doctor or nutritional consultant if you have serious difficulties.

CONCLUSION

Nutritional responsibility calls for maturity and self-sufficiency. There are no shortcuts to health. The logical, natural intelligence of the body is increased when it is generously provided high-quality nourishment. It is childish and detrimental to continue to feed on the pulp of the profit machine.

In this article, I have tried to guide you through the process of changing from a traditional modern diet to a modern traditional one. Along the way, basic nutritional and self-healing precepts have been offered, in order to provide new mental supports to replace any pillars of habit or belief that may be about to fall.

Don't stagnate! Keep the past behind you as a lesson—a reminder. Move in your own fine way to take greater nutritional responsibility. In the words of Lao T'zu, the Taoist poet/philosopher: "A journey of 3,000 miles begins with a single step." It's never too late to begin.

Edward Bauman is a holistic health educator and nutrition consultant at the Berkeley Holistic Health Center, and the Breema Center of Healing Arts. He is the originator of Dietwise Nutrition, a program to instruct individuals with diet planning, natural foods cookery, and appropriate supplementation. He is also a co-editor of the Holistic Health Handbook *and the* Holistic Health Lifebook.

Enjoying Natural Foods
Patti Nikolić

In the mid-1960s a number of health-food stores opened in the United States for the first time. They sold natural foods that had been grown in soil free of chemical fertilizers, and that was marketed in a whole, unprocessed state. Many people called natural foods a fad, a fraud, or at the least, an unnecessary expense. As time has passed, more and more people are finding that this food tastes richer and is more satisfying than the commercial fare.

Many of us have heard about the "miracle" of brown rice, but we have never been able to cook it right, or to combine it with other foods in order to turn it into a balanced, nutritious meal. Ms. Nikolić discusses how to shop for and prepare natural foods in a simple and enjoyable way. Her good experience with fresh vegetarian food is reflected in her delightful commentary and zesty recipes.

"In the early 1900s, almost 40 percent of our caloric intake came from fruits, vegetables, and grain products. Today only a little more than 20 percent of our calories come from these sources."

Senator George McGovern
Chairman, Senate Select Committee
on Nutrition and Human Needs

The Select Committee on Nutrition published a report in January 1977 entitled *Dietary Goals for the United States.* It is the first comprehensive statement on the risk factors in the American diet. This report was further substantiated by the Surgeon General's *Report on Health and Nutrition* in July 1979.

Simply stated, the Senate Committee's recommendations were that we increase consumption of fruits, vegetables, and grains; decrease consumption of meats and dairy products; and minimize the intake of foods containing high concentrations of fat, sugar, and salt.

Many Americans are beginning to change their eating habits to incorporate a greater variety of healthful foods into their diet. The following information and recipes will assist you in cooking naturally, for fun and for better health.

SHOPPING CUES: HEALTH-FOOD STORES AND CO-OPS

Healthy food does not necessarily have to be more expensive. Careful shopping can help you to make the most out of your food dollars and cents. Many of the food items mentioned in recipes are available in supermarkets, but some must be purchased in health-food stores. A health-food store is basically a specialty store, and it may be a new adventure for you to shop in one. Going with a friend who is familiar with a store may be a great help. It can be very frustrating (and expensive) to impulsively buy foods you don't know what to do with. Your friend may also know the stores in your area which have the best prices and selection.

In the beginning, choose a few basic staples to experiment with. Go slowly! Keep in mind that your goal is to incorporate more simple, whole foods into your diet. Buy a few things at a time, especially if you are feeding a family or household that is already set in its eating habits. Too many dramatic changes in the daily fare, you may discover, will raise a lot of resistance.

Beware of small stores selling primarily pills (food supplements) and packaged items. Generally speaking, they are higher priced. Also, be conscious of freshness. In smaller stores with less traffic, foods may stay on the shelves longer. Be especially careful when shopping for items such as raw nuts and seeds, raw milk,

SUGGESTIONS FOR FURTHER READING

Rudolph Ballentine, M.D., *Diet and Nutrition.* Himalayan Institute, 1978.

Bubba Free John, *The Eating Gorilla Comes in Peace.* Dawn Horse Press, 1979.

Kurt Donsbach, Ph.D., *The Nutritional Approach to Super Health.* International Institute of Natural Health Sciences, 1980.

Bernard Jensen, N.D., *Nature Has a Remedy.* Jensen Publications, 1978.

Nutrition Search Group, *Nutrition Almanac.* McGraw Hill, 1979.

specialty bean flours, wheat germ, and oils. All these have a relatively short shelf life.

Cooperative stores have become more and more popular in the last ten years. Basically, they are consumer-owned stores, and operate on the principle of providing food as a service rather than for profit. Their markup reflects this. Whereas most stores have a 50 percent or higher markup (over wholesale), co-ops usually are between 20 and 30 percent. This can mean considerable savings. Many of these stores have different systems: some require you to pay a small membership fee; some ask for volunteer time. Ask the cashier for information.

Most co-ops and many health-food stores require that you bring your own bags and jars. Keeping a shopping basket containing these items in your car is a simple habit to get into. Your basket can be refilled with bags and jars as you are putting groceries away.

Sometimes single people with busy lives find that there is less regularity in their eating schedules. Food waste can become a real problem. It can be very helpful and time-saving to buy staples in larger quantities and store them in glass jars. Then, more frequent shopping trips can easily be made to buy such perishable items as fruits, vegetables, or dairy products.

GRAINS AND COMPLETE VEGETABLE PROTEIN

The easiest way to decrease the intake of fat is to cut down or eliminate meats or dairy products from the diet. For thousands of years people of the world have relied on plant sources for protein (grains, beans, nuts, and seeds). It has only been since the turn of the century that wealthier countries have relied so heavily on meats and dairy products for protein.

Natural protein complements to grains are brewer's yeast, tofu, soy grits (add 2T. to the cooking grain), all beans, and dairy products.

COOKING TECHNIQUE

Bring 2 cups water to a boil. Add 1 cup brown rice to the pot with ¼ tsp. salt (optional) and a small amount of cooking oil, which will help keep grain from sticking to the pan. Reduce to simmer. Cook 20-30 minutes.

CASHEW RICE

3/4 C. sesame seeds
½ C. cashews
½ package tofu, cubed
1 small onion, chopped fine
grated ginger to taste
garlic to taste
soy sauce

Sauté onions, tofu, garlic, and ginger. Add sesame seeds and cashews. Serve on top of rice.

Leftover grains are especially handy to have available in the refrigerator for quickie meals. Leftover brown rice can be refried with raisins, sunflower seeds, cinnamon and nutmeg for a great snack or quick breakfast.

Millet can be rewarmed for breakfast with milk and any of these: sunflower seeds, ground sesame seeds, dates, raisins, or bananas; add a little honey.

Tomato Rice Soup in a Hurry. Sauté some onion, green pepper, and other vegetables you may have available. Add to a large can of tomato juice with leftover rice. Thin with water if necessary. Add spices and simmer.

Bulghur Salad. Last night's leftover salad, bulghur (1 cup soaked in hot water for 20 minutes), and some lemon juice, soy sauce, and oil for dressing. Refrigerate and serve.

EAT YOUR VEGETABLES!

Have you ever grazed leisurely in a garden on a hot August afternoon? Or have you ever picked a tomato fresh from the vine? Have you ever picked an ear of fresh corn—so tender

(continued on p. 82)

(continued from p. 81)

you'd never think of cooking it? For most people who grew up in America, eating vegetables ran a close second to washing dishes in the race for the most painful punishment. It is no wonder that the canned or frozen vegetables most often found on the dinner tables of America are but distant relatives of those ripe on the vine.

GUIDELINES FOR CREATING GREAT VEGETABLE DISHES

(1) Buy vegetables that are in season. It is your greatest guarantee of quality and economical price.

(2) Buy local vegetables, if possible, or grow your own.

(3) Usually vegetables that are in season at the same time will taste good together. Combine them, using your own imagination and sense of color.

(4) A wok is great for stir-frying but not totally necessary; a fry pan will do. A steamer is an excellent investment. It fits in the bottom of a saucepan to keep vegetables from sitting in water.

(5) Use the minimum amount of water and the least amount of time. Cook vegetables until softened, but still crisp.

SUMMER VEGETABLES

green peppers
onions
squashes
garlic
garbanzo beans (optional)
tomatoes
basil, oregano, and thyme
soy sauce

Cut all vegetables to bite-size pieces. Saute onions, garlic, green pepper, and spices. Add tomatoes and squashes. Cover and let simmer. Top with nutritional yeast or parmesan cheese. Serve with brown rice or bulghur.

GREEK BROCCOLI

broccoli, cut into bite size pieces
sliced onions
garlic
olive oil
black olives
lemon juice

Sauté garlic and onions in olive oil. Add the black olives and broccoli. Cover and steam until done. Add a little liquid from can of olives if necessary. Dress with lemon juice or parmesan cheese.

SOUPS

I especially enjoy making soups, because they are usually around for a few days, ready to be served at the slightest hint of hunger. They are also a creative cook's delight—anything goes! And they are a great way to get rid of the many too many vegetables I bought at the market last week and need to use up very soon.

Good soup begins with good stock, although stock is not absolutely necessary if you don't have the time. Finding a convenient way to make stock is important; I find I don't do it unless I make it easy for myself. The most convenient way to make stock is to put all the washed vegetables in a big pot and let it simmer on a back burner while I am preparing and eating dinner, and by the time the dishes are done, the stock is ready to refrigerate for later use. (Strain out the vegetables. If you have simmered the stock at a low temperature with a lid on it, all the vitamins and minerals will be in the water.)

CREAM OF CAULIPOT

1 cauliflower, cooked
3 potatoes, cooked
1 cup instant dry milk
4 cups stock, including the liquid from cooking potatoes and cauliflower
2 T. butter
1-3 tsp. soy sauce
1 medium onion, chopped
optional vegetables
garlic
cayenne and nutritional yeast, to taste

Heat the stock in a large saucepan; stir in the milk powder, butter, and soy sauce. Put about a cup of this liquid in a blender with part of the cauliflower and potatoes (which have been cooked until very tender). Continue using this liquid and blending the cauliflower and potatoes until most of the vegetables are smooth. Return the soup to a saucepan and simmer it while you add the minced onion.

WINTER VEGETABLE SOUP

        1½ qt. vegetable stock or tomato
            juice
        3 carrots
        ¼ head cauliflower
        broccoli, cut into bite size pieces
        3-4 Tbs. olive oil
        1 medium onion
        1 cup cooked beans
        handful broken noodles
        garlic, basil, sage (to taste)
        2-3 Tbs. lemon juice

Heat olive oil in a large kettle and add the onion, garlic, and all the vegetables. Sauté lightly. Turn to a lower temperature, adding stock, herbs and cooked beans. Add broken noodles 10 to 15 minutes before serving and cook *al dente*. Garnish with fresh chopped parsley or nutritional yeast and serve hot. Serves 6-8.

CHILDREN AND SWEETS

Children and sweets! What playwright could have created a better drama? I often think of my own taste buds as being like small children: not having fully developed their own good sense, they constantly need gentle guidance toward choices that are nutritionally sound. Many of us, even as adults, live by the whims and passing fancies of the taste buds.

It is important to understand that sweets (especially white sugar) are subtly addicting. It is only natural for the body, when depleted by erratic or nutritionally deficient eating habits, to crave the quick energy that sweets provide. This is very deceiving, however, because the body is further depleted by the intake of more sugar. The best protection against this cycle is to eat regular balanced meals and keep sweet intake at a minimum.

The earlier a child is exposed to good nutritional habits, the better. If the child's likes and dislikes are firmly established before he or she is exposed to the subtly seductive affects of television advertising and the influences of other children at school, you will find it much easier to develop harmonious agreement with your child concerning foods.

In working with children of various ages, I have found it most helpful to enthusiastically present a new food, making the nutritional information fun and interesting to the child. It can be very self-defeating to overemphasize the "it's good for you" aspect. (That phrase still gets a rise out of the rebellious child in me.) It is also helpful not to present a food as a substitute for an already well-established favorite, such as honey for sugar, or carob for chocolate.

Children are great cooks! They take a great pride in being responsible for feeding themselves or other members of the household. These snack recipes are so easy anyone could make them.

CAROB NUT FUDGE

        1 C. honey
        1 C. peanut butter
        1 C. carob powder
        1 C. sesame seeds
        1 C. sunflower seeds
        ½ C. coconut or raisins
            (optional)

Measure everything out ahead of time. In a large saucepan, melt gently (on a low flame) the honey and peanut butter. Add the carob powder, stirring until blended. Quickly stir in sesame and sunflower seeds. Spread on a cookie sheet or baking pan. Cut when slightly cooled.

I especially like to use this recipe at Christmas time, serving it to visitors who are not used to eating a fudge that's so nutritious. For variety, ½ tsp. of coriander blends its flavor with that of carob quite nicely.

CAROB SUNDAE SAUCE

        ¼ C. butter
        ¼ C. carob powder
        ¼ C. honey
        Enough milk and/or water to
            thin to desired consistency

Melt together on a low flame the carob, honey, and butter. Slowly stir in enough milk and/or water until desired thickness is reached.

YOGURT BANANA SPLIT

(1) Starting with a bowl of plain yogurt, slice bananas and place along the sides.

(2) Garnish with fresh fruit, raisins, and walnuts and/or sunflower seeds.

(3) Top with carob sundae sauce, molasses, maple syrup, or honey fruit preserves.

It's a winner!

(continued on p. 84)

(continued from p. 83)

SUGGESTIONS FOR FURTHER READING

Anna Thomas, *The Vegetarian Epicure*. Vintage Books, 1972.

Frances Moore Lappe, *Diet for a Small Planet*. Ballantine Books, 1972.

Laurel Robertson, Carol Flinders, and Bronwen Godfrey, *Laurel's Kitchen*. Nilgiri Press, 1976.

U. S. Senate Select Committee on Nutrition and Human Needs, *Dietary Goals for the U. S.* United States Government Printing Office, 1977.

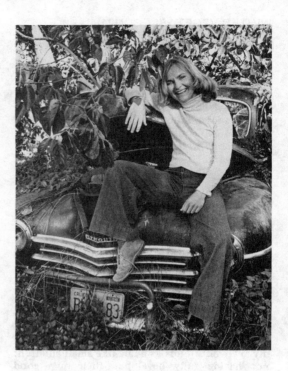

Patti Nikolić has spent several summers working as a cook's apprentice at Ananda Meditation Retreat. She received a Bachelor of Science degree in Home Economics at the University of Illinois, and a Bachelor of Arts degree in Expressive Arts from California State University at Sonoma. She has also studied various holistic health practices at the Garden of Sanjivani, a school in Santa Cruz, and has been a student of the teachings of Paramahansa Yogananda.

Patti has taught natural foods cooking classes in Sonoma County, and participated in various community health awareness projects there.

She has lectured throughout northern California, and was a founder and editor of Focus on Health *newspaper in Santa Cruz. She is currently teaching and doing freelance writing.*

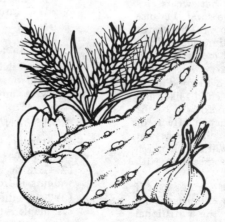

Hypoglycemia:
Paying Dues for Sugar Blues
Edward Bauman
and Mary Claire Blakeman

If you wake up tired, experience erratic mood swings, and cannot focus your attention, you are probably experiencing a low blood-sugar condition called hypoglycemia. This condition, which affects all of us to varying degrees at different times, is a signal of physiological havoc within the body. This disturbance is the price one pays for a high-stress lifestyle in which real nutritional needs are continually unmet. When the roof falls in on your mental, emotional, and physical health, hypoglycemia, or "sugar blues," has caught up with you.

The word hypoglycemia is explained by its root syllables. "Hypo" means low; "glyc" indicates glucose, the major sugar transported to the cells; and "emia" refers to the blood; so the entire meaning is "low sugar in the blood." Contrary to the assumption that a high sugar intake raises one's energy levels (which it does for only a short time), the over-all effect of sugar is to lower energy drastically, as the body rallies to stave off glucose saturation.

In a condition of optimal health, the body's glandular system secretes hormones that hold the level of glucose in the blood relatively constant. Among the biggest affronts to this naturally balanced system are refined carbohydrates, especially granulated sugar. Refined sugar is difficult for the body to metabolize properly, and poses an acute problem for those in a low blood-sugar condition.

When a blast of glucose enters the bloodstream, the pancreas responds by secreting the hormone insulin to absorb excess sugar. This action stimulates the liver to take the glucose from the blood, in order to return the insulin level to normal for that person. If there is a continual intake of refined carbohydrates, the pancreas becomes overactive, and then depleted. A pattern is created in which the pancreas releases too much insulin, which, rather than stabilizing the blood-sugar level, causes it to become dangerously low.

At such a time a person feels weak, shaky, or tired, and so he or she may reach for a candy bar, cup of coffee, or a soft drink, in hope of a quick pickup. (According to the U.S. Department of Agriculture, the average American consumes more than 90 pounds of sugar per year.)

Ingesting sugar in a hypoglycemic state is like pouring gasoline on a dying fire. The result is a brilliant, but short-lived blaze, and subsequent exhaustion. The sufferer craves sugar, but the more he or she eats, the worse the symptoms become, and the further the system is thrown out of line. Not only are the pancreas and liver affected, but so are the adrenal cortex glands, which produce anti-insulin factors.

When these glands, which are important in handling stress, can no longer do their job, the cortex becomes worn out. At this point hypoglycemia affects the mind. Brain waves become abnormal, the person becomes more sensitive to noise, becomes depressed, and often is unable to relax or sleep. Insufficient glucose in the blood contributes greatly to neurotic behavior. Other symptoms of hypoglycemia include nervousness, exhaustion, dizziness, and hunger. In extreme cases, convulsions and coma occur.

Hypoglycemia may remain at an undetected, yet mildly troublesome level for years, growing steadily worse, until it can no longer be ignored. Medical authorities disagree on the incidence of hypoglycemia, but some estimates put the number of sufferers at one in five Americans, with higher figures for children. Alan H. Nittler, M.D., a specialist in hypoglycemia, finds it to be a common condition. "In fact," he writes in his book, *A New Breed of Doctor,* "I assume it to be present until proven otherwise."

The most accurate method to discover if one has hypoglycemia is the five-hour glucose-tolerance test. Such a test can be conducted by nutritionally minded doctors at hospitals or clinics. During the first two or three hours, blood-sugar levels may be very high, only to fall later. Thus, if the test is conducted for only three hours, a misdiagnosis of diabetes is possible. Such a mistake could lead to a dangerously inappropriate therapeutic program.

You can get a rough idea of your glucose tolerance by a self-administered test which uses orange juice. On an empty stomach, drink a glass of orange juice, and notice your energy levels for a period of several hours. If your energy peaks and then drops quickly, your tolerance for sugar is low. This reaction is a

(continued on p. 86)

(continued from p. 85)

danger signal from your body/mind, like the oil light on a car, warning you to take care.

Dietary suggestions for hypoglycemics include high, complete protein food combinations taken frequently in moderate portions; fresh, low-carbohydrate vegetables; grains; legumes; unsaturated fats (in seeds, nuts, and cold-pressed oil); occasional fresh fruit; and a complete vitamin/mineral supplement program, strong in the B-complex group. When preparing a diet program, remember that hidden sugar is almost always present in commercial, canned, frozen, or restaurant food.

Besides diet, the reduction of stress is an integral part of the treatment of hypoglycemia. Stress is any extra burden placed on your body: anxiety, fatigue, stimulants, pollutants, chemical additives, change, injury, or surgery. Stress raises the body's requirements for most nutrients. If these requirements are not met and sugar is substituted for quick energy, the hypoglycemic pattern is reinforced, along with its depleting side effects.

Chocolate and coffee (which contain caffeine), salt, tobacco, and alcohol all cause stress in the body. Their relation to hypoglycemia is like that of sugar. Craving any of these substances indicates a low blood-sugar condition, which is only temporarily relieved and then worsened by partaking of these "treats."

If you suspect you suffer from hypoglycemia, consult a holistically oriented physician or a nutritional consultant. Begin to make improvements, and follow your own natural impulses toward health. Don't worry—it only aggravates your condition.

By heeding the signal of hypoglycemia and responding positively, you can correct this pattern, and save yourself more serious health problems in later life.

SUGGESTIONS FOR FURTHER READING

Paavo Airola, Ph.D., *How to Get Well.* Health Plus, 1974.

Ben and Sarah Colimore, *Nutrition and Your Body.* Light Wave, 1974.

Ford Heritage, *Composition and Facts About Foods.* Health Research, 1971.

Hans Kugler, M.D., *Dr. Kugler's Seven Keys to a Longer Life.* Stein and Day, 1978.

Laurel Robertson, Carol Flinders, and Bronwen Godfrey, *Laurel's Kitchen.* Nilgiri Press, 1976.

Max Warmbrand, M.D. *Encyclopedia of Health and Nutrition.* BJ Publishing Group, 1974.

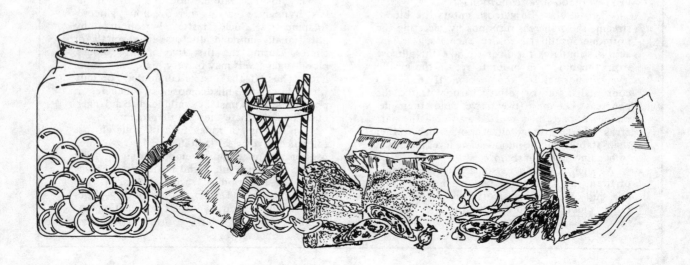

Are Vitamins and Food Supplements Really Necessary?

Paavo Airola, N.D., Ph.D.

Although many of us shop and eat carefully, and do what we can to steer clear of environmental pollutants, the question is often raised, "Do supplements really help to protect against disease and promote health? Are they a vital health-insurance investment?"

Dr. Paavo Airola, America's foremost nutritionist, responds with an emphatic yes. *He reviews the benefits of individual vitamins, and suggests nutritionally concentrated food supplements that he believes will be a blessing to anyone who tries them. Such data on the quality and quantity of supplements and how they work for us is valuable information for people struggling with stress and contamination factors that are beyond the control of the individual.*

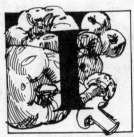deally, all vitamins, minerals, and other nutrients should be obtained from foods, without the addition of concentrated vitamins in pill or tablet form. This was possible 100 or even 50 years ago, when all foods were grown on fertile soils, were unrefined and unprocessed, and contained all the nutrients nature intended them to contain. But today, when soils are depleted, when foods are loaded with residues of hundreds of toxic insecticides and other chemicals, and when the nutritional value of virtually all foods is drastically lowered by vitamin-, protein-, and enzyme-destroying practices (such as harvesting the produce before it is ripe), the addition of vitamins and food supplements to the diet is of vital importance. Nutritionally inferior and poisoned foods of today cause many nutritional deficiencies, derangement in body chemistry, and lowered resistance to disease.

The prime purpose of food supplementation is to fill in the nutritional gaps produced by faulty eating habits and by nutritionally inferior foods. But vitamins and food supplements can also be used therapeutically, and, as such, can be of tremendous help in fighting disease and speeding recovery.

USES OF VITAMINS

Vitamins can be used in four distinctly different ways.

1. *Prophylactically, for preventive purposes.* Since it is almost impossible in today's denatured and poisoned world to obtain high-quality, poison-free foods, vitamins and food supplements will help to assure that your diet is adequate in all needed nutrients; thus, diseases related to vitamin and mineral deficiency can be prevented.

2. *For correcting deficiencies.* When a specific vitamin or mineral deficiency is indicated, the prescribed vitamins or minerals can correct the deficiency and cure the condition caused by it.

3. *For protection against toxic environment.* The damage to your body by certain common poisons in air, water, food, and environment can be minimized and even prevented by the regular use of certain vitamins, minerals, and other food substances, as I will show later.

4. *Therapeutically, as drugs or biological medicines.* Many avant-garde practitioners around the world are now using vitamins in massive doses, doses *that are far above the actual nutritional needs,* in the treatment of all kinds of conditions of ill health. It has been found that, in large doses, many vitamins have a miraculous healing, stimulating, and protective effect on a variety of body functions—an effect that is totally different from the usual vitamin activity as nutritional and metabolic catalysts.

Here are a few examples.

VITAMIN C

You need 100 mg to 200 mg of vitamin C a day for the maintenance of normal, healthy body functions. But when you take the same vitamin in huge doses, let's say 5,000 to 10,000 mg a day, it will perform totally different functions, such as the following.

1. Killing pathogenic bacteria, acting as a harmless antibiotic.

2. Preventing and curing colds and infections, having a natural antihistamine activity.

3. Effectively neutralizing various toxins in the system, being a most potent antitoxin.

4. Speeding healing processes in virtually every case of ill health.

5. Increasing sexual virility.

6. Preventing premature aging, by strengthening the collagen and preventing the degenerative processes in organs, blood vessels, and cells.

VITAMIN E

For normal, healthy functions of all your organs and glands, you need, perhaps, 100 IU of vitamin E a day (the official estimation is only 45 IU). But, when you take large doses of vitamin E, such as 600 IU to 1,600 IU or even more, it assumes a drug-like role and can perform the following activities.

1. It markedly decreases the body's need for oxygen.

2. It protects against the damaging effects of many environmental poisons in air, water, and food.

3. It saves lives in cases of atherosclerotic heart disease by dilating blood vessels and acting as an effective antithrombin.

4. It prevents scar-tissue formation in burns, sores, and postoperative healing.

5. It has a dramatic effect on the reproductive organs. It prevents miscarriage, increases male and female fertility, and helps to restore male potency.

VITAMIN A

The official recommended daily allowance is set at 4,000 U.S.P. Units. But when taken in such large doses as 100,000 U.S.P. Units per day, vitamin A has been known to have the following effects.

1. To cure many stubborn skin disorders.

2. To cure chronic infections and eye diseases.

3. To increase the body's tolerance of poisons.

4. To prevent premature aging, particularly of the skin.

NIACIN

The official recommended daily allowance is 10 mg, but many doctors around the world have been using large doses of niacin (up to 25,000 mg) to treat schizophrenia, actually achieving dramatic cures with this so-called megavitamin therapy.

These few examples show that vitamins, in addition to their common use as food supplements to prevent or correct deficiencies, can also be used successfully in large doses therapeutically, *instead* of many commonly used drugs. Although drugs are always toxic and have many undesirable side effects, vitamins are, as a rule, completely nontoxic and safe.

PREVENTIVE USE OF SUPPLEMENTS

When no specific disease is present, but a person needs a strengthening, health-building diet to achieve *optimum health,* more vitality, and greater resistance to disease, I recommend optimum nutrition (as outlined in my books and articles), supplemented with the following food supplements and vitamins. This supplementation is also advised for all those who are recuperating from disease and wish to restore health and vitality as fast as possible.

1. *Vitamin C,* preferably in natural form from rose-hip concentrate or other natural sources: 1,500 to 3,000 mg a day; even more in acute conditions of ill health, such as colds. Vitamin C is nontoxic in the above-mentioned preventive dosages.

2. *Vitamin A,* natural, from fish-liver oil, or lemon grass: 25,000 U.S.P. Units per day. Under a doctor's supervision, it can be taken in doses up to 100,000 units a day for shorter periods.

3. *Vitamin E,* natural d-alpha-tocopherol from vegetable oil: 600 IU per day. If you have not used vitamin E before, start with 100 IU and increase by 100 IU each week. If you are suffering from high blood pressure or rheumatic heart disease, consult your doctor on the proper dosage for your condition.

4. *Vitamin B-complex, with B_{12},* natural, from yeast concentrate: 1 to 3 tablets per day. (The usual strength of *natural B-complex* does not exceed 10 mg per tablet for B_1, B_2, and B_6.)

5. *Brewer's yeast:* 1 to 3 tbsp. a day.

6. *Kelp:* 1 tsp. of granules per day, or 3 tablets.

7. *Fish-liver oil,* unfortified, for vitamins D and A: 1 tsp. per day.

8. *Lecithin:* 1 to 2 tsp. of granules per day.

9. *Multimineral supplement,* such as 100 percent natural "Nature's Minerals": 4 to 6 tablets per day.

VITAMINS AND OUR TOXIC ENVIRONMENT

No longer can anyone doubt that poisons in our environment cause all kinds of serious disorders, disease, and death. These disorders range from the vague, subclinical conditions, such as headaches, irritability, chronic mental and physical fatigue, and digestive disorders, to our most dreaded killers: heart disease and cancer.

There is much talk today about environmental pollution. Even the President of the United States has said, "We must clean our environment—or perish!" But, if you think those responsible for our health will take swift action to clean our air, water, and food supplies of disease-producing and killing poisons, you are in for a big surprise. Nothing of decisive value will be done for a long time. You should be prepared to see things get much worse before they get better. Not until real mass tragedies begin to occur, when millions of people will be dropping dead, will any effective measures be taken. Let's face it: the real powers that run our country are the financial and industrial big boys from the chemical, drug, medical, food processing, auto, oil, and other vested interests. They will see to it that nothing is done that can hurt their profits. The fact that all these poisons in air, soil, water, and food are making Americans the sickest people in the world does not bother them. The whole economic structure of the American chemical, drug, medical, and hospital industry is based on one principle: "The more sickness, the more profit!" Moreover, the government agencies which are supposed to protect us from the toxic dangers in our food, drug, and other environmental sources are largely controlled by these interests.

Therefore, if you want to be protected against ever-increasing amounts of deadly poisons in your environment—in the air you breathe, in the water you drink, and in the food you eat—*you must do it yourself;* no one else will.

WHAT CAN YOU DO?

I have made a thorough study of what one can do, and have found many means you can employ for your protection. The damage to your body by certain common poisons in air, water, and food *can* be lessened, minimized, or even prevented by the regular use of certain vitamins, minerals, and other food substances. Certain minerals and vitamins neutralize or counteract the effects of toxins. Certain foods can help the development and growth of beneficial bacteria in your intestines, and these can help to detoxify and neutralize certain toxic residues in food. Certain vitamins and food substances can increase your body's tolerance and resistance to toxins. Some other vitamins can help your body to excrete ingested poisons from the system. Here is a list of specific foods and food supplements that can minimize the damage to your body from common poisons in air, water, and food.

Yogurt and other soured milks. It has been found that sour-milk bacteria neutralize most poisons, specifically DDT, strontium-90, and toxic drugs, and make them "safer," that is, minimize their damaging effect on the body: 1 pint to 1 quart a day.

Kelp. An excellent protector against radioactive fallout substances such as strontium-90 and radioactive iodine: 3 to 5 tablets or 1 tsp. of granules a day.

Lecithin. Lecithin neutralizes all body poisons. It also helps to counteract the effects of radiation and X-rays; 1 to 2 tsp. of granules a day.

Brewer's yeast. This, the best natural protective food against pollution, helps your liver in its detoxifying work. Use generously: 2, 3, or more tbsp. a day.

Vitamin B-Complex, high potency. B-vitamins protect you against many toxic residues in foods.

Vitamin B_1. Specific protector against damaging effects of lead; 25 mg a day.

Vitamin B_{15}. Effective protector against air pollution and smog, particularly against dangerous effects of carbon monoxide; 100 to 200 mg a day.

Pantothenic acid. Protector against radiation injuries, etc.: up to 100 mg a day. Brewer's yeast is an excellent source.

Vitamin C. The best general antitoxin; specific against lead and cadmium. It will help your body to withstand the toxic assault better, and it will prevent damage. It will protect all your organs and glands: large doses, up to 3,000 mg per day. In acute cases of poisoning from any source, doses of 1,500 mg every hour, up to 10,000 mg per day.

Vitamin E. Effective protector against poisons in polluted air, especially ozone, nitrogen dioxide, and carbon monoxide. Helps liver in its detoxifying work. Protects you against most poisons in food, water, and air: up to 600 IU per day. (For higher dosage, or if suffering from rheumatic heart disease, or high blood pressure, consult your doctor.)

Vitamin A. Improves your body's oxygen economy; thus, protects you against damaging effects of smog. It helps activate enzymes that are involved in detoxifying lead poisons: up to 25,000 U.S.P. Units per day.

Vitamin D. Improves the utilization of calcium, one of the most important antitoxin minerals: up to 2,500 U.S.P. Units per day.

Calcium and Magnesium. Help your body to neutralize and pass off many toxic substances, such as lead, mercury, strontium-90, radioactive iodine, and cadmium. Calcium up to 1,000 mg; magnesium up to 500 mg a day. Bone-meal tablets (with bone marrow) and dolomite are good sources of calcium and magnesium.

Garlic. Japanese studies showed that the regular use of garlic can help in eliminating lead, mercury, and cadmium from the body. "Kyolic Formula 101" (sold in health-food stores) is the best form of garlic for this purpose, because it is fortified with algin, another effective detoxifier.

TIPS ON TAKING VITAMIN SUPPLEMENTS

1. As a general rule, all vitamins and food supplements should be taken with meals, or immediately after meals, because they are better assimilated when in combination with foods.

2. Divide all the suggested daily amounts equally between three meals, or at least between two meals.

3. Take *all* vitamins and food supplements *continuously*, with the exception of high potency synthetic B-complex vitamins, large doses of synthetic isolated B-vitamins, and large doses of vitamins A and D. These should be taken for 4 to 6 weeks; then after a one-month interval, taken for another 4 to 6 weeks; and so on. These vitamins are cumulative and may cause vitamin imbalances in the system if taken in large doses for a prolonged period of time. Also, the continuous ingestion of certain isolated B-vitamins in large doses may cause deficiencies of other B-vitamins, and may interfere with the body's own synthesis of these vitamins in the intestines. Naturally, brewer's yeast (B-complex) and plain fish-liver oils (A and D) can be taken continuously.

4. Special medicinal supplements, such as digestive enzymes, hydrochloric acid, special vitamins and minerals *in massive doses,* should be taken only on recommendation of a doctor or nutritionist who can assess your actual need and dosage. These should be taken only during the treatment, or for about one to three months, *then discontinued.* After a one- to

three-month interval, treatment can be repeated, if necessary. Between treatment periods, vitamin- and mineral-rich natural food supplements should be used, such as brewer's yeast, bone meal, lecithin, fish-liver oils, and rose hips. Vitamin C can be used continuously in reduced dosage. When vitamin E is used for a heart condition, it should also be used continuously.

5. Although vitamin E in the form of mixed tocopherols is perfectly safe for a healthy person to take for preventive purposes, those who take vitamin E for therapeutic purposes or for treatment of specific conditions should take only the *pure d-alpha-tocopherol capsules* (possibly supplemented by mixed tocopherols). Only the alpha-tocopherol fraction of the E vitamin complex is now known to be effective in treatment of disease.

6. As a rule, all vitamins and food supplements should be taken *together.* Being synergistic in their action, they work best that way, and complement each other. There is, however, a notable exception to this rule. Vitamin E and synthetic iron supplements are *antagonists.* Iron tablets have an adverse effect on the metabolism of vitamin E. Therefore, when iron tablets are taken (for example, in treatment of anemia), they should be taken 8 to 12 hours *after* or *before* taking vitamin E. For example, take the total daily dose of vitamin E for breakfast, and iron tablets at dinnertime. Natural *iron-rich foods,* however, have no adverse effect on vitamin E utilization.

7. Although in my book *How To Get Well,* I list specific vitamins for the biological treatment of most ailments, and in most cases list the commonly used therapeutic doses, *there is no such thing as a common or average person or patient.* As Dr. Roger J. Williams stressed so expertly, "Individual human beings have great diversity in human nutritional needs." There is also a great difference in every person's *response* to vitamins and other therapeutic substances, depending on his health condition, nutritional status, the quality of the foods he eats, his ability to assimilate nutrients, the mineral content of the water he drinks, the toxicity degree of his environment, and his emotional health. Because of many physical and mental disorders, vitamins may not be assimilated properly. Poor teeth, diarrhea, the lack of digestive juices, intestinal parasites, infections, colitis, gall bladder or liver disorders, mental stresses—these are just a few of the conditions that interfere with vitamin utilization. Then there are the countless vitamin antagonists that destroy or interfere with ingested vitamins, such as smoking (vitamin C), alcohol (vitamin B), rancid foods (vitamins E and A), chlorinated water (vitamin

E), laxatives (vitamins C and B), aspirin and other drugs (vitamin C).

Therefore, since every individual's needs are different, your doctor, after a careful examination and nutritional and metabolic evaluation of your condition, must decide the *exact dosage* and the *duration* of the vitamin therapy *for you.*

8. When possible, all vitamins should be *natural,* not *synthetic.*

NATURAL VS. SYNTHETIC VITAMINS

Most drugstore-quality vitamins are made from synthetic chemicals—they are not derivatives of natural food substances. Although this is also true of some brands sold in health-food stores, most vitamins sold in health-food stores are concentrations of nutrients from such natural sources as rose hips, green peppers, and acerola berries (vitamin C); brewer's yeast, liver, or rice polishings (vitamin B); fish-liver oil or lemon grass (vitamins A and D); vegetable oils (vitamin E); kelp (iodine); bone meal, egg shells, and milk (minerals); etc.

There is a great deal of controversy about the differences in usefulness of synthetic vs. natural vitamins. Natural-health authorities usually claim that synthetic vitamins are useless, ineffective, and extremely harmful. Most orthodox doctors and nutritionists claim that synthetic vitamins have a molecular structure identical to that of the so-called natural vitamins, and that they are just as effective. Who is right?

In Sweden, two groups of silver foxes were fed identical diets, but one group received a food supplement in the form of all the known synthetic B-vitamins; the control group received vitamins in the form of brewer's yeast and liver. The synthetically fed animals failed to grow, had bad fur, and acquired many diseases. Animals fed the natural vitamins grew normally, developed beautiful fur, and enjoyed good health. Approximately similar results were demonstrated in other animal studies in various countries. "On the whole, we can trust nature further than the chemist and his synthetic vitamins," explained Dr. A. J. Carlson of the University of Chicago.

We must keep in mind that in nature, vitamins are never isolated. They are always present in the form of vitamin complexes. There are 24 known factors in the vitamin-C complex. There are 22 known B-vitamin factors. E vitamin, as we know it, is composed of at least nine natural tocopherols. And so on.

When you take natural vitamins, for instance, in the form of rose hips, brewer's yeast, or vegetable oil, you are getting *all* the vitamins and vitamin-like factors that occur naturally in these foods—that is, all those that have already been discovered, as well as those that have not yet been discovered. Also, our knowledge of vitamins is not complete. New vitamins are discovered frequently. For example, it has been clinically demonstrated that foods which are naturally rich in B vitamins, such as brewer's yeast and liver, contain some potent, *but as yet unidentified or isolated,* B-vitamin factors. When you take your vitamins in the form of vitamin-rich supplements or in the form of "complexes," you are getting the benefit of all the known and all the unknown vitamins.

Does this mean that synthetic vitamins are useless? Not necessarily. The rightful place of synthetic vitamins is in their therapeutic use, where extremely large doses of easily soluble and fast-acting vitamins are necessary. For example, Dr. W. J. McCormick, the world-famous authority on the therapeutic uses of vitamin C, has successfully used huge doses of ascorbic acid (vitamin C) in acute cases of poisoning or infection, preferably intravenously. His treatments have brought spectacular results and often saved lives. You cannot very well inject rose hips intravenously and get such results. Dr. Linus Pauling has used synthetic ascorbic acid to successfully prevent or cure the common cold. Recently, vitamin C was used successfully in the treatment of cancer. In huge doses, synthetic vitamins perform as fast-acting drugs. Their action is often more rapid than the action of natural vitamins, especially since they can be injected intravenously. This fact can be invaluable in acute conditions of poisoning or ill health.

Vitamin E is another good example. Proponents of natural vitamins advise taking vegetable oils rich in vitamin E, particularly wheat-germ oil, instead of isolated vitamin-E capsules. Or, if capsules are used, they advise taking vitamin E in the form of mixed tocopherols, as it occurs in nature. But Drs. Evan and Wilfrid Shute, the world's foremost authorities on therapeutic uses of vitamin E, used only an isolated alpha-tocopherol in their successful practice and research work. They contend that alpha-tocopherol is the only active part of the vitamin-E complex and that the other tocopherols are not necessary in therapeutic use.

The intelligent solution to the controversy over synthetic vs. natural vitamins seems to be as follows:

The isolated and synthetic vitamins and minerals in large doses have their rightful and indispensable place in the short-term treatment of acute conditions or severe deficiency diseases, or where only the isolated fractions of a vitamin complex are needed for specific therapeutic purposes. But those who do not suffer from any specific disease or deficiency, but are interested in food supplements and vitamins mainly for preventive purposes—that is, to protect their health and to prevent disease and premature aging —should use natural vitamins in the form of food supplements, such as brewer's yeast, rose-hips concentrate, kelp, bone meal, fish-liver oil, vegetable oils, etc. In these supplements, all the vitamins and other nutritional substances are present in their natural, balanced combinations, which is essential for better assimilation, synergistic action, and maximum biological effect.

TO AVOID CONFUSION

For those who are confused about which vitamins are synthetic and which are natural (since even most health food stores carry and sell both), I advise reading the labels. As a rule, if the formula on the bottle does not say that the vitamin is natural or is derived from natural sources, it is synthetic. Manufacturers of natural products are always eager to advertise their natural sources. Occasionally, fancy chemical names are used which the consumer doesn't understand; thus, it is difficult to make an intelligent choice. Also, some manufacturers employ clever wording, or even by colorful pictures of fruit or berries try to make you believe that theirs is a 100 percent natural product, when it actually is not. For example, if the label reads "Vitamin C—Rose Hips," it does not necessarily mean that the product is made from rose hips. It may only mean that ascorbic acid has an added rose-hip concentrate with it, perhaps 95 per cent ascorbic acid and 5 per cent rose hips. If B-complex formula contains more than 10 mg of each major B per tablet, it is *not* 100 per cent natural, and sometimes even potencies less than that are synthetic. You have to be an expert label reader!

CONCLUSION

Many health writers and nutrition experts are still clinging to the outdated and antiquated belief, popular in the early decades of this century, that the diet of healthy people does not need to be supplemented with extra vitamins and minerals—that we will get all the vitamins, minerals, and other nutritive substances that our bodies require from the foods we eat.

In fact, perhaps more than half the books on a typical health-food store shelf today—those by the proponents of natural hygiene, macrobiotics, mucusless diets, fruitarianism, Eastern-oriented vegetarianism, to name a few—expound the view that it is "unnatural" to take tablets and pills, and that if we eat proper high-quality foods, we don't need them. Although, in principle, they are, of course, right, they forget that what was true 50 years ago is not relevant today.

It is virtually impossible to obtain high-quality foods that are grown without agricultural chemicals on fertile soils, foods that are whole, unprocessed, unadulterated, and poison-free. Even so-called organically grown produce is grown in a polluted environment, is watered by polluted waters, and transported long distances, which lowers its nutritional value. Therefore, vitamin supplementation is a must—not only for the average American who subsists on a diet of devitalized, overprocessed, and nutritionless supermarket foods, but even for those of us who make heroic efforts to eat so-called natural foods. If you add to this the fact that none of us can escape toxins in polluted air, water, and environment, and that many vitamins have a neutralizing and protective effect against these poisons, the conclusion will be obvious: dietary vitamin supplementation is a *must* in today's poisoned and denatured world.

SUGGESTIONS FOR FURTHER READING

Books by Paavo Airola, Ph.D., published by Health Plus Publishers, P.O. Box 22001, Phoenix, AZ 85028.

Are You Confused?
Cancer: Causes, Prevention, and Treatment—The Total Approach
Everywoman's Book
How to Get Well
How to Keep Slim, Healthy, and Young With Juice Fasting
Hypoglycemia: A Better Approach
Rejuvenation Secrets From Around the World That "Work"
Stop Hair Loss
Swedish Beauty Secrets
The Miracle of Garlic

Paavo Airola, Ph.D., N.D., is an internationally recognized nutritionist and naturopathic physician, educator, and award-winning author of thirteen widely read books, notably his two international bestsellers, How To Get Well, *and* Are You Confused? *His latest book,* Everywoman's Book, *firms Dr. Airola's unchallenged leadership in the field of nutrition and holistic healing, and, in addition, demonstrates his genius as an original thinker and profound philosopher.*

Dr. Airola is President of the International Academy of Biological Medicine and is engaged in extensive educational work with both laymen and professionals. He has been a visiting lecturer in many universities and medical schools, including the Stanford University Medical School.

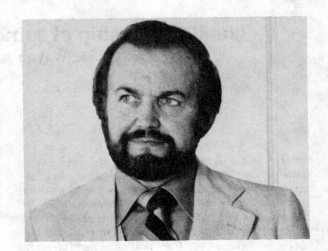

The Relationship of Minerals to Health and Disease

De Wayne Ashmead, Ph.D.

If you are feeling rundown, sluggish, and out of tune, a mineral deficiency or imbalance may be at the root of your problem. Minerals are the pure metal ions that spark our internal cell combustion. Dr. Ashmead points out that less is known about the role of minerals in the body than the role of vitamins. Even small departures from normal mineral composition within our bodies may result in many different types of disease.

Mineral supplements are now being chelated, or combined with complementary amino acids, to help the body metabolize them. The anecdote that begins this article attests to the restorative powers of chelated mineral therapy when used in conjunction with an appropriate diet and tender loving care.

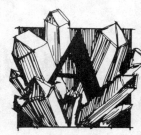 bout five years ago Rosy had a stroke. My mother was distraught. Rosy, a little dachshund, had been part of the family for years. Now the dog was completely paralyzed. The veternarian who attended her suggested that Rosy be put to sleep. It was the only humane thing to do.

"No," my mother cried fiercely. "Rosy has been with me too many years. She doesn't want to die anymore than you do."

"But look at her," the veterinarian argued. "She can't even stand up to go to the bathroom, let alone walk outside when she needs to go. It would be better for the dog if she were put to sleep." Then he added, "Rosy will never get any better."

In spite of these arguments, my mother's wishes prevailed. The dog lived even though she couldn't walk. To pick the animal up apparently caused excruciating pain, so Rosy was slowly slid onto a two-foot square board and then carried outside. Once on the grass, she was slid off the board so she could

Reprinted from *Bestways Magazine* (April 1977), 400 Hot Springs Road, Carson City, Nevada 89701.

go to the bathroom. Then she was slid back onto the transport board and returned to the house.

At first Rosy was force-fed, but later she was able to eat and drink without assistance. In addition to her regular food, my mother gave Rosy high levels of chelated minerals, minerals which had been attached in a special way to amino acids. Many researchers have shown that when this process is done correctly, the ingested minerals are more compatible with the body, and therefore are absorbed and metabolized in much higher quantities.

At first the minerals had no effect on Rosy. Then one day she lifted her head up. About four weeks later Rosy slowly pulled herself up and stood on her four shaky legs. After taking two or three steps, she collapsed. The next day she took a few more steps. As the weeks went by, Rosy became stronger and stronger. Soon she was walking around the house. But the great day came when the dog wanted to go outside all by herself. When the door was opened Rosy bounced down the three steps to the ground. Later my mother heard Rosy scratching at the back door. She had hopped back up the three steps and was waiting to come in.

In time Rosy became very frisky, and she lived several more years before finally succumbing to old age. If her age is equated to human years, Rosy lived to be more than 100 years old.

The veterinarian who had attended the dog was amazed at her recovery. He conceded that mineral nutrition did play a major role in Rosy's health, but he wanted to know why the effect was so dramatic.

I sat down with him and explained. "To understand the importance of mineral nutrition to health, let us break the body up into the simplest unit, the cell."

"OK," he replied.

Continuing, I said, "Rosy, you, and I are made up of many systems. One such example is our digestive system. Each one of these systems is composed of several organs. For example, your digestive system contains the following organs: the mouth, esophagus, stomach, intestine, pancreas, liver, and gallbladder.

Each one of the organs in a system is made up of tissues; such as muscles, connective tissue, epithelial tissue, and nerves. These make up one organ in the digestive system: the intestine. Finally, each tissue is composed of various cells. The epithelial tissue is made up of argentiffin cells, globlet cells, paneth cells, and absorptive cells.

"As you know, each type of cell in your body has a specific function. When it and all the other billions of body cells carry out their assigned roles, they work together to form you.

"Now, Doctor, if we examine those cells under the microscope, we will discover that each one of them is only about 1/3000 of an inch in diameter. That means approximately 600,000 billion of them all work together to build an average adult. As each second of your life passes, 50 million cells throughout your body die and are replaced by new cells, provided your nutrition is adequate to support regeneration. You see, all these billions of cells in your body live out their useful lives and die in amazingly short periods of time.

"Because the human body is so complete, most cells are interdependent, and as such are varied in structure. Despite this dependence, each minute cell carries out a number of continuous chemical processes within its structure. In fact, each cell may be thought of as a chemical factory which utilizes enzymes to bring about the chemical reactions. In a single cell, for example, there may be up to 50,000 enzyme units. All of these chemical reactions caused by the different enzymes are what keep the cell, and us, alive. Indeed, it has been estimated that as many as two million enzyme reactions must take place in certain cells each minute."

The veterinarian glanced at his watch. "You have given me a course in physiology," he said impatiently, "but you still haven't told me what all this has to do with mineral nutrition."

"I was just getting to that," I explained. "Most enzymes within the cells cannot work alone. They need an activator, which in most cases is a specific mineral. For example, in the liver cells there is an enzyme called butyryl dehydrogenase. This enzyme breaks down fats into simpler units. But it won't digest protein down into amino acids or build these amino acids into new protein structures such as skin; one of the enzymes involved in this process requires manganese. Carbohydrate metabolism in your body cannot take place unless molybdenum activates a specific enzyme. In red blood cells, oxygen is brought in, and carbon dioxide given off, only if the enzyme carbonic anhydrase is present. Zinc must activate that enzyme.

"Many of these enzymes are absolutely vital for life. If they are inhibited, you will die. For example, transmission of nerve impulses along the nerves to and from the brain takes place only when acetyl choline is broken down by the enzyme cholinesterase. If the enzyme is prevented from functioning, which can take place when you come in contact with certain insecticides, a nerve block will occur. This is followed by rapid death due to paralysis of your respiratory center. Cyanide can kill because it combines with the iron in the heme enzyme (such as the heme in hemoglobin) and permanently blocks that enzyme's activity. This enzyme is needed to help carry oxygen throughout your body. The iron can no longer activate the enzyme in hemoglobin because it is tied up; so you die of suffocation."

I went on to explain to the veterinarian that the roles of specific minerals in activating specific enzymes is a very complex subject. For example, Schutte, in his book *The Biology of the Trace Elements,* lists 202 identified enzymes that are influenced by minerals. In many instances, if the activating mineral is absent or is replaced by another mineral, the enzyme will not function. And as I had explained to the doctor, if that specific enzyme doesn't work, even though it is present in the cells, the whole body can die. Even if enzyme blockage doesn't cause death, it can cause serious health problems.

In their five-volume treatise, *Mineral Metabolism,* Doctors Comar and Bronner wrote that some diseases are characterized by only slight alterations in the concentration of specific minerals in the fluids surrounding the billions of body cells. The mineral levels of these fluids can affect the mineral composition inside the cell, where many of the enzymes work. These researchers found that even very small departures from the normal mineral composition within our body cells may result in many different types of diseases without making any appreciable difference in the mineral makeup of our bodies as a whole.

Although some diseases are directly related to a mineral deficiency (such as iron deficiencies and anemia), most diseases are indirectly related. In other words, when the right minerals are present to correctly activate the cellular enzymes in their proper sequences, the body usually has a natural defense mechanism which is able to overcome or resist the effect of most causative disease agents. Thus mineral deficiencies in and of themselves are not always the direct cause of a health problem, even though the deficiencies may set up conducive conditions for that illness.

To illustrate, iron is needed not only to prevent anemia, but also to activate a specific enzyme that makes white blood cells. In the body, white blood cells attack and destroy invading infections and infectious diseases. If body iron levels are low or even lacking in the tissue area where the white blood cells are made, so that specific enzymes cannot be activated, production of white blood cells stops. If this happens at a time when an infection or disease has invaded the body, death to the entire body can result. In a study conducted by Dr. Hopson and myself, and reported in a medical journal, we found a significant relationship between the amount of iron in the tissues and the amount of diseases.

In their book, *Modern Nutrition in Health and Disease,* Doctors Goodhart and Shils point out that we should recognize that not all mineral disorders result in specific and charactersitc clinical signs or pathological changes which are easily recognized, even by a competent physician. This is especially true when the disorder is mild. There are many factors, including: age: sex: the timing, duration, and severity of the mineral deficiency: and the nature of the mineral; and its relationship to the other elements or other constituents of the diet. The authors also stated that many of us, because of various problems, do not absorb adequate amounts of a needed mineral, even though it is found in the diet. Even after absorption, some of us fail to synthesize these minerals into biologically active components for enzyme systems, etc. Still others of us, for one reason or another, excrete excessive amounts of minerals from our bodies. All these problems play crucial roles which may affect human nutrition, and this in turn affects the health of the person involved.

Thus, it should be painfully obvious that we are not products of what we eat, but of what we absorb and retain. Foods differ from batch to batch in their mineral contents. For example, spinach, a vegetable long thought to be high in iron, may vary between 1,584 parts per million down to 19 parts per million of iron, according to research done at Rutgers University.

Many people feel the answer is in mineral supplements. But even the swallowing of numerous pills or capsules doesn't assure mineral absorption. There are seven, and possibly eight, specific barriers within our bodies which may reduce the amount of minerals we are able to absorb from our intestines. Because these barriers can effectively prevent absorption of the minerals, research at Albion Laboratories has shown that the majority of the minerals we swallow are never absorbed.

Realizing that there is a very real possibility that the minerals swallowed are not absorbed, many people have turned to chelated minerals for a solution. Unfortunately, this may not solve the problem either, because chelation does not guarantee mineral absorption. Many mineral supplements, although chelated, are not chelated as the body chelates. This means that absorption of certain non-compatible amino-acid chelates may be lower than that of many nonchelated minerals, as university research has shown.

On the other hand, research by many investigators has shown that when a mineral is chelated in a specific way, then mineral metabolism usually increases, because the mineral is properly protected from the absorption barriers. Other investigators have found that when these correctly chelated minerals were supplemented to diseased animals who had specific mineral deficiencies, the responses to that type of supplementation were much more positive, when compared with responses from other forms of the same mineral supplementation.

I should not wish to convey the impression that every disease known to man is related to a mineral disorder. Perhaps research will bear that out, but for the present we don't know it to be true. I personally believe that less is really known about the roles of minerals in the body than about the roles of vitamins. What we state today may be revised by future research.

In 1975, Professor Valkovic wrote that the majority of the minerals in our bodies serve chiefly as activating components of our enzyme systems. If the mineral is removed from the enzyme, the enzyme usually loses its capacity to function. "Many clinical and pathological disorders arise . . . as a consequence of trace-element deficiencies and excesses for which there are no acceptable explanations in biochemical or enzymatic terms. This suggests either that there are many trace-element-dependent enzymes of great metabolic significance which have not yet been discovered, or that these elements participate in the activity of other compounds in tissue. This might suggest that there are some important facts still to be discovered about the role and interrelations of metal ions in nutrition and in health and diseases."

Dr. De Wayne Ashmead is Executive Vice-President of Albion Laboratories. He is a prolific author, publishing the results of research in the field of chelated minerals in a variety of scientific and nutritional journals. He has lectured extensively on chelated mineral nutrition throughout the world. He has worked with several government agencies worldwide, including the United Nations, to help establish nutrition programs in their countries.

Macrobiotics: Living in Harmony with the Universe
Michio Kushi

Throughout the world, hundreds of thousands of people are now practicing macrobiotics, which can be defined as a way of life according to the order of the universe. Translated literally, macro is the Greek term for "large" or "great," and bios is the word for "life." Macrobiotics means the way of life according to the macroscopic, or largest possible, view.

This seemingly abstract philosophical concept can be applied to everyday life by means of the unifying principle of yin and yang. The practice of macrobiotics involves understanding and applying this universal order of change to our lifestyle, including the selection, preparation, and manner of eating our daily food.

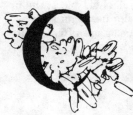ooked whole grain cereals have constituted a large part of humanity's diet for hundreds of thousands of years, and up until relatively recent times, cereal grains were eaten as staple foods throughout the world: rice in the Orient, wheat in Europe and America, buckwheat in Central Europe, and corn in the Americas. In fact, the English word *meal* is also the word for ground grain, and in Japanese, the term used for a meal is *gohan*, which means rice.

The first principle in the selection and preparation of food, according to long biological tradition, is to eat unrefined cereal grains and cooked vegetables as our main foods.

A second principle to consider is that we should eat in accordance with our immediate environment, specifically, the climatic conditions in which we live. Ideally, we should eat foods that have grown within a radius of several hundred miles from where we are living, in order to maintain natural physiological

This is an excerpt from the booklet, "Macrobiotics: Experience the Miracle of Life," copyright © 1978 by the East West Foundation.

balance with our local climatic area. However, if foods of proper quality are not available in our immediate environment, it is possible to import foods from other areas, provided they are grown under climatic conditions similar to those in which we live. Generally, foods grown in the same latitudes, brought in from either east or west, would be suitable for this purpose. However, foods which are imported from areas with climates noticeably different from those in which we live are not suitable for maintaining adaptation to our native climate, and thus when eaten in large enough quantities often result in illness.

For example, for people living in the northern part of the United States, pineapples grown in Hawaii, sugar from Cuba and South America, citrus fruits from Florida and southern California, coffee from Colombia, and spices from the Near East and India would be far removed from their natural climate, and therefore not beneficial for the maintenance of health. Before the advent of modern techniques of food storage and transportation, foods from outside the local environment were eaten much less frequently. For example, people living in warm tropical climates traditionally eat a more *yin* diet than people living in cold northern climates. If we move from one climate to another, our method of cooking should also change, but we should always keep whole grains and cooked vegetables as our principal foods, since they grow in almost all climates.

Within a particular climate, we experience various seasonal changes, and should vary our diet accordingly, primarily using foods which either are naturally available during a particular season or can be naturally stored. This third principle of macrobiotic eating is based on flexible adaptation to the changing seasons. During the summer, fresh vegetables in the form of salad and fruits are naturally available, and can be used from time to time as supplements; whereas in winter, they are not naturally available. In traditional cultures, vegetables were usually pickled in salt or stored in a root cellar for use in winter.

Cereal grains, beans, seaweeds, and other foods which can be naturally stored in winter and summer should be the mainstay of our diet throughout the year. Also, when cooking during winter, we accentuate *yang* factors, such as fire, salt, and pressure, in order to create balance with our more *yin* or cold environment; in summer, the emphasis on these factors would be less. Nowadays, however, particularly in the modern industrial nations, most people eat a uniform diet throughout the year. For example, ice cream and citrus fruits are consumed both in winter and in summer; and, as a result, chronic illness is reaching epidemic proportions.

When we are selecting and preparing our foods, individual differences need also be considered, with variations according to age, sex, amount of activity, occupation, original constitution, previous eating patterns, and social environment. The fourth principle of macrobiotic eating involves modifying our diet to suit individual differences.

YIN AND YANG IN DAILY FOOD

In general, animal foods exert a *yang*, or contractive, influence, and vegetables produce a more *yin*, or expansive, influence. External factors, such as pressure, fire, salt, and time (aging), produce a more contractive influence; whereas less pressure, water, oil, and freshness (less time) result in expansion. Within the vegetable kingdom, we can consider as being more *yin* all plants which are larger in size; grow above the ground in an upward direction or below the ground in a horizontal direction; are juicier, softer, longer, or more delicate; and are produced in a warmer climate. *Yang* vegetables are those which are smaller in size; grow in a downward direction below the ground, or horizontally above the ground; are drier, harder, shorter, or stronger; and are produced in colder climates. Also, we can classify vegetables according to color, from the more *yin* colors—violet, indigo, green, and white—to the more *yang* colors—yellow, brown, and red. In addition, we should also consider the ratio of various chemical components, such as sodium, which is *yang,* to potassium, which is *yin,* in assessing the *yin/yang* qualities of vegetables and other foods.

Proceeding along the scale from *yang* to *yin,* we can generally classify foods as follows: eggs, meat, poultry, and fish; then cereal grains, which generally maintain an approximate 1:7 ratio of sodium to potassium; then beans, seeds, root vegetables, leafy round vegetables like cabbage, nuts, leafy expanded vegetables, fruits, sweeteners like maple syrup and honey, sugar, and drugs.

Since we continually need to maintain a dynamic balance between *yin* and *yang,* when we eat foods from one extreme, we are naturally attracted to the other. For example, a diet consisting of large quantities of meats, eggs, and other animal foods, which are very *yang,* requires a correspondingly large intake of *yin* foods, such as fruits, sugar, alcohol, spices, and in some cases drugs. However, a diet based on such extremes is very difficult to balance, and often results in sickness, which is an imbalance caused by excess of one of the two factors.

GENERAL YIN AND YANG CATEGORIES OF FOOD

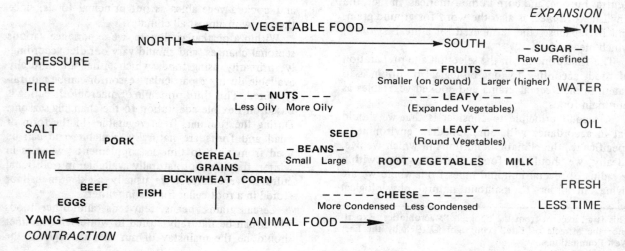

Within each category of foods, there are *yin* and *yang* variations. For example, red-meat fish, such as swordfish, is more *yang* than white-meat fish, such as flounder. Among grains, buckwheat is the most *yang* and corn the most *yin*, with brown rice generally in the center. Smaller beans containing less oil, like azuki beans, are more *yang* than larger beans, like lima and soybeans, which contain more oil. The same is true for nuts, with smaller and less oily varieties being more *yang* than those which are larger and contain more oil.

THE WAY OF EATING

In order to reflect the over-all order of biological evolution in our eating, as well as to maintain a 7:1 *yin/yang* balance, we need approximately 50 per cent of our daily food to be unrefined cereal grains. These include brown rice, whole wheat, millet, oats, rye, barley, corn, and buckwheat, and can be varied according to individual need or desire. When preparing brown rice, use a pressure cooker made of either stainless steel or enamel. Pressure-cooked rice is far superior to boiled rice for everyday use, since many desirable nutritional components are lost in boiling. Whole wheatberries are rather tough and somewhat difficult to chew; so they are usually ground into flour, which is baked into bread. Bread should ideally be baked from freshly ground flour without the addition of yeast. In general, creamy or floury cereals should be avoided, even if they are made from unrefined grains.

Along with cereal grains, about 20 to 25 per cent of our daily food should consist of cooked vegetables, which can be prepared in a wide variety of cooking styles, such as sautéing, steaming, boiling, baking, and pressure-cooking. Among root vegetables, carrots, daikon (white radish), turnip, radish, burdock, lotus root, and jinenjo (mountain potato) are excellent. When preparing root vegetables, cook both the root and green portion; you will achieve the proper *yin/yang* balance if you use the whole vegetable. Among ground vegetables, cabbage, onions, fall and winter squash, cauliflower, broccoli, and chinese cabbage are quite nutritious. Some leafy vegetables, watercress, kale, parsley, scallions, dandelion, collards, carrots, daikon, turnip greens, and others are fine for regular use. Vegetables such as cucumbers, mushrooms, lettuce, parsnips, stringbeans, and celery can be used occasionally.

In addition to grains and vegetables, about 5 to 10 per cent (one or two cups) of soup can be included in daily intake. Soup broth can be made with miso

---

Seven Principles of the Order of the Universe
Michio Kushi

1. Everything is a differentiation of One Infinity.
2. Everything changes.
3. All antagonisms are complementary.
4. There is nothing identical.
5. What has a front has a back.
6. The bigger the front, the bigger the back.
7. What has a beginning has an end.

(which is prepared from fermented soybeans, salt, and grain), to which may be added several varieties of vegetables, including seaweed. Broth can also be prepared with tamari, a naturally processed soy sauce. Soups, of course, can also contain grains and beans, to which several kinds of vegetables may be added.

The remaining 10 per cent of our daily food intake can include beans, sea vegetables, and occasionally salad, with locally grown fruits (in season), animal food (preferably fish or shellfish), and seeds and nuts, depending on climate, season, and individual need. Among beans, those which are smaller and contain less oil, such as azuki beans, chickpeas, and lentils, are preferable, although other beans may also be eaten on occasion. In general, soybeans contain too much oil and are too *yin* for daily use; therefore, traditionally they were aged with sea salt (*yang*) to produce miso and tamari for daily use. Among sea vegetables, hiziki, arame, wakame, kombu, nori, and dulse can be eaten regularly as a side dish, in addition to their use in soups.

Since fruits are generally very *yin*, it is preferable to serve them dried, or cooked with the addition of salt. A moderate amount of animal food is allowable, particularly during winter or in more northern climates, but the ratio of animal foods to vegetable foods should usually not exceed 1:7. With animal foods, it is preferable to eat more of the *yin* varieties, and those which are farthest removed from us on the scale of evolution, such as shellfish, or white-meat fish, instead of red-meat fish or poultry. Again, as with fruits and salad, for some conditions, animal foods may need to be avoided for a certain period.

Twelve Theorems
of the Unifying Principle
Michio Kushi

1. One Infinity manifests itself into complementary and antagonistic tendencies, *yin* and *yang*, in its endless change.

2. *Yin* and *yang* are manifested continuously from the eternal movement of one infinite universe.

3. *Yin* represents centrifugality. *Yang* represents centripetality. *Yin* and *yang* together produce energy and all phenomena.

4. *Yin* attracts *yang*. *Yang* attracts *yin*.

5. *Yin* repels *yin*. *Yang* repels *yang*.

6. *Yin* and *yang* combined in varying proportions produce different phenomena. The attraction and repulsion among phenomena is proportional to the difference of the *yin* and *yang* forces.

7. All phenomena are ephemeral, constantly changing their constitution of *yin* and *yang* forces: *yin* changes into *yang*; *yang* changes into *yin*.

8. Nothing is solely *yin* or solely *yang*. Everything is composed of both tendencies in varying degrees.

9. There is nothing neutral. Either *yin* or *yang* is in excess in every occurrence.

10. Large *yin* attracts small *yin*. Large *yang* attracts small *yang*.

11. Extreme *yin* produces *yang*, and extreme *yang* produces *yin*.

12. All physical manifestations are *yang* at the center, and *yin* at the surface.

Among beverages, those which are generally balanced between *yin* and *yang* are to be preferred, including bancha tea, cereal-grain coffee, and tea made from roasted grains, such as rice or barley. In general, drink only when thirsty. If you need to urinate more than three or four times each day, or if the palms of your hands or your feet perspire during normal activity, you are drinking too much liquid.

For cooking, oils which are more *yang*, such as sesame or corn, are preferable, but should not be used excessively. The best seasonings are white sea salt, tamari soy sauce, miso, and umeboshi (a variety of wild plum naturally processed in salt), and these should be used in moderation.

There are several condiments which can be added to cooked grains and other foods. The most widely used is *gomasio*, or sesame salt, which is a combination of roasted sesame seeds and sea salt. Depending on whether you need a more *yin* or more *yang* preparation, the proportion of sesame seeds to salt can vary between 8:1 and 12:1. Ideally, gomasio should be freshly prepared every few days in a small earthenware bowl called a *suribachi*. Another convenient condiment is roasted seaweed powder, easily made by roasting seaweed in the oven until it is burnt, then crushing it into a fine powder. This condiment can be used in place of gomasio, particularly by people who feel they have been eating too much salt.

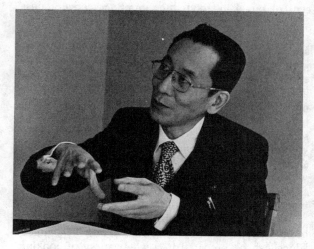

Michio Kushi is the world's foremost teacher of macrobiotics and Oriental medicine. He is the author of The Book of Macrobiotics *and* The Macrobiotic Way of Natural Healing.

Mr. Kushi was born in Kokawa, Wakayama-ken, Japan on May 17, 1926. His early years were devoted to the study of international law and world peace. He studied at Tokyo University, where he received his Master's degree in Law. He came to the United States 30 years ago to pursue graduate research work at Columbia University.

Michio Kushi is the founder of Erewhon, Inc. a natural-foods distributor; East West Journal; Sanae Restaurant, Inc.; the East West Foundation; and the Kushi Institute. He has conducted world-wide seminars, and given lectures and consultations guiding thousands of people toward the restoration of their physical, mental, and spiritual health and happiness.

Mr. Kushi currently resides in Brookline, Massachusets.

Fat Liberation
Alan Dolit, with Sandy Brown, M.D., and Leah Maggie Garfield

Think how much power we give to food. Lonesome, scared, feelings hurt? How about an ice cream sundae, a beer, or a bag of chips? Food is the most abused substance in this country, says Alan Dolit, originator of Fat Liberation weight-control groups.

Fat Lib is not based on nutritional guidelines. It offers no diet or exercise program. It is an awareness approach, wherein individuals express their feelings and fantasies in group sessions, in order to work through behavior problems related to food and weight control.

Fat Liberation works because it deals with the cause of being overweight, not the external symptom. And, in 90 percent of the cases Dolit reports, the weight that is lost stays off.

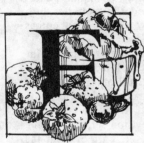 at Liberation was primarily born because I was too fat. Four and a half years ago, I weighed 230 pounds, and I didn't like it. From the time I was 19 to the time I was 36, I was battling the weight problem. I had lost weight several times doing traditional kinds of dieting, but I would gain the weight back within a year. I never enjoyed dieting; it's a drudge, like doing repetitive exercises.

Until four and a half years ago I was involved in all sorts of groups, both as participant and as facilitator. I adapted the group methods to my own weight-reduction needs and they began working. Within a three-month period I lost about fifty pounds without ever dieting, primarily by being aware of what I was doing.

When I started my first group, I didn't have a name for what I was doing; it was just a weight-control group. Then one night during the first group we heard a male voice in the hall say, "Is this where the fat ladies are meeting?" There were audible groans from the people in the group. At that time gay lib and women's lib were getting started; so I said, "Let's call this group fat lib." I've stayed with the name ever since.

During the first year I was learning to develop exercises and awareness techniques oriented toward losing weight. The things that worked, I kept and refined; and the things that didn't work I threw away. Basically, what the group is all about is using an awareness approach to discovering who we are. I tell people that losing weight is really a fringe benefit of Fat Liberation. Most people, by the end of the eight-week session, stop smoking and stop abusing people, and start experiencing all kinds of positive changes.

EXERCISE

I used exercises as a key to understanding how we are abusing ourselves by abusing food, and to explore what options we have. We do relaxation and pragmatic meditation. We do a lot of dream fantasies, gestalt awareness, and role playing. We role play not only with other people, but with food. We become the candy bar or the chocolate cake. We talk to the food, play with the food, and write poetry to it. We kiss the food. One of the exercises I developed is to say "I love you" to whatever food you're going to eat. If you can't say "I love you" to it, maybe you don't really want that food. A woman in one of my groups did that exercise. She took an apple to a field one night and started caressing it. She talked to the apple, petted it, and said "I love you" to it. And then she broke down and started crying, as she realized she hadn't said "I love you" to anybody in a meaningful way in years. She was unable to say it to her husband. She realized the lack of communication in her marriage. The irony was that she leads women's groups, and was still playing little girl to her husband, which caused a lot of resentment. She hadn't discovered that before.

These exercises have a tendency to open up all kinds of vistas to people. For example, one woman was having bad asthma attacks when she started the group. By the time the group was over, her asthma didn't bother her any more. In addition to losing weight, she had worked through many of her problems, and her asthma was so managable she didn't have to take medicine for it.

Some people who come to the workshops are not overweight at all by any criterion, but they are unhappy with their eating habits, and they feel they are fat psychologically. If they had a slower metabolic rate, they probably would be fat. I have grossly fat people too, maybe a couple of hundred pounds overweight.

Our approach is not to repudiate food; we get more into the taste of it, into the texture of it, and into the whole sensory awareness approach to food. If people have the urge for chocolate cake, I say, "Fine, plan to eat it; plan to eat the whole chocolate cake." One of the things people discover is that they think they'll have a little sliver, and about two minutes later they go and have another piece. By the time the night's over, they'll have eaten the whole cake. They'll feel guilty as hell, too. So I say, "Plan to eat the whole thing." I mean, take the chocolate cake, put it right there where you can see it, and talk to it. Really communicate with it. Most people tell me that if they pay attention to it, by the time they have eaten one-fifth of the cake or less, they don't want any more. But had they not been conscious of what they were doing, they'd have eaten the whole thing.

I think most people are fat because they don't pay attention. They'll be doing other things, like reading the newspaper, and before they know it, all the cake is gone. In fact, most fat people, I have discovered, do not enjoy food. I tell people to bring their favorite foods to the workshop. Usually they discover after doing some sensory awareness with it that they don't really like it. In one group about 90 per cent of the people who brought their favorite foods discovered that they didn't even like the food. And if they don't like their favorite food, what about all the other crap they've been eating?

GROUP DYNAMICS

In the group, we do homework assignments from my book. I'll also give individual assignments to people. Usually somebody will bring up something that he or she discovered by doing one of the assignments. For example, in one of my groups a woman was talking about going on a peanut-butter binge. For a whole week she was eating great big jars full of peanut butter, and she gained a lot of weight. So I said,

"Let's have an instant replay. Bring whatever happened into the present, and we'll reenact it." What had happened to her was that she had just received a phone call from her mother, who, it turned out, was coming to visit. She hadn't seen her mother for a long time, nor did she want to see her. In reenacting the call, she literally got into her childhood, and she realized that when she got into heavy things with her mother as a child, she would eat peanut butter. She made the connection right there about her mother and the peanut butter, and just by making that connection, she was able to swear off peanut-butter binges for good. In another exercise, I'll say, "Give yourself a time limit, half an hour or fifteen minutes, and observe what happens during that time limit when you have the urge to eat. Localize where you have that feeling of hunger." When people really get into it, they discover that it's not really hunger, but something else, some kind of tension, perhaps. But if, after we go through all these observations, the person says, "It's truly hunger that I feel right now," I'll say, "OK, give yourself fifteen minutes more, and see what happens." That specific exercise aims at avoiding immediate gratification.

What people take away from the group and keep is basically the awareness. It's like getting an education. Once they've incorporated the exercises into their own psyches, they know them. Then comes the change in attitude.

There are two universals I've discovered among fat people. One is that fat people are looking for a certain kind of magic—a pill, a diet, a shot, or hypnosis—to lose weight. The other is that they play victim; if it weren't for my husband, if it weren't for my mother, if it wasn't for the television set, if it wasn't for the Vietnam war, or whatever. Part of what fat lib does is get people out of the victim role to a power role, reclaiming the power they've given to food. Through the group process, power is transferred to the group, then back to the person himself. It's successful when the person is able to reclaim power, and take responsibility for his or her behavior. I think that's the dynamic, and why it works.

The beauty of fat lib is that everybody's out front from the beginning. They see through all the games. They're aware of their own defenses, and when they get together as a group, they recognize a common purpose. They know more about themselves and each other after two hours than they know about people they've been seeing in other contexts for many months. Right off the bat, people are up front, trusting, and supportive. I think it's the support more than anything else that gets people off on the right track.

YOU CAN'T GET FAT
IF YOU DON'T OVEREAT

I find nutrition theories boring. Most of the people who come to the fat lib classes know just about everything there is to know about nutrition. Even nutritionists come to my group, and if they don't know about nutrition, who does? It's a paradox. They are food-conscious, and yet they're fat.

I've seen many flyers for workshops on substance abuse with drugs or alcohol or cigarettes, but never for food. I think food is the most abused substance there is in this country. Even skinny people abuse food, but with fat people it's more obvious. They have the Pinocchio effect. When Pinocchio tells a lie, his nose betrays him by growing larger. With fat people, their bodies immediately betray them by growing larger.

I keep hearing from fat people that "I don't eat any more than Mary," and then they'll talk about Mary, or someone else in the office, who eats more than they do. I say, "Well, check it out." I'd bet there probably is a very small percentage of people who can eat almost anything they want to and still not gain weight. Maybe this is one of them. I tell the person to become a fly on Mary's wall, become invisible, follow her around, and watch everything she eats. I'll be willing to bet they find that, although for one particular meal she might eat more than they do, she doesn't eat when she's bored, angry, or frustrated; whereas they're eating at all these times. Watch Mary. When she's not hungry any longer, she'll stop eating, no matter how much food is left on her plate. Fat people will be eating until the food's all gone, whether they're hungry or not.

Aside from some people who may have hypothyroidism, I think very few people are organically fat. Everybody has a particular way his or her body metabolizes food, but one can allow for that; so anybody who doesn't want to be fat doesn't have to be. I've discovered that people are fat because they choose to be. They gain a lot from being fat. Until they realize this they'll never be thin.

Food is always convenient. It's always there, whereas a lover isn't. One of my techniques is the Mary Poppins approach to obesity. To refresh your memory, "A spoonful of sugar makes the medicine go down." You know that song? Well, with fat people it's a little bit of food makes the anger go down, and the hurt go down, and the frustration go down. You swallow all these things with the food. The problem is that it doesn't go away. It stays with you in little balls all over your body, and it's disguised; so you're not in touch with the pain, the anger, and the hurt. As you start losing weight, they come to the surface like an air bubble. You really get in touch with the pain and the hurt as you start losing weight. I think that's the major reason other approaches don't work, because most people aren't willing to deal with these hurts and frustrations. It takes a lot of energy to deal with these things.

There are other reasons that I've heard over and over again. One is that some women are afraid to be too thin because they would have to deal with their sexuality, and that takes a lot of work. Then there's, "What if, even after I lose weight, people still don't like me? I'll have nowhere to hide, then." Another reason for being fat is for protection against the world. You feel more solid, more secure; if you lose weight, you fear losing your grounding, floating away. Fat people don't have to deal with their loneliness; they have a reason for being lonely. These are some of the things people gain by staying fat, or by becoming fat in the first place.

THE GOAL IS TO STAY THIN

My work is still evolving, although it continues to work as it is. I'm always finding new things, and I think that anybody who persists in this is going to discover things too. People don't have to come to me, although I feel it would facilitate their own growth if they did. I've already learned through my own and other people's mistakes; so I have some short-cuts. I also think that these basic techniques would work without much modification in any modality, for drugs, alcohol, cigarettes, sex, television, or whatever self-destructive behavior people are hung up on.

I think the reason diets don't work is because they only deal with the symptoms. It's like hacking away at blackberry bushes by cutting away the stems and the leaves. Until you get to the roots, the blackberry bushes are going to keep growing back. Diets are effective as long as you do them, but the moment you stop, the weight, which has been waiting there all the time, catches up again. What fat lib is really doing is dealing with the roots of overweight rather than the stems and the leaves.

Based on correspondence, evaluation forms, phone contacts, running into people, or hearing about them, I can say that 90 per cent who go through our group are retaining their weight loss. That's really a high success ratio.

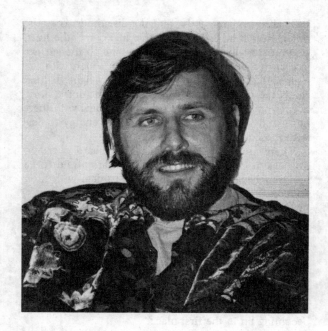

When he's not being a social worker or group leader, Alan Dolit is daddy to three girls, husband to Kay, and active in the Unitarian Fellowship. That, along with following his own advice, is how he continues to be liberated from excess fat.

Leah Maggie Garfield is a psychic healer, teacher, and reader who has been in private practice for the past 12 years. Her background includes American Indian training, barefoot doctoring, herbology, Chinese medicine, and various disciplines in bodywork. She is currently in practice at Rainbow's End Farm in Sebastopol, California.

Sandy Brown, M.D., practices family medicine in Fort Bragg, California, and is the founder of The Mendocino Foundation for Health Education (P.O. Box 1377, Mendocino, CA 95460).

A Self-Styled Physical Fitness Program
Eleanor Glorioso

Incorporating an exercise program into your life is one of the most rewarding things you can do for yourself. Designing your own exercise program allows you to decide what areas of your body you want to strengthen, as well as where you would like to develop flexibility or muscle tone. It allows you to mix and match to your own taste. In this article, Eleanor Glorioso tells us about the various attributes of physical fitness, and what parts they play in our lives. She examines three important types of popular exercise: calisthenics, aerobics, and yoga, presenting the principles and benefits of each, and she gives some important guidelines to follow, regardless of what exercise program you might choose.

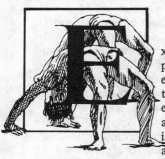

Exercise affects us not only physically, but mentally and emotionally as well. In nature, the human organism is essentially active. Inactivity and the stress of modern living can cause many physical and psychological disorders, anything from heart ailments to anxiety and depression. In essence, a body that isn't used simply deteriorates. All the working components become weak, leaving the organism less efficient and more vulnerable to disease. Since the mind, body, and emotions interact with one another, any disorder is reflected both psychologically and physically. Regular exercise provides an outlet for daily tensions and natural aggressions, so that mental and emotional faculties can function with clarity. And, of course, it also keeps you fit and healthy.

THE BENEFITS

The benefits of exercise are innumerable. It is used by medical professionals in therapy and rehabilitation programs to promote general good health. For the individual who just wants to get in shape, exercise offers a new perspective on life. It strengthens a person's physical, mental, and emotional stamina. People who exercise regularly seem to be less nervous, and better able to handle the stress problems of daily living in a more relaxed manner. It can make you more vital, alert, efficient, self-sustaining, and confident.

Unfortunately, our present mode of living doesn't naturally integrate enough exercise to maintain sound health. One hundred years ago, the demands of daily living made physical fitness a necessity for survival. But today, the average lifestyle has become quite sedentary. Consequently, there is a growing concern and need for us to supplement our daily routines with an adequate amount of exercise.

PHYSICAL FITNESS—WHAT IS IT?

Physical fitness is made up of four basic elements: flexibility, muscular strength, muscular endurance, and cardiovascular-respiratory fitness. Each aspect of fitness is unique in its function, yet all are interdependent if over-all physical fitness is to be achieved.

Flexibility is the range of movement possible at the joints (bending or folding, for example), and it is essential for fluidity and locomotion within the body frame. A simple way to test your flexibility is to stand with your feet together and legs straight. Slowly bend forward from the waist and try to touch your toes with your hands. If you can't do this, then you need to develop more flexibility at the hip joints.

Muscular strength is measured by the amount of force it takes to contract a muscle. It involves any kind of lifting or pushing movement, and it is necessary for sustaining physical performance. Yet it can be maintained for only brief periods of time. Body building is a perfect example of how muscular strength can be developed, and it also shows the limited duration of such strength.

Muscular endurance, unlike muscular strength, is the ability of a muscle, or a group of muscles, to perform a task for a certain period of time. Sit-ups and push-ups are frequently used to measure this type of endurance. It is necessary, for instance, if you're standing or sitting for long periods of time at a job.

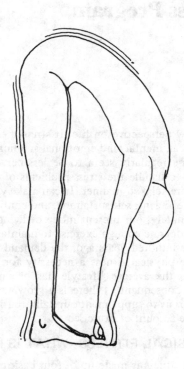

Flexibility is the range of movement at the joints such as bending forward to touch your toes.

Cardiovascular-respiratory fitness is the most important of the four physical-fitness elements. It involves the body's capacity to take oxygen into the blood stream, and it determines how well the lungs, heart, veins, and arteries supply oxygen to the cells, in order to remove wastes and produce energy. All activities, even sleep, require energy, which is produced when oxygen combines with foodstuffs in the body. Since the body cannot store oxygen, it needs to replenish the supply continually.

It's confusing nowadays, trying to find an exercise program that develops the four elements of physical fitness equally. Most programs tend to emphasize the development of one or two elements, but not all of them. For a well-rounded program, calisthenic, aerobic, and yoga exercises should be practices and selected according to what they develop. Since cardi bic, and yoga exercises should be practiced and selected according to what they develop. Since cardiovascular fitness is the most important element, it should be the foundation around which an exercise program is built. The other elements should be emphasized with equal importance.

CALISTHENICS

Calisthenic exercises made up a large portion of the physical-education programs offered in public schools from the 1940s to the 1960s. These programs consisted of exercises like sit-ups, push-ups, and jumping jacks. The principle of calisthenics is to repeat an exercise, gradually increasing the number of times you do it within a certain amount of time. For example, how many sit-ups can you do in two minutes? There are several advantages to calisthenics, but the most important aspects are that it develops almost all muscles or muscle groups, and it allows you to correct specific problems.

There are numerous calisthenic programs a person can undertake. Each develops the four elements of physical fitness, but in varying degrees. People interested in developing body tone and physical strength, and in conditioning major muscle groups, will find calisthenics helpful.

AEROBICS

Aerobic or cardiovascular exercise has been studied, discussed, and written about by medical professionals for years. But not until 1968, when Dr. Kenneth Cooper's book *Aerobics* was published, did the public become aware of it. In his book, Dr. Cooper presented clear and simple arguments in favor of cardiovascular fitness, and he backed everything up with carefully documented research.

Aerobic means literally "with oxygen," and the key to aerobic exercise is oxygen consumption. Any repetitive, steady, rhythmic exercise performed for two or more minutes without producing undue fatigue is probably aerobic. Jogging, swimming, cycling, and jumping rope are some good examples. Since aerobic exercise increases the volume of air input in the body, it improves the capacity and efficiency of the lungs, heart, veins, and arteries to bring in and deliver oxygen to the cells. If you want to burn calories, build over-all physical stamina, and develop muscular endurance, then aerobics can help accomplish this.

YOGA

Yoga is a segment of the Hindu philosophy. Although it is made up of many branches and divisions, it can be broken down (roughly) into two broad categories: the meditative, which includes Karma yoga, Jnana yoga, Bhakti yoga, and Raja yoga (the ruling yoga); and the physical, which is Hatha yoga. Yoga means to join together, and even though many of the branches differ in their approach, all strive to achieve the same goal: union with the supreme consciousness. For those who regard yoga as a religion, this consciousness is Brahma, the universal spirit. For those who regard it as an art or science, it means a deeper knowledge of self.

Hatha (physical) yoga is one of the more passive approaches to physical fitness. It deals with conserving energy in order to have a ready reserve, whereas calisthenics and aerobics are based on the principle that the more energy you spend, the more you create. Physical yoga involves getting in and out of a number of body postures called *asanas,* breathing exercises (*pranayama*), and relaxation techniques. The main body postures include head stands, shoulder stands, balancing, stretching, and sitting positions. Each posture, slowly and deliberately placed, and combined with concentration, enacts the union of body and mind that is yoga. It aids in developing physical and mental discipline. Psychologically, yoga strengthens a communion with self by allowing one to *feel* one's movements slowly and completely.

Opinions vary on the benefits of Hatha yoga, but those most commonly claimed are increased flexibility, relaxation, and endurance; strength of the vital organs and glands; improved circulation; alertness; body control; and taut, smooth skin.

TIPS AND POINTERS
FOR GETTING STARTED

It's wise to have a physical examination before starting a regular exercise program, unless you're under thirty and have had an examination within the last year. This way you'll know what your overall physical condition is before you start. An examination also safeguards you against any unnoticed or potential problems that might come up along the way. The program you decide to follow should progress slowly, demanding only a minimal amount of exertion at first, and increasing gradually. This allows you to build physical stamina and achieve your goals at a safe and progressive pace. The following important guidelines should be followed when doing body work.

Warm-up exercises lubricate and prepare the body for more vigorous and demanding activity, thereby minimizing the possibility of injury. Start with something simple and work slowly, familiarizing yourself with disciplined and placed movements. This enables the body's metabolic rate to accelerate gradually, supplying more oxygen and blood to the cells. Increasing the oxygen and blood supply creates energy;

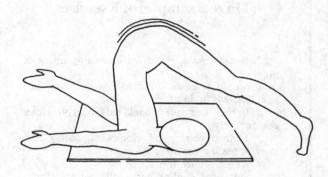

Regarded as a means to a deeper knowledge of self, Hatha (physical) yoga is one of the more passive approaches to physical fitness.

the heat produced "warms up" the muscles and joints, allowing more fluidity and better locomotion.

Listen to your body. Feel and observe your body's reactions to any given exercise. Pay attention to your "body limit." It can be found by bending or stretching to the point where you just "can't go any further," but not to the point of undue pain. Extreme pain is a warning that you've exceeded your "body limit," and you've increased your chances of sustaining an injury that could keep you from doing any kind of body work until it heals.

Keep moving. It can be dangerous to start or stop moving abruptly when exercising. Continuous movement between exercises, and for a short time afterward, should always be a part of any exercise routine. Continual movement that keeps pace with the body's rhythm during exercise will maintain a safe and even increase or decrease in the pulmonary and respiratory systems. This prevents unwanted strain on the lungs, heart, veins, and arteries.

Incorporating an exercise program into your life is one of the most rewarding things you can do for yourself; however, the rewards are not gained quickly or easily. Be gentle with yourself. Have respect for your body. It takes time and patience to attain health and well-being at a safe and progressive rate. But in the long run, exercise can redefine and make clear one's values by deepening knowledge of self. It introduces a special element of joy that comes only from feeling alive and able.

(Text continued on p. 110)

Three Examples of Exercises
Lorin Piper

This exercise is good for loosening up neck muscles.

1. Sit in a chair, or stand with your feet shoulder-width apart.
2. Bend your head back as far as you can comfortably.
3. Rotate your head clockwise, softly and slowly, feeling the stretch.
4. Repeat twice more.
5. Do three similar head rolls counterclockwise.

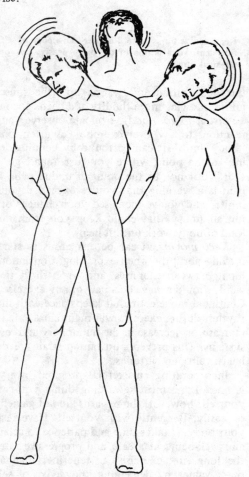

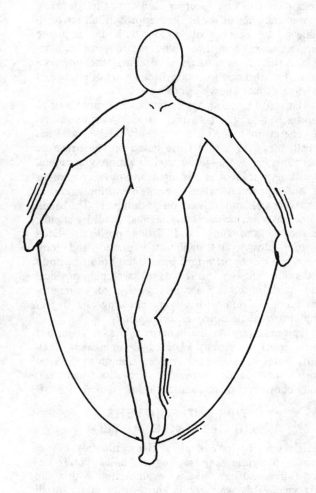

Jumping rope is aerobic because it is steady, repetitive, and rhythmical, and it increases oxygen consumption. Start with two or three minutes of slow jumping, and work up to more. Some of the side benefits of jumping rope are that it:

(1) reduces fat on legs, thighs, and hips;

(2) increases agility and improves balance;

(3) strengthens muscles all over the body, including the heart.

A very complete book on jumping rope is *The Perfect Exercise: The Hop, Skip, and Jump Way to Health,* by Curtis Mitchell (Simon and Schuster, 1976).

This footlift pose is a yoga exercise that develops balance.

1. Stand up straight and pick up your left foot with both hands.

2. Place it on your right thigh as high up as it will go.

3. Hold it there with your right hand. (Try to keep your spine straight and your left knee from bending.)

4. Stand steadily on your right leg for as long as you can, and breath deeply.

5. Repeat this exercise with your right foot on your left thigh.

Naturally, standing steadily in this posture is easier said than done. Expect to hop around for a few days. But it can be accomplished, and it's a good way to improve your balance.

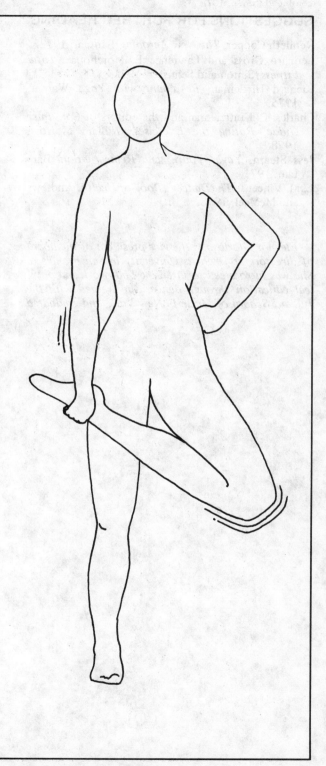

(continued from p. 107)

SUGGESTIONS FOR FURTHER READING

Kenneth Cooper, *The New Aerobics.* Bantam, 1972.

Leonard Gross and Lawrence E. Morehouse, *Total Fitness.* Simon and Schuster, 1975.

Richard Hittleman, *Be Young with Yoga.* Warner, 1975.

Charles T. Kuntzleman and the editors of *Consumer Guide, Rating the Exercises.* William Morrow, 1978.

Jess Stearn, *Yoga, Youth, and Reincarnation.* Bantam, 1971.

L. M. Vincent, *The Dancer's Book of Health.* Andrews and McMeel, 1978.

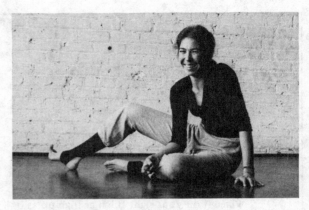

Eleanor Glorioso is the vice-president of the board of directors at Orpheus University in San Francisco. She was introduced to intensive bodywork and physical education through dance. She trained with the Julliard School of Music in New York, and graduated from the Peabody Institute in Maryland in 1967. Not fully satisfied with the mechanical and performing aspects of body work, Eleanor went on to study primal and bioenergetic therapy techniques. She is currently developing a dance-therapy program and is a full-time dance and exercise instructor in San Francisco.

Creative Running: Tips from a New Age Coach
Dyveke Spino, M.A., M.S.W., with Ann Spence

Twenty minutes of running four to five times a week, plus twenty minutes of flexibility exercises, can transform your body into a vitally alive, physically fit organism. Running exercises the cardiovascular system, balances the endocrine system, and harmonizes the hemispheres of the brain.

Dyveke Spino, a coach who trained under master Olympic coach Percy Cerutty, views athletic discipline as a vehicle for integrating masculine and feminine aspects of being, for releasing inner power, and for experiencing transcendence. In this article Dyveke gives us lots of inspiration, pointers, insights, exercises, and images to use in running.

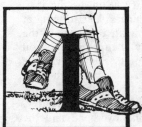'm coming to you today with the spirit of Mount Tamalpais, which has been my guide and teacher. This gentle, mysterious mountain, with twelve hundred miles of trails, waterfalls, forest paths, and rocky ridges, overlooks the San Francisco Bay area as a sentinel and keeper of the spirit. Each morning at dawn I run to the West Point Inn, four miles up a 6 per cent grade on the old fire trail.

Each morning at dawn I face my mentor, for each step reveals my level of inner peace or inner stress. And as I pass the waterfalls, rocks, and gates that guard the fire trails, I dream of someday seeing hundreds of women and men beginning their day on the trails.

There's more to running than putting one foot in front of the other with some degree of speed and rhythm. There is the possibility of transforming the ability of your consciousness to transcend physical limitations, to reach toward magical spaces of ecstasy and oneness with the universe, toward structural harmony and internal flow.

This article originally appeared in the *New Age Journal*.

GETTING STARTED

When you first start to run, be very gentle and kind to yourself. Let the feminine side of yourself nurture, protect, and care for you. Be sensitive to feelings. Most people don't train this way. They tear up in their cars, jam on the brakes, jump out, and take off at full tilt around a track—or worse, on pavement. This is the *yang* energy—they want to get there, and work as fast and as hard as they can. They get shin splints, pulled Achilles tendons, and all kinds of injuries, because they don't realize what they are doing. They don't integrate running with the rest of their lives. How often I feel a quiet pain when I watch crumpled runners banging on pavement, taking in lead poisoning, thinking they are getting "fit," when just a few hundred yards away is a beautiful grass field where they could undulate their spines, take in the *prana* of the grass, and fill their lungs with fresh oxygen.

The best time to run is early dawn, just as the sun is rising, when the *prana* is at the apex, the air cleaner, and your mind uncluttered by the demands of the day.

Ideally, run in a beautiful place—on soft grass, through the woods, or around a lake or reservoir. Be especially careful to *avoid being chilled*. It's best to wear loose cotton (rather than synthetic) clothing and to dress on the warm rather than the cool side. Especially at the beginning, wear long pants to keep the muscles warm. Pay attention to the obvious. If you've worked up a big sweat, don't stop to chat with a friend. Elevate your training to a feeling of becoming an artist with your body. Treat it with extreme care and delicacy. Wear good running shoes: nylon is preferable to leather, because it holds its shape and doesn't retain water.

Before starting your run, spend at least ten minutes doing gentle stretching exercises or the yoga sun-worship series.

Setting the mood and tone of your feeling state before training takes only a few minutes, and can evoke the heroic and transcendent parts of you. Imagine waking up to an inspirational scroll with affirmations and desires implanted in your consciousness, or allowing the swell and vibrance of the music of Mozart to descend into your cellular system as you start each day. This may be as important as putting one foot down in front of the other. When I get my runners doing this, their compulsive drive throttles down into an inner calm and personal reverence.

Once you have set the mood for your run, go out and explore your environment. Find a grassy field or a soft dirt track that is flat. Start by running slowly, lightly on the feet, going from the heel to the toe, slightly toeing in. Start doing what is called the "shake-up." Dangle the body from the shoulders, through the hips and ankles. Keep your pace at the nine-minute-mile pace, slightly above a fast walk. Work yourself at a pace where you are breathing hard but are not out of breath, or straining anything in your body. Do this for fifteen or twenty minutes, three times a week; in six weeks you will naturally increase your time, distance, and frequency, and will have laid a long, slow distance base. There's no need to constantly push yourself past your limits; just go out and start moving. In order to increase the intake of oxygen in the body, use the "talk test"—if you can carry on a conversation, you are in an aerobic state.

You don't have to run with a competitive spirit, either with yourself or with another person. As you run along very slowly, doing the shake-up, the layers of tension and deep holding begin to loosen and re-form into more harmonious patterns of "flow." For the experienced athlete or jogger, consciously slowing yourself down for long periods of time is imperative. Sense the alignment of your body, the fluidity of your skeletal-muscle frame, the deep relaxation of all the muscle sets, and open your mind to the edges of your own personal ecstasy. The actual incremental time increase is much less important than over-all mental, spiritual, and physical health.

Once you are running, start to play with the recesses and reserves of your inner self. Imagine that there's a sky hook lifting you up, or that you're standing under a waterfall, and there are beautiful, radiant beams of water streaming down your back. Then start to imagine a tube going from your throat down to the abdomen, and feel the breath going up and down the tube. "Sense" pools of water around your knees, and imagine your feet are coming down on air puffs. When running up a hill, imagine there is a giant hand pushing you from behind, or connect an imaginary "light streamer" to a tree and let it pull you up.

While running, let your eyes become soft and slightly out of focus. When you release your eyes, you release the lower part of the spine. Running with "soft eyes" also opens up the sensitivity of your other means of perception and intuitive sense. Look about thirty feet ahead of you, and let your feet begin to find their own way.

If running with a partner, imagine a stream of energy connecting your shoulders to each other's, and take turns being in the lead and being equal. The dance of energy exchange breaks down patterns of power. When running with a group, visualize a sunstar over your heads, and then send out a network of light-streamers to hook up to that imaginary sunstar. This sets up an energy field, and actually can pull along the weakest members of the group without strain or injury. It can create a sense of joy and inner connectedness between the group. You can also use imagery such as a phalanx, feeling like birds flying in formation, or sled dogs running in a team.

Play with your environment as you run. Visualize a white dot of iridescent light spinning in your forehead, then loop it around your head and project it onto living things at a distance. Look at a tree in the distance. Feel the energy of the tree, and let that energy pull you toward it. Look at a delicate leaf and feel its fragility, its vulnerability. Run to the leaf, touch it gently, go inside. Imagine a deer running at your side, connect your energy with the grace of the deer, and become the deer as you run. Imagine you are an Indian running in complete silence over the soft grass, as if the people you pass can neither see nor hear you. Let the wind gently push you along, and the sun fill your body with soft, golden energy. Run along with the birds flying overhead and the squirrels scampering along the ground.

Become the leaf and grow with the branch. Look into the eyes of an animal and feel its soul. Allow the song of a bird to ripple through your muscles as you run. Why shouldn't we know the ultimate oneness with all things?

About 80 per cent of your training should be long, slow distance running. The other 20 per cent might involve rhythms, tempos, percussions, and accelerations. For instance, run backwards, sideways. Jump and twirl. Shout out your ideals or release them as mental pictures in balloons. Do short, fast steps, pumping your arms up and down, focusing your energy on fast step repeats, loudly making the sound of a bee (beeeeeeeeeeeeeee!). Feel the explosive and percussive effects of your accelerated energy flow. It's no different than the exultation of brilliant Bach or the harmonies of Bartok. Run with your hands on your hips, lifting your knees high in front of you, feeling the grandeur of a prancing horse.

Lift your shoulders high as you breathe in deeply, and exhale quickly by dropping the shoulders, making a loud gutteral noise as the air is released. Make noise; hear yourself. Touch your primordial, primitive self, and allow your unconscious to explode into your body.

Run asymmetrically, galloping or loping like a horse. This tends to extend normal thought patterns, getting you out of the "groove," and brings creative reintegration.

After any percussive or energetic movements, return to the calm rhythm of the shake-up, and recover gracefully and flowingly. The purpose of these techniques is to sensitize and awaken both the male and the female energies in the psyche, and to experience them directly and simultaneously.

Always end your training with another ten minutes of stretching, for instance, the yoga triangle pose, forward bends, or hanging over an elevated leg. Do not bounce. Breathe into the stretch, find the edge, and relax into it. Steam baths and massage are a good adjunct to physical training, greatly accelerating the elimination of toxins and new cell growth.

The most important aspect of this type of training program is to learn to get in touch with yourself at all levels. The distance, the pace, the variations, will all evolve naturally and organically once the cardiovascular system becomes exercised and detoxified, the endocrine system starts functioning in balance, and both hemispheres of the brain are purring harmoniously. Twenty minutes of running, four to five times a week, plus twenty minutes of flexibility work done in a state of reverence and relaxation, can transform your life.

A NOTE ON RITUALS

Rituals are a great aid in training your will or directing your intentionality to a repetition of desired behavior. Rituals also reinforce your spirit and help you retain a sense of dedication to your training.

Give a daily greeting to certain trees or beautiful places along your running trail. Circle around a particular tree each day to feel its energy, and treat certain rocks or shrubs as friends welcoming you on your way. Each day, place a rock at a special place and watch them multiply—a testament to your steady progress (one such pile helped me run high up on Mount Tam every day). Find a beautiful spot along the way to stop and meditate. Find different trees, representing different aspects of yourself, to meditate on. If you run by water, take five minutes to become one with the water—allow your consciousness to drift

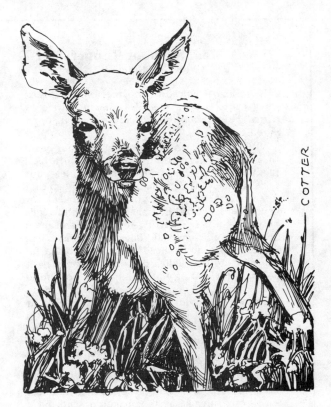

Imagine a deer running at your side, connect your energy with the grace of the deer.

into a drop of water and become everlasting life. On my morning runs I often sit on a rock overlooking the ocean and touch the curled bark of a eucalyptus branch. It reminds me of ancient parchment and Gregorian chants. From this ritual I return home to my Steinway, and sometimes original music comes forth from the inspiration of the ritual.

Creative expression is a natural result of this kind of training, and you can finish your ritual off with time to write in a journal or play a musical instrument. The fresh oxygen to all cells, the pageantry of nature, the sense of personal integration may bring forth the dormant artist in you.

In any case, allow yourself to indulge in a "reward" as part of your ritual, be it a special juice you like to drink after running or a special-smelling soap or talcum powder. After all, you deserve it.

MEN AND WOMEN ATHLETES

There are as many kinds of athletes in the world as there are individuals—certainly we can no longer define an archetypal "male" or "female" athlete.

(Text continued on p. 116)

A Meditation for Runners
Dyveke Spino

With a soft voice, dictate the following very slowly into a tape recorder. Listen with eyes closed before running, to create a calm, open mood.

Relax. Lie down on the floor on your back. In a state of relaxation, stretch out both legs. Let your palms be open to the side, let your arms stretch out. Try to align your body so that it feels balanced, so that your feet are over your knees, over your hips. Imagine that all the cells of your body are starting to expand and open up. Begin to sense an imaginary sunstar six inches above your head. Feel this beautiful whirr of bright light, starting to come right down to the top of your head, down your forehead, into your neck, into your chest, streaming down into your heart and lungs. Feel your own cellular structure, your whole beautiful biochemical system, starting to open up and expand. Feel a white light starting to stream down your shoulders and pour out the ends of your fingers, almost as if that beautiful white light were allowing your whole body to open up. You feel all your energy starting to connect with your sunstar, as if you could send out a beam of energy and connect with the energy around you.

Now, start to spin that energy around. As your sunstar begins to whirr and create a force field of energy six inches from the top of your head, start to imagine now that spiraling rivulets of white light are moving down your body. Feel it gyrating and expanding and sending out energy. Feel it going down your left leg, right around your kneecap, your ankle, right out through the end of your foot. Now it is going down your other leg. You are beginning to feel very light and very airy and very joyous, as if you are more than your physical body. You are becoming aware that you have an energy body, or a force field, that is around you, that is of your own creation.

You are beginning to be lifted now, as if your own energy were able to lift you right off the ground in your own consciousness. And you can sense now what is beyond where you are now. Send your consciousness outside, and begin to feel the bark of a tree, as if your skin could become the bark of that tree. Go inside the tree; begin to feel what it would be like if your spine were inside that tree. Your hair could blow like the leaves. Feel the sun and the wind and the grass. Feel yourself swimming in an ocean, running over a beautiful field, running without a physical body, as though you were just a beautiful leaf, flowing over the grass effortlessly, your joints and ligaments and tendons completely aligned and balanced, your whole psyche opened up and connected with all living things.

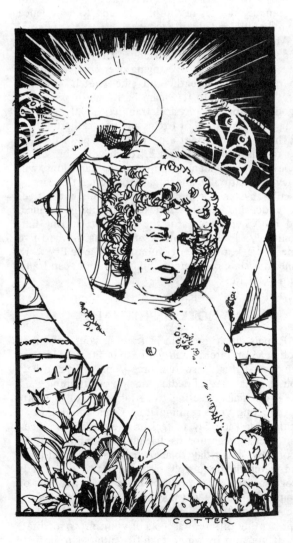

Before the Run: Strrrretch!
Dyveke Spino

This set of exercises stretches the spine in seven directions. Dictate the following very slowly into a tape recorder, then listen and follow the instructions.

1. Lie on your back. Close your eyes and relax deeply. Go inside your body and sense the holding patterns on the right side and left side of your body. Feel how each foot turns outward.

2. Slowly lift both legs over your head and allow your knees to fall beside your ears. Breathe and hold, relaxing into the stretch.

3. Very slowly uncurl your spine, coming back down on the floor one vertebra at a time.

4. Lift your right leg to a knee-to-chest position, then place it to the right side of your body. Slowly roll the bent leg across your body and place it on the floor on the opposite side. Extend your right arm straight up above your head, on the floor, and turn your head to the right. Once you are in this position, imagine that there is a golden ball in the center of the Earth, spinning rapidly and pulling you deeper and deeper into the Earth. Allow your shoulders and knee to sink into the ground. Breathe deeply, then uncurl yourself slowly, coming back to a prone position.

5. Repeat the same stretch on the left side: left leg over the body to the opposite side, left arm up straight over the head, look to the left. Uncurl back to the prone position.

6. Place both hands behind your neck and slowly curl up to a sit-up position. Lean forward over your legs with knees straight. Relax into the stretch, but don't bounce.

7. Very slowly uncurl your spine again, coming down to the floor one vertebra at a time, starting from the small of the back.

8. With bent knees, slowly tilt up the pelvic area and lift up, with head and neck remaining on the floor. Slowly come back down, one vertebra at a time, starting from the neck.

9. Close your eyes and once again sense the alignment of your body, left and right. Notice any changes that may have occurred since you began the stretches.

10. Let yourself be in a calm, quiet space, aware of yourself—of the inner alignment and feelings of your body. With this quiet awareness, slowly get up and begin your run.

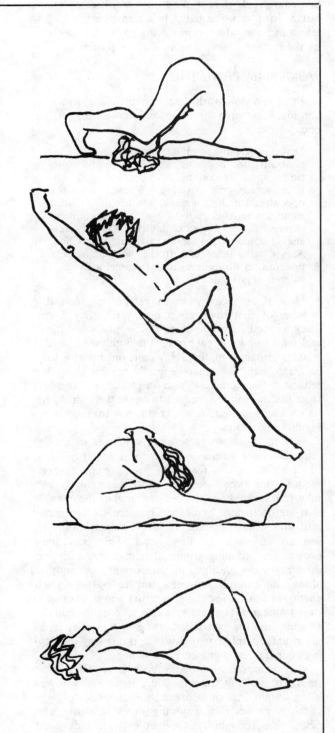

(continued from p. 113)

Someday, such stereotyping may vanish completely, but as long as we're living in a transitional era, athletes (and non-athletes) are going to be slowed down by the restrictive sexual models of the past.

WOMEN IN TRAINING

Ernst van Aaken, the great German doctor/coach, considered women the true endurance athletes. He once wrote:

> "Psychologically, men are more explosive, inconstant, not enduring, and in pain and exertion—especially among high-performance athletes—somewhat sniveling. Women are the opposite: tough, constant, enduring, level and calm under the pain to which their biology exposes them (during childbirth). On the average, [women are] more patient than men. Armed with these advantages, women are in a position to do endurance feats previously considered impossible."

Most of the women I coach are not in touch with a sense of their own endurance when they begin. They generally feel helpless and overly self-critical, and tend to have a real problem maintaining a regular training program at first. However, once past a trial-and-error period, women generally exhibit incredible tenacity. They are less eager to put undue stress on their bodies, and are content to enjoy the training for its own sake, rather than breaking records or improving distance or time.

Setting up a strong support system is of crucial importance for women in the initial stages of training. In order to have a feeling of progress and success, record your experiences in a journal regularly and take time to make a positive appraisal of the changes that are occurring. You can also reach out to others—husbands, lovers, friends, children, or neighbors—for support in your training ritual. This sometimes evolves into training groups that meet regularly for dinner or celebration, to encourage one another along. Be careful, however, not to put so much energy into inspiring the group that you neglect your own training. Make sure you also take time to do the training just for yourself. Setting up a regular training ritual, complete with rewards, is one way of keeping your training going on your own.

A new appreciation of the body is one of the first results of starting training. This, combined with ensuing weight loss or improved muscle tone, is inextricably woven with enjoying one's sexuality and developing the ability to manifest one's dormant capacities in the world. Psychologically, the increas-

ing sense of self-mastery helps one to overcome possible patterns of self-denial, masochism, and weakness that so many of us unfortunately still find deeply imbedded in our psyches. Giving up these negative patterns can have as great an impact on health and vitality as the physical effects of the training. I often see women who feel victimized by overpowering men in their lives take a quantum leap in their level of self-expression and career almost immediately, once they physically take charge of disciplining their bodies.

MEN IN TRAINING

Most of the men I coach have a natural inner discipline that needs to be balanced by awakening their "feminine" instincts. I find that corporation executives or overextended professionals (physicians and psychiatrists, for example) welcome the sensitivity of a woman coach with whom they can share their fears, dreams, competitive struggles, and feelings of inadequacy—concerns that they have "so little time" to take care of themselves.

Having been well-taught in the ways of competition, men are usually driven by the numbers—systems, logs, schedules, and linear left-brain mechanics—and often have a driving compulsion to compete against themselves and others. Wanting to get "the most the fastest," they drive through injuries, and train when exhausted; many believe that "If it doesn't hurt, it isn't doing any good."

Before starting a training program, it's a good idea to take time to do a lifestyle reflection. Take a look at your life, your schedule, your passions, fears, silent dreams, your family gestalt, and your state of health. I find the self-report system often reveals the mode of training. Look for the missing links in your life, and then see how you can balance them. Often, extremely knowledgeable athletes in national competitions have absolutely no flexibility program; others know nothing of nutrition.

In order to deemphasize competitive tendencies, take time with your running; using visualizations, get into being where you are running rather than "getting there." When running with others (especially less-experienced athletes), let the others take the lead, fall behind a bit, and let yourself be pulled along, rather than having to be strong in the lead. Put emphasis on stretching exercises before and after running, and use visualizations to get in a calm and quiet state before getting out on the turf. While running, think in terms of developing a soft power, running with the graceful strength of a deer. Let your shoulders unlock and flow, move them about.

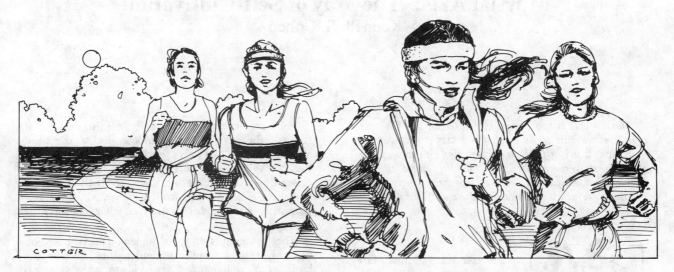

Setting up a strong support system is of crucial importance in the initial stages of training. Join with spouses, friends, lovers, children, or neighbors in a daily training ritual.

Alternate your running with non-weight-bearing exercises, such as swimming or hanging, so that your body can find its natural alignment.

Above all, don't push yourself too hard. If injuries do occur, treat yourself kindly. Have the injury checked by an osteopath or chiropractor, rather than trying to run it out, possibly harming yourself further.

Body work such as chiropractic adjustments, rolfing, shiatsu massage, or acupuncture all help to stabilize the *chi* flow and the bodily alignment. Many of the athletes I've worked with have had years of serious injuries that they have "trained through"; in a month of work, with proper orchestration of mental tension, healing techniques, and release, incredible breakthroughs occurred naturally and harmoniously.

THE COACH OF THE FUTURE

The coach of the future will be a creative artist of the soul, a true shaman. The coach will operate with the "feminine" principle—receptive, intuitive, "field-force," embodying eros (as Jung speaks of it), and relationship-oriented. This will be balanced with the "masculine" sequential and linear principles of mechanistic efficiency—specific stretching exercises, log of training miles, schedules.

However, the dominant mode will shift to the feminine. The coach must become knowledgeable in the vast array of natural, holistic healing arts available, and realize that most communication comes through "presence." The lifestyle and spirit of such a coach will be an example to emulate. The coach will not hold up a stopwatch or control through authoritarian measures or threats, but will tend, with love, to the growing of a psyche to the next level of reawakening. The purpose of competition, seen as an outmoded value of an industrial age, will be transformed: the goal will be to awaken the spirit to higher and higher levels of personal transformation.

The coach will be the muse—the inspirer of the soul—to awaken the dreamer, the poetic, the heroic, the transpersonal.

Dyveke Spino is a clinical psychologist, tennis professional, champion long-distance runner, and concert pianist. As co-founder and co-director of the Esalen Sports Center, she was the only woman certified to teach the training methods of master Olympic coach Percy Wells Cerutty. Formerly Assistant Professor of Psychology at Sonoma State University, she holds M.A. and M.S.W. degrees, and has also taught at the University of California at Davis and the University of California at Berkeley. She is currently a lecturer and consultant to educators, business executives, and industrial groups, for whom she organizes intensive physical-fitness programs. She is the author of the recently published New Age Training for Fitness and Health *(Grove Press, 1979).*

Martial Arts: The Way of Self-Cultivation
Kenneth S. Cohen

Martial arts is more than self-defense. The Chinese consider wu shu *to be one of the arts of the gentleman. It is a way of self-understanding and expression through movement. It is an ideal exercise of the body, mind, and spirit, leading to vibrant health and the deep harmony that the Chinese call "The Way."*

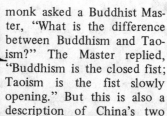 monk asked a Buddhist Master, "What is the difference between Buddhism and Taoism?" The Master replied, "Buddhism is the closed fist; Taoism is the fist slowly opening." But this is also a description of China's two great systems of martial arts: *wai chia,* the Buddhist-inspired martial arts, emphasizing static postures, hard, linear movements, muscular conditioning, and endurance; and *nei chia,* the Taoist-inspired "internal" school, emphasizing slow, fluid movement, economy of strength, and the cultivation of vital energy (*ch'i*). The two schools are like the *yang* and *yin* of movement, and thus comprise a whole system of physical education and culture. And like *yin* and *yang,* the distinctions are not rigid. The Chinese say, "Within *yin* there is a drop of *yang;* within *yang* there is a drop of *yin.*" Each school of martial arts borrows techniques from the other, and each has a common origin in the ritual dances of the ancient Chinese shamans.

Chinese mythology tells of a battle between the famous Yellow Emperor (Huang Ti) and a horned monster named Chih Yu. In order to defend himself, the Yellow Emperor had to invent the sword, battle-axe, spear, and other weapons. Chih Yu responded with techniques which are said to be the basis of Chinese wrestling. Thus, the most ancient word for martial arts, *chiao ti,* literally "horn goring," probably originally meant the ritual enactment of this battle. Chiao Ti dances are still practiced by tribes in Northern China and Manchuria.

Scholars have also found references to an ancient festival, the *No* (definition unknown), of the third millennium B.C. Twelve participants, dressed like the twelve animals of the Chinese zodiac, would dance down the streets of a town, under the direction of a bear-masked shaman. This was a kind of exorcism rite performed to purify a village before the new year.

The movements of these ancient dances, based on Gods, folk heroes, animals, and nature, became the basis of Yoga-like exercises.[1] These were systematized by the famous Taoist physician, Hua T'o, in the first centuries A.D. His "Five Animal Frolicks," imitating the deer, crane, ape, bear, and tiger, became part of the regimen of Taoist and Buddhist monks. At first these exercises were practiced solely for their healthful benefits. They balanced the organs, relaxed the body, and relieved the legs after long sittings of meditation. When China was besieged by "barbarians," the monks quickly learned to convert these passive exercises into self-defense techniques. The crane standing on one leg could be a preparation for a kick. The gesture called "Ape Steals Fruit" could be used to pluck an opponent's eyes. The clawing movements of the tiger could be used to literally claw one's enemy. Sometimes famous military men, such as General Yueh Fei (to whom an entire system of martial arts is attributed—Yueh Fei Boxing), would seek refuge in a monastery and help the monks to refine their martial arts.

Two men, in particular, are responsible for the present systems of martial arts: Bodhidharma and Chang San Feng. Bodhidharma was the Indian Buddhist monk who brought Zen to China in the fifth century A.D. He settled in the *Shao Lin* Monastery in Honan Province and taught his monks a series of 12 exercises (the *I Chin*) to strengthen the muscles, and an additional 18 (the *Lo Han*) to acquire the basic skills needed for self-defense. Bodhidharma's exercises were often very hard and vigorous, such as doing push-ups on the fingers of one hand, or touching the chin to the anklebone! The boxing method he created was expanded to 170 gestures, all embraced within five basic styles: the Dragon, Tiger, Leopard, Snake, and Crane. These five styles, usually called *Shao Lin K'ung Fu* or simply *K'ung Fu,* are still practiced to this day.[2]

Each style consists of many choreographed dances, or "forms," based on the methods of attack and defense of the respective animals; individual postures are linked together in rapid, staccato-like rhythm. Individual techniques of self-defense are also practiced —blocks, punches, kicks. The advanced student learns to wield the four basic weapons—sword, broadsword, staff, and spear—with the same dexterity as his hands. Eventually he practices free-style self-defense, during which he can draw upon his vast reservoir of techniques as needed.

K'ung Fu is also called *wai chia,* literally "outer family," because it has its origins outside of China, and because it emphasizes outer, that is muscular, strength, as opposed to the power of breath.

Chang San Feng, the well-known founder of *T'ai Chi Ch'uan* (the most widely practiced martial art in the world) was a Taoist monk of twelfth-century China. He is believed to have studied Taoism on Mount Mao, the home of meditative Taoism, and later as a recluse on Mount Wu Tang. One day while walking through the woods he observed a battle between a hawk and a snake. Every time the hawk would come close, the snake would just move gently out of the way. Finally the hawk had to give up in despair. Chang San Feng noted how the aggression of the hawk was "neutralized" by the suppleness of the snake. By moving out of the way of attack, the snake not only defended itself, but left the hawk in a vulnerable position. This was like the joining of opposites, the *yin* and *yang.*[3] In Chinese philosophy, this union is known as *T'ai Chi* (literally, "Great Ridgepole"), the peak of the mountain where the shady slope (*yin*) and the sunny slope (*yang*) meet.

The *T'ai Chi Ch'uan* (*Ch'uan* means "boxing") created by Chang San Feng is a series of 108 relaxed postures connected one to the next without break.[4] Each gesture is inspired by some aspect of nature; thus the practicioner feels himself to be "a small Heaven-Earth," that is, a microcosm of the universe. The movements are practiced so slowly, fluidly, meditatively, that they give the appearance of swimming in the air. Unlike *K'ung Fu,* the stance is narrow and high, the breath slow, deep, long, and fine.

T'ai Chi Ch'uan is part of the *nei chia,* literally "inner family," of martial arts. Like its sisters *Pa Kua Chang* (a coiling, spiraling exercise) and *Hsing I Ch'uan* (a linear, spirited series of rising and falling gestures), it may be practiced solely for health and

peace of mind, or individual postures may be speeded up and used for self-defense. The same gesture which is used to cultivate one's reserve of vital energy may, in another context, be used to deliver a devastating blow.

The *nei chia* also has its weapons and free-style sparring. But, unlike *K'ung Fu,* there is equal devotion to Taoist meditation, and sensitivity exercises such as "sticking," during which one tries to adhere gently, and with even pressure, to one's partner's hands, no matter where or how they move; and "neutralizing," in which one moves completely out of the way of oncoming force, without letting it touch one's body. It is unfortunate that in China's Boxer Rebellion many *T'ai Chi* Masters thought they could also neutralize bullets, and found out they were wrong!

STRENGTHENING BODY AND MIND

The Buddhist deity, *Manjusri,* symbol of wisdom, is usually depicted with a sword in his hand. Most people associate the sword with violence, but the highest stage of martial arts is when the sword is used to prevent aggression rather than foster it.

A *samurai* was once journeying on a boat when he was noticed by another, a ruffian who used his swordsmanship only to bolster his own ego. This braggart came over to the samurai and said, "You wear a sword; what school of swordsmanship do you belong to?" The samurai answered, "The No-Sword School." This angered the man, and he said, while fondling the hilt of his sword, "Let's see you use your no-sword." The samurai replied, "Don't you think this boat is a bit too small? Why don't we take a small rowboat to that island we are passing. We can duel on the beach, and the winner can row back out to the mother ship when it reaches the other side." The braggart agreed, and the samurai insisted that he enter the rowboat first. But just as he did, the samurai gave the boat a shove and sent it trailing behind the mother ship by a rope. The samurai laughed, "I'll be seeing you. This is my No-Sword School!"

There are four kinds of boxing.

1. The best never takes place because, by exercising compassion, one can make the enemy one's friend.

2. If that is impossible, the martial artist can, by recognizing the early stages of aggression, avoid it altogether.

3. If that is impossible, the martial artist should counter aggression before it is serious.

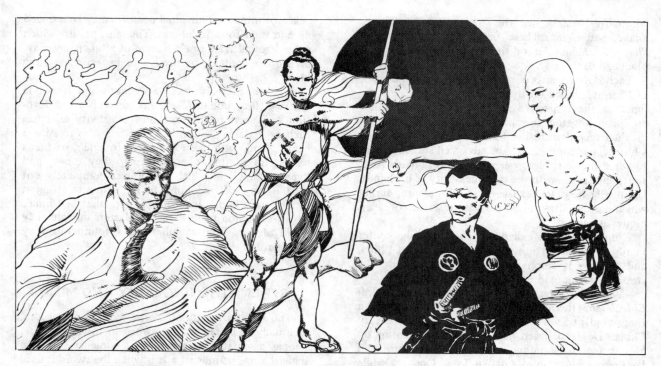

Each school of martial arts borrows techniques from the others, and each has a common origin in the ritual dances of the ancient Chinese shamans.

4. Finally, in the event of a sudden attack, it is best to deal with one's foe as quickly and efficiently as possible. And then one might have to minister to his wounds!

Most practice the martial arts simply for the superb physical and psychological conditioning they demand. The *wai chia* and *nei chia* together constitute an all-round plan for health and well-being.

Wai chia has some of the finest aerobic exercises. To stand in a low "horse stance" for an hour, punching the hands alternately in the air, is equivalent to an equal time of jogging. And how excruciating if, as in the old days, one has to stand with a cup of water balanced on the thighs, shoulders, and head! The punch has to be so controlled, the musculature so differentiated, that the water will not spill. *K'ung Fu* is also excellent for stretching the joints and ligaments; the various kicks gradually loosen the hamstrings and allow a full rotation of the femur. The author has seen one *sifu* (Master) escape a sword thrust to the solar plexus by bending straight back under the blade! But the Western student should exercise caution in all of this. Orientals begin with more supple bodies and are in less danger of injuring the spine, hips, or knees.

Some techniques require a fantastic control of body weight and balance. A legend says that Bodhidharma once crossed a river by balancing on a floating reed! In his Shao Lin monastery, students would train this "lightweight energy" (*ch'ing kung*) by jumping across a stream on logs floating in the water. Or they might simply jump up and down with successively heavier weights attached to their waists and ankles. The latter is still considered a practical way to develop the springiness needed for sudden, unrehearsed movements, or very high kicks.

The *nei chia* was the first to explore *ideo-kinesis,* the relationship between image and movement. The *T'ai Chi Classic* says that *i* (idea, image, intent) must precede *li* (force). If the mind stops, then the movement will stop. A well-known example of this is the board-breaking "karate chop." If the mind stops at the wooden board, it will not break. But if the mind thinks *through* the board, then it will break easily. Furthermore, if the mind can form no clear idea of the movement to be performed, then it cannot be done. But once idea and movement are in harmony, the idea alone may bring the same benefits as the actual movement. One *T'ai Chi* Master cured himself of a serious ailment by simply imagining that he did the *T'ai Chi* exercise every day. Similarly, precise awareness (another meaning of *i*) is often sufficient to open a blockage.

The *nei chia* emphasize two principles: relax (*sung*) and sink (*ch'en*). By "relax" is meant to make the whole body soft, supple, light, and nimble, to use the minimum effort necessary for any movement (and, as this implies, to allow stress, or as the Chinese say, *ch'i,* to distribute itself as evenly as possible over the entire body). By "sink" is meant to let the weight sink easily down through the feet, to trust the support of the floor, to let the abdomen go, and thus allow a fuller, more natural breathing.

It is this which gives the *T'ai Chi* player an appearance of swimming in the air, or the *Pa Kua-ist* of a dancing, coiling dragon. The body is so light that "if a fly alights on the shoulder, the shoulder bends with its weight." Naturally such relaxation has a profound effect on the health. All shaking and nervous twitches are quickly eliminated: the heartbeat becomes slower, the veins and arteries are cleared of all debris. Digestion is regulated; ulcers caused by tension and worry quickly disappear. Abdominal breathing "inspires" atrophied muscles in the lungs; the abdominal muscles are massaged, and the sexual glands stimulated. As the inner connective tissue, the fascia, are relaxed, displaced organs can return to their natural positions. There is room to breathe.

Relax and sink have further, technical, meanings in Taoist alchemy. The psychic energy (*shen*), which the Chinese pictures as an actual fire-like force continually moving upward, can begin to flow down. The water-like sexual energy (*ching*), which normally flows down through the genitals, can flow up. They meet in the lower abdomen, the "crucible," and there mix with the life-breath (*ch'i*) in order to create the pill of immortality.

It should be remembered that the *nei chia* was originally part of a holistic system of healing. The ancient Taoist lived very simply on breath, roots, sunlight, and mineral water. Eventually, he would "transmogrify" his body (*hua shen*); the Taoist would be released from his heavy, physical body into a lighter, etheric body, like a butterfly emerging from a cocoon. Then he could either remain on earth, or float up to the heavens as a divine immortal.[5]

DYNAMIC AWARENESS

"Meditation in movement is a hundred times better than meditation at rest." It is one thing to practice choreographed forms or pre-set self-defense techniques, and it is quite another to engage in free-style

---

Cultivating the Vital Energy
Kenneth S. Cohen

Stand with the feet parallel, shoulder width apart. There should be some bend in all the joints, especially the knees, so that the weight of the body passes easily down through the feet. Tuck the hips gently under so that the lower back is straight, and feel this straight line passing all the way up to the crown of the head. The abdomen should be loose, the chest, shoulders, and neck soft and relaxed. The head feels as if it is held from above by a string.

Hold the hands in front of the chest, facing slightly inwards, as if they are embracing a giant ball. The fingers should be gently extended so that the arms make a semicircle, with one even line running from shoulders to fingers. While holding this posture, bring the attention down to the lower abdomen. See if you can feel both the lower abdomen and the lower back moving with the breath, as if you have a balloon in your torso. Then shift your attention to your fingers. Can you sense the movement of the breath in them?

Gradually begin to move the hands slightly away from each other with every inhalation, and slightly toward each other with every exhalation, as if your hands are your lungs. The movement should be slow and even. Can you feel the breath doing the movement for you? After a few minutes, return to simply standing and watching the breath. Then lower the hands and relax.

---

sparring. Now the problem is how to use all one's knowledge creatively; how to express oneself through what has been learned; how to use technique and yet keep the mind empty, ready to react quickly, freely, to the changing play of the opponent. Here self-defense is a paradigm for the problems in life itself.

Boxing requires a subtle coordination of foot, hip, and shoulder. The *T'ai Chi Classic* says, "The vital energy begins at the feet, is controlled by the waist, and is manifested in the hands." When striking, the foot must step first and root firmly into the ground. Then the waist is twisted quickly, so that the momentum of the turn throws the hand out and delivers the punch. In neutralizing or blocking, the action is reversed. One steps back or to the side, away from the incoming strike, turns the waist, and guides the strike

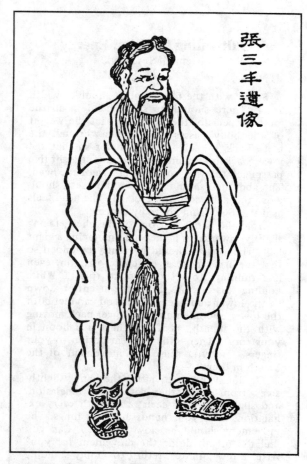

張三丰遺像

Chang San Feng, mythic founder of T'ai Chi Ch'uan. A stone rubbing from Hsuan T'ien Monastery in Wu Tang Mountain, China.

away. Most martial arts techniques follow this principle. Those that do not, though they may be aesthetically pleasing, will not carry enough of the body weight to be effective.

All this requires one to stand in a very particular posture. The back must be kept straight, "plumb erect," as the *Classic* says. The shoulders must be kept relaxed. If they lift up in a desire to protect oneself, they only have the reverse effect of exposing the ribs. The knees must be slightly bent, to prevent sudden movements from shocking the lower spine. The abdomen must stay relaxed, so that one does not stop breathing at the very time when breath is needed.

The face should have a calm, tranquil expression—strength is concealed within, "like steel wrapped in cotton," so that the opponent does not know what to expect, and cannot fathom one's movements. The eyes are soft and unfixed, so that one can use the peripheral vision. Some *Kung Fu* stylists still train their eyes by standing in the center of four heavy, swinging sand bags. One must avoid their collisions, not allowing the gaze to be captured by any particular bag, lest one be crushed! Even the ears must be trained to hear changes in the opponent's rhythm, or to hear an attack from behind. It is said that Bodhidharma's hearing was so acute that he could hear the conversations of the ants.

In most *kwoons* (martial-arts schools) the student either spars without making contact, or wears a full suit of protective armour. This allows him to practice without fear (or with less fear), and to enjoy martial arts as sport. When he faces his opponent, his awareness must be all-pervading. If it wanders for an instant, he is hit! Ideally he is in such harmony with his opponent that defense and offense are simultaneous.

Suzuki describes the strategy of the martial artist most succinctly. He must avoid "the six diseases: (1) the desire for victory; (2) the desire to resort to technical cunning; (3) the desire to display all that he has learned; (4) the desire to overawe the enemy; (5) the desire to play a passive role; and, lastly, (6) the desire to get rid of whatever disease he is likely to be infected with."[6] The latter is, of course, the crux of the problem. If only one can stop using the mind to pursue the mind, everything else will fall into place.

THE WAY

As in all arts, the boxer must first master the medium. But once the techniques are understood, they must be left to the unconscious. "You forget the belt when it fits. You forget the mind when it's comfortable," says the Chinese philosopher Chuang Tzu. When force comes, the master moves with it; response is immediate, that is, without mediation. The acquired has become the spontaneous.

Confucius was once strolling along the banks of a great waterfall when he saw a man jump in and go swimming down the rapids. Thinking the man in danger, Confucius ran downstream to help him out. But the man emerged unscathed and began to sing. Confucius asked, "Do you have a way to stay afloat?" The man replied, "Why, yes! I just go in with a swirl and come out with a whirl. I follow the way of the water and don't think of myself."[7]

Kabir says that spiritual transformation is the result of intensity. In the martial arts, all one's faculties must be at their optimum. The body/mind, taken to the limits of its endurance, must turn back to its own depths to find a new source of power. Then every blow will flash out of the void, unprepared and unrehearsed. One gradually learns to trust this dimension more and more. Boxing frees the mind from its ruts, and brings one to a kind of freshness and intimacy that is unparalleled.

NOTES

[1]Known as *tao-yin* in Chinese, *do-in* in Japanese, some of which are mentioned by name in the *Chuang Tzu Classic*, third century B.C.

[2]The number of styles has greatly proliferated, to include such animals as monkey, bear, dog, and even the praying mantis. Others are classified according to a family tradition, notably Hung, Liu, Tsai, Li, and Mo. In general, *K'ung Fu* styles developed in northern China emphasize leg techniques. Those from the south emphasize the hands.

Chinese boxing has exerted a very wide influence, since it is probably the oldest and most refined of the Asian martial arts. *Karate*, meaning literally "Chinese Hands," is derived from *K'ung Fu*. *Judo* and *Ju-jitsu* were influenced by Chinese grappling (*ch'in na*) and wrestling (*shuai chiao*).

[3]In world mythology, the bird is a common symbol of solar consciousness, the mind "disengaged from the field of time and space," as Joseph Campbell says. The snake, which sheds its skin, as if reborn, is a common symbol of the regenerative powers of nature. It is earth-bound, lunar consciousness. Thus, this old *T'ai Chi* story acquires a new dimension; it is the *unio mystico* of *God* and *Nature*, of the eternal and the temporal.

[4]Interestingly enough, there are 108 beads on the Buddhist rosary. It is as if one thread runs through all the *T'ai Chi* postures. But 108 is also important in Taoist numerology: $1 + 0 + 8 = 9$, the number signifying immortality.

[5]A word should be said about the relationship between the weapons and health. According to Chinese philosophy, there is a correspondence between the five elements, the five organs, and the five weapons. The sword corresponds to water; its use benefits the kidneys. The broadsword corresponds to metal, and benefits the lungs. The staff is wood, for the liver. The spear is fire for the heart, and the empty hand or fist is the Earth element, which benefits the spleen and aids in distribution of *ch'i* throughout the body.

[6]Daisetz Suzuki, *Zen and Japanese Culture* (Princeton University Press, 1970), p. 153-54.

[7]*Chuang Tzu*, chapter 19, trans. Alan Watts, as spoken to the author.

SUGGESTIONS FOR FURTHER READING

F. Donn Draeger and Robert W. Smith, *Asian Fighting Arts*. Berkley Publishing Corp., 1974.

Wen-shan Huang, *Fundamentals of T'ai Chi Ch'uan*. South Sky Book, 1979.

Pierre Huard and Ming Wong, *Oriental Methods of Mental and Physical Fitness: The Complete Book of Meditation, Kinesitherapy and Martial Arts in China, India and Japan*. Funk & Wagnalls, 1977.

Robert W. Smith, *Chinese Boxing: Masters and Methods*. Kodansha, 1974.

Daisetz Suzuki, *Zen and Japanese Culture*. Princeton University Press, 1970.

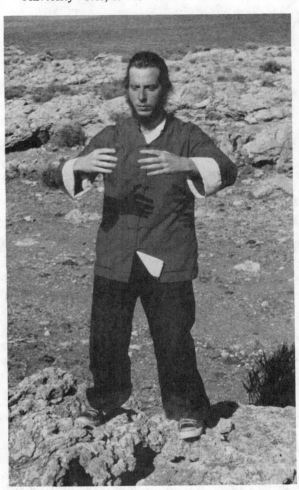

Kenneth S. Cohen is a scholar of Chinese Buddhism and Taoism. His articles on poetry, religion, and education have appeared in Dragonfly Quarterly, Interface Journal, Yoga Journal, Chanoyu, *and other scholarly journals. He collaborated with Alan Watts on his* Tao: The Watercourse Way.

Mr. Cohen trained in Chinese Boxing for ten years with Masters William Ch'en, P.B. Ch'an, Paul Gallagher, and others. Former co-director of the Montreal Center for the Healing Arts, he is currently teaching T'ai Chi Ch'uan *and Japanese Tea Ceremony in Berkeley, California.*

Dance
Summer Brenner

Dance is one of the oldest forms of re-creation known. All over the world, different peoples have used dance to express themselves, transcend their pain, and merge with the infinite. Somehow, in our sophistication, we seem to have lost this innate ability. Ms. Brenner shares with us her experience of dance as both self-expression and discipline, thereby helping us all to transform our own self-consciousness into consciousness of self.

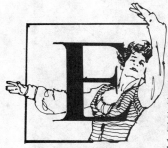

Every movement offers the possibility of communication. Every act is a motion. Almost by definition, life is movement. Whether we are speaking, driving, walking, making love, fishing, typing, or doing yoga, the bond between the inner feeling of movement and the outer expression of motion applies unceasingly. So first I want to say that dance is what we do and how we do it—no matter what it is. That is where we begin.

Starting with this realization, we come to dancing as the application of certain principles of movement which govern the body, principles which derive from physics, biology, aesthetics, and religion. The fact is that we are already moving through our lives, through space and time, through rhythms created by our various activities: we are already dancing. This is the quintessential understanding.

So many people tell me their secret: that they always wanted to be a dancer. Many of them never dance, and are convinced they can't. A major factor in their decision to "sit this one out" is self-consciousness. The really important twist is to turn self-consciousness into consciousness of Self. Do you really want to be that "closet dancer"—or is that the only kind you dare to be? Do you really believe you're too old, too busy, too fat? Do you want to move through the world with ease; to do your daily chores with a different physical attitude; to teach your children to love dancing; to take your sport and realize it as a dance? There are many choices for all of us.

Your choice can start with one moment of awareness. Breathe in. Now breathe out.

You have taken your first step.

A PASSIONATE RECREATION

In 1974 I found myself in the San Francisco area, 29 years old and the mother of an infant. Having just somersaulted through the physical and emotional changes of pregnancy and childbirth, I felt ready for action, ready to become fit and trim and active and light. I wanted to affirm that parenting is not a restriction, and that children in no way kept their folks from growing and moving on in their own lives. The time had come for my first formal dance class in twenty years.

I began with a weekly modern dance class. Fortunately I found a teacher who could convey her beliefs about life along with her techniques of movement. She started us with very simple things—walks, sitting postures, gentle bends—and told us that these were the most elemental, and the most important.

Soon my casual recreation became a passionate one. I must say something here about the concept of recreation. Often we fail to take our playtime seriously enough, unless we are motivated by a contest. Very often, we only allow ourselves to re-create our harmony and balance in the world for a short time out of every year: a vacation. I do not have to be paid for my dancing in order to consider it a part of my daily life, as necessary to me as a vocation or a job. We need to realize that our play is as essential and important as our work, and strive to love and learn from both.

I have gone through the typical laments: why didn't I continue dancing when I was seven, or resume at 15, and so on. But one finds the time when the time is right. Now I'm here, a woman over 30, a mother, practicing dance one hour per day.

There are common objections to starting a physical activity past the "normal" age for it. Everyone has heard of the exceptions—the 70-year-old novice skiers or mountain climbers or scuba divers. I would like to encourage everyone to become that exception. It is true that the body is more reluctant to move as it grows older. But biological change doesn't entirely cease when the adult body stops growing. What really matters is changing your mind. You must believe you can do it, no matter how clumsy the beginning feels to you.

I needed encouragement to take up dancing as a vital, frequent activity. When my one class per week jumped to four, I heard the voices of others added to the small inner voices of my own, asking what all this dancing meant anyway. I was 30, after all. I was too old to be a "dancer," and it was taking a lot of time and money away from my home, my family, my other work and pursuits. This kind of criticism brought me some doubts.

Well, I knew dancing made me feel good, and I knew feeling good about myself made everything else a lot better. Was I indulgent and selfish? Those anxieties seem a long way off now. Every part of my life has been positively affected by dance. My increased health, the facility of movement I share with my child and his friends, the passion and enthusiasm which have unfolded within me, the students and teachers I've been fortunate enough to work with—all these have convinced my skeptical friends and relatives. In fact, many of them have taken up dance themselves.

MATTER AND MOTION

That we are constantly in motion is a deep physical fact. Motion is what we define as change. Each atom in our body is moving, each molecule, each cell. There is nothing in our natural world that is static. Matter and energy transform and transfer and translate the condition of our life. Going across the street, the yard, the hall, the rug, the carseat. The whole concept of motion takes us to the deeper side of matter.

When I began to consciously and conscientiously dance, I also began to consciously move. In trying to learn how to properly breathe and sit and walk, I have begun to touch the depths within the most rudimentary gestures. Consequently I can practice dancing at the kitchen sink.

Once we begin to move through our lives with the awareness that we belong on the Earth and in our bodies, every activity takes the shape of a dance. There you are, the manifestation of billions of molecules, orchestrating the whole magnificent show that

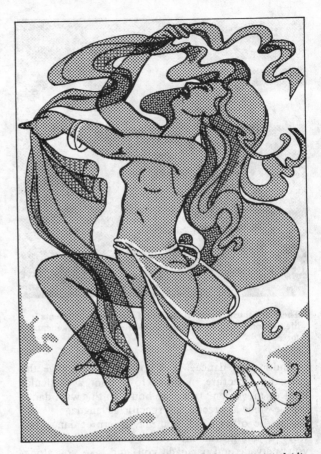

You may interpret dance as a way to feel movement: to let it pervade and persuade you, to be willingly led by it.

is you. Your thighs carry you well, your arms soar, your neck cranes, your fingers energize, your eyes account for space, your buttocks pull you around. You're dancing.

MIND AND MOTION

The body is a marvel. It both asks questions and gives answers. It can bring us to the formulas that rule all creation. Watch the waves. They're all very similar. They roll and break and give at the same point. But each time each one is utterly unique—utterly perfect, changeless, in tune.

There are two ways to approach the paradigm of the wave in dancing. One is to become absolutely *conscious* of every part of your being. The other is to *feel* every part of your being. The first demands an exact training, to infuse certain well-defined attitudes of grace, certain forms, into the body. (This is the purpose of the bar in ballet, and of strenuous massage

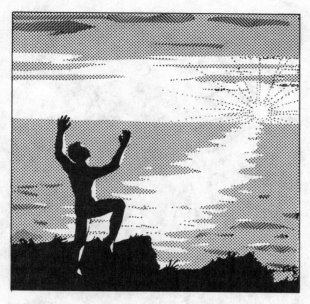

There are those places in the world, and those moments in life, when everything we feel is an expression of an elemental force.

in Indonesian dance.) The goal is to rearrange the muscular structure in order to extract a particular kind of movement from the body. In this way, dance can be made as precise and specific as language.

On the other hand, you may interpret dance as a way to *feel* movement: to let movement slide into you, pervade and persuade you, and take you along, to be willingly led by it. This attitude is closer to that of my African dance teacher, who told me I looked at her too much. She wanted me to get the feeling, the general direction and rhythm of the steps, rather than become anxious about the precise combination.

Sometimes I feel my mind is too tight and needs to let go. Sometimes I really need the structure of exact discipline.

THE DANCE OF LIFE

There are those places in the world, and those moments in life, when everything we feel is an expression of an elemental force. Everything that touches us is part of the kindling for the living fire. At this very

moment, my back is resting up against the most crystalline blue sky, and the wind is jagging my hair. What can I say? I feel wonderful! Everything around me adds to it. There are children gurgling under the back stairs. The strong winds of this day dance me back to leaves on sidewalks, smells in cloakrooms, New York in September, northern Pacific summers, corn in Kansas . . . we all sometimes lodge in these breathless moments.

For me it is dancing that leads me again through to these moments. By means of a conscious understanding about my own movements, I have come to realize that dance can be as reflexive, as unconscious, as breathing. I have seen this realization demonstrated on the stage, in country and western bars, at bus stops, in check-out lines, on beaches and in ports.

The more intimate we are with our physical being, the closer we come to our animal grace. Dance was the original communication that linked instinctual and habitual gesture with emotional and social concern. This became ritual, and ritual eventually developed into particular dance forms.

Now we are winding our way through the forms to the seeds of the original inspiration for dance. The spiral leads us inward to the breath and heartbeat, our internal rhythms. The path follows the coordinate points of our physical and emotional necessities. In the deepest seat of the body, we find the deepest seat of the psyche. The return trip begins the marriage of all the dancing aspects of our selves.

Summer Brenner was born March 17, 1945. She grew up in Atlanta, Georgia, studied in Boston and in Europe, and lived in New Mexico for several years before moving to California in 1973.

Two books of her poems, Everyone Came Dressed as Water *(1973) and* From the Heart to the Center *(1977), and a novella,* The Soft Room *(1978), have been published.*

Since 1974 she has studied modern dance (Hawkins), flamenco, African, and improvisation. She also teaches Creative Movement for Children, and is currently editing an anthology of essays by dancers called No Plain Feet.

Summer Brenner has recently moved to the Berkshires in Massachusetts with her husband and son.

Stress Reduction
L. John Mason, Ph.D.

Stress is a natural occurrence in all our lives. Our bodies are equipped with the ability to respond to stressful situations, and then to relax when the emergency is over. The problems of stress and tension occur when you don't know how to relax after a difficult experience, or when there is an accumulation of tense situations, with no time for relief in between. In this article, Dr. Mason gives us a clear understanding of how we can learn to approach the difficult situations that come up in our lives, as well as some suggestions for stress-reduction techniques that can be put to use every day.

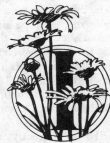

In order to define and describe stress reduction, we need a basic understanding of stress. Stress is inherent in every healthy form of life; it is the force exerted by any one thing against another. A person could not maintain an erect posture without the tension of opposing muscles that balance each other and keep the skeletal system erect. Eating puts some stress on the digestive system; exertion puts stress on the cardiovascular system. We are not concerned with such *essential* stress or tension, but with undesirable, excess tension which threatens the body's well-being. Each individual has a unique response to stress, and needs to discover techniques that will alleviate unnecessary stress.

Let's look at the historical source of the stress response. The body responds most extremely to the most extreme stress: threat to the survival of the organism. If placed in a life-threatening situation, an organism responds with the fight/flight response, identified by Dr. Walter Canon in the 1930s. Imagine that you are coming home from work late one evening. It is already dark. As you go to unlock your door, you realize that it is open. Your heart begins to pound, and sweat starts to drip down your forehead.

From *Guide to Stress Reduction*, copyright © 1980 by L. John Mason, Ph.D. Reprinted by permission of Peace Press.

Someone has been in your apartment. Who could it have been? As your mind races through the possibilities, your breathing quickens; your hands are clammy on the doorknob as you push open the door. You flick on the lights. The lamps are knocked over; your grandmother's porcelain figurines are not in their place—the living room is a disaster. You have been robbed. The robber may still be in your apartment. Your knees are weak, and there's a knot in your stomach as you grab a bookend to defend yourself. Or should you run? This scenario describes the fight/flight response.

A variety of physiological changes occur with dramatic suddenness, to help you to survive, either by fighting off the threat or by fleeing from it. What typically happens?

1. The heartbeat increases, in order to pump blood throughout the necessary tissues with greater speed, carrying oxygen and nutrients to cells, and clearing away waste products more quickly.
2. As the heart rate increases, the blood pressure goes up.
3. Breathing becomes rapid and shallow.
4. Adrenalin and other hormones are released into the blood.
5. The body releases stored sugar into the blood to meet the energy needs of survival.
6. The pupils dilate to let in more light; all the senses are heightened.
7. Muscles tense for movement, either for flight or protective actions, particularly the muscles of the thighs, hips, back, shoulders, arms, jaw, and face.
8. Blood flow to the digestive organs is greatly constricted.
9. Blood flow increases to the brain and major muscles.
10. Blood flow to the extremities is constricted, and the hands and feet get cold. This is protection from bleeding to death quickly, if the hands or feet were to be cut in fight or flight.
11. The body perspires to cool itself, since increases metabolism generates more heat.

The major stress response can occur if you are in a life-threatening situation, or experiencing an exciting, highly stimulating activity, such as racing a car or riding on a roller coaster. After the danger has passed, you stop, assess your survival, and then breathe a "sigh of relief." (You may go to the other extreme and collapse in shock.) The surge of energy subsides, and your metabolism slows down. Some people are actually addicted to this adrenalin rush, and need to do dangerous things in order to get their "kicks." Others who are addicted to the rush will eat a lot of sugar quickly, which raises the blood-sugar level. During the fight/flight response, the body releases stored sugar into the blood. When ingestion of large quantities of sugar raises the blood-sugar level, the body responds as if under threat, and triggers the fight/flight response. Eating a hot fudge sundae may trigger the same response as a roller-coaster ride.

The "sigh of relief" that you automatically breathe when climbing out of the roller coaster actually does give relief. The long, slow, complete breath and accompanying sigh releases tension from the rib cage and throat, and allow for natural, relaxed breathing to begin again. This is an innate form of stress reduction.

The chronic stress that we suffer daily is probably not a reaction to a real life-or-death threat. Human consciousness has developed to the extent that stress responses can be triggered by our emotions, thoughts, and social expectations. Unfortunately, the increase in our brain's capacity may have dire side effects on our total well-being. The lower, or primitive, parts of the brain have not changed much in the last million years. But abstract thought produced in the sophisticated, higher centers of the brain can trigger the autonomic survival reflexes that are located in the lower centers.

Over the years, the continual triggering of the stress response for inappropriate situations causes wear and tear on the body. We may not be conscious of the stress until we are confronted with pain. Recognizing your unique stress response is the first step in the journey toward stress reduction.

Let me draw a clearer picture of the mind/body connection in stress-related dysfunction. Tension headache is common, and relatively easy to explain. As we become anxious and face a difficult task, we brace ourselves by holding our skeletal muscles tight. This tightness may occur in the forehead, face, eyes, jaw, neck, or shoulders. After a long siege of rigidity, these muscles go into spasm (extreme contraction). If we just stop and relax, resting our muscles briefly during the day, and realize that we do not need to brace ourselves physically against a nonphysical threat, our tension headaches may be prevented.

Ulcers, allergies, asthma, high blood pressure, colitis, and headaches are recognized as psychosomatic disorders. In these disorders, mental or emotional states contribute to or cause the illness. How can infections, hormonal imbalances, or even cancer be related to the stress response? As much as 90 per cent of all disease may be caused, directly or indirectly, by stress.

Hans Selye, an endocrinologist and the world's leading researcher into the effects of stress on the body, states his theory in *The Stress of Life*. When the brain perceives stress, either consciously or unconsciously, the message is transmitted to the hypothalamus. This "switching station" carries signals in and out of the brain. The hypothalamus sends impulses to parts of the pituitary gland, the master endocrine gland. The pituitary releases hormones which stimulate other glands, such as the adrenals, which, in turn, release other hormones, such as adrenalin. A life-or-death situation may trigger this response, but the brain may respond in a similar way to persistent lower levels of stress. Even though you may not be constantly experiencing the full-fledged fight/flight reaction, some of its characteristics may be present. If a stress response is chronic, the constant presence of stress hormones begins to wear down the body's immunological system. Selye calls this the general adaptation syndrome. The body becomes more susceptible to infections, diseases, and even cancer. In the case of cancer, the body might normally eliminate a mutant cell, but if the system is weakened, the cell may take hold and develop into a tumor. This general adaptation may also upset the balance of the hormones, so that the body overcompensates when it swings back from the stress response, turning against its own healthy tissue. The result of such an imbalance is called an autoimmune ailment; many consider rheumatoid arthritis such a disease.

Thus, stress is related, directly or indirectly, to many, maybe even most, diseases. Stress-reduction techniques will not only prevent or alleviate a tension headache, but also act to prevent future diseases.

Life changes can be stress-producing, whether they are negative or positive. Two researchers, Holmes and Rahe, statistically developed the patterns of certain typical life events and the proportionate degree of stress they elicited. The numbers given in the following chart are relative to the number and degree of health changes (disease) that occurred in the group of 7,000 people in the survey.

The list indicates the relative numerical values of stress production for some common life changes. Check off the events which you have experienced in the past 12-18 months. Add up your score. If the total is over 150, you have experienced a lot of stress, requiring a high degree of adaptation. Offset the negative effects of this stress by beginning to practice some stress-reduction techniques.

The principles for stress reduction are relatively simple. Once you identify your own unique stress response, you can reverse this tendency and evoke the

Stress-Reduction Techniques
L. John Mason, Ph.D.

Stress affects people in different ways. Some people respond positively to stress, and it motivates them to achievement; others are negatively affected by stress. It is important to be aware of your own unique response to stress. When your body signals stress or tension, it is a warning that should not be ignored or buried in your mind. Pay closer attention to your body's SOS.

To help alleviate tension I recommend a simple, but very powerful relaxation technique: deep breathing. Breathing is the easiest physiological system to control. You can consciously slow and deepen your breathing, and have this relaxation generalize to the rest of your body. Breathe slowly from your diaphragm, pause for a moment after inhaling, and then exhale fully and completely, ending with a slight sigh. While you are exhaling, allow your muscles to loosen (drop your shoulders and jaw, relax your arms and legs).

Take at least forty deep breaths every day. To remind yourself to practice deep breathing, associate it with something commonly done during the day. If you are in a busy office, and the telephone seems to ring incessantly, don't grab the phone on the first ring. Let it ring an extra time and take a deep breath. Exhale fully and completely, and pick up the phone— relaxed and free of nervous tension.

All the time you spend driving from place to place can make you tense and edgy, and if you find yourself in a traffic jam, you may be grinding your teeth by the time you arrive home. If you drive a great deal, try taking a deep breath and relaxing at each stop signal, or use billboards and highway turnoff signs as reminders. Every time you inch forward in rush-hour traffic, instead of frantically beeping your horn at every stop, take a deep full breath and exhale fully and completely. As you breathe, check your shoulders and forehead to see if they are tense. You really don't need to drive with your shoulders or your forehead.

A dramatic, but not unusual story was told to me by a man who attended one of my stress-reduction lectures. He had a very high-pressure job and was also going through a custody fight for his son. The added pressure of the legal battle made it almost impossible for him to function well at work. He was having difficulty meeting deadlines, and relationships with his coworkers were rapidly deteriorating. After signing up for the entire ten-week course, he attended the introductory lecture. I didn't see him at the second and third lectures and began to wonder what had happened to him; the course had been closed, and he had been very insistent that I allow him to enroll. When he didn't show up for the fourth lecture I decided to call him at work. He told me the following story.

I had recommended that clock-watchers put a piece of tape on the office clock; every time they turned to check the time, they would be reminded to take a deep, full breath. After the first lecture, he realized that he was constantly looking at his watch while working. He placed a piece of tape (in his case it was bright blue) on his watch, and took a deep breath when he checked the time. Exhaling fully and completely, at first very difficult for him, became easier with each day. Even though he couldn't attend the second lecture because of work responsibilities, he continued to practice deep breathing. On the ninth day of practice he actually counted the times he took a deep breath, and was amazed to discover that he had taken 53 deep breaths in just one work day. On the tenth day of practice he was approached by an office secretary who commented on the change in his personality; she wanted to know what drug he was taking, because it had obviously helped him so much. She didn't believe that deep breathing had affected such a radical change, but when he showed her the tape on his watch she finally believed him. Breathing cues, combined with proper deep breathing, had worked for him; he apologized for not returning to class, but he felt that deep breathing exercises were enough to keep him relaxed and free from tension.

Another easy and effective breathing technique is counting backwards from ten to one while breathing very slowly. Practice this when you feel tension beginning to take hold, or do it once an hour as a preventive measure. It is important to picture the number in your mind clearly as you slowly count backwards. Allow yourself to become more relaxed with each exhalation. Remember, the battle for stress reduction is 50 per cent awareness of your own stress response, and 50 per cent letting go. Find a way to give in to relaxation.

STRESS CAUSED BY LIFE CHANGES

Event	Value
Death of spouse	100
Divorce	73
Relationship or marital separation	65
Jail term	63
Death of close family member	63
Personal injury or illness	53
Marriage	50
Fired from work	47
Relationship or marital reconciliation	45
Retirement	45
Change in family member's health	44
Pregnancy	40
Sex difficulties	39
Addition to family	39
Business readjustment	39
Change in financial status	38
Death of close friend	38
Change to different line of work	36
Change in number of marital arguments	35
Mortgage or loan over $10,000	31
Foreclosure of mortgage or loan	30
Change in work responsibilities	29
Son or daughter leaving home	29
Trouble with in-laws	29
Outstanding personal achievement	28
Spouse begins or stops work	26
Starting or finishing school	26
Change in living conditions	25
Revision of personal habits	24
Trouble with boss	23
Change in work hours, conditions	20
Change in residence	20
Change in schools	20
Change in recreational habits	19
Change in church activities	19
Change in social activites	18
Mortgage or loan under $10,000	17
Change in sleeping habits	16
Change in number of family gatherings	15
Change in eating habits	15
Vacation	13
Christmas season	12
Minor violation of the law	11

relaxation response. This term was coined by Dr. Herbert Benson, a cardiologist who has studied stress and its effects on the heart and circulatory system. Benson believes that you can learn to reverse the stress response, and elicit instead a feeling of deep relaxation and calm. For example, if you have a tendency to hold tension in your vascular system, and to manifest stress in cold hands and feet, you can learn how to warm your extremities with a stress-reduction technique. People who hold tension in their skeletal

muscles can become more sensitive to this tension and practice techniques which offer almost instantaneous relief. If your heart races and your mind is full of anxious thoughts, relaxation exercises will teach you greater control over your mind and body. *A Guide to Stress Reduction* describes a wide variety of relaxation techniques and exercises. You can find those that work best for you, and then, with practice, you can really learn how to relax and control your unwanted stress and tension.

I am sure you can find ways to learn deep relaxation, and to handle your stress in a more positive way. To make this process work, you must *do* these exercises, not just read about them; you might want to tape them to experience their value more fully. The time you put into this will be well-spent. Researchers believe that 20 minutes of deep relaxation a day may take the place of two hours of sleep. You will use your energies more efficiently. Your relaxation will lead to deeper, more peaceful sleep. You can release previously wasted energy for work; for your family, for yourself. Your attitude toward life will become more positive, and annoyances which may surround you now will not plague you. Your whole body and mind will be on a more even keel, not on the roller coaster of life, with its traumatic ups and downs. Twenty minutes of deep relaxation a day will do this and probably more for you. It will aid your mental, physical, emotional, and even spiritual growth. It is really worth the investment, if you want to start doing something positive for your life, and to grow with health, happiness, and efficiency.

Remember that these tools are for you, and if you want them to, they will give you great power.

L. John Mason, Ph.D., author of Guide to Stress Reduction *(Peace Press, $6.95), is a stress-reduction and biofeedback therapist at the Stress Education Center in Sonoma County, California. He is affiliated with the Department of Psychophysiology at Brookwood Hospital in Santa Rosa, where he practices biofeedback therapy at the Pain Clinic. Mason is a certified member of the California State Biofeedback Society.*

L. John Mason conducts lectures, workshops, and classes in stress reduction, biofeedback, and visualization techniques for the public and health-care professionals. Guide to Stress Reduction *includes a chapter on how to conduct stress-reduction classes. Cassette tapes of stress-reduction exercises led by Dr. Mason are also available for $8.95 from Peace Press, 3828 Willat Avenue, Culver City, California 90230.*

Learning to Relax
Andrew Michaels, Ph.D.

How many times have you been told, "Just relax, and everything will be all right"? Then you say to yourself, "Sure, just relax, but how?" *The following exercises are offered as a sampling of the many relaxation techniques now available. There are exercises to relieve both mental and physical tension. Twenty minutes a day of deep relaxation will contribute to better performance in whatever you do. To really benefit from the exercises, try them—just reading them won't be enough. You can make a tape recording of them and listen to them. Experiment to find the ones that most suit your needs.*

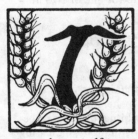

ake a moment to think about the last new skill you gained. Initially, you may have felt self-conscious or awkward. You may have had to make adjustments in your schedule to permit you time to practice. You may even have had to push yourself to get past an initial resistance.

Whether the skill you thought of was playing tennis, learning a language, or learning to drive, you probably found that the more you did the activity, the more fluid your experience of it became. If you continued the process, chances are the activity became "part of you," until it eventually felt like second nature.

Learning to get into a deeply relaxed space is just such a skill. At first it may feel awkward taking the phone off the hook, and asking those around you not to disturb you for awhile. It may seem strange to say phrases to yourself, or give yourself a face massage. But soon *you will find your body reminding you* that it's time to take care of yourself, and those around you will adjust easily enough. At that point,

This article has been reprinted by permission of the author from a holistic stress-management workbook entitled *Why Do You Think They Call it a Deadline?* The workbook can be ordered from Andrew Michaels, 1820 Hopkins, Berkeley, California 94707, for $3.95.

doing some form of stress reduction technique on a daily basis will involve little more decision-making than whether to brush your teeth; you'll do it because it feels natural and healthy. And, like most skills, the more you do it, the easier it becomes, and the sooner the subtleties of the skill become apparent.

PREPARATION
PURPOSE

To provide an appropriate physical and psychic environment in which to do all of the following stress-reduction techniques.

CONCEPT

The feeling of being centered and grounded is optimal as an orientation point for these exercises.

CAUTION

Think of the preparation as part of the exercise itself, rather than as something "extra" which can be disregarded.

PROCEDURE

1. Find a quiet place where you will not be disturbed. Those around you will need to learn to accept this time as "your time," when you should not be bothered except for an emergency. It may help to place a small sign on your door.
2. If possible, take the phone off the hook. To prevent the phone's "off-the-hook" signal, turn the dial and then place a matchbook or some other object between the dial and the phone, thus preventing it from returning to its usual position. Callers will get a busy signal.
3. Find a comfortable place to lie down or sit.
4. Take off your glasses; take out contact lenses if necessary.
5. Loosen any constrictive clothing, especially belt, shoes, and collar.

6. Allow your arms to find a comfortable position, and allow your eyes to close.

7. Pay attention to your breath, allowing your abdomen to rise on the inhale and descend on the exhale; imagine that you can breathe energy into your mind.

8. Imagine a screen on the inside of your forehead —a screen on which you can project images. Then draw a line down the center of your body from the top of your head to a point directly between your feet.

9. Check to see that your weight is evenly balanced on both sides of that line. Make whatever physical adjustments are necessary to bring your body into symmetry.

10. Optional. Simply continue to be aware of your breath. Allow yourself to "watch your thoughts" without becoming involved in them. This step is the essence of *Vipassana,* or insight meditation. Witness; breathe; observe.

AUTOGENIC TRAINING

PURPOSE

Over-all mind and body relaxation; to introduce the understanding of tapes and suggestions.

CONCEPT

Our mind and body functions can be controlled by what we tell ourselves and how we see ourselves.

CAUTION

Suggestions should always be phrased in short, positive sentences, such as "I feel relaxed," rather than "I do not feel any tension." Be *certain* to do part five of this exercise. Failure to cancel (all but the personal) suggestions is counterproductive.

PROCEDURE

1. Preparation.
2. Bring your attention into your (*part of body*) and say to yourself, "My (*part of body*) feels (*appropriate phrase*)."
 (a) right arm—heavy and warm.
 (b) left arm—heavy and warm.
 (c) right leg—heavy and warm.
 (d) left leg—heavy and warm.
 (e) abdomen and chest—relaxed and warm.
 (f) "My breathing is gentle and rhythmical."

(g) "My heartbeat is calm and regular."

(h) shoulders and back—heavy and warm.

(i) neck and head—heavy and *cool.*

Note: Be sure to say each phrase to yourself slowly, and to repeat each phrase twice.

3. Now that you are completely relaxed, repeat your personal suggestions several times. (See the procedure for developing your personal suggestions following this exercise.)

4. Take several moments to simply drift, float, and sink.

5. To bring yourself back to a relaxed and fully conscious state, count backwards from three to one, using the following phrases:

"Number three—My entire body feels relaxed and refreshed." (Repeat)

"Number two—I am at peace." (Repeat)

"This is the number one."

When you say "the number one," take a deep breath, flex your hands and your feet, and then slowly open your eyes. Remain there for one or two minutes before getting up.

PERSONAL SUGGESTIONS

PURPOSE

To be used with autogenic training or other deep relaxation exercise, as a means of helping to improve self-image, helping to control habitual patterns of behavior or reactions to particular situations, increasing relaxation in specific parts of the body, and alleviating psychosomatic conditions.

CONCEPT

Deep but conscious relaxation is the optimal psychic environment in which to reprogram the maladaptive messages we tell ourselves, and to stimulate new, more adaptive messages.

CAUTION

Suggestions should always be phrased in short, positive sentences. No more than two personal-suggestion sentences should be used in a single relaxation period. Each suggestion should be repeated two or more times.

PROCEDURE

1. Specify, as much as possible, the personality characteristic, behavior, or psychosomatic disorder

which you want to change.

2. Consider how you *would* like to be, do, or feel (e.g., confident, able to enjoy a good night's sleep, or clear-headed). Do *not* consider phrases that are descriptions of how you *wouldn't* like to feel (e.g., not so crabby, less restless, or pain-free).

3. Choose one or two adjectives for each suggestion, and put them into a sentence such as: "I see myself as a (*confident*) and (*relaxed*) person." Now visualize yourself as that person for several moments. "I see myself as an individual who (*remains centered in difficult situations*)." Visualize yourself behaving that way. "My (*mind*) feels (*healthy*) and (*peaceful*)." Visualize what you look like when you feel that way.

PROGRESSIVE RELAXATION

PURPOSE

To release muscular tension, and to facilitate overall relaxation.

CONCEPT

Muscles are tightened and then released into a state of deep relaxation.

CAUTION

Tighten down less heavily on areas with recent strain or sprain.

PROCEDURE

1. *Preparation.*

2. *Four-part breath*—Inhale through abdomen; hold for five seconds; release all at once through the mouth; sink as you breathe easily.

3. *Right arm*—Inhale; hold breath and tighten entire arm by making fist; tighten fist, wrist, forearm, and bicep as you lift entire arm six inches into the air; release breath all at once, as arm flops down; allow arm to sink; roll arm slightly and compare to left arm. Repeat.

4. *Left arm*—Repeat procedure with left arm twice. Note how arms feel in comparison with the legs.

5. *Right leg*—Inhale; hold breath and tighten entire leg by pointing toe; tighten toes, foot, calf, thigh, and right buttock as you lift entire leg into the air; release breath all at once, as leg flops down; allow leg to sink; roll leg gently and compare to left leg and arms. Repeat.

6. *Left leg*—Repeat procedure with left leg twice.

7. *Abdomen*—Inhale (less fully); hold breath and tighten by making a "hard stomach"; release breath all at once; compare to arms and legs. Repeat.

8. *Chest*—Inhale deeply, allowing chest to rise; hold breath and tighten the muscles below the armpits (pectorals); release breath all at once; compare to abdomen. Repeat.

9. *Shoulders and back*—Inhale; hold breath and tighten shoulders by raising them up as if to cover the ears in shrugging gesture; release breath all at once, as shoulders return to original state of rest; allow shoulders to widen and lower by reaching hands gently for feet; sink; compare to torso. Repeat.

10. *Neck*—Inhale; hold breath and tighten by raising head up six inches and *gently* tensing back neck muscles until mild trembling is felt; release breath all at once, as head flops gently to original position; sink; compare to shoulders and back. Repeat.

11. *Face*—Inhale; hold breath and tighten by bringing entire face to a point at the tip of the nose, as the eyes squint and lips pucker in a kissing gesture; release breath all at once; allow face to expand and relax; sink; compare to neck. Repeat.

12. *Conclusion*—Gently allow hands to move, and give yourself a face massage. Take care of yourself, giving attention to your hairline, forehead, eyebrows, eyes, temples, ears, nose, cheeks, mouth, and chin. Work your way back up the face, checking each of these areas; run your fingers through your hair from the roots all the way out, as you pull any remaining tension out of your body, through your scalp, and into your hands; "throw" tension far away by shaking hands vigorously; sink, float, drift . . . .

MANTRA MEDITATION

PURPOSE

To enable the mind to clear, center, and rest; to facilitate a bodily relaxation response.

CONCEPT

Consciousness sinks from surface awareness to the "source of thought," and then returns refreshed and rejuvenated.

CAUTION

If you find yourself caught up in thoughts instead of the mantra, do not get frustrated and stop; instead, let the thoughts go and gently return to repetition of the mantra.

(Text continued on p. 136)

(Descriptions for these exercises appear in the text on pages 136-139.)

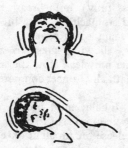

1. Neck Roll

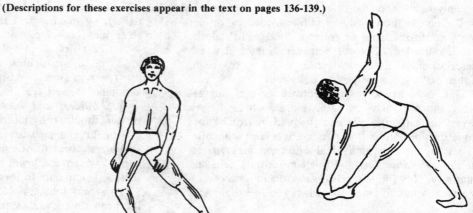

4. Inner Groin Stretch

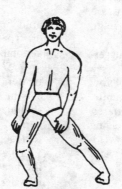

6. Side Triangle Twist

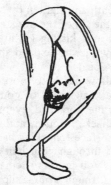

2. Forward Bend

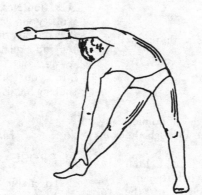

5. Side Triangle Bend

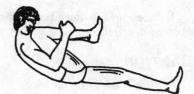

7. Head Knee

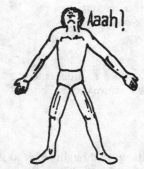

3. Spread Eagle Back Bend

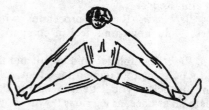

8. Split Forward and Side Bending

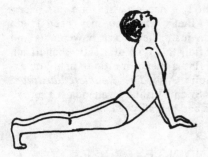

9. Simple Cobra

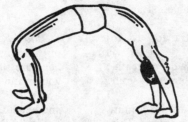

12. Backbend Wheel

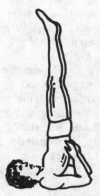

15. Shoulder Stand

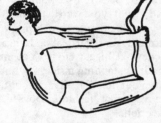

10. Bow

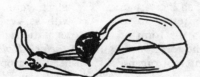

13. Ear Knee

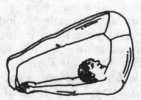

16. "The Plough" pose

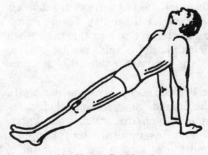

11. Simple Backbend

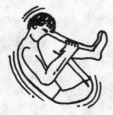

14. Spiral Roll

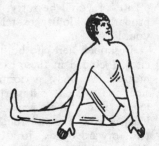

17. Sitting Twist

(continued from p. 133)
PROCEDURE

1. Choose a very short phrase or word to repeat to yourself. Examples of common mantras are the words "one," "Om," *"shanti"* (peace), or the phrase "I am relaxed."

2. Preparation.

3. (a) Repeat the phrase to yourself over and over. Some people like to forget about their breath and just meditate with the mantra. Others prefer to coordinate their mantra with their breath, e.g., inhale—"I am"—exhale—"relaxed" . . . .

(b) Continue repetition of mantra for 15 to 20 minutes.

(c) Bring yourself back by taking a deep breath, flexing hands and feet, and then slowly opening your eyes.

(d) Allow yourself to remain seated for a minute or two before resuming your activities. This transition time is very important.

Note: If you fell asleep, next time sit in a more upright position.

FLEXIBILITY

As you no doubt have experienced, an increase in muscular tension is one of the body's responses to stress. This may affect you directly in the form of sore, achey muscles, or indirectly, in the form of excess or unbalanced pressure on the internal organs, nerves, joints, or spine. The following series of exercises, which are derived from the disciplines of *T'ai Chi Ch'uan,* bioenergetics, and yoga, are designed to help you release some of the tension your muscles are holding, as well as tone and rebalance your entire body.

A word to the wise . . . Caution must be taken while *learning* and *doing* all these exercises. Remember, your body is its own best healer. It knows how much you can do, and how far you can stretch. Listen to it—do not overstretch yourself with heroic effort, or you'll be sorry. On the other hand, done properly, flexibility exercises can be a daily joy in your life.

Described here are both standing and floor exercises. Included in these exercises are three types of motion the body performs: forward-back, side to side, and twist. It is important to become more flexible in each of these ways. It is also essential that you balance your exercise routine. That is, after one or two forward bends, do a backward bend to reverse the stretch; if you twist in one direction, be sure to do the opposite twist. Choose those exercises best

suited to your body's needs (which are *not* necessarily the easiest—that's why you may need to do them!). These are just a few basic movements and positions. If you find this type of practice beneficial, you may want to find a friend or class to help you expand your repertoire. Also, *The Complete Illustrated Book of Yoga* by Swami Vishnudevananda is a superb guide to positions and overall yogic philosophy.

STANDING EXERCISES

Body Rope I. With your feet together and hands on hips, imagine that your feet and the top of your head are the ends of a rope. Now slowly begin to revolve your body around that vertical axis, as if your body itself was a rope held stationary at your feet and head. Do several revolutions in each direction.

Body Rope II. Now separate your feet, placing them shoulder length apart. Be sure that your feet are pointed straight ahead, as if you were standing on railroad tracks. Place your hands on your hips. Now revolve your body around that vertical axis again, this time making a somewhat bigger circle. You may wish to think of yourself as standing inside a cylinder which your waist (not your head!) stays in contact with as you move in rope-like fashion. Do several revolutions in each direction.

Neck Roll. With legs apart for balance, allow the head to drop forward as far as possible, then revolve head toward your right, so that your right ear approaches lying on your right shoulder. Let the head continue to revolve around, so that your head now leans directly back, then around so that the left ear lies on the left shoulder. Do not raise your shoulders up to meet your ears; let them stay down and relaxed. Revolve a couple of times to the right, then reverse in similar fashion. Do this exercise only as part of a larger routine, not habitually, as some people do.

Forward bend. Breathe normally as you stand with feet solidly on the ground. Now, as you exhale slowly, lean forward until you can touch your knees, calves, ankles, or feet. Remain bent over for approximately five seconds, or as long as feels comfortable, while holding onto that part of your body as you *gently breathe into your back.* Do *not* bounce up and down. Allow yourself to bend over farther after your breath has helped your back muscles to stretch out. You may feel some trembling in your body. Allow that trembling to happen. Return to an upright position by bending your knees slightly and stacking your vertebrae up one at a time. Let your head be the last part of your body to come back into position. Repeat two to four times.

Spread Eagle Back Bend. Begin with a brief forward bend. Then, as you come back up, inhale and spread your fingers wide apart. Open your eyes widely, and stick your tongue out (as in the lion yoga pose). Continue to bend backward until your arms are fully extended away from your body, thus stretching the chest muscles. Again, allow any trembling to happen. Now exhale the breath with a long, loud, "Aaaah!" Finish with another brief forward bend, returning to an upright position by stacking the vertebrae. Repeat.

Inner Groin Stretch. Separate the legs farther than shoulder width. Feet should be straight ahead. Now, while keeping your torso vertical, bend your right knee so that you stretch the inner groin muscles, as you give most of your weight to your right foot. Move with the exhale. Hold position for a few moments or as long as feels comfortable. Reverse. Repeat both sides. Be especially careful with this exercise at first so that you don't pull or overstretch any sensitive muscles.

Side Triangle Bend. Stand erect with feet slightly farther apart than shoulder width. Turn your right foot 90° toward the outside. Now slide your right hand down your right leg towards your ankle, as you bend *directly* over your right hip. The left arm is brought directly overhead until it is against the left ear and parallel to the floor. Hold for 5 to 10 seconds as you breathe. Reverse. Repeat two to four times.

Side Triangle Twist. This one may be a little harder. Stand as in side triangle bend. Twist body, bringing the left hand over to the right foot. Look back and up as the right arm swings straight up in the air, forming a straight line with the left arm. Hold as long as feels comfortable. Stand up and rest. Reverse. Repeat.

FLOOR EXERCISES

FORWARD BENDING

Head-Knee. Sit on the floor with your legs straight out in front of you. Breathe into the abdomen. Now, on the exhale, begin to bend over so that your head moves toward your knees. Let your hands hold onto your legs wherever they can, under the knees, calves, ankles, feet, or toes. Hold the position for a while as you *breathe into your back.* Use the natural expansion of your body as you inhale to gently stretch the back muscles. Sit up. Repeat two to four times. Follow with a backward bending position.

Split Forward and Side Bending. Sit on the floor with your legs straight and your feet as far apart as possible. Now as in the head-knee position, hold onto your legs as far down as you can lower your head and torso toward the floor. This will probably be more difficult than the head-knee position, but will get easier with practice. This position provides a stretch to the groin muscles in addition to the legs and back. Relax. Now lean over the right leg, moving both hands toward the right ankle. Breathe. Now lean over the left leg, moving both hands toward the left ankle.

BACKWARD BENDING

Simple Cobra. Lie on the floor face down with the palms of your hands down and near your shoulders. Now as you inhale, lift your head up and back bending your spine back and pushing your torso up off the floor as much as possible. This is *not* a calisthenic "push up," because your pelvis and legs stay on the floor. Breathe at the top of the stretch. Return to original position slowly. Repeat. Follow with a forward bending position.

Bow. Lie on the floor face down with your arms at your sides. Now bend your knees and grab your ankles with your hands as your torso is lifted up. Arch your back so that your thighs are held up off the floor as much as possible. Breathe and stretch. Return.

Simple Backbend. Sitting with your legs straight out, place your hands at your sides and slightly behind you. Now by arching your back and supporting yourself with your hands, lift yourself up on your heels, and let your head go back as far as possible. Hold five to ten seconds. Repeat.

Backbend Wheel. Lie on your back with your knees up and feet flat on the floor, shoulder length apart. Place your palms on the floor next to your ears, so that your fingers point toward your shoulders. Now, by pushing with your arms and legs as you arch your back, lift yourself off the floor as much as possible, and let your head go back. Hold for five seconds as you breathe. Repeat if desired.

OTHER BACK AND NECK STRETCHES

Ear-Knee. This easy position is useful for stiffness of the lower back (proceed with caution!) and for relieving intestinal gas. Lie flat on your back. Now bend your right leg so that you can hug it to your chest, lifting your head up and forward. Optimally, you can touch your knee to your right ear. Hold for five seconds. Reverse. Repeat.

Acu-Yoga
Michael Reed Gach

Acu-Yoga is a system of exercises that integrates the knowledge of two ancient methods of health maintenance, acupressure and yoga. Increased effectiveness is the result of combining these two complementary practices of self-treatment. Both systems relax muscular tension and balance the vital life forces of the body. In yoga this is accomplished by controlling the breath while holding the body in certain postures. In acupressure body energy is directly manipulated by means of a system of points and meridians. In yogic terms this energy is called *prana*. Acupressure uses the Chinese name of *chi*, as in "Tai Ch'i," or the Japanese term *ki*. The meridians are the pathways that the vital energy flows through, and the points are places where you can tap into that energy.[1]

When tension accumulates around these points, it prevents the energy from flowing properly, creating an excess of energy in one area of the body and a deficiency in another. Each Acu-Yoga posture naturally presses and stretches certain nerves, muscles, and acupressure points, awakening the meridians and releasing the tension in the points, so that the energy can circulate freely. This process balances the body as a whole, and also stimulates its natural ability to heal itself.

NECK TENSION

The Chinese have called the neck the "pillar of heaven," because in a healthy person the mind is calm and at peace. The neck, however, is also the *first area* of the body where tension hits. Therefore, whenever a person is under any sort of stress, whether from personal, social, or work demands, the neck is one area that always becomes tense.

THE NECK AND THE MERIDIANS

Many meridians travel through the neck within a small area. When there is tension in the neck, these meridian flows can intermingle

---

[1]It should be noted that acupressure and acupuncture are based on the same principles, points, and meridians.

and cause complications, such as stiffness, sore throat, or swollen glands.

The acupressure points in the neck are known as "windows of the sky." When the neck is strong, flexible, and in proper alignment, these "windows" are clear and open— that is, we are open to the flow of life, and experience its harmonious nature. When tension interferes, however, it can affect us in many ways, and we become more closed physically, emotionally, mentally, and spiritually. Since the neck is such a key area, and so prone to tension, it is especially important to practice techniques to unblock it.

EXERCISES FOR THE NECK
PILLAR OF HEAVEN POSE

1. Kneel on the floor and sit on your heels.
2. Inhale, and clasp your hands together behind your neck.
3. Lean forward as you exhale, and place your head on the floor. Tuck the chin into the chest.
4. Raise your buttocks up and gently move forward on the top of your head, stretching the neck muscles.
5. Breathe long and deep.
6. Slowly turn your head to each side and gently lean forward, so that other areas of the neck are stretched. The sore points on the top of the head facilitate the release of chronic neck tensions.
7. Continue, stretching both sides and the middle of the neck, for two minutes.
8. Inhale and return to a sitting position.
9. Relax for a few minutes on your back.

WINDOWS OF THE SKY POSE

1. Lie on your back.
2. Clasp your hands together behind your neck.
3. Exhale, and slowly pull the head up, using your arm muscles. The heels of the palms should be firmly pressing the sides of your neck.
4. Breathe deeply, keeping the head up in this manner. Eyes are closed. Relax into the pose.
5. Continue for three minutes.
6. Bring the elbows together, stretching further. The shoulder blades remain on the floor.

7. Inhale and slowly lower the head to the floor.

8. Relax with your arms by your sides.

BOAT POSE

1. Lie on your stomach, feet together and arms at your sides. Rest your head on your chin.

2. Stretch your arms so that they are straight in front of you, on the floor.

3. As you slowly and deeply inhale, arch your back, lifting your arms, chest, head, and legs off the ground.

4. Begin long, deep breathing. Push beyond the time you think you can hold the pose, working up to one minute.

5. Inhale deeply and stretch up, then exhale and relax down. Let your arms be by your sides, and turn your head to the side.

6. Relax for at least three minutes.

This exercise is also beneficial for developing stamina and concentration, strengthening the lower back, improving circulation, and balancing the abdominal area.

Michael Reed Gach is the director of the Acupressure Workshop of Berkeley, a California State-approved massage school. Michael teaches various forms of Acupressure: Jin Shin, Shiatsu, Acupressure Massage, Reflexology, Do-In and Acu-Yoga. He is the author of Acu-Yoga: The Acupressure Self-Help Manual for Stress Management, *published by Japan Publications. His book and information about the programs he conducts are available by writing the Acupressure Workshop, 1533 Shattuck Avenue, Berkeley, California 94709.*

Spinal Roll. Bring *both* knees and head up as in the ear-knee position, with arms holding your knees against your chest. Now gently rock and roll along your spine. Be certain you have sufficient padding or carpet under you.

Shoulder Stand. Lying flat, first bend the knees as you slowly raise your feet directly overhead. The weight of your body should rest on your shoulders, with your back supported by your hands. The chin locks and presses against the chest. *Breathe.* This pose is held for one-half minute by beginners, and 15 minutes or more by more advanced students. For a variation, from this position bend the legs so that the knees are next to the ears. Follow with a backward bending position.

"The Plough" Pose. This is one of the more difficult positions; so go gently and build up to it. From the shoulder-stand position, allow the feet to continue moving directly overhead until the toes touch the floor in line with the head. The hands move from supporting the back to nearly touching the feet. Hold as long as feels comfortable. Do not attempt this exercise unless you are already fairly flexible. Follow with a backward bend.

Sitting Twist. Sit with your legs together and straight out in front of you. Now flex your left leg so that your left foot is to the right of your right knee. Then place both your hands on your left side and *twist* to the left as if you were trying to look behind you. Hold for five to ten seconds as you breathe.

Reverse entire procedure (i.e., right leg flexed). Repeat.

For a more difficult variation, begin the same way, then twist more, so that you are able to reach with your right arm to the left of your left knee, and grab the right side of your right knee with your right hand. Reverse. (Sound impossible? It's not.)

SUGGESTIONS FOR FURTHER READING

Alan Lakein, *How to Get Control of Your Time and Your Life.* McKay, 1973.

Kenneth Pelletier, *Mind as Healer, Mind as Slayer.* Delta, 1977.

Synthesis Magazine (Redwood City, Calif.: Synthesis Press, 1974, 1975, 1977).

Swami Vishnudevananda, *The Complete Illustrated Book of Yoga.* Pocket Books, 1960.

Anthony Zaffuto, *Alphagenics.* Warner, 1974.

Andrew Michaels has had extensive experience in clinical practice and as a teacher of stress management in the San Francisco Bay Area. His approach involves helping the client learn how to deal more effectively with the sources of his or her stress, using deep relaxation, biofeedback, and diet/exercise counseling in order to strengthen the body's ability to cope with stress. Dr. Michaels earned his Ph.D. in Clinical Psychology at Pacific Graduate School in Palo Alto.

Water: Nature's Elixir
Amelia Wright

Most of us realize how relaxing it is to enjoy a hot bath, or how refreshing a shower can be. Water is a natural healer. We acknowledge it as such constantly, in ways as simple as a relaxing cup of tea, or as complex as a trip to the ocean, where we immerse ourselves in the atmosphere it creates. We can use water as a healing agent more consciously in our daily lives as we learn more about its different uses. The benefits of different water temperatures, how to use compresses to relieve headaches, how to use herbs in baths and teas, and many more practical ideas and recipes are presented in this article.

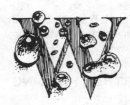ater is truly a virtuous element, as precious to life as the sun, air, and earth. What is more refreshing than a clean, cool glass of water to quench a thirst?

In this article I will illustrate some of the uses of water for soothing and relaxing the body, mind, and soul.

More than 80 per cent of our body consists of water. It is not only the vehicle by which nutrients are delivered to every cell throughout the body, but also the main factor in the removal of wastes in the elimination process. Water fills the double task of replenishing *and* cleansing. Our bodies need a constant supply of clean water to keep this cyclic nourishing and cleansing process in balance.

The amount of clean water you drink will directly affect how your body is able to eliminate toxins and wastes. All the eliminative organs (liver, kidney, colon, intestines, etc.) need water to perform. Our skin, the largest eliminating organ of all, needs water to help in the constant job of flushing out toxins and wastes through our pores. A steady supply of clean water helps to keep the skin open and clear.

BATHS AS WATER THERAPY

Baths have been used for soothing, healing, and cleansing the body for centuries. They can be relaxing and stimulating, and can aid in eliminating toxins and bacteria, as well as in healing the skin.

WATER THERAPY, HOT OR COLD?

The effects of water therapy can be explained in terms of the sympathetic nervous system, which is a delicate system of nerves that runs down the back on both sides of the spinal cord. These nerves are connected to every organ and area of the body. When these nerves are stimulated, soothed, or irritated, so is the rest of the body.

In general, *heat* increases surface circulation, dilates pores, and increases elimination through the skin. Prolonged heat is sedating, and may lead to sluggishness. *Cold* stimulates internally as well as superficially. It also increases the circulation while contracting the blood vessels and pores of the skin. The two used simultaneously will produce the most beneficial overall toning effect.

Water therapy can be used to stimulate the nervous system and brain. It acts as a toner, increases vitality, enhances all forms of elimination, and eases pain and fevers.

The following water treatments have been used for ages, and are powerful aids for restoring and maintaining health.

COMPRESSES

An excellent headache reliever is a hot compress on the back of the neck and a cold one on the forehead. Just take two washcloths or any other soft, absorbent, *natural* fiber material, and dip one in hot water and the other in cold. Wring them out and apply them to the skin. The warm cloth on the back of the neck has a soothing effect on the central nervous system throughout the body, and the cold cloth on the forehead has a clearing and refreshing effect

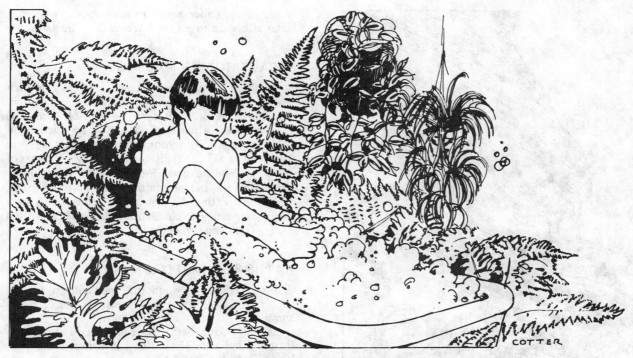

The peacefulness of the tub can be very mind-clearing as well as physically soothing.

on the head itself. The combination of relaxation and stimulation is a great aid in the relief of headache.

THE HIP OR SITZ BATH

Baths of alternating hot and cold water help restore health to all the organs of the lower back and pelvic area. Fill the bathtub at least half full with cold water, then sit in the water with your feet resting on a towel out of the water at the end of the bath. This bath should only last a few minutes. Follow the cold one with a hot one. Then follow with a cold again.

This combination of hot and cold stimulates and increases the tone of the nerves and organs of the entire pelvic and lower abdominal area.

THE FOOT BATH

The foot bath is a great source of pleasure as well as therapy. Using alternating pans of hot and cold water, just submerge your feet. Start with some warm, soapy water. This is good for sore, tired feet, calluses, and varicose veins. Let the water melt the tensions away. Follow with a short cold bath to restore energy and tone. Then briskly dry the feet with a towel. For a real treat for yourself or someone

else, follow the bath with a soothing foot massage, using light oil to soften and soothe your touch.

FULL BATHS

Hot baths are excellent for relieving aches and pains of tired muscles. They are particularly helpful for insomnia. A nice warm bath before bed can help to induce a peaceful sleep and pleasant dreams.

Remember any hot or warm bath should be followed by a cool shower or rinse-off to increase the benefits and restore muscle tone and circulation, which get sluggish during a warm or hot bath.

BATH ENHANCERS

The following additions to your bath water have been used for centuries.

Oils

Add your favorite kind of oil to your water. I suggest olive or almond oil. You don't need much; just add two or three tablespoons to your bath and soak it up. This treatment nourishes the skin by restoring the oil often lost during bathing, and leaves your skin feeling moist and silky smooth.

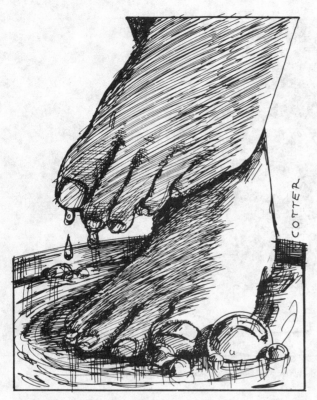

The foot bath is a great source of pleasure as well as therapy.

Herbal Combinations

A combination of chamomile, comfrey, and peppermint added to bath water is relaxing to the body, healing to the skin, and a mild decongestant in the steam. Mix two parts of chamomile to one part each of peppermint and comfrey. Add this to a quart of water that has boiled. Turn off the heat, and let it steep for 15 to 20 minutes. Then strain the water into your bath, relax, and enjoy.

Baking Soda, Epsom or Mineral Salts, and Apple Cider Vinegar Baths

All of these have been used for the relief of muscle pain, for dry, itchy skin (particularly from sunburn, poison oak, or poison ivy), for inducing perspiration (therefore eliminating toxins), preventing colds after a chill, and generally for relaxing and soothing: an all-round remedy for just about anything that may ail you. One cup of any of them is good for a general effect. Up to three cups can be used for more therapeutic purposes. Make the water hot enough to relax you, but warm enough to allow you to stay in for a

while. Again, remember to rinse or shower with cold water afterward to get the full benefit of the bath.

A SALT RUB OR MASSAGE

A salt rub or massage is excellent before your bath to clear away dead skin, and to increase circulation. Sea salt is the most effective, because of its mineral content. Make a paste of salt and water, then vigorously massage it into your skin. This should feel very invigorating. Do not apply to cuts or any rash areas of the body, and leave on for only about ten minutes. To remove the salt, slip into a warm bath or shower, and follow with a cool one. This treatment is especially stimulating to circulation, and should leave you feeling fresh and invigorated.

BATHS FOR CHILDREN

Warm baths are a wonderful, tried and true way to enable children who are overtired and/or overstimulated to mellow out and relax Just supply some simple, fun bath toys and perhaps some non-irritating bubbles. The water and its nurturing qualities will do the rest. I have seen *many* cranky moods transformed into happy ones by the soothing effect of water.

LUXURY BATHS

This is my favorite. Choose your favorite addition to the bath: bubbles, oils, herbs, salts, or whatever combination you prefer. Turn off the light and light up a candle. Light some incense, and put on your favorite music to relax to. Then treat yourself to a nice slow soak. Keep the water at a temperature that is comfortable and soothing. Just let the water wash away your tensions, worries, and extra thoughts. This bath is also doubly enjoyable when shared with a friend.

HOT TUBS

Hot tubs are merely the latest expression of a very old practice of bathing, healing, and socializing.

Many ancient cultures—Roman, Egyptian, Greek, Turkish, and Japanese—have histories of communal bathing. For the wealthy, it was a luxurious accomodation for the enjoyment of the home owner and family and friends. In a more practical sense, for poorer communities the bath was a place to share the luxury of bathing water.

Relaxing Teas and Foods
Amelia Wright

Chamomile tea. Mix three tablespoons chamomile with one tablespoon peppermint tea to one quart of boiling water. Do not boil the herbs. Let them steep for ten or twenty minutes. This tea calms the nerves, aids digestion, and helps produce a peaceful sleep.

Skullcap is a strong nervine that not only calms the nerves, but also feeds and nourishes them. One teaspoon to one cup boiling water will do the trick.

Vervaine is also a strong nervine, especially good for sleep. One tablespoon to boiling water is the recommended dose.

You can experiment with any of the herbs mentioned above by combining them to find the right balance to suit your needs. You can increase the proportions, make a larger amount, and sip it all day. *Honey* and *peppermint* are good for producing the flavor that suits your palate.

Foods that are high in *calcium* are also good for the nerves. Some of these are sunflower seeds, carrots, cucumber, yogurt, parsley, and comfrey tea.

Salt is a stimulant, and we Americans eat far too much of it. If you have trouble resting at night, eliminate or reduce the amount of salt in your evening meal. There are many salt substitutes that are also nourishing. A trip to your local health-food store will show you a wealth of foods, teas, and vitamins that will help you to change your diet pleasantly, and convert to eating habits that are pleasurable as well as beneficial to you.

Therapeutically, all the benefits previously ascribed to hot baths followed by a cool rinse are true with hot tubs as well.

The hot tubs offer the opportunity to soak at leisure in warm water deep enough to fully submerge your whole body. Most home bathtubs are just not deep enough to allow you to sit with water up to your neck. Hot tubs are usually big enough to allow some form of floating, giving the relaxation that only total buoyancy and weightlessness can provide.

Hot tubs are not used for cleansing; always rinse off before entering one. Many individuals with

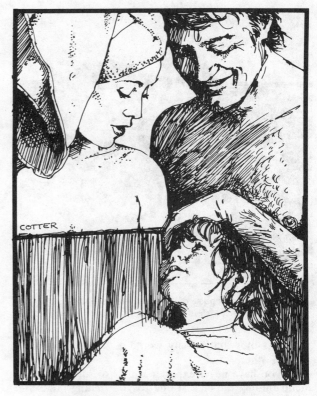

A hot tub is a beautiful way for family and friends to relax, and share time together.

chronic physical discomfort because of arthritis, poor circulation, or damaged muscle tissue have hot tubs in their homes or on their property to experience the daily relief from their aches and pains.

A hot tub in any home for the aging would be of great service. Many older people stay away from regular bathtubs because of the danger of slipping, but most hot tubs are made of wood and have comfortable benches for sitting on. With the correct application of warm water, the time spent in the hot tub will give an older person (or anyone, for that matter) great pleasure and relief from stress or pains.

The peacefulness of the tub can be very mind-clearing as well as physically soothing.

Communal bathing is a beautiful way for family and friends to relax, be nourished, and share intimate time in a nonthreatening way. Hot tubbing can make some very positive contributions to family relations. Parents and children very often have such different schedules of activity that it is hard for them to share even mealtimes, let alone relaxation and recreation. But the shared pleasure of the hot tub is appreciated by everyone, and I have seen families gathered around

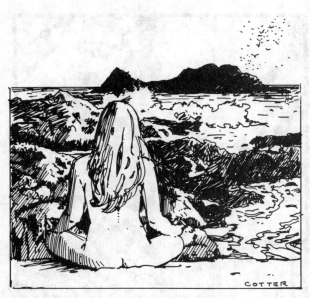

Meditating on the pulse of the ocean—where water and sky, spirit and Earth, meet—offers a feeling of peace and rejuvenation.

their hot tubs that usually would be seeing very little of each other.

If you have never experienced a hot tub, I recommend finding the closest one to you, taking yourself and anyone else whose company you enjoy, and finding out what a pleasure they can be.

WATER AS A SPIRITUAL SYMBOL

Water has been used as a symbol for the subconscious, the female principle, psychic perception, intuition, and countless other metaphors throughout literature and art. In the *I Ching*, water is suggested as personal power. It is water's nature to fill up a vessel and to continue to spill over. In times of turmoil or inner confusion, it is good to become still and silent. This resting period gives one a chance to quietly sort things out and regain perspective. Then the sense of

purpose and personal power is allowed to grow and become clear again. Just like the constantly overflowing water from the full vessel, the strength from within is allowed to flow out.

I would like to suggest the following simple meditation to use for relaxing the body, mind, and spirit.

OCEAN HORIZON MEDITATION

When at the ocean, just simply gaze at the perfect line of the horizon; the place where water and sky, spirit and Earth, meet. This meeting represents the perfect balance and harmony in nature. Imagine your own body rhythms matching the evenness of that line. Take your time, and let your breathing become deep and calm. You will start to feel a rhythmic dance between your breathing and the pulse of the ocean. Stay with this feeling as long as it is comfortable. You will walk away with a quiet mind and a great feeling of peace and rejuvenation.

SUGGESTIONS FOR FURTHER READING

Jethro Kloss, *Back to Eden.* 1939, 1976.
Fr. Kneipp, *My Water Cure.* 1886.
Vincent Priessnitz, *The Cold Water Cure.* 1843.

These books, plus others on hydrotherapy, are available from Health Research, P.O. Box 70, Mokelumne Hill, CA 95245.

Amelia Wright, co-editor of the Holistic Health Handbook *and the* Holistic Health Lifebook, *is a former administrator at the Berkeley Holistic Health Center. As an expression of her longterm interest in all aspects of health, she has lectured and taught introductory classes in holistic health; she is now a minister with the healing Church of the Gentle Brothers and Sisters in San Francisco.*

Art and Relaxation: Recreate Yourself
Cathryn M. Keller

Art and creative expression come from the inside out, from our private feelings out to visual expression. The following article addresses the expression of art as a means of relaxation. As a healing outlet for tension and hidden feelings, creative expression is a tremendous tool for learning at very deep levels. Ms. Keller suggests a variety of techniques and exercises to be used for fun, self-realization, and relaxation.

"I grew up pretty much as everybody else grows up, and one day . . . found myself saying . . . 'I can't live where I want to, I can't go where I want to, I can't do what I want to, I can't even say what I want to.' School and things that painters have taught me even keep me from painting as I want to. I decided I was a very stupid fool not to at least paint as I wanted to and say what I wanted to when I painted, as that seemed to be the only thing I could do that didn't concern anybody but myself—that was nobody's business but my own. So these paintings and drawings happened. . . . I found that I could say things with color and shapes that I couldn't say in any other way —things that I had no words for."

Georgia O'Keefe, 1923

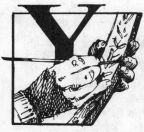ou don't have to be an artist to experience the healing powers of art, nor do you have to strain and stretch your salary at expensive weekend workshops. Whether it's at home, in a museum, or outdoors, you can refresh, revitalize, and renew yourself by means of the process of creative expression. Involvement in artistic exploration is inherently therapeutic and holistic, because it offers a unique opportunity to unite the mental, emotional, physical, and spiritual aspects of being.

The art projects described here offer a variety of ways to explore the dynamic tensions between chaos and order, spontaneity and control, mastery and letting go. By tuning in to your creative sources, you can discover your vision of yourself and your world. Since art is an intuitive means of symbolic speech, it can reveal feelings and conflicts, and problem-solving may result, in both predictable and unpredictable ways.

Getting started on any kind of artistic endeavor can be somewhat difficult for anyone whose earlier attempts were squelched by those familiar criticisms; *"That's* not what a tree looks like!" "Who taught *you* to draw?" We need to unlearn those rigid, structured "rules" about what is or isn't art. The personality traits that play a central role in creativity are spontaneity, imagination, intuition, originality, perception, excitement, and inspiration. Those traits exist in all of us and are closely associated with what many refer to as the "free child" part of us, rather than the "adapted child"—the part that learned to be good and color within the lines. Acknowledging that you want to let your expressive aspects flourish and grow will, at the very least, lead to some refreshing, stimulating experiences. The following art projects will help stimulate creativity. The main point, however, is to have fun and enjoy the relaxing, unfolding process.

SUPPLY SOURCES

Depending on what you're doing—drawing, sculpture, various crafts—important supply sources include art-supply stores (the larger the better); hardware stores for inexpensive brushes; and the local butcher, print shop, or computer center for paper. Five-and-ten or discount stores (the junkier the better) can be a terrific source of unexpected treasures—fingerpaints, watercolors, glitter, gold stars, colored construction paper. Drafting supply stores carry a wide variety of unique pens and pencils, rulers, paper; and great rubber stamps. In the beginning you might want to stock up on some crayons, oil pastels, or powdered tempera (it's easy to mix and you only need the basic colors—red, yellow, blue, black, and white). You'll also need paper in the largest size possible (butcher or wrapping paper, or newsprint pads). You might also want to start thinking about collecting things to use in a collage, mobile, weaving, or sculpture. Let your imagination really go crazy here. You can use just about anything—shells, rocks, seeds, roots, rusty metal, rubber from an old tire, springs from a bed, the label off a can, the can itself. Look for things at the beach, in a park, an empty lot, trash cans, salvage and wrecking yards, your own front yard. Explore familiar and unfamiliar environments with new eyes.

WARM-UP EXERCISES

If you can't wait to get your hands into the paint or clay, by all means go to it. Otherwise, you might want to quiet your mind first and let go of troublesome thoughts. Relax, turn some music on, swing your arms around, and feel the blood tingling in your hands. You might want to try some meditation techniques that help enhance creativity. Some good examples can be found in the chapter on "Autogenic Training" in *The Holistic Health Handbook*.

Some simple exercises for getting started require only paper and crayons, oil pastels, or paint. Select a color that represents the way you feel right now. Don't plan on drawing anything specific, just move the crayon or brush around on the paper in time to some music or your own inner rhythms, in whatever pattern feels right. If you're angry or happy about something, express those feelings on the paper. You might want to try writing your name in a special way that expresses who you are, or maybe you wish you

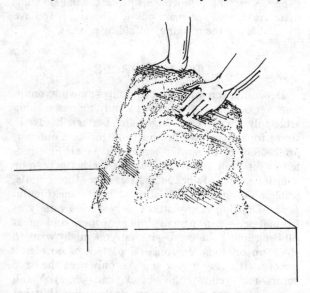

Clay is one of the easiest and least expensive sculpture materials to work with, and it feels so good to touch.

had another name. Write it. If you're righthanded, try drawing with your left hand, and vice versa. This will bring you right back to being a child. After drawing or painting like this for awhile, observe how you feel and what you learn.

YOUR BODY, YOUR SELF

You'll need paper large enough to lie on for this project, and help from a friend. (If you can't find large wrapping paper, tape sheets of newsprint together.) Lie down on the paper and have your friend trace an outline of your body on it. Do this again on another piece of paper. Now color in one of the outlines according to how you feel. Tune in to your body. Be especially aware of any areas of discomfort or illness, and select colors and symbols to express them. Where do you feel especially good, strong, sexy, warm, cold, hungry, sad, hurt? Set the first drawing aside and think about what you've just done. Maybe some problems surfaced as a result of the drawing—problems that existed before, but now you're more aware of them. You might want to do something to make yourself feel better. Maybe moving around for awhile would help, or maybe you feel like screaming or pounding some pillows. Maybe you'd just like to forget the whole thing and curl up and take a nap.

Get out the second outline and color it in, once again observing your feelings and expressing them. (Ideally, if your friend is still around, have him or her trace a new outline. Notice how you position yourself on the paper this time. Are you any looser or less tense than before?) Now put the "before" and "after" outlines side by side and compare them. What have you learned about yourself?

CLAY

This is one of the easiest and least expensive sculpture materials to work with, and it feels so good to touch. You can pull it, sock it, shove it, smooth it, and squeeze it through your fingers. Whether you use colored modeling clay from the five-and-ten, or potter's clay from an art store, let the sensations in your hands guide you. Do you feel like making simple baskets, pencil holders, or hand prints? Or do you just want to pound for awhile?

Making an image of yourself out of clay can be a revelation. Don't be concerned about making an exact replica; symbolic or abstract images may be the best way to express who you are right now. What do you or don't you like about your self-portrait? If you're dissatisfied with some aspects, change them.

FOOD SCULPTURE

There are many ways to use food to create sculpture. (Think about the physical images fruit and vegetables bring to mind.) One of the easiest and most enjoyable types of food sculpture is cake art—cakes shaped and decorated in just about any image you like. Do your face, or a friend's, or a part of your body you're proud of—a breast, a long leg, a muscular arm. Just bake a large sheet cake and carve out the desired image. (You don't have to carve a perfect image, since you can create shapes by dabbing frosting here and there.) You can use food coloring in the frosting or on shredded coconut for the hair, or carrot curls for red hair; cherries for a mouth; white Chiclets for teeth. This is an especially rewarding thing to do with children. Their ideas for cake decorating are quite often completely unorthodox and totally wonderful, although not always edible (uncooked macaroni for curly blonde hair!). Also, if the two of you are sculpting your face, a child's perception of what you look like can be very revealing.

SOFT SCULPTURE

Three-dimensional, sewn, stuffed sculptures are wonderful to look at and touch. If you know how to use a sewing machine, then you might want to give it a try. Start with something easy like a quarter moon out of silver satin, or gold lamé stars. Simply draw the image on paper and use that as a pattern on the material. Stuff it with dacron or fiber-fil. Later you might want to try something more ambitious like a giant, smiling red mouth; a huge crayon or pencil; a rainbow, or fluffy white clouds to hang from the ceiling; a cactus; or a life-size doll of yourself.

BATIK AND TIE-DYE

It's easy to achieve spectacular results with minimal effort when you do batik or tie-dye. Whether it's a wall-hanging or a T-shirt, the process more or less takes over, and you don't have to worry about how well you draw. Simply dip a brush into melted wax, swirl it around on the material, and watch fluid, sensual shapes emerge. When you dye it, the color goes where there isn't any wax. There are numerous how-to books on these fiber crafts and those that follow.

WEAVING

The ancient craft of weaving isn't nearly as difficult as it seems. In fact, you don't even need an elaborate loom. You can make your own by winding

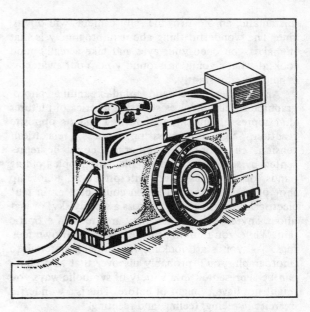

The wonderful thing about photography is that it makes you open your eyes and take a good look at what's around you.

yarn around a door frame, a bamboo hoop, or nails hammered along the edges of a wooden crate. Instead of yarn, you might want to use rope or twine from boating supply stores, or tightly twisted pieces of material. Explore the endless possibilities for incorporating shells, driftwood, seeds, copper wire, or even nuts and bolts in the weaving. You can also dye your own yarn with flowers, grass, berries, coffee grounds, tea, artichokes, radishes, onions, or even weeds from the yard. These natural dyes provide much softer and more muted colors than commercially-dyed yarn.

KNITTING, CROCHETING, EMBROIDERY, AND NEEDLEPOINT

The relaxing and sanity-restoring qualities of these more "common" fiber crafts have been known to women for centuries. If some of them appeal to you, yarn stores are invariably staffed by people who are happy to show you how to get started. If you're the type of person who has a hard time justifying "just" relaxing in front of the TV or sitting around listening to music, then you might find that by getting those knitting needles going, the puritanical demon inside who is telling you to produce will relax!

PHOTOGRAPHY

You don't have to have an expensive Nikon or Ansel Adams' touch to enjoy photography. An

Instamatic, an old Brownie—any camera—will do just fine. The wonderful thing about photography is that it makes you open your eyes and take a really good look at what's going on around you. Your awareness is heightened instantly.

An excellent eye- and mind-expanding photographic exercise involves shooting a series of pictures that represent any kind of feeling and its opposite reaction, e.g., loneliness/togetherness, relaxation/tension, chaos/order. Togetherness could be represented by something obvious, like two people holding hands, or, for a less literal interpretation, a close-up shot of peas in a pod. Tension could be seen in taut electrical wires suspended across a stormy sky, or just about anyone's face when they are stuck in a traffic jam. While you're doing this, examine your own feelings. As you start looking for subject material to photograph, you'll probably discover that all feelings can be represented in a variety of symbolic ways you might not have thought of before. This is a wonderful exercise in seeing, feeling, and reacting.

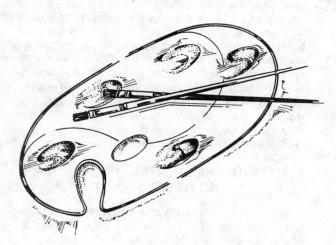

CREATE A NEW ENVIRONMENT FOR YOURSELF

We sometimes forget how relaxing and satisfying it can be to redecorate and do little things around the house. Beautifying and improving the spaces you spend a lot of time in gives a sense of accomplishment, and it says a lot about who you are or who you've become. Think about how colors and images affect you. You might want to paint your bedroom in a soft, soothing, sensual color, or indulge in your secret desire for a room in bold, Chinese red. You might want to build some shelves, perhaps for displaying collections or mementoes. If you have boxes full of old photographs, scrapbooks, or sketchbooks, display them on a shelf or mount some of the pictures and hang them on the wall. Spending some time reordering the images and tokens you've saved from the past can be a profoundly moving experience.

RELAX

As you learn to value relaxation more and more, you will probably realize that you don't always have to be "doing." Absorbing inspiration from external sources can be extremely revitalizing. One way to do this is by going to art or science museums, zoos, and planetariums. Out-of-the-way historical museums in small towns are often rich with unique folk art. If you're looking for design ideas or are intrigued by a certain type of art, take a sketchbook along, make yourself comfortable, and draw. You can also check out a stack of art books from the library and treat yourself to hours of continued pleasure at home.

Artistic endeavors can be thoroughly enjoyable and relaxing, especially if you don't take them too seriously. Despite what the teacher said about your purple tree with the striped leaves back in the first grade, there's really no one way to interpret art. So indulge, play, create, and enjoy!

SUGGESTIONS FOR FURTHER READING

Anthea Callen, *Women Artists of the Arts and Crafts Movement*. Pantheon Books, 1979.

Robert McKim, *Experiences in Visual Thinking*. Brooks-Cole, 1973.

Carla Needleman, "Potter's Progress, Self-Understanding and the Lessons of Craft." *Psychology Today*, June 1979.

Kimon Nicolaides, *The Natural Way to Draw*. Houghton Mifflin, 1969.

Janie Rhyne, *The Gestalt Art Experience*. Brooks-Cole, 1973.

Cathryn M. Keller is a filmmaker, editor, writer, and occasional art teacher.

Section III:
Mind/Spirit
Psychological, Spiritual, and Ontological Well-Being

"Man is made by his belief. As he believes, so he is."
Bhagavad Gita

"Disease is a kind of consolidation of a mental attitude, and it is only necessary to treat the mind of a patient and the disease will disappear."
Dr. Edward Bach

"There is now incontrovertible evidence that mankind has just entered upon the greatest period of change the world has ever known. The ills from which we are suffering have had their seat in the very foundation of human thought. But today something is happening to the whole structure of human consciousness. A fresh kind of life is starting."
Pierre Teilhard de Chardin

"The kingdom of God is within you."
Luke 17:21

"Take responsibility for your every thought, your every feeling, your every action."
Fritz Perls

"The most beautiful experience we can have is the mysterious. It is the fundamental emotion which stands at the cradle of true art and true science; whoever does not know it and can no longer wonder, no longer marvel, is as good as dead, and his eyes are dimmed."
Albert Einstein

Introduction
MIND/SPIRIT: Psychological, Spiritual, and Ontological Well-Being

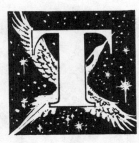

The basis of Holistic Health is the philosophy of an integrated body/mind/spirit. Yet people who accept and talk about the connection of bodymind sometimes are confused by how to fit spirit into the picture. This section could just as easily have been called body (physical and environmental), mind, and spirit, because it is truly impossible to separate one from the other. These aspects of self are all interwoven, and any divisions are simply an attempt to be a bit more specific. The feeling of well-being that comes from a healthy body is a mental and spiritual experience. And often the most spiritual experiences of a lifetime come through a recognition of the beauty of nature, or the miracle of physical life.

In this section we deal specifically with the aspects of the inner life that we call mind and spirit. We have tried to present material that will give you different vantage points for viewing the mind/spirit, thus giving you different vantage points for viewing the mind/spirit, thus giving you fresh insights, as well as practical information and exercises to enable you to experiment with some of these approaches.

All the great spiritual teachings of the world have reminded us in countless ways that the kingdom of God is within us. The richness of our inner lives is what gives meaning to the outer. "All is one" is the great Buddhist maxim. Holism is basically a spiritual concept, one of its underlying principles being the interdependence and interrelatedness of every aspect of life. Everything exists in relationship to everything else. The more consciousness and awareness we can cultivate, the more wholeness and interrelatedness we can experience in our lives. In this section we present different approaches to aspects of the mind/spirit. The psychologies, philosophies, research on right/left brain and holographic theory, psychic counseling, and various spiritual approaches represented here can all offer us a tool of fresh insight for the further evolution of our own consciousness, our own mind/spirit.

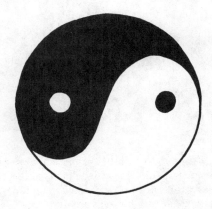

151

Mind/Spirit Survey
How well does each statement describe your patterns
of thought and action?

1. I experience peace of mind.
2. I am not irritable or annoyed by little things.
3. I am not at the mercy of my emotions.
4. I find constructive ways to express my feelings.
5. I have a positive self-image.
6. I can hear and evaluate criticism for what it's worth.
7. I feel a balance in giving and receiving energy.
8. I use some form of mental techniques that are helpful to me.
9. I feel a spiritual base and purpose in my life.
10. My religious affiliation is a source of inspiration in my life.
11. My background has given spirituality a positive connotation.
12. I view life's lessons as opportunities to gorw in spiritual understanding.
13. I believe the planet is currently undergoing a spiritual transformation.
14. There are many paths that lead to heightened spiritual awareness.
15. Material comfort is not as important to me as spiritual understanding.

Practical Metaphysics: Attuning the Mind
Lorin Piper

Implicit in holistic health is the idea of self-responsibility, the belief that we are the creators of our own lives. This may seem like an impractical and abstract concept if you have no idea how your own reality is created. However, we create our realities very simply, by our thoughts and beliefs. A healthy mental attitude will produce a healthy life. In this article Lorin Piper presents information to give us a deeper understanding of how our beliefs create our reality, as well as some exercises and suggestions to help us experience this relationship directly and consciously.

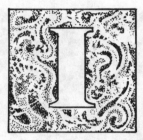nside each of us is the knowledge of how special and unique we are. We treasure our own individual consciousness and the life that has formed it. Each of us desires to take his or her uniqueness and express it in the world, to live life to the fullest extent imaginable. Often we find that what keeps us from doing so are our thoughts and beliefs about ourselves, others, and our relationship to the world. In this article I will offer some ways of uncovering and working with these thoughts and beliefs by the use of practical metaphysics, and I will present the idea of a spiritual basis for life as the source of meaning and motivation for our existence.

WHAT IS METAPHYSICS?

The term metaphysics is translated from the Greek as "after physics," and is commonly used to mean "beyond the physical." By "practical metaphysics" I mean to show how theories about what lies beyond the physical can be used in a practical and tangible way in our lives. As one of my teachers once said, "The purpose of meditation is to have a happier life, not to meditate better or longer." The purpose of metaphysics is the same. We can use metaphysical techniques to rid ourselves of any self-imposed limitations, and to express our lives freely and naturally. Just as the laws of physics and gravity are built on theory, but can be used to send rockets to the moon, we are able to use certain mental techniques to create tangible realities right here on Earth.

WE CREATE OUR OWN REALITIES

The first time I heard the idea that we create our own reality, I was puzzled. I felt as though I'd been told that my problems were all my fault. Up until that time, I thought my problems were basically caused by sources outside myself—my parents, my boyfriends, and society in general. So it was quite a jolt to be told that I had created this life that I wasn't so happy with. Fortunately, there is a great advantage to this belief. If you have the power to create something that has made you unhappy, you also have the power to create what makes you happy. This all made sense to me one day when I heard someone say, "There are two kinds of people in the world. There are happy people, and there are people looking for reasons to be happy." At that point I chose to be a happy person. As soon as I realized I had a choice in the matter, things could change. Changing old negative beliefs about ourselves is a way to change our lives, and to consciously create our own reality.

A belief is an assumption about reality that we hold as an absolute truth. Our beliefs are our personal truths, the foundations of our lives. Belief is the creator of experience; the mind is the creator of our beliefs. Therefore, the mind is the determiner (and chooser) of our experience. We can learn to attune the mind. We may not always be able to control it, but we can choose where we focus it, what power we give it. A basic metaphysical principle is, "As you attune, you receive." A very common way of saying this is, "What you see is what you get." This simply means that what you focus on, give your attention to, is what will appear in your life. We create our lives by our thoughts and words, beliefs and imaginations. What we hold in our minds becomes the reality of our lives. We attract to ourselves naturally what we have in our minds. If we see something in our lives that we don't like, we can look within, and examine our thoughts and beliefs about it.

THE SUBCONSCIOUS MIND

Our belief creates our physical reality by means of the subconscious mind. The subconscious mind does not reason. It accepts and acts on whatever is put into it. For this reason it is sometimes called our willing servant. And for this reason, what we put into it is very important.

When modern psychology first told us about the subconscious mind, it was envisioned as a dark, murky place full of uncontrollable fears and desires. People tried either to avoid it completely or, if they couldn't avoid it, to confront it by means of psychoanalysis. It was seen as a kind of battle between the clear and rational, and the unclear and uncontrollable. But our subconscious is a valuable and creative aspect of ourselves. It acts as a meeting place for our inner and outer lives. Thoughts and beliefs from the conscious mind are impressed on the subconscious and become the underlying cause of our life. Deeper knowledge and desires from universal mind appear in the subconscious, to be seen and examined in the form of dreams, images, and feelings.

The subconscious creates by means of the universal mind. The universal mind is the result of the synergy of individual consciousness, which creates a super-consciousness, another dimension of mind. We are constantly creating and receiving through the universal mind, which is a constantly evolving body of all accumulated knowledge, thoughts, and energies. It is the energy field through which thoughts or ideas are transmitted nonverbally, or through which psychic events occur.

This is how our belief creates our physical reality: when we accept or formulate a belief in our conscious mind, our subconscious, our willing servant, accepts it, and puts it into the universal subconscious, which manifests it. A very simple example of this is a person with self-confidence, who believes in himself, and who expects to be liked by others. Of course, people do like such a person. People intuit the confidence and liking of the person and act accordingly. A more subtle example is someone who says, "I catch a cold every January," and does. The belief creates the experience as precisely as the other person's self-confidence generates positive responses.

Thus, our reality is not an elusive experience. It is something we create, either mindfully or uncon-

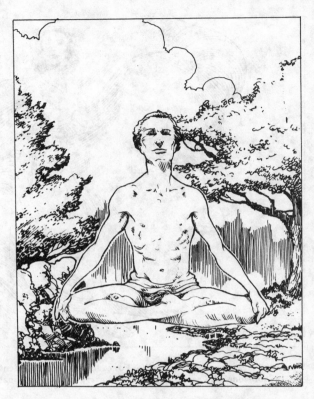

The purpose of meditation is to have a happy life, not meditate better or longer.

sciously. As we look at our outer life and see how we are creating it, we can assume responsibility for ourselves. With this responsibility comes power, the power to choose and create freely. We become the authorities in our lives.

At the same time we are experiencing this authority in our outer lives, many of us are learning to experience receptivity in our inner lives. We are finding deep within ourselves the stillness, the transcendence, and the creative energy we are seeking.

We are arriving at this from many different paths. From jogging, relaxation techniques, the various mental and psychological approaches, art forms, crafts, as well as meditation, yoga, and psychic exploration, people are reporting varied but similar experiences. These experiences all seem to share a state of consciousness wherein a person knows himself as a being in union with what feels like "the infinite." People who experience this union consider it one of the most inspiring and fulfilling moments of their lives. We've heard it spoken of many times, in many words. Transcendence, the Tao, cosmic consciousness are some of the terms that have been used for it. But this

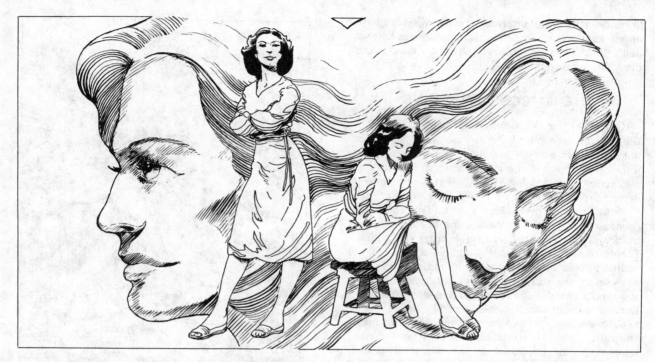

Belief creates our physical reality. For example, a self-confident person who believes in himself can expect to be liked by others—
or, someone who says, "I catch a cold every January," probably will get sick.

is not a state of consciousness reserved for "an enlightened being." It is available to all of us who are willing to open up and be receptive to our inner selves.

The inner self is always available to us. It is our source of guidance, inspiration, motivation, and creative energy. We can cultivate it by any of the previously mentioned ways. My personal favorites are meditation and dream journals. But the most important thing to remember is to listen to it and respect it. The thoughts, images, dreams, and intuitions that pass through our minds are not meaningless. We can pay attention to them and learn to know ourselves. To unify the inner and outer lives, to carry out into the world that transcendence and unity we find within, is to be truly a unified and whole being.

A MEDITATION FOR CONTACTING THE INNER SELF

This meditation can be used to contact the inner self in whatever form you desire. You can receive guidance from the inner voice, experience peace, or feelings of love, or power. Only two things are necessary for this. One is the willingness to believe that this is possible, and the other is a quiet place. Find a place where you won't be disturbed, and sit in a comfortable position with your spine straight. The basic steps are very simple.

1. Close your eyes.

2. Make peace with the noises, lights, and sensations of your environment. Do this by making statements like "I make peace with noises. They do not disturb me."

3. Relax the physical body. You can use autogenic techniques or deep breathing exercises.

4. Relax your conscious mind. Say to your thoughts and ideas, "Peace, be still, peace, peace."

5. Relax the subconscious mind. Say to your pictures, feelings, emotions, and memories, "Relax, relax, be still."

6. Move your attention to the silence within. You can say, "deeper, deeper." Ask your inner self to unify with you. State what it is you want (the answer to a problem, a feeling of support) and relax into the experience.

When you feel finished, say "thank you" to your inner self. To come back, work through the sequence in reverse order, thanking and giving your attention to the subconscious and conscious minds, the physical body, and finally, the environment. I like to ritualize the end of my meditation by taking three breaths, opening my eyes, and saying "I am aware and alert."

Don't be disappointed if it doesn't all happen at once. Be willing to take your time, and be patient. At times I'll ask a specific question and think nothing has happened. An hour later, the answer jumps up to consciousness. Also, don't worry about time. Meditate for the amount of time that is perfect for you, be it five minutes or an hour. And use your conscious rational mind to examine what happened. If you received guidance to do something that doesn't make much sense, use your rational mind to decide if it's nonsense, or something you really want to do. After all, it's your inner self.

UNDERSTANDING THE EMOTIONS

Our emotions are our reactions to our mental processes. They are what move us mentally, impel us into action, and cause change. A healthy mental-emotional balance is the ability to experience one's emotions, as well as the ability to examine the thoughts causing them.

Often people think that getting in touch with and experiencing their emotions is the primary healing experience. Some people think of emotions as being stronger and more real than thoughts. But it is our thought that creates our emotion. As Seth (a personality channeled through Jane Roberts) says, "As you think, so you feel, and not the other way around." Although it is essential to know the emotional self, the emotional self is not the true essence of who we are, any more or less than the body or mind.

An example of thought creating emotion would be to think of something sad. The normal reaction is to feel sad. For years I would cry every time I remembered my dog dying when I was little. If you think of a sad time, you can experience sadness. If you think of something that makes you happy, you can likewise experience feeling happy. One thought will usually be associated with another, so that if you are thinking of a pleasant experience, you will probably go on to think of other pleasant experiences. Our thought and emotions magnetize similar thoughts and emotions, within as well as without. Try saying something nice about yourself (that you can believe) and experience your feeling. Say something unkind about yourself and experience that feeling too. It is the conscious mind and our belief that generates our emotions.

Experiencing and expressing our emotions freely is always a healing experience, something that makes us more whole, and that creates a fuller expression of

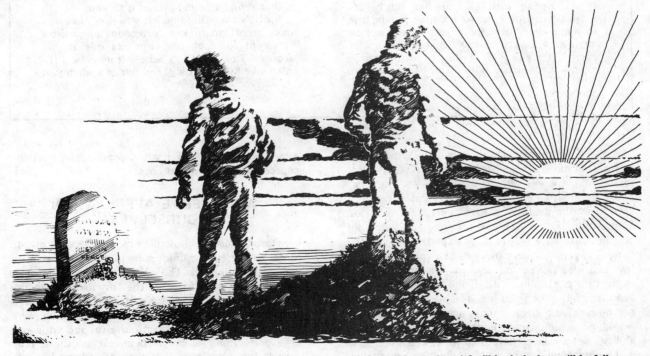

If a person allows himself to grieve and mourn freely over the death of a loved one, the grief will heal, the love will be fully experienced, and the bereaved person can move on to experience more love and life.

Examining Our Beliefs
and Reprogramming Them
by Affirmation
Lorin Piper

Examining our beliefs can be an infinite process, but let's start now with this simple exercise. Sit down with a pencil and paper, and begin to write down what you believe. Do this by saying, "I believe," and finishing that sentence. Write down everything that comes into your mind that you believe. Consider your beliefs about everything—yourself, others, the world, the physical, mental, spiritual, and environmental aspects of reality as you believe them to be. Consider your moral concepts, your ideas about childhood, old age, and money. When I first tried this exercise, I wrote down about twenty beliefs, ranging from "I believe the world is round," to "My father is an insensitive bully," to "I believe it must be difficult to be 80 years old." They all came off the top of my head, without much thought, and they gave me plenty to think about. These beliefs about reality are not the truth. They are only our beliefs, our personal truths. As we hold them to be true, we make them true for ourselves, and our experience is created by our belief. For example, when I perceived my father as an insensitive bully, a five-minute phone call became a gross imposition, instead of a simple five-minute phone call. When I thought it must be difficult to be 80, I dreaded the idea of my being 80. And so on, and so on, ad infinitum.

After you've made your list, look at it to see what makes you feel good and what doesn't. The beliefs that you like, and that seem to work for you, you can keep. The ones you don't like, that don't work for you, you can change.

"In order to dislodge unsuitable beliefs and establish new ones, you must learn to use your imagination to move concepts in and out of your mind."

Seth, in Roberts,
The Nature of Personal Reality

One way of reprogramming your beliefs is to introduce new beliefs into the conscious mind by means of affirmations. An affirmation is a positive statement that we tell ourselves in order to create the statement as a reality in our lives. For example, if you have been having financial problems that you want to solve, you could affirm (state) that you are abundantly provided for by the universe. Your mind will then attune to that abundance and attract it to you.

So let's take those beliefs you don't like and make an affirmation—a corresponding positive statement for each one. For example, if you wrote (as I once did), "I believe it must be difficult to be 80 years old," and felt bad when you

life. When we repress our emotions, we remove ourselves from life and becomes less of ourselves. For this reason many people differentiate between "primary" and "secondary" emotions. An example of this is grief over the death of a loved person. If a person allows himself to grieve and mourn freely, the grief will heal, the love will be fully experienced, and the bereaved person can move on to experience more love and life. The person who doesn't experience and express his grief holds onto it, and in holding onto it, keeps himself back from life. The possible confusion, nervousness, or bitterness that might result in this case would be a secondary emotion, caused by the inability to experience grief, the primary emotion.

Our emotions are the motion, the life of our being. We cannot deny or transcend them. We can, however, experience them, and try to identify and heal the source of any unpleasant ones.

WE DESERVE AFFIRMATION OURSELVES

Deep inside we know how special we each are. In order to express our uniqueness in the world, we must value it in ourselves. The only true motivation comes from a sense of self-worth. The only love we can give to others is the love we have in ourselves. We are all involved in a process, the process of becoming more fully ourselves. As we affirm ourselves and know our own perfection, we can recognize it in others. True love is the knowledge that each of us is on his own special journey to know himself more fully. Love is

read it, you could write out an affirmation that said, "Being 80 years old is a joyful, productive time." Give your beliefs the power to work for you, instead of against you.

GUIDELINES FOR AFFIRMATIONS

Here are some basic guidelines for writing out affirmations.

1. State your affirmation in the positive sense. State it without negatives (like "no," "not," "un-," or "without") and without conditions (like "if" or "but"). For example, say, "I am free from the desire or habit of smoking cigarettes," instead of, "I don't smoke."

2. State the affirmation in the present tense, as if it were happening right now. Don't put it in the future, or "someday." For instance, say, "I am perfectly healthy now," instead of, "I will get well in time for the party tomorrow."

3. Don't make comparisons with other times, places, or people. For example, say, "I make money easily," instead of, "I make money more easily than before," or, "I make money more easily than most people."

4. State the affirmations personally, in terms of yourself. Don't make them general, or oriented toward someone else. Try, "My life is full of interesting, loving friends," or, "I attract to myself the relationships I desire," not, "John realizes how great I am."

5. Take any negative reactions you have to your affirmations and turn them into new affirmations. This clears your mind of any "buts" or doubts.

Say your affirmations with all the conviction you have. Realize that this is the truth for you. I love to say affirmations, because it feels so good to experience the sensation of knowing that this is really the truth, this beautiful positive statement.

Some people write out each affirmation twenty times. Some put them on small file cards and carry them around with them, reading them several times a day. I like to put the affirmations I'm currently working with in a place where I'll see them every day, such as next to the mirror where I brush my hair. The idea is to impress these statements in your mind, thus letting them become the truth in your life. You don't have to look far and wide to consciously create your life. Just look at what you've created already. Look at your physical body, your relationships, your environment. Are you happy with them? Everything in your life that looks like a problem (illness, poverty, moodiness, contention), can be transformed. You can examine your beliefs to see what's causing you this grief. You can make every problem a growth situation, and get what you really want out of it, by having the courage to examine your beliefs, and work on changing the ones that are limiting you.

another word for the creative force of the universe, for what people call God. We may not be able to relate to all the words, but we all know what love is in one form or another. Love is outgoing, life-affirming; it sees the beauty in the world and in others. We all deserve appreciation and affirmation. One could start every day positively by saying, "I love myself," or by affirming one's being as simply as saying, "I am." As we affirm ourselves and our desires, we can create the lives we desire. It has been said that the purpose of life is to bring the unconscious up into consciousness. The many mental, psychic, psychological, and spiritual techniques available to us at this time can all be of help in fulfilling this purpose.

SUGGESTIONS FOR FURTHER READING

Aldous Huxley, *The Perennial Philosophy*. Harper and Row, 1970.

Ann and Peter Meyer, *Being a Christ*. Dawning Publications, 1975.

Jane Roberts, *The Nature of Personal Reality*. Prentice-Hall, 1974.

Lorin Piper holds a degree in prayer therapy through the Teaching of the Inner Christ, a nonsectarian metaphysical teaching. She has studied and worked with various types of meditations, psychic trainings, and metaphysical groups. She has served as an administrator for the Berkeley Holistic Health Center, and is a co-author of this book.

Jungian Psychology
Strephon Kaplan Williams, Ph.D.

The work of Swiss psychiatrist Carl Gustav Jung (1875–1961) is not easily summarized or explained. The most brilliant of Freud's early disciples, and often referred to by Freud as his successor, Jung finally broke with Freud about 1913 because he could not accept the central Freudian doctrine of repressed infant sexuality as the basis for neuroses.

Jung developed a highly complex theory, too transcendent for most psychologists, of basic human types, and of the collective as well as personal unconscious. Although Jung's collected works of more than 60 years fill more than 20 volumes, he disdained the idea of summarizing it, either in conversation or writing. The main focus of Jung's work was on the development of personality, the search for meaning, and the use of certain media (dreams, images, symbols, and journals) in order to know the inner and outer selves.

We are fortunate here that Strephon Williams has presented to us, simply and clearly, the basic concepts of Jungian psychology, as well as exercises to enable us to understand and make use of this great work.

"Everything good is costly, and the development of personality is one of the most costly of all things. It is a matter of saying yea to oneself, of taking oneself as the most serious of tasks, of being conscious of everything ·one does, and keeping it constantly before one's eyes in all its dubious aspects—truly a task that taxes us to the utmost."

Carl Jung

G. Jung was a monumental personality, in both his life and his work. Indeed, what is most important about Jung's personal psychology is his courage in dealing with his *own* unconscious. He transformed his personality, and lived the rest of his life deeply and spiritually attuned with his own archetypes, the energy centers of his essential being.

During Jung's lifetime he developed an extensive private practice, using his great healing powers for those who came to him from all over the world. He taught his psychology to many, and wrote more than twenty volumes on his approach.

Today Jungian psychology seems to be growing in influence in American cultural centers, but not in the psychology departments of universities. Could the increasing interest in Jung be due in part to a new openness to individual spiritual and psychic experience, which Jung's theories of the unconscious go a long way toward explaining? Jung's model, with his emphasis on wholeness, broadens psychology to include myth and other cultural arts. Many, besides therapists and their clients, are intensely interested in exploring archetypes. Such people include artists, writers, dancers, poets, cultural historians, as well as others from all walks of life.

JUNGIAN ANALYSIS, THERAPY, AND GROWTH

The ultimate goal of Jungian analysis is not to get a better job or relationship, or to solve a drinking problem (to use some typical examples). These and other everyday problems may be involved, but the central focus is the *realization of personality* as the key to life's meaning.

To realize one's personality is to develop one's abilities and personal characteristics, and to participate in the major life stages and experiences, as fully as possible. It is to follow the unique thread of one's own destiny, and to integrate all of oneself, by conscious activity, into a single whole.

Each individual is, of course, unique, but the following would be some of the central characteristics of a man actively realizing himself, using the Jungian approach.

JUNGIAN PERSONALITY VALUES

He would devote a certain part of each day and week to inner processes, such as working with dreams, with parts of himself, reflecting upon himself, using perhaps art work, and certainly journal work. This would become habitual, as a way of becoming conscious of the patterns or archetypes that underlie his behavior.

Included within the arena of what gradually undergoes examination would be his "myth of childhood," of how archetypal patterns formed, and what now needs changing and resolution. He looks at how he projects inner material from the unconscious into his environment, relationships, work situation, and so on. The result of this examination would be a developing sense of what he must do in order to integrate material evoked from inner and outer worlds.

Gradually there would develop a sense of center, of the unfolding of the central archetype of the Self by means of dreams and other primary intuitions. This would become at some stage a *spiritual* process, in the sense that the ego, or choice-maker, would become more and more devoted to manifesting "the other," or what the Self, the God within, wants in terms of meaning and direction in life.

Not everyone in Jungian analysis achieves this, of course, or is meant to. But somewhere along the line the initial *therapy* changes to *analysis.* Therapy deals primarily with problem solving, crises, and giving support and reflection to the client. Analysis deals with these concerns in terms of the underlying patterns within the psyche which produce the outer behavior. In addition, most people in analysis, as happened with Jung himself, must let go of many inadequate personality structures, and therefore come to face the full force of the unconscious. This may even precipitate what almost seems to be mental illness. When this stage is worked through, the individual emerges much transformed, and often with a profound religious sense, having found personal symbols and meaning for his life.

For those who do not go through the long-term process, there is still much that is healing in Jungian work. Processing childhood material to get free of parental problems and emerge into mature adulthood

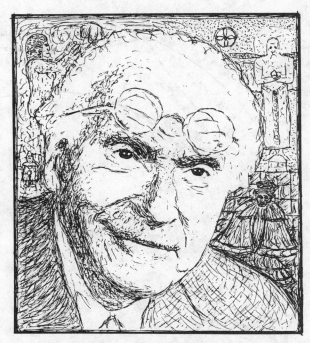

C. G. Jung in his later years. The brightness in his eyes and the warmth of his expression show the personal integration which was also the core of his psychology.

is one satisfying result of the Jungian approach. Getting unblocked and tuned in with sources within one's own unconscious can be one of the short-term goals. Discovering what we project onto our friends and lovers can go a long way in developing more effective relationships. Personal creativity and the sense of meaning are often enhanced. Major changes, crises, and stages of life all have their archetypal bases, and the Jungian model offers much toward making successful transitions.

A primary emphasis in the Jungian approach is on the search for meaning. In practical terms this means the developing of inner guides and directions by means of on-going dream work and other techniques for exploring the unconscious.

ARCHETYPAL STAGES RELATED TO MENTAL ILLNESS AND PERSONAL GROWTH

In terms of the stages of archetypal manifestation, the psychotic, or severely disturbed person, is generally fixated at an early symbolic level. Such a person's behavior is largely symbolic, full of bizarre and hallucinatory material, and lacks emotional feeling and conscious awareness. Treatment involves eliciting the

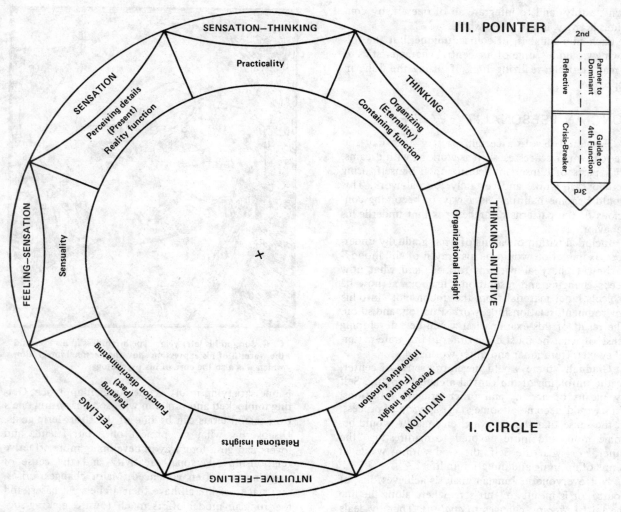

III. POINTER

I. CIRCLE

II. SQUARE

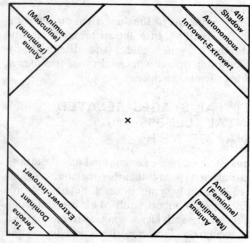

The Jungian Type and Function Wheel is a quick and reliable way to begin to understand one's typology, or predisposition to action. Trace or photocopy this page and cut out the square and pointer and pin them to the center of the wheel. You can move the square and pointer to various qualities on the disc to test out which might be your natural dominants. By applying this type and function wheel to yourself you will better understand the more natural way for you to approach relationships, careers, conflicts, or personal creativity. This can foster greater acceptance of yourself as you really are.

symbolic inner world of the psychotic, and working with him or her to get the symbols translated into emotional experience. Being imprisoned by a three-headed giant is translated into "What monsters in your own childhood and life today are dominating you?" The severely disturbed person is encouraged to experience the archetypes as feelings, and to build a stronger ego for dealing with these feelings. This leads to the final attainment of emotional, conceptual insight and action.

Many of us are merely somewhat self-defeating, because we suffer from only the most attenuated versions of the archetype. We are mostly overrational, fixed on overconceptualizing and on trying to control everything. The so-called "normal neurotic" usually experiences archetypes closer to the original source only in bouts of drunkenness, hypnagogic drug use, crises, sexual frenzy, religious ecstatic experiences, or some other type of heightened behavior.

People go into therapy and analysis when their rational systems of abstraction and control no longer work, and they suffer incursions of uncontrolled archetypal energy which endanger or overwhelm them. Suicidal urges, depressions, uncontrolled anger, failures of choice-making, inordinate fears, and a host of physical symptoms all point to a person's being out of relation to the archetypes, and therefore dominated by them.

The Jungian therapist and analyst works with such people to support them in reexperiencing their archetypal roots, and then bringing the experience back up the continuum into consciousness as a motivation for personal action and change.

Usually Jungian therapy and analysis happens one or two hours each week. The analysand, or client, sits face to face with the therapist-analyst, and brings up dreams, fantasies, feelings, and other inner experiences. These are then related to personality attitudes and dynamics and to outer situations of relationship, job creativity, and so on.

Reflection on what is happening may be combined with the use of active imagination processes applied to dreams and visionary experience. The therapist-analyst will also be receiving projections (the traditional transference) from the client's unconscious, and these are worked with as the dreams are.

At its best, Jungian psychology seeks to aid each individual in his or her own development, not to impose beliefs or judgments about what a person should or should not do or be. There are no dogmas in Jungian psychology. Each individual is unique. In the final analysis, an individual's "authority" comes from a place very deep within, which Jung has termed the archetype of the Self.

This uniqueness characterized Jung himself. He reportedly said several times, "Thank God I am not a Jungian!" It is this kind of openness which shows that one is securely in relation to one's own center rather than following someone else's authority.

THE ARCHETYPES AND HOW THEY OPERATE

At the base of all existence are energy clusters, or *archetypes* of innate character, energy, and function. The most primary of these may be arranged in a crystal (Figure 2) with the Self, the central archetype, at the center. Surrounding the Self in pairs of opposites are the other primary archetypes: the Feminine, the Masculine, the Adversary, the Heroic, Death-Rebirth, and the Journey (see also Figure 3).

An archetype is an innate pattern within the psyche and within all life. We see the archetypes play themselves out, mostly automatically, in our lives. People go through a developmental journey process all their lives, yet also fall into crises, death-rebirth, and new directions. At times of real clarity and growth, we choose to integrate and transform our lives, as is the nature of the Self.

All great myths and stories are about archetypes and how they function. We experience archetypes in movies and novels. We experience them also in our own lives, in conflicts, love, and religious experience—in fact, in all the experiences of our lives.

An archetype manifests in the following sequence, starting at the most primal level.

1. The archetype in itself as original *matrix,* or form and its *energy,* which functions in certain characteristic ways.

2. Next, the archetype manifests as *symbol,* or images invested with diffuse energy. Naked bodies of young men and women "glow" when idealized with life force and their respective archetypes. Mandalas, or sacred circles, such as the rose windows of Christian cathedrals, "glow" with energy. This is the level of *secondary archetypes,* which manifest from the primary archetypes.

3. Then we have the archetype still manifesting as symbol, but also functioning as *feeling and emotion.* This is the level of the *complexes,* or semi-autonomous personalities in the personal unconscious. The anima as complex not only is the image of the feminine for the man, but also functions to excite and inspire his life. *Feelings* are momentary energy reactions, either positive or negative, which motivate

actions. "I like you; so I will do this for you." *Emotions* are sustained feeling states of long duration that are not easily within conscious control. These include grief, falling in love, enthusiasm, passion, depression, inflation, and anger.

4. The final major level of archetypal manifestation is at the most conscious level of *feeling-emotion* and *concept*. "I am not only angry. I know why I am angry, and I know what I think about it, and I know what it means."

THE SEVEN BASIC ARCHETYPES

THE SELF

The Self is the separative, integrative, transformative center within the psyche from which dreams, visions, and other inspirations originate. At its center are the light and the dark, the primary opposites of the universe. The *individuation* process originates here. The *opus,* the wholeness process, the work of one's life, is to continually live from this center, so that much or even most of one's totality becomes separated, integrated, and transformed. *Transformation* is total revolution in the psyche; it is the creation of a new, evolving point out of the separation and unifying of opposites. It is the essence, perhaps, of most personal spiritual experience.

The Self shows itself symbolically as the *coniunctio,* or divine union; the philosopher's stone of alchemy; the Divine Child; the Uroborous, or snake eating its tail; the butterfly; the stove; the ring; the tapestry.

Besides dreams and visions, the Self manifests especially in the life experiences of *synchronicity,* or meaningful coincidence, sexual and spiritual ecstasy, and moments of absolute clarity and action for consciousness. Its sacred objects and events include the mandala, the temple, the treasure, the book, gifts, the bridge, the star, seeds and eggs, the lit candle, the rainbow, the lotus, Christmas, and weddings.

THE FEMININE

The all-inclusive quality of the Feminine creates relationship and acceptance. It says "yes" to things. It creates also the cave: the womb from which life flows, and the tomb to which life returns.

In the woman the Feminine expresses the dominant qualities of her own soul. This is a Feminine somehow different from the man's own Feminine, or anima, which is to him an opposite, rather than his own true nature. In both, the in-dwelling of the Feminine rests in substance, in matter itself.

The Feminine is vessel, cave, womb, queen, princess, the goddesses of love and fertility, the well, lake, bed, throne, spider.

In life the Feminine operates to create relationship, flow, beauty, and birth. It can also destroy, by devouring and formlessness. It nurtures as well as suffocates, and is seemingly irrational, or without logic. It is mystery. Its festivals celebrate fertility, the erotic, family, and divination.

Its sacred objects include the vessel, the gate or the doorway, the scabbard, the throne, the moon, and the veil.

THE MASCULINE

The Masculine imposes structure; it says "no" when needed. It thrusts, penetrates, asserts itself, gets the job done. It is decisive and discriminating, and tends toward the rational and perfection.

For the man the Masculine expresses his dominant life force, or soul, his being out of which he habitually acts and accomplishes. For the woman her decisiveness and discrimination are expressed through her animus, her own form of the Masculine, which is colored differently from that of a man. In both sexes it is the realm of the spirit, of ideas and values.

Symbols of the Masculine include sword, king, Unicorn, phallus, and sun, and the sacred manifestations of sceptre, tool, tower, and sword.

In life the Masculine shows itself in fathering, making, directing, organizing, and building of structures. It initiates and rules the day. It propagates the new life without actually manifesting it. Its rites are for the creation of power and cohesiveness, for "firming up," planning, and accomplishing goals.

THE HEROIC

The Hero or Heroine always faces the difficult and even the insurmountable: the adversary itself. In the great myths and stories, it often conquers, at least temporarily. The Heroic functions to achieve victory and healing, to bring resolution to that which is in conflict and chaos. Its energy is positive, or outgoing. It surges with nobility, truth, and goodness. Its symbols are youth, triumphal marches, the garland, the spoils, the great heart, the shield, the battle, the message, the hospital, and the healing balm.

In life the Heroic manifests in battle, struggle, saviour religions, and all the general's, the entrepreneur's, and the physician's tasks. It saves and embod-

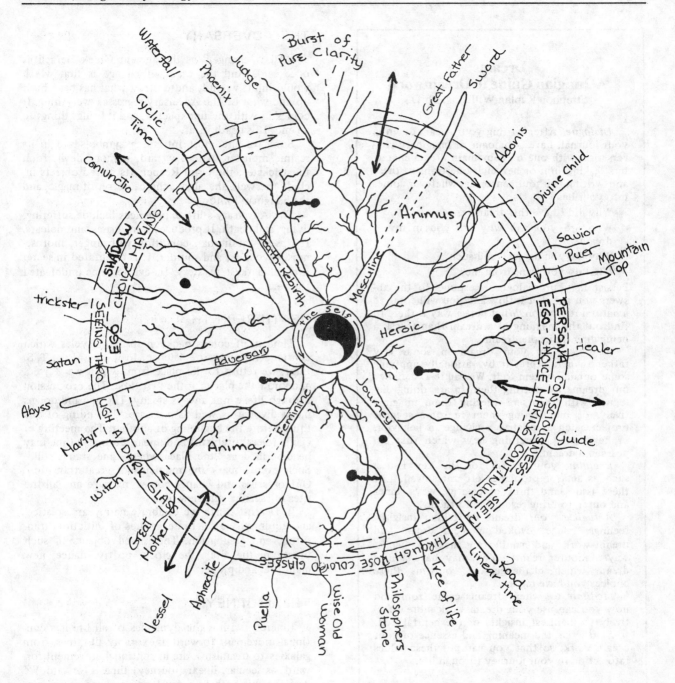

This Mandala of the Psyche provides another model of the human psyche, with its seven primary archetypes and the manifesting secondary archetypes and complexes. The Self is the central, integrative archetype uniting all the other archetypes. The animus and anima complexes emerge out of their primary archetypes to constellate the sexual characteristics of the psyche. Included also is the ego, and how it functions as a continuum relating all the archetypes. We see how the ego's consciousness functions through either the persona (bright positive image) or the shadow (negative dark awareness). The psyche, like the physical body, is organic, and therefore interrelated and moving in a constant play of opposites. In essence, this shows the holistic nature of the psyche and what it might mean to express all these parts in one integrated whole.

Dreams:
A Jungian Guide to Dreamwork
Strephon Kaplan Williams, Ph.D.

Dialogue. After writing your dream down in your journal, have a dialogue or imaginary conversation with one of your main dream characters, asking him or her such questions as these and writing, without censoring, whatever comes into your head:

Why did I have this dream?

Who are you and why are you in my dream?

Why did you do such and such?

What do you want from me?

Persist in your dialogue. Respond to the answers you get. Let it flow and you will come to a natural resolution. What better way is there to find out the meaning of a dream than to ask a being directly in the dream?

Re-experience your dream in some way rather than interpret it by rationally applying some outside system to it. We can re-experience our dreams by putting them in art, doing dialogues with them, re-entering them imaginatively, or manifesting them in some specific project, such as poetry, a change in behavior, or developing something new which first appears in a dream.

Examine your dream for the key issues, such as acts or problems left unresolved. List these issues and think of creative ways, inner and outer, to bring resolution to them.

Actualize your dream by taking insights, feelings, images evoked in your dream and dream work, and manifesting them in specific ways in outer reality. You may have a new dream which challenges or confirms these choices you have made.

Meditate on where dreams come from, and how you can use your dream work more effectively to manifest insights of the central Self.

Synthesize the meaning and essence of your dream work, so that you can put these values into action in your journey through life.

THE ADVERSARY

"All is change," as the ancient Greek Heraclitus once said. And the agent of change is that which would limit, wound, and destroy what has been built up and what is. The Adversary regresses everything. It comes in with the unexpected, and it brings things to an end. It is death itself.

Some of the most intriguing symbols are in its realm: monster, witch, wizard, demon, devil, fool, the trickster, the Grim Reaper. Its sacred objects include the wall, the abyss, the cauldron of magic, and the hangman's knot.

The Adversary's life experiences include suffering, dying, and death. It produces wars, crises, and defeats. It upsets the human condition with anger, moroseness, psychosis, and murder. It is celebrated in secret rites of darkest mystery, Its evil remains undefeated forever.

DEATH-REBIRTH

Time itself comes back on itself in cycles which continue throughout existence. In the words of T. S. Eliot, we return to the place from which we started, and know the place for the first time. The progression through life is not always steady. The ups and downs mean divorce as well as marriage, the ending of one thing before the beginning of another. The meeting of cyclic (Death-Rebirth) and linear (Journey) time may be described as "the place where time stands still." Such events mark the moments of great transition. Out of crisis and change comes marriage and all the rites of sacrifice and new life.

In Death-Rebirth we celebrate new years, solstice, and equinox. We celebrate in rites of initiation, transition, and graduation. The sacred objects of such times are the altar, the clock, poetry, dance, new plant life, and prayer.

THE JOURNEY

Inherent within the dynamics of all life is a continual movement forward. Inexorably all things, from galaxies to organisms, are in continual movement forward, as secular, linear (journey) time is forward. We describe this both as a developmental and as a diminishing, or aging, process. Thus within linear time is also the rising and decline of Death-Rebirth.

Birthdays and anniversaries celebrate the intersections of these linear (historical) and cyclic (sacred) times. Each stage of the Journey is built upon what went before, but always the direction is toward the

ies the upright life. Its festivals are the victory celebration and the return to healthy life. Great teachers and explorers create new knowledge from its energies.

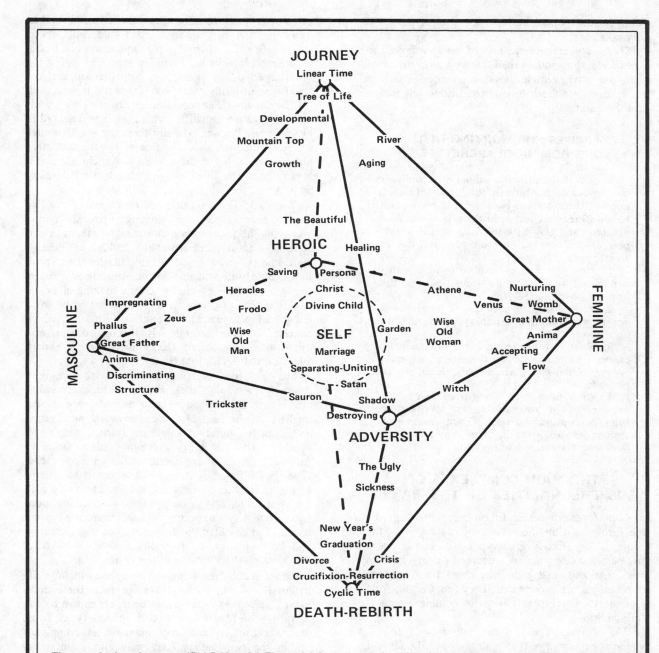

The seven basic archetypes unified field model. The model shows the relationships of the archetypes to each other, and how they manifest as secondary archetypes. Each of the seven basic archetypes has an inherent set of characteristics, or essence, and each stands in a relation of opposition or reciprocity to another. The Self stands at the center, equidistant from the other six primary archetypes, illustrating how it is the unifying, separating, transforming point for the other archetypes. These secondary archetypes (e.g., wise old woman, great father, trickster, Christ) are here placed between the primary archetypes from which they gain their characteristics. With this model it is possible to see how archetypes, or energy centers of unique character, underlie the major images and characteristics of the psyche and of life. The crystal is itself the universal symbol for total and balanced interrelatedness.

future, except when the regressive pull of the Adversary takes over.

Sacred objects and symbols of the Journey are the tree of life, the winding road, the ascent up the mountain, the staff, vehicles, guides, rivers, and streams.

We celebrate the Journey in vacations, pilgrimages, and the quest.

EXERCISES FOR WORKING WITH YOUR DOMINANT ARCHETYPE

Usually one primary archetype dominates our development through childhood into adulthood, although some people experience a shift to a different archetype in the transition. When you look and play with the diagrams, their symbols and concepts, what do you find has the greater energy for you?

1. What did you most have to deal with in childhood? In adulthood? Write a page on this, or paint how you feel this.

2. After doing the above, look for the opposite to your dominant archetype, and describe how you feel about it.

3. What actions can you take in your life to create a balance between these opposite archetypes? Perhaps you are already doing so. Describe how.

4. What have been the three most central experiences of your life so far? Write down brief descriptions of them. Then describe the archetypes dominant in these experiences, and the effect they have had on you.

THE MAIN COMPLEXES OR SUBPERSONALITIES OF THE PSYCHE

Complexes, or semiautonomous subpersonalities, are formed within the individual psyche, with their roots in the primary archetypes. The complexes are the personal unconscious aspects of the psyche. They are functional, and gain their character from childhood and adult experiences. They function like other secondary archetypes. The main complexes are the following:

The Anima: The feminine component in males which is projected onto females or onto the feminine in other males or the environment. (This projection is the basis for the "falling in love" experience.)

The Animus: The masculine component in females which is again projected onto the opposite sex, or onto the masculine within the female, as in the case of same-sex experiences.

The Persona: The bright or positive side of ourselves that we generally show to the world in order to

get along. We most often get paid for our Personas. The Persona is the good therapist, friend, mother, etc. It originates out of the Heroic, and serves as a buffer to the world. Thus in Figure 3 it is seen as half of the outer layers of the psyche. As such it colors the consciousness in terms of the way the world is perceived.

The Shadow: The repressed side of ourselves, made up of "negative" qualities which we have rejected in building our Persona. Usually these are qualities such as anger, instinct, or ordinariness. Yet the criminal's Shadow might be of the upright judge who sentences him or her. The Shadow has roots in the Adversary archetypes.

The Ego: The two primary functions of the Ego are choice-making, or the directing of psychic energy, and being the focus of consciousness by means of perception, memory, and processing. In Figure 3 the Ego continuum goes full circle, because ideally the creative Ego makes itself available for manifesting any appropriate part of the psyche. In choice-making, the creative Ego uses as guides its own attitudes or personal laws, memory, perception, and information which comes from the central Self through dreams and other primary intuitions. Occasionally the Ego experiences a burst of absolute clarity.

The Ego's most creative functions are to strengthen its own inherent abilities, and to make choices that manifest the separative-integrative-transformative qualities of the Self. Most Egos grow up, however, in childhood by building a *defense system,* which prevents the true flexibility the Ego needs in order to function. The defensive Ego identifies with one archetype, gets inflated by it, and is thus unable to get free to manifest other archetypes. An Ego identified with the Heroic will always be trying to be good and positive in one way or another, and will therefore neglect to manifest so-called "bad" qualities of anger, cruelty, and instinctuality, or even qualities of other archetypes, such as the flowing of the Feminine.

Other much less dominant complexes include the parental and child complexes. In fact, these complexes, as well as other minor ones, are shown on the periphery of Figure 3 as secondary archetypes. Thus, secondary archetypes may manifest as complexes within the personality. They may also manifest as characters in myth, art, theater, or in outer roles in society.

EXERCISES FOR WORKING WITH THE ANIMA OR ANIMUS

1a. If you are a woman, describe all the qualities of your "ideal man," or "ideal masculine woman."

1b. If you are a man, describe your "ideal woman," or "ideal feminine" in a man.

2. List ways these qualities are actually inside yourself.

3. Describe, using your love relationships, what happens to you when the object of your love denies or no longer carries these qualities for you.

4. To integrate your masculine, withdraw the projection by putting these qualities and feelings into poetry, art, dance, and specific life projects in which you express these qualities yourself. List specific things you will do.

5a. If you are a man, describe what you do or don't do to capture the woman's animus. Evaluate!

5b. If you are a woman, describe what you do or don't do to capture the man's anima. Evaluate!

EXERCISES FOR WORKING WITH THE SHADOW AND PERSONA

Note: Do not worry whether certain qualities belong more to the Anima or Animus, or to the Shadow or Persona. For clarity, refer back to the basic archetypes that underlie them.

THE PERSONA

1. Describe the chief positive qualities about yourself, the things you most like, your positive images of yourself.

2. Have a friend describe your positive qualities without having seen your list. Then compare lists and evaluate.

3. A creative Persona is a necessity for interacting with the world. Describe specific things you will do to improve your Persona in terms of looks, dress, behavior, and conversation.

YOUR SHADOW

1. Describe the chief negative things about yourself that you don't like, or that others find hard to take.

2. Describe the negative qualities you really do not like in others. Compare with the above.

3. Have a friend, or an enemy (our enemies are our best friends), describe your negative qualities. Which are in you, and which seem to be projections onto you? Why do you get such projections?

4. Take your beginning Persona list from above, and list the opposites to these qualities. How would you compare this Shadow list with your other ones?

5. List some specific ways you can enact your Shadow qualities positively in your everyday life. Wholeness means accepting and integrating the totality of one's personality.

EXERCISES FOR DESCRIBING YOUR EGO

Using Figure 3, which areas of the Ego continuum do you see as stronger? In other words, how has your Ego or choice-maker manifested or not manifested the underlying archetypes? Write answers to these questions.

1. Describe your Ego's defense system as a reaction to certain archetypes (primary or secondary).

2. Where have been, if any, the points of absolute clarity for your Ego?

3. What qualities of the archetypes help you make strong choices?

4. Which qualities of the archetypes weaken your choice-making ability?

5. What archetypes do you most remember? Which do you least remember?

If you have worked through the material, you should now have a basic grasp of some of your psyche and how it functions. This has been an exercise in consciousness. You can now begin to apply this scheme to your everyday life, including dream work, and thereby increase the depth and level of your choice-making and action. Glimpsing the underlying qualities of things produces meaning and excitement for many people.

JUNGIAN TYPOLOGY

Typology is the science of describing general differences in personality types. Jung has formulated these differences as follows.

The Extrovert: One who is other-directed, who bases choices on the reactions of or about other people, objects, events, and things. The extrovert is usually more interested in what others think and feel than in what he or she feels. Extroverts generally find it harder to be alone, and base their opinions of themselves on what others think.

The Introvert: The introvert is inner-directed, generally more interested in his or her internal reactions to things than in the things themselves. Introverts prefer one-to-one or small-group situations to those involving large numbers of people.

Along with being either introverted or extroverted, a person develops certain predispositions about *how* he or she makes choices. Much conflict exists among people because these differences are not recognized. As you read the following descriptions, see which one most appeals to you, and which appeals the least.

Sensation Person: One whose main focus is on the details and concreteness of reality. Such a person gives

The New Dimensions of Psychology: The Third and Fourth Forces

Roberto Assagioli, M.C.

Let us take a look at humanistic psychology, which is also known as the Third Force. It differs from other psychologies in its principal characteristic purposes, which are: to study the nature and qualities of the healthy human being, with particular attention to his higher aspects; to discover his latent potentialities; and to develop and use techniques for actualizing these potentialities, giving them practical expression in every sphere of life and human activity.

HUMANISTIC PSYCHOLOGY

The eminent psychologist William James, a pioneer in this field as in others, early recognized the existence of the immense stores of energy and valuable potentialities in the human being, and expressed his conviction in very definite terms:

"I have no doubt that the great majority of people live, in both a physical and an intellectual and moral sense, using but a limited part of their potentialities. . . . The so-called normal man, the one we may term the 'healthy Philistine,' is only a fraction of what he could be, while we all possess reserves of life to draw upon which we do not even dream of."

A number of researchers, therapists, and educators, most of them American, have produced a series of books and articles reflecting this humanistic orientation.

Reprinted by permission of The Human Dimensions Institute from *Human Dimensions Journal*, 3 (no. 1), 4–5.

The most articulate and ardent advocate of humanistic psychology has been Abraham Maslow. He presents a general survey of it in his book, *Toward a Psychology of Being*. The title of the book clearly indicates the author's approach to the study of the human being. He considers man in terms of the centrality of his existence, in which are inherent the truly human values, and from which they stem. Maslow calls these values B-values, a term derived from the word being, and he enumerates them as follows.

(1) Wholeness: unity; integration; tendency to one-ness; interconnectedness; simplicity; organization; structure; dichotomy-transcendence; order.

(2) Perfection: necessity; just-rightness; just-so-ness; inevitability; suitability; justice; completeness; "oughtness."

(3) Completion: ending; finality; justice; "it's finished"; fulfillment; finis and telos; destiny; fate.

(4) Justice: fairness; orderliness; lawfulness; "oughtness."

(5) Aliveness: process; non-deadness; spontaneity; self-regulation; full functioning.

(6) Richness: differentiation; complexity; intricacy.

(7) Simplicity: honesty; nakedness; essentiality; abstraction; skeletal structures.

(8) Beauty: rightness; form; aliveness; simplicity; richness, wholeness, perfection; completion; uniqueness; honesty.

(9) Goodness: rightness; desirability; oughtness; justice; benevolence; honesty.

(10) Uniqueness: idiosyncrasy; individuality; noncomparability; novelty.

great attention to detail, to getting things just right, ignoring the larger perspective, or the feeling level of a situation. Engineers, rule followers, lawyers, office workers, accountants, and perfectionists fall generally within this type. The present is their predominant orientation.

Intuitives: The intuitive is the opposite of the sensation person. Intuitives cannot be bothered with details, and are concerned only with perceiving the whole, with having great insights, and with unlimited creativity. They will often start many projects, but finish very few because of their lack of ability to deal with details. Sudden insights and creative ideas out of the blue are their forté. Theoretical physicists, innovators, creators, therapists, esoterics, psychics, and the slightly bizarre number in the ranks of the intuitives. The intuitive is always focused on the future. The present is never good enough, and the past is quickly forgotten.

Thinking Types: The organizers of society, with

(11) Effortlessness: ease; lack of strain; striving or difficulty; grace; perfection; beautiful functioning.

(12) Playfulness: fun; joy; amusement; gaiety; humor; exuberance; effortlessness.

(13) Truth: honesty; reality; nakedness; simplicity; richness; oughtness; beauty; purity; completeness; essentiality.

(14) Self-sufficiency: autonomy; independence; not needing other than itself in order to be itself; self-determining; environment transcendence; separateness; living by its own laws.

We have here a very dffferent image of the human being from that presented by current psychologies, and from that held by modern man of himself. This is no "idealistic" portrait, but one based on the lived experience of many persons, and on man's primary, intrinsic tendencies. In order to accentuate the "naturalness" and authenticity of these tendencies, Maslow has used the appropriate neologism "instinctoid," meaning that they are innate, and as genuine as the other instincts.

It might be thought that humanistic psychology constitutes the avant garde—the spearhead, so to speak, of the new scientific psychology. But it is not so: another kind of psychology is being developed on the basis of the Third Force, a psychology no less empirical, that is, one that remains experimental and scientific. Its concern is with the higher aspects of the human being, those aspects of his nature and life that are generally called "spiritual."

But this is too general a term, and it continues to lend itself to confusion and misunderstandings, arising out of its too-close association with the fields of religion and philosophy. Therefore the term "transpersonal" was rightly proposed, and is used to denote this new field. It possesses the advantage of being neutral; it simply indicates a plateau (or "height") above the "normal" one. Called the "Fourth Force" in psychology, it has had various precursors, among them William James and Dr. Richard Bucke, author of the classic book *Cosmic Consciousness*. Abraham Maslow has been its courageous advocate and exponent.

FOURTH FORCE

The rapid and vigorous development of this current is evidence of the extent to which it is fulfilling a real need. It already has its own journal, the *Journal of Transpersonal Psychology*, and an Association for Transpersonal Psychology has been formed, whose prospectus contains the following definition of the Fourth Force:

"Transpersonal psychology is the title given to an emerging force in psychology and other fields by a group of men and women who are interested in ultimate states. The emerging transpersonal orientation is concerned with the empirical scientific study and responsible implementation of the findings relevant to: spiritual paths, becoming, metaneeds (individual and species-wide), ultimate values, unitive consciousness, peak experiences, B-values, compassion, ecstasy, mystical experience, awe, being, self-actualization, essence, bliss, wonder, ultimate meaning, transcendence of the self, spirit, oneness, cosmic awareness, individual and species-wide synergy, theories and practices of meditation, sacralization of everyday life, transcendental phenomena, cosmic self-humor and playfulness, and related concepts, experience, and activities."

either facts, ideas, or people. Thinking involves making or discovering conscious links between people or things. Mathematicians, some teachers, executives, lawyers, bridge players, and the somewhat cool and objective are generally among the thinking types. Thinking bridges time past, present, and future. Writers and consciousness bearers can often be seen in this category.

Feeling Types: Feeling is the relational function. Feeling is the expression of positive and negative energy. "I like this and I don't like that!" As with thinking, its opposite, feeling organizes reality. It does not perceive it, as does intuition. Feeling types are the harmonizers and socializers who work well with people. These are teachers, therapists, the compassionate, and the perceptive. Feeling types are great gossipers and dancers, who love body contact. Yet others will also be the ones who experience the greatest "freakouts." They seem to live the relational life at double the intensity for the rest of us.

(Text continued on p. 175)

One Head, Two Brains
Kathleen L. Hawkins, M.A.

According to split-brain research, the two halves of the human brain correspond to two potentially separate "minds," which differ in content, organization and thinking skills.

Your left brain is analytical, verbal, and sequential. Your right brain is timeless, visual, and intuitive.

Working in harmony, the two halves can provide you with infinite creative capacities and a more balanced personality. The challenge, then, is to tap the reserves of both sides of your brain, and to develop cooperation between these two very powerful, highly individual hemispheres for a more dynamic, expressive life.

LEFT BRAIN: INTERPRETER

Your left cerebral hemisphere is the interpreter of experiences. It has a powerful capacity for analytical functions, and well-developed abilities for verbal expression, writing, languages, higher mathematics, and science.

It concerns itself with objects and labels, categories and abstractions. Temporal sequence, outcome, and consequences are very important to the left hemisphere, because it perceives cause-and-effect relationships.

If you are a left-brained thinker, you think in words rather than pictures. You love concepts and abstractions, and will be attracted to subjects such as philosophy, criticism, and languages. Your extremely efficient, logical left brain has many attributes of the assertive, objective, conscious mind.

Some people, however, can be too objective. If you are one of these, there are many things you can do to develop your intuitive, visual nature, for a more perfect balance between hemispheres.

Experience your experiences. Because the left brain organizes its world in linear sequence, if you are entrenched in left-brain thinking, you may be overly concerned with causes and consequences, with the past and the future. Learn to enjoy the moment, without immediately analyzing it. If you must analyze yourself, reserve it for a later time.

Dishabituate yourself once in a while from the verbal-analytical mode of thinking. If you love to spend all your time discussing philosophy with friends over coffee, go to a symphony for a change, and enjoy your vacation from words. Alter your spatial orientation by sitting on the opposite side of the bus, or in a different place in a room than you normally do. Try writing with your left hand.

Learn to relax by means of medidation. Don't submerge yourself in safe intellectual exercises in order to avoid your feelings. Free your feelings by practicing meditation. Begin to incorporate visualizations in your meditations.

Associate occasionally with emotional, intuitive people. Experience what they are doing and saying, as if you were doing or saying it. This will help you to establish rapport with such people, to gain insights, and to "hitch a ride" on a right-brained transport system for a change.

Cultivate your hunches. Begin with the safe ones, by playing games such as, "What color is the next car around the corner going to be?" and working up to important decisions.

Incorporate sketches into your note-taking. In order to exercise your right brain, illustrate what you are thinking and hearing. You will find that the pictures and diagrams you come up with will be very personal to you, and will therefore help you remember the material better. It is also easier to recall a picture than pages of linear, verbal notes.

Keep a dream journal. When you travel in right-brain country, it is best to speak the language. By means of a dream journal, investigate the symbols and images that are personal to you, and therefore necessary for your right-brain expression.

RIGHT BRAIN: DREAMER, BRIDGER OF GAPS

Your right brain is the dreamer, bridger of gaps, and pattern maker. It thinks in images rather than words, and these images will be rich in detail, movement, sounds, and other sensory qualities.

Information comes into your right brain rapidly and automatically, thereby enabling it to perceive experience directly. Because its style of thought is holistic and spontaneous,

(continued on p. 174)

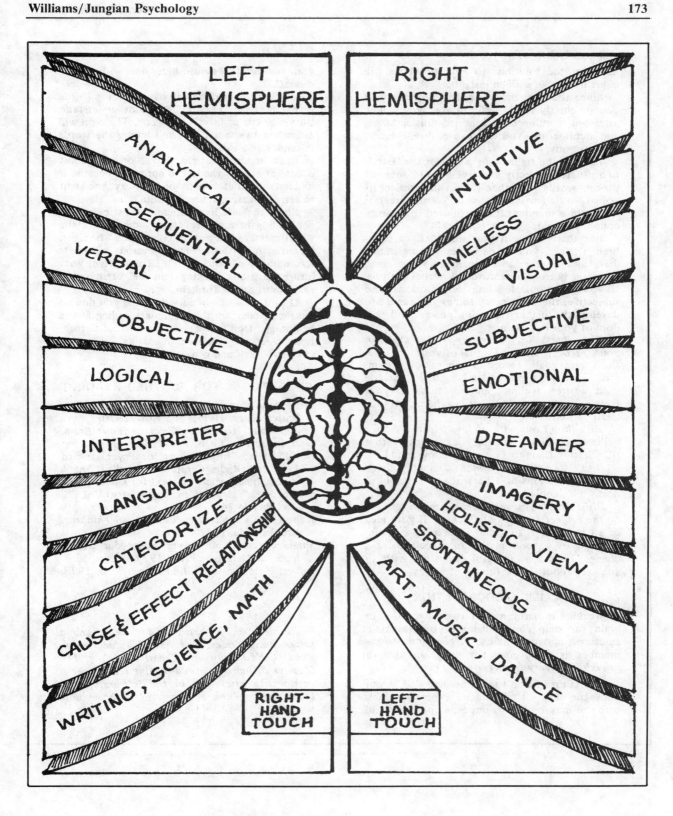

LEFT HEMISPHERE

ANALYTICAL
SEQUENTIAL
VERBAL
OBJECTIVE
LOGICAL
INTERPRETER
LANGUAGE
CATEGORIZE
CAUSE & EFFECT RELATIONSHIP
WRITING, SCIENCE, MATH

RIGHT HEMISPHERE

INTUITIVE
TIMELESS
VISUAL
SUBJECTIVE
EMOTIONAL
DREAMER
IMAGERY
HOLISTIC VIEW
SPONTANEOUS
ART, MUSIC, DANCE

RIGHT-HAND TOUCH

LEFT-HAND TOUCH

(continued from p. 172)
many of the solutions to your problems will come by way of sudden insights.

Since the right brain is spatially oriented, if you are chiefly a right-brain thinker, you will be attracted to subjects such as art, music, dance, and architecture. You will love beauty, balance, and harmony.

Because the right brain perceives the Gestalt of a situation directly and visually, and does not process words other than those which reflect its holistic style (metaphors, double entendres), it thinks in a manner often attributed to the sub-conscious mind.

For this reason, if you are chiefly a right-brain thinker, your experiences will be immediate and intense, as opposed to experiences that have been once-removed by verbal analysis. If you find yourself being too emotional and subjective, there are many things you can do to develop the higher reasoning powers and wisdom of your left brain.

Discipline your feelings by relying more on your intellect. Keep a journal of your long- and short-term goals, recording when you accomplish each step toward attaining them. Include your desires, feelings, and reactions. If your feelings are confused, write them out for clarification.

Talk things out with a close friend. Practice explaining and interpreting your feelings, rather than letting them pile up and become muddled.

Don't take things personally. Detach yourself from the opinions of others. It's not your business what people think of you.

Dishabituate yourself from too much reliance on the subjective mode of thinking. If your idea of a good time is to spend an evening at a concert, go to a book review or a lecture for a change. Have a meaningful discussion with an analyzer about the usefulness of words.

MAXIMIZE COOPERATION

Working in harmony, the two halves of your brain can help you to balance your thinking, emotions, and personality. A good rule to remember is: *A feeling for every thought, a thought for every feeling.*

"Of course I don't mind helping you," your colleague says, but his facial expression indicates he may be feeling imposed upon. How do your two cerebral hemispheres deal with double messages?

The left hemisphere will pay attention to the verbal message, because it cannot understand the visual cue of facial expression. The right will assimilate the visual cue, and ignore the words it cannot process.

Each hemisphere may decide on a different course of action: the left to approach because it understands that help is on the way; the right to retreat because it sees conflict.

Since the left hemisphere is most often the controlling hemisphere, it may disconnect the visual message the right is conveying. The right, however, in spite of being repressed, still holds the memory of conflict. This could affect your future decisions, making you feel vaguely uneasy about asking for help.

If you suspect someone is giving you double messages, clear up the misunderstanding at the beginning. Don't repress it. Keep the perceptions clear in your own mind, as well as between yourself and others

SUGGESTIONS FOR FURTHER READING

Edward de Bono, *Lateral Thinking: Creativity Step by Step.* Harper and Row, 1970.
Tony Buzan, *Use Both Sides of Your Brain.* E. P. Dutton, 1976.
David Galin, "Implications for Psychiatry of Left and Right Cerebral Specialization; A Neurophysiological Context for Unconscious Processes." *Arch. Gen. Psychiatry,* Vol. 31 (October 1974).
Robert McKim, *Experiences in Visual Thinking.* Brooks/Cole, 1972.
Sheila Ostrander and Lynn Schroeder, *Superlearning.* Delacorte Press, 1979.
Robert Sommer, *The Mind's Eye.* Dell, 1978.

Kathleen L. Hawkins is a novelist and a prize-winning poet. She has M.A. degrees in Reading Education and Creative Writing. The founder of her own speed-reading school, she is particularly interested in the left-brain/right-brain phenomenon as it applies to the reading process.

(continued from p. 171)

SOME GENERAL PRINCIPLES ABOUT JUNGIAN TYPE AND FUNCTION

1. Each person has all characteristics, yet certain ones predominate.

2. These predispositions often express themselves in combinations, such as an introverted-feeling body therapist, or a thinking-intuitive group leader.

3. Different predispositions may apply in different situations. Sensation-thinking is needed to do the income tax; feeling-intuitive is needed for working intimately with people's problems.

4. Acceptance of different types and functions can turn conflictive relations into complementary ones.

5. The least developed function usually acts autonomously, and is loaded with negative and positive energy.

6. It is absolutely necessary to develop a dominant type and function in order to act decisively. Inability to make choices can often be traced to ambivalence about what is one's natural disposition, in need of development.

7. Many people have been forced by environmental factors to develop dominants other than their natural one. Thus they get into occupations and relationships not really suited to them. This produces crisis in life, and people then undergo self-exploration to find out and live their natural predisposition.

8. The holistic approach means developing our natural dominants, but also developing all sides of oneself. When should one be introverted, when extroverted? When should one do what one is least good at, as well as most good at, in the interest of wholeness?

EXERCISE: FINDING OUT YOUR TYPE AND FUNCTION PREDISPOSITIONS

1. Look over the different descriptions, and decide, even if only tentatively, which most apply to you as your dominants. Add qualities of your own to the description. From Figure 4, decide also your least-developed function, as the opposite to your dominant.

2. Check your typing of yourself by typing your partner in an intimate relationship. Is he or she generally an opposite to you, or the same as you?

3. Pick a difficult relationship you are having, and use the type and function model to help explain the personal nature of the conflicts. Then list remedies you will use based on type and function. You might choose to understand and accept the situation, rather than push your own point of view. Or you might choose to get out of the relationship because you clash too much.

THE JOURNEY TOWARD WHOLENESS

Who knows what will be the habits of future ages? We are still evolving. Perhaps for many living in our time, there is a journey, at once personal, conscious, and connected to the deepest sources within being, a journey using many of the habits of consciousness, such as dream work, journal work, and profound centering, a journey in which the Ego, the choice-maker, grows strong in cooperation with the far greater and more meaningful center, the Self. Such a journey may be worth every sacrifice. The rewards are nothing less than the life vitality which comes with the development and transformation of personality.

SUGGESTIONS FOR FURTHER READING

J. Campbell, *The Portable Jung.* Penguin, 1977.

C. G. Jung, *Man and His Symbols.* Doubleday, 1976.

_____, *Memories, Dreams, Reflections.* Vintage, 1965.

F. Wickes, *Inner World of Choice.* Prentice-Hall, 1963.

Strephon Kaplan Williams, *Jungian-Senoi Dreamwork Manual.* Journey Press, 1980.

Strephon Kaplan Williams, Ph.D., is a practicing analyst/therapist in Berkeley, California and the author of the Jungian-Senoi Dreamwork Manual *and* Transformations-I: Meditations in a New Age. *He is an instructor at John F. Kennedy University in Jungian psychology and transpersonal dreamwork, and studies Aikido, a Japanese martial art.*

Gestalt Therapy
Deborah Weinstein, M.A., L.M.F.C.C.

Gestalt (the whole picture) therapy offers us simple techniques that can cut to the heart of complex problems. For this and other reasons, it has become an important tool for human growth.

Fritz Perls, the founder of Gestalt, described it as an action approach to deepening awareness and living in the here and now. In this article, Deborah Weinstein explains the principles of Gestalt therapy, and provides us with some easily usable techniques.

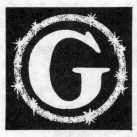

estalt therapy was developed by Fritz Perls in the late 1940s, and since then has slowly gained profound influence in the humanistic psychology movement. The Gestalt approach carries with it both a descriptive psychology and a holistic philosophy. It is a unique way of perceiving and understanding human process and conflict, and has its own body of therapeutic interventions and emphases.

Fritz Perls was trained as a traditional psychoanalyst, but grew disenchanted with the limitations he saw in the medical orientation of the psychoanalytic model. Perls saw the need for a more growth-oriented system of psychotherapy, and drew from various disciplines in order to develop Gestalt therapy. Wilhelm Reich's work with the body and muscular armoring; Jacob Moreno's use of psychodrama; the Yiddish theater; the Gestalt psychologist Goldstein— all had powerful effects on Perls' thinking. He combined these disciplines into a therapy he called Gestalt, meaning "the whole picture."

In this system, an individual is seen as composed of many Gestalts, or pictures, some of which are confused and in conflict. These incomplete situations from the past interrupt the freedom of the individual, hampering his ability to enjoy his life in the present. In the Gestalt therapy session, the incomplete Gestalts emerge from the background, and, with work, become resolved or completed. This "unfinished business" from the past provides the content for the session. The process of the Gestalt therapy session emphasizes the "here and now." In the face-to-face, heart-to-heart contact between therapist and client, careful attention is paid to the client's awareness of his five senses, so that he can recapture his vitality. As unfinished Gestalts are resolved, the whole spectrum of emotions becomes increasingly available to the individual.

Gestalt therapy is practiced in different styles and modes. In a workshop, group, or individual session, the individual can be seen at any moment like a holographic image—any part of which contains the whole within it. The individual can represent his life situation at any moment in the way he speaks, breathes, or uses his body. The skilled therapist notices these things, and uses her observations to facilitate awareness for the client in the "here and now."

"Right now I notice you are looking away from me, breathing shallowly, and tapping your foot when you talk about your boss," could be the beginning of an exploration based on the most obvious things in the moment. These can lead to feelings and thoughts the client was not aware of before, but was unconsciously reflecting in his voice, his foot, and his breathing. The three zones of awareness—the inner zone (our internal bodily sensations and emotions); the middle zone (where we think, analyze, fantasize, and rehearse); and the outer zone (our five senses, where we contact the physical world)—are all important in Gestalt therapy. In many other therapies only the middle zone is explored, leaving much of the whole person excluded from awareness, or aliveness. After asking the client to notice his foot-tapping, a Gestalt therapist might ask the client to exaggerate this previously unconscious gesture, and then to follow whatever happens next.

This may develop into full-scale kicking and anger at the boss, or into a decisive, self-assertive stamp, or into a flirtatious game of "footsy." The excitement of Gestalt lies in liberating all of this suppressed energy, and in following the always new, often surprising process of the client as he attains new understandings or experiences. Perhaps this client never realized how flirtatious he felt with his boss. Perhaps he has never before expressed that playful side of himself in front of another person. Not only is he meeting a suppressed or repressed part of himself in the session, but he is experiencing *being this part of himself* in the company of a caring human witness, who acts as a guide and companion, helping him enter uncharted ground. The client is not merely alluding in general terms to flirtatious feelings. He is not *talking about* feelings; he is encouraged to give himself permission to *demonstrate* this side of himself in the session. This invitation to experiment and to "act through" feelings is the unique aspect of Gestalt. It is a qualitatively different experience to consciously be a flirtatious person in the session than it is to talk about being flirtatious. It is riskier, livelier, and more self-revealing.

By paying attention to language, the Gestalt therapist can also encourage more feeling in the client "It's sad that one often misses out on the good things in life," a client could say wistfully. A Gestaltist would ask him to "own" this statement, not to abstract or generalize by saying "it" or "one," instead of "I." "I feel sad that I often miss out on the good things in life" has a more powerful impact on the speaker—as well as the listener—than the former statement. It is more personal, revealing, and direct. The risk of self-disclosure is experienced instead of avoided. In addition, the client can feel empowered by owning his statements.

"I *can't* seem to listen to my wife," when changed to "I *won't* listen to my wife," shifts the responsibility from something outside of the client to the client himself. Once responsibility is taken, choice and change are possible.

So far we've said that Gestalt therapy enlivens and empowers the individual by focusing on the whole person, and by constantly demanding that the client own and take responsibility for his feelings. But what about conflict resolution? How can Gestalt help a person resolve issues, or confusion, or better understand his dreams and fears?

A person is composed of many different parts, some of which are unrecognized, some of which are in conflict with each other. The Gestalt therapist encourages the client to give a voice to each of these parts, and to carry on dialogues between the parts.

"I can't decide if I should leave my girlfriend or not. I want to make it work between us, but I resent her so much I can't stand it." The therapist might ask the client to become the part of himself that wants to leave, and to give this part a voice. The client will imagine that the side of him that wants to stay with

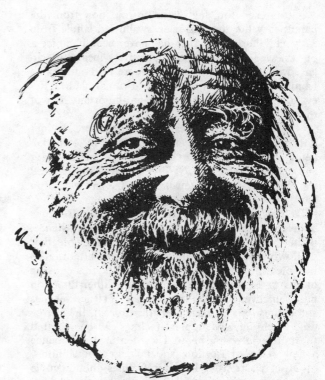

Fritz Perls, the founder of the Gestalt approach to therapy perceived the need for a more growth-oriented system of psychotherapy.

his girlfriend is sitting on an empty chair opposite him, and that that side also has a voice. After "the leaver" expresses himself, the client will get up and move to the empty chair, sit down, and become "the stayer," answering and arguing with the conflicting side. As this dialogue progresses, what has previously been a confusing mass becomes two clear polarities. Many discoveries can follow from this initial dialogue. After listening to himself, the client may discover that his resentful side sounds just like his father, who would leave situations when he felt threatened. Or he may discover that the part of him that wants to stay sounds guilty, weak, or more depressed than he had realized.

In another dialogue, the client can represent his own critical side, called the "top dog," as it berates his "underdog," or victimized side.

T: "Why can't you work harder and get better grades? You're just lazy and undisciplined. You should study harder!"

U: "Oh, God, I don't want to. I feel burdened already, and I don't want to study any harder. You make me feel nervous and stupid."

Often the "top dog" is an introjection from the parent—a value that has been swallowed whole from early childhood, and that has never been examined, or "chewed over." It sits oppressively inside the client, who is often unaware of where this value came from, and how much it rules (and ruins) his life. Re-evaluating these introjections is an important part of therapy.

The Gestalt dialogue can take other forms. It does not have to involve conflicting sides of a human being. The participants in a dialogue can be the client and his tight stomach: "Why are you so tense all the time?" "Because you mistreat me and work too hard!"

This awareness of what we unconsciously do to our bodies is a unique emphasis in Gestalt. For instance, if the therapist notices that the client often breathes shallowly, she may ask the client to pay attention to this breathing and either to exaggerate this choking or to try to deepen his respiration. Either direction might uncover very early memories of stifled feelings and expression. By means of this process, the energy used to chronically suppress feelings can be liberated for more creative purposes. The client may experience a new sense of freedom and increased possibilities.

Often we transfer left-over feelings about people from our pasts (often our parents) onto others in our current lives. For instance, if a client is troubled by an incident with a teacher, the therapist may suggest he have an empty-chair dialogue with this teacher. If the therapist notices such a strong feeling of sadness that it doesn't seem to fit the current situation, she may ask the client, "Who else might have treated you this way?" The client may respond, "I felt this way when I was six and my parents split up. I was ignored after that."

At this point in more traditional therapies, the client would talk about his feelings when he was six. In Gestalt, the therapist might say, "Be that six-year-old boy right now, and put your parents on the empty chair. Tell them how you feel about their separation." Thus, a far deeper opportunity to ab-react and experience these hurt feelings is provided in Gestalt. By imagining the parents in the room and speaking to them from the six-year-old's perspective, the client can bring these long-held, painful feelings to the surface, and can release them in the safety of the therapeutic hour.

Dreams can also be explored in this way. Often we project parts of ourselves that we cannot accept onto other people, or onto objects in our dreams. For example, the client might say, "I dreamt I was carrying a hammer around aimlessly in a park." Even though the tone of the dream reflects no anger, when asked by the therapist to "become the hammer," the client may discover he feels very angry. "I am metal and I love to pound on things and I sound like this . . ." Then, by acting out the part of the aimless stroller, the client might discover a truth about the lack of direction in his life.

Facing and reowning all of these parts of ourselves is the emphasis in Gestalt dreamwork. By giving a voice to different parts of ourselves, we are able to experience our multifaceted depth. The exaggeration of gestures and feelings gives us permission to examine the whole spectrum of our feelings—even the "unacceptable" ones. In dialogues, we clarify and reclaim our whole selves. With thoughtful work, we can integrate our fragmented parts into a more harmonious, whole person.

Gestalt therapy can allow for a more equal relationship between client and therapist than in medical-model therapies, where the therapist remains more hidden. The relationship between client and therapist is complex, and varies greatly with different therapists. Because Gestalt does not see things in pathological terms, the therapist is freer to treat her client as an equal, thus empowering the client, and providing a model of political equality or cooperative endeavor, rather than the more rigid hierarchical relationship between a doctor and his patient.

In more recent years, Gestalt has evolved beyond the individualistic perspective of Fritz Perls. In attempting to make his point about individual responsibility, Perls wrote, "I do my thing and you do your thing. I am not in this world to live up to your expectations, and you are not in this world to live up to mine." A San Francisco-based collective of seven Gestaltists, called the Gestalt Community Action Project, is evolving a theory and practice of "Social Gestalt." Social Gestalt sees the individual in the context of his environment, interrelated to each person and the surrounding world, responsible to and for the well-being of the whole. The "Gestalt" of a person is not just his body, mind, and spirit, but includes his social class, race, heritage, values, past, present, and future.

By examining these aspects of himself and understanding the societal influences on his introjections, projections, and conflicts, a client can feel more deeply related to his whole context. He can also see how his beliefs were formed, and he can work to change the parts of his environment that negatively affect his health, vitality, and wholeness. The truth is, that as each of us integrates more of our personal gestalts, we will naturally see ourselves as affected by, and part of, a larger context. Thus, one's "whole picture" can expand to include the whole human condition.

SUGGESTIONS FOR FURTHER READING

Fritz Perls, *Gestalt Therapy Verbatim.* Real People Press, 1969.

_____, *The Gestalt Approach and Eye Witness to Therapy.* Science and Behavior, 1973.

_____, *Ego, Hunger and Aggression.* Allen and Unwin, 1947.

Fritz Perls, R. Hefferline, and P. Goodman, *Gestalt Therapy.* Dell, 1951.

E. and M. Polster, *Gestalt Therapy Integrated.* Brunner/Mazel, 1973.

Frank Rubenfeld, *Social Gestalt: A Response to Illusions of Freedom and Powerlessness.* Psycho-Political Pamphlets, 1978.

John O. Stevens, *Gestalt Is.* Real People Press, 1975.

Deborah Weinstein, M.A., L.M.F.C.C., is a psychotherapist in private practice in San Francisco. She combines an analytic Gestalt approach with bioenergetics in her work with individuals, families, and groups. She is co-founder and a training staff member of the Gestalt Community Action Project, a collective that teaches Social Gestalt to minority therapists and community workers. Ms. Weinstein has taught at Antioch University, and is a graduate of the Bioenergetic Society of Northern California.

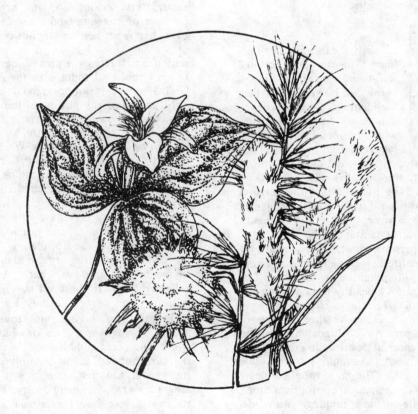

Enjoyment is Health
Murray Korngold

What is mental health? Murray Korngold thinks of it as the ability to experience enjoyment. In this article, he tells us that there are no professionals in the field of living happily. If there were, Murray would be one of them, for he seems to be one of the happiest and most enjoyable people we know. Here he presents his insights and knowledge on such subjects as mental attitudes, learning aptitudes, psychic work, the importance of gratitude, attachment and nonattachment, and much more.

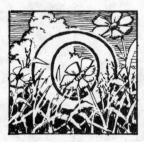

Ordinarily, health and the feeling of mental or emotional well-being are seen as related. I propose, however, that they are identical. Consider the example of Norman Cousins, who described his remarkable recovery from a serious illness by the use of laughter. He watched *Candid Camera*, Marx Brothers films, and did all kinds of things to make himself laugh. The point is that the laughter didn't simply lead to health; it *was* health. To laugh, or sing, or experience a strong positive effect doesn't lead to mental health; it *is* mental health.

Of course, the repertoire of a healthy person's behavior includes the entire range of negative and positive responses. Grief, disappointment, anger, and fear are just as appropriate for a healthy person as joy and laughter, provided that: (a) the person doesn't get stuck in any particular feeling, whether negative or positive; and (b) the person's life is goal-directed and purposeful, taking a cheerful positive direction.

For example, a mechanic would say the same about your car's alternator. The gauge should indicate that the alternator is discharging at appropriate times, and charging while the engine is running. This model could have many applications—neurohormonal, psychodynamic, physiological, psychic, etc.—but the point is simple: in order to live reasonably happily and to deal appropriately with difficulties and adversities, one needs to have free access to positive thoughts and feelings, and to avoid getting stuck in negative ones.

There are no professionals on the subject of living happily. In that department we are all amateurs. There are those who teach the doctrines of great teachers, saints, and sages, and who seem to wear the mantle of true professionalism, but don't be deceived. There are no pros when it comes to living.

It seems to me that some people mix up two separate matters: seeking God and being happy. The experience of knowing God is rare, but living right and being happy are neither rare nor contingent on finding or seeking God. I know, dear reader, that this last sentence is sure to stir up a hornets' nest somewhere. I don't mean to indulge in theology, but knowing God, I believe, is not up to me. It's up to God. Living right and using my powers of mind and body in the service of my own happiness is up to me.

If we use these powers the way that children do, we will be on the right track. When Jesus said that in order to enter the kingdom of heaven one had to become as a child, he was describing a practical reality. In my associations with children, and particularly when teaching them, I'm constantly struck by the marvelous ability they have with absurdity. Children play with the absurd, and just for the joy of it turn ideas upside down and inside out. They seem to care less about what's true or false than they do about enjoyment. They'll deny what's obvious to me, and vehemently assert the most outrageously far-fetched notions. And of course they learn incredibly fast.

Ernest Jones, Freud's biographer, once described genius as being skeptical about what others are gullible about, and being gullible about what other people are skeptical about. This is certainly a description of a small child. Children are born geniuses, and then are taught how to be dull and dreary. They're taught how to sit still for hours every day, and how to pay attention to what bores them silly. What an incalculable waste of beautiful human resources!

We're all geniuses and children at heart, or we wouldn't be playing this game of reading and writing about such an elusive subject. With all due credit to

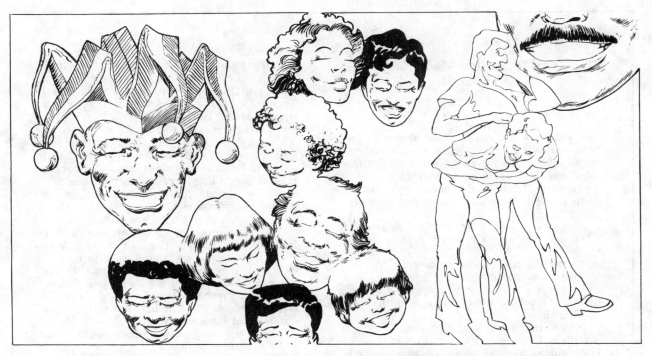

To laugh, or sing, or experience a strong positive effect doesn't lead to mental health—it *is* mental health.

those who have devised and marketed methods and technologies for swiftly teaching hundreds of thousands of ordinary people how to deal with powers of mind creatively, I have to confess that their ways no longer appeal to me; not only because these ways usually harden into dogma and jargon, but also because they concentrate too much attention on technique, and don't leave one free enough to improvise in the service of one's own peculiarities. If you can use psychic power in one way for one purpose, you can use it in another way for another purpose. You can use it for healing, solving problems, and also for staying serene. The evidence is conclusive. It works for me, and I'm a lifelong neurotic.

Now what does it take to learn to do psychic work efficiently, matter-of-factly, and regularly? In talking with Lawrence LeShan (author of *The Medium, the Mystic, and the Physicist*) about his workshops in psychic healing, I learned two interesting things—one political and one psychological. The first thing was that New York City still has a medical superego. The view there is that psychic healing should be medically supervised according to law (which seems a narrow view to me).

The second thing came when I asked Dr. LeShan if he found it easier to teach psychic healing to women than to men. His response delighted me because it was simple, and it sounds true. He said that there were no significant differences that way, but it did seem that the best psychics were the people who liked a lot of different foods, and who had very few aversions.

In other words, people who enjoy trying new things also enjoy learning new things. People who approach new things with fear and trembling will learn with fear and trembling. So it would seem, then, that the point lies somewhere in the neighborhood of enjoyment.

Of course, we intuit that enjoyment doesn't mean pleasure. Although it may include pleasure, "enjoy" is best understood and practiced as a transitive verb. Enjoy: to charge with joy. So, people who are charging around in search of new taste treats, in contrast to those who rarely deviate from their ritual menus, are charging their experience with joy.

I want to deal briefly now with three points: (1) the attitude of seriousness; (2) the importance of gratitude; and (3) the clearing of negative tapes by means of humor.

At this point I interrupted the writing of this piece to read what I had written thus far to a dear friend. This man, who is an accomplished healer and

Transformation Made Easy
Art Buchwald

I was in New York the other day and rode with a friend in a taxi. When we got out, my friend said to the driver, "Thank you for the ride. You did a superb job of driving."

The taxi driver was stunned for a second. Then he said, "Are you a wise guy or something?"

"No, my dear man. I'm not putting you on. I admire the way you keep cool in heavy traffic."

"Yeh," the driver said and drove off.

"What was that all about?" I asked.

"I'm trying to bring love back to New York," he said. "I believe it's the only thing that can save the city."

"How can one man save New York?"

"It's not one man. I believe I made the taxi driver's day. Suppose he has 20 fares. He's going to be nice to those 20 fares because someone was nice to him. Those fares in turn will be kinder to their employees, or shopkeepers, or waiters, or even their own families. Eventually the good will could spread to at least a thousand people. Now, that isn't bad, is it?"

"But, you're depending on that taxi driver to pass your good will to others."

"I'm not depending on it," my friend said. "I'm aware that the system isn't foolproof, so I might deal with ten different people today. If, out of ten, I can make three happy, then eventually I can indirectly influence the attitudes of three thousand more."

"It sounds good on paper," I admitted, "but I'm not sure it works in practice."

First published as "Love and the Cabbie." Reprinted with the permission of the author.

"Nothing is lost if it doesn't. It didn't take any of my time to tell that man he was doing a good job. He received neither a larger tip nor a smaller tip. If it fell on deaf ears, so what? Tomorrow there will be another taxi driver whom I can try to make happy."

"You're some kind of a nut," I said.

"That shows how cynical you have become. I have made a study of this. The thing that seems to be lacking, besides money, of course, for our postal employees, is that no one tells people who work for the post office what a good job they're doing."

"But they're not doing a good job."

"They're not doing a good job because they feel no one cares if they do or not. Why shouldn't someone say a kind word to them?"

We were walking past a structure in the process of being built, and passed five workmen eating their lunch. My friend stopped. "That's a magnificent job you men have done. It must be difficult and dangerous work."

The five men eyed my friend suspiciously.

"When will it be finished?"

"June," a man grunted.

"Ah. That really is impressive. You must all be very proud."

We walked away. I said to him, "I haven't seen anyone like you since *The Man from La Mancha.*"

"When those men digest my words, they will feel better for it. Somehow the city will benefit from their happiness."

"But you can't do this alone!" I protested. "You're just one man."

"The most important thing is not to get discouraged. Making people in the city become kind again is not an easy job, but if I can enlist other people in my campaign . . ."

"You just winked at a very plain-looking woman," I said.

"Yes, I know," he replied. "And if she's a school teacher, her class will be in for a fantastic day."

---

teacher, listened, giggled, then cleared his throat and commented uneasily that it all sounded too easy. I suppose you could say that my friend has the attitude of seriousness. From this angle, life is no laughing matter. But the attitude of seriousness, that man is born into suffering, can also be seen as the original mystification. It's more accurate to see life as a laugh-

ing matter, since enjoyment is the prior and primordial state. We humans are the only beings I know of who are obsessed with the survival program, with the concept of original sin and of life as insolubly problematic.

Conscious people see themselves as the causes of their problems, and not as the effects. To be aware of oneself is to be aware that one creates one's own problems. To be sure, we don't create our problems out of the whole cloth, so to speak, but rather out of the fabric presented to us at every turn. Yet, we do create them. There are no problem-free lives, since problem-solving seems to be the format within which we all operate. However, our freedom to choose whether or not to enjoy our problems is no illusion. It's the most real thing we've got. It's the most real thing we are. If the only choice we have is between enjoying or not enjoying our problems, then it seems to me irresistibly logical and appealing that we should see all life as play. Indeed, there are hundreds of millions of Indians who at least give lip-service to the concept of play (*Lila*) as being the only cosmic reality, although everyone I've ever heard preach this doctrine seems to take himself very seriously, quite unlike Mark Twain, who could not have been taking himself very seriously when he defined play as "very serious activity without any purpose." Sometime you might try listing the names of people you know under two separate headings: those who take themselves very seriously, and those who don't. Honestly. In which group of characters do you feel the greatest trust?

The single emotional polarity that I regard as the most fateful in one's life is gratitude versus envy. The biblical saying that to him who hath it shall be added, and from him who hath not it shall be taken away, strikes me as precisely accurate. If you start from the assumption, as I do, that mind and its contents *create,* then a preoccupation with not having is a recipe for not having. Contrariwise, being absorbed with having is a recipe for having. The emotional states that correspond to these two modes are envy and gratitude. These are two extremely powerful emotional triggers, and they appear to operate effectively in all aspects of creating new realities or re-creating old ones. If I want to "create" that my day will be a successful one, it's not enough for me to visualize or imagine it vividly. The imagining is necessary, but not sufficient. What makes it sufficient is to experience the desired outcome with gratitude. The more profound the gratitude, the more effective the outcome.

One needs to be reminded now and then that the mind isn't logical. On the contrary, from a rational point of view, the mind is an imbecile, and operates entirely on the basis of emotional imagery and valences. It's the feeling behind it that counts, as the saying goes.

The happy irony about the use of gratitude as an emotional tool is that regardless of objective outcome, the frequent experience of gratitude is very healthy, and is absolutely guaranteed to improve digestion, bowel function, blood pressure, and relationships with others. It's not necessary to discuss envy, since all of us are already well-acquainted with that subject.

Despite the fact that it's generally healthier to think about and pay attention to what you want, rather than to what you don't want, there are aspects of mind which are deeply ingrained in highly charged negative tapes, all very inconveniently connected with strong survival programming. This wretched side of our natures has been called by many names, including Satan, childhood conditioning, original sin, karma, reactive mind, repetition compulsion, human nature, and so on. By one means and another, conscious beings are eternally engaged in clearing these tapes. What all effective clearing procedures seem to have in common, whether they are metaphysical, physical, psychological, or spiritual, are the following:

1. Whether by yantras, mantras, or breathing exercises, whether by neutralizing unconscious resistance, bypassing bad habits, or transcending old tapes, there is always, always, always an inducing of slower and more regular rhythms in the whole personal field. This includes the slowing down of brain-wave output, heartbeat, breathing, and most bodily processes. Clearly, any diagnostician who is feeling pulses or reading auras is really inquiring into our rhythmic state in order to discover the current state of health. This is what relaxation is all about. Relaxation equals openness, nongrabbing, accessibility, and slowing down. Relaxation equals enjoyment.

2. All of us have had the experience personally and with clients in which there is a sudden release into humor. After repeating the same old lamentation over and over, we suddenly arrive at the illuminating flash: "Wow. Is that what I've been hassling myself for all this time? What a joke." The true "Aha!" is usually accompanied by humor, by a realization of the inherent comedy, even ludicrousness, of our situation. What was experienced the first time as a tragedy, then reiterated tediously as drama, melodrama, and boring suffering is all of a sudden seen as a joke, as a farce. It can no longer be taken seriously, and is now, at long last, believe it or not, finally enjoyed. It really seems to happen that way.

Democritus, that sweet old Greek who discovered atoms, wasn't just whistling Dixie when he said that the main task of human intelligence is to take life, which is presented to us as tragedy, and transform it into comedy.

The litmus paper test, then, of whether, indeed, we are proceeding correctly is enjoyment.

A New Perspective on Reality
Marilyn Ferguson

> The brain is a hologram,
> interpreting a
> holographic universe.

Neuroscientist Karl Pribram of Stanford and physicist David Bohm of the University of London have proposed theories that, in tandem, appear to account for all transcendental experience, paranormal events, and even "normal" perceptual oddities. The implications for every aspect of human life, as well as for science, are extremely profound.

This breakthrough fulfills predictions that the long-awaited theory would (1) draw on theoretical mathematics; and (2) establish the "supernatural" as part of nature.

The theory, in a nutshell: *Our brains mathematically construct "concrete" reality by interpreting frequencies from another dimension, a realm of meaningful, patterned primary reality that transcends time and space. The brain is a hologram, interpreting a holographic universe.*

Phenomena of altered states of consciousness (which reflect altered brain states) may be due to a literal attunement to the invisible matrix that generates "concrete" reality. This may enable interaction with reality at a primary level, thereby accounting for precognition, psychokinesis, healing, time distortion, rapid learning, experiences of "oneness with the universe," the conviction that ordinary reality is an illusion, and descriptions of a void that is paradoxically full, as in the Taoist saying, "The real is empty and the empty is real."

For several years those interested in human consciousness have been speaking wistfully of the "emerging paradigm," an integral theory that would catch all the wonderful wildlife of science and spirit. Here, at last, is a theory that marries biology to physics in an open system: it is the paradoxical borderless paradigm that our schizophrenic science has been crying for.

Reprinted from *Brain/Mind Bulletin*, published twice monthly, $15 per year ($19 first-class mail) in North America, $22 (airmail only) all others. $1.50 for two back issues. P.O. Box 42211, Los Angeles, CA 90042.

In the 1963 book *You and Your Brain,* Judith Groch observed that paranormal events could not be ignored just because they were inconvenient to the framework of our knowledge. Einstein, unable to reconcile inconsistencies within Newton's physics, "unlocked a theoretical door through which scientists then poured in pursuit of the knowledge that lay on the other side." Groch suggested that the brain awaited its Einstein.

It is appropriate that this radical, satisfying paradigm has emerged from Pribram, a brain researcher-neurosurgeon who was a friend of the Western Zen teacher Alan Watts, and Bohm, a theoretical physicist, who was a close friend of Krishnamurti, and a former associate of Einstein.

WHAT IS HOLOGRAPHY?

Holography is a method of lensless photography in which the wave field of light scattered by an object is recorded on a plate as an interference pattern. When the photographic record—the hologram—is placed in a coherent light beam like a laser, the original wave pattern is regenerated. A three-dimensional image appears.

Because there is no focusing lens, the plate appears as a meaningless pattern of swirls. *Any piece of the hologram will reconstruct the entire image.*

Physicist David Bohm says that the hologram is a starting point for a new description of reality: the *enfolded* order. Classical reality has focused on secondary manifestations—the *unfolded* aspect of things, not their source. These appearances are abstracted from an intangible, invisible flux that is not composed of parts; it is an inseparable interconnectedness.

Bohm says that primary physical laws cannot be discovered by a science that attempts to break the world into its parts.

There are intriguing implications in a paradigm that says the brain employs a holographic process to abstract from a holographic domain. Parapsychologists have searched in vain for the energy that might transmit telepathy, psychokinesis, healing, etc. If these events emerge from frequencies transcending time and space, they don't have to be transmitted. They are potentially simultaneous and everywhere.

Changes in magnetic, electromagnetic, or gravitational fields, and changes in the brain's electrical patterns would be only surface manifestations of seemingly unmeasurable underlying factors. J. B. Rhine, who pioneered modern parapsychology, was skeptical that an energy would be found. Psychologist Lawrence LeShan, author of *Alternate Realities,* believes that energy is a less useful concept in psychic healing than a certain merger of identity, perhaps a resonance.

PRIMARY REALITY MAY BE FREQUENCY REALM

Is reality the product of an invisible matrix? "I believe we're in the middle of a paradigm shift that encompasses all of science," Karl Pribram said at a recent Houston conference, *New Dimensions in Health Care.* He went on to spell out a powerful multifaceted theory that could account for sensory reality as a "special case," constructed by the brain's mathematics, but drawn from a domain beyond time and space, where only frequencies exist.

The theory could account for all the phenomena that seem to contravene existing scientific "law," by demonstrating that such restrictions are themselves products of our perceptual constructs. Theoretical physics has already demonstrated that events cannot be described in mechanical terms at subatomic levels.

Pribram, a renowned brain researcher, has accumulated evidence that the brain's "deep structure" is essentially holographic—analogous to the lensless photographic process for which Dennis Gabor received a Nobel Prize.

Pribram's theory has gained increasing support and has not been seriously challenged. An impressive body of research in many laboratories has demonstrated that the brain structures see, hear, taste, smell, and touch by sophisticated mathematical analysis of temporal and spatial frequencies. An eerie property of both hologram and brain is the distribution of information throughout the system, each fragment encoded to produce the information of the whole.

Although the holographic model generated fruitful answers, it raised a question that came to haunt Pribram. Who was looking at the hologram? Who was the "little man inside the little man," what Arthur Koestler called "the ghost in the machine"?

After agonizing over this problem for some time, Pribram said, he decided that if the question had stymied everybody since Aristotle, per-

haps it was the wrong question. "So I asked, 'What if the real world isn't made up of objects at all. What if *it's* a hologram?'"

Pribram's conversations with his son, a physicist, led him to the recent theories of David Bohm. To his great excitement he found that Bohm speculated that the nature of the universe might be more like a hologram, a realm of frequencies and potentialities underlying an illusion of concreteness. Bohm pointed out that ever since Galileo, science has objectified nature by looking at it through lenses.

Pribram was struck with the thought that the brain's mathematics might be "a cruder form of a lens. Maybe reality isn't what we see with our eyes. If we didn't have that lens, we might know a world organized in the frequency domain. No space, no time—just events. Can that reality be 'read out of' that domain?" Transcendental experience suggested that there is access to the frequency domain, the primary reality.

"What if there is a matrix that doesn't objectify unless we do something to it?" The brain's own representations—its abstraction—may be identical with one state of the universe.

Pribram pointed out the extraordinary insights of mystics and early philosophers that preceded scientific verification by centuries. One example is the metaphysical description of the pineal gland as the "third eye." Recently it was found that the pineal may be something of a super master gland, since its secretion of melatonin regulates the activities of the pituitary, long considered the brain's master gland.

The eighteenth-century philosopher Leibniz described a system of "monads" that coincides strikingly with the new paradigm. His discovery of integral calculus enabled Gabor to invent the hologram two hundred years later.

"How did these ideas arise for millennia before we had the mathematics to understand them?" Pribram asked. "Maybe in the holographic state—in the frequency domain—4,000 years ago is tomorrow.

"Eastern philosophy has come into Western thought in the past. Every once in a while we have these insights that bring us back to the infinite," he told his audience. "Whether it will stick this time, or we'll have to go around once more, will depend on you. The spirit of the infinite could become part of our culture, and not 'a little far out.'"

Clairvoyant Counsel

Helen Palmer, M.A., Ph.D.

Clairvoyance, or clear vision, is the ability to see vibrational forms that cannot be seen with the human eye, such as visions, auras, and energy patterns.

A clairvoyant reader has the ability to visualize and report information about situations in other people's lives. Often this takes the form of forgotten events, inner thought patterns, the internal logic in outwardly bizarre behavior, unrecognized options, and future possibilities.

In this article, Helen Palmer, a noted clairvoyant, explains clairvoyance in language we can all understand. She describes the clairvoyant-client relationship, and gives us a good set of exercises for developing our own clairvoyant capacities.

We are also very fortunate to have here a portion of a transcript of one of her clairvoyant or "psychic" sessions. This session focuses on bringing up the underlying cause of the client's experience. It is an example of clairvoyant counseling at its best: the client is introduced to an aspect of himself he had not formally known before, and is given insights to help him deal consciously with that aspect in a life situation.

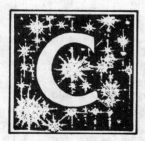 lairvoyance is a voluntary dream. It is the ability to discriminate between times when the brain is thinking, and times when it is visualizing. These two internal functions are deeply intertwined, but we rarely think it important to distinguish between them. A clairvoyant is a person who, by either aptitude or training, is able to distinguish when she or he is thinking, as a separate mental experience from when she or he is "seeing" an internal image that is independent of personal thoughts. To use clairvoyance as a source of information for daily life, you need a strong visual imagination, and enough personal determination to perform the mental practices that separate thinking from visual imagination.

The thinking function of the brain allows us to examine issues from the point of view of known information. We can think out different approaches and solutions to an issue by examining what we know about it, and hypothesizing the missing pieces of information. Imagination allows us access to unknown information, because we can imagine people and events that we have never personally experienced, even if they are located far away, or in the past or future.

In psychological work, the imagination has been traditionally viewed as a suspect vehicle for information. Imagination is unrepeatable, very hard to quantify, and the repository of a personality's daydream avoidances, projections, and unfulfilled desires. Although imagination is useful in artistic life, and for exploring the deep patterns of personality by means of dream recall, psychologists have considered the training of imagination to be antithetical to understanding one's mental and emotional patterns in terms of an ordered, societal reality, to which one must adjust. Until quite recently, imagination was seen merely as a difficult-to-measure "creative" factor that was present in artistic types.

New therapeutic approaches have placed the training of imagination in the role of opening communication with the parts of the self that are not easily contacted by thinking. Visualization is especially used in viewing and directing changes in the physical body, and in clarifying mental and emotional patterns. Among the recent therapies that use imagination for clarification and change are: self-hypnosis, for reprogramming, by visualizing a corrected situation; Gestalt, for identifying and acting out the conflicting parts of personality; guided fantasy, for uncovering unrecognized inner patterns; and dream journal work, for the deciphering of messages from the voiceless parts of ourselves.

These visual techniques are not psychic, because they use images to connect to situations that "belong" to the visualizer. Obviously, one's internal body organs and forgotten memories are still included in one's system, even though they may be difficult to locate, or to remember. However, in the growing group of people who habitually visualize as a meditation practice, or as a self-help tool for personal change, the clairvoyant property of imagination can suggest itself. This is the use of images as nonverbal communication channels between the self and people or "unknowable" situations outside the self.

A visualization has no psychic content when the images are directly guided by a person's personal thoughts. If a person thinks "beach scene," and his brain produces a visual counterpart of sand dunes, waves, and people wearing swimsuits, we can only infer that the brain moves easily back and forth between thoughts and images. The same person might also think "remember last night's dream," and sure enough, he is likely to recover visual sequences from that dream. However, as a person gets used to visualization for dream recall, and as that person gains access to his or her inner life, an interesting situation emerges: from time to time, images appear that contain information which clearly could not have come from personal thoughts. "Unknowable," or psychic, information appears in the imagination, along with images that are counterparts to personal thoughts. The most common example of psychic information coming through visual imagination is the precognitive dream. People commonly report accurate dreams of "unknowable" future events that are later played out. Another common experience is that of resolving an intellectual problem by the indications received in a dream. These are examples of clairvoyance, because a *clear view* of information that was unavailable to the thoughts of the person was obtained by the inner eye—the eye of the imagination.

All the mechanisms of clairvoyance are present in a dream. The personal thoughts stop in sleep, and a state of visualization begins, to be remembered only when the dreamer wakes and starts to think again. Thought stops; a vision appears; and, last of all, the thoughts remember what has already been seen. The sequence of actions in psychic perception is: first, thought is suspended; second, information is received through the imagination; and, last of all, the thoughts come back to interpret the sequences of imagination that have already gone by. This is an action of first seeing, then thinking, which is the reverse of the action that appears in guided imagery: think first, then see.

Although dreams indicate that there are physical receptors for psychic information, dreams have great liabilities; it is difficult to choose the topic of a dream; dreams come and go sporadically; they are

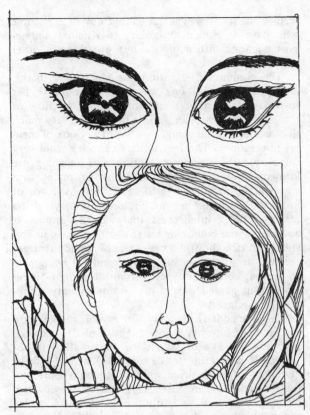

To use clairvoyance as a source of information, you need a strong visual imagination and the ability to distinguish the difference between internal visual images and personal thoughts.

hard to complete and recall; and they are heavily loaded with personal imagery, which often obscures the psychic content. The psychic task remains that of obtaining voluntary control of the mechanism of the dream. That means, being able to choose the topic of a dream, and to separate the visual imagination from the biased images that are guided from personal thoughts.

In principle, every person who has ever dreamed and awakened to remember the message of the dream has access to the physical mechanism of clairvoyant information for daily life. In practical terms, it is difficult to suspend personal thoughts and attain a separate state of visualization, especially when dealing with your own emotional material. We want so much for a certain answer to appear, that the danger of guided imagery, powerfully directed by personal wishes, is very strong. It is difficult to get a clear view of loaded material when we strongly desire or fear a particular outcome. It is for this reason that people have historically sought clairvoyant counsel from those people who have developed the ability to visualize and report accurate information about situations in other people's lives.

The common designation for a person with this ability is "reader," one who can focus his or her imagination to receive and understand the flow of images coming from an outside target. It is very much like reading the meanings in a wordless book of mental impressions. The impressions can vary from very literal pictures, wherein picture and meaning are known simultaneously, to highly abstract pictograms, wherein the meaning has to be derived by force of intellect, much like a symbolic dream that yields its message under intellectual analysis. The important abilities of the counselor are (a) being able to understand and talk about the messages contained in images received from the outside target, and (b) being able to prevent personal thoughts from intruding into the reading, as guided images that are mistakenly attributed to the target.

The tremendous advantages of psychic readings are the kinds of information that they provide access to, and the speed with which the information is obtained. It is possible to visualize all kinds of hidden material—forgotten events, inner thought patterns, the internal logic in outwardly bizarre behavior, unrecognized options, and future possibilities. A reader generally gives an hour-long view of situations that took years to play out in real life, and probably took months of therapy to understand.

The most common situations that a counselor is asked to visualize are health, relationships with people, work situations, sexual patterns, progress in meditation, and the outcome of projects. People want a clairvoyant to provide access to information that is hidden from themselves. They want a view of hidden, repeating patterns in their relationships, of blind spots in their thinking, of possibilities that they cannot see.

In this form of counsel, the burden is on the reader to produce information pertaining to the client's questions. The client presents questions, and the reader reads. This is obviously a very different interaction from what happens in a therapy session, wherein the therapist facilitates the client's insight. Properly used, therapy and psychic counsel are highly complementary, because the insights of both intellect and intuition can converge on a client's situation. The reading adds the kinds of information that are unavailable to intellect; for, no matter how intelligent or well-trained a therapist might be, the limits of intellectual connection confine the understanding of the client to a dialogue of close analogies.

For example, a client might say, "When I'm in love, it's like a roller-coaster ride. It's out of control and thrilling for me."

And the therapist might think, "When I'm in love, it feels like a glassy calm. However, I have ridden on a roller coaster, and I have been in love in my own way."

In attempting to understand each other, these two are constrained, by the limits of intellect, to take the other's statement, and glue it on to an internal experience of their own.

Because a clairvoyant's personal thoughts and experiences are temporarily suspended during a reading, the client is not understood as a close analogy. During the time that a reader has focused her visual brain on an outside person, she does not see a stereotype of the outsider, a projection, or a close approximation; she sees the other as he is to himself. The reader is viewing situations of love from the single perspective of the ups and downs of a roller coaster. A reader's vision is not limited to the personal point of view of the client; he or she can also visualize any objective situation in which the client is involved. This objective situation can be read from any point of view.

Because there is so little interaction between clairvoyant and client, a reading is best used as an adjunct to therapy, so that the client has a place in which to move psychic information into actions for daily life.

The clearest situation of psychic counsel is the absent reading. A common example of this is in family counseling, when a client is interested in clarifying relationships with several family members who are not physically present. Another example is when a therapist seeks psychic clarification of the progress of treatment of patients not present during the reading.

I give next a set of focusing exercises that demarcate the mental terrain of an absent reading. The set can serve as a guide in developing the ability to receive and understand information from a distance, without the presence of physical cues or any prior knowledge of the distant target. The evidence of accuracy in any reading is the recognition of self by the target person. Moreover, they will be described as they exist inside themselves, rather than in general terms, from an outsider's perspective, or as an attempt to imagine what it might be like to stand in someone else's place. The point of focusing exercises to develop clairvoyance rests on the idea that, once identified, any capacity improves with training. Although individuals vary in their aptitude, most people can identify and learn to maintain a state of visual imagination.

EXERCISE FOR THREE EYES

The first expectation about clairvoyance is that a brand-new mental experience is going to be activated; an inner eye is going to be found and opened that was never there before, rather than distinguishing the already active imagination of the inner eye from the visual information entering through the physical eyes.

Seat yourself at a distance of several feet from a blank wall. Project an image of a green triangle from your head, until it stabilizes on the wall.

Notice: (1) The green triangle is obviously not really tacked to the wall, but is proceeding from your inner imagination onto a spot in the real world. It seems to exist there as long as you exert the effort of concentration to keep it present. (2) The triangle is very tenuous compared to the solid wall, and the edges of other solid things, like furniture, that you will catch with the corners of your eyes.

Rest. Close all three eyes. No visual objects for the physical eyes, and no imagination for the third eye.

Again, project a stable green triangle. Move your concentration between seeing only the wall (two physical eyes), and only the triangle (third eye).

Notice: (1) It is difficult to keep both the wall and the triangle present at the same time. (2) The triangle is hard to get started, but relatively easy to maintain, once it is projected against the wall. (3) You are concentrating in a slightly different spot in your head when the triangle is present. Identify this spot, close all three eyes, and press the spot with your finger. This is the location of the third eye, or the spot where the sensations connected to visualization are usually felt.

Again, project the green triangle. It is probably still tenuous, but present enough to describe. "Description" here means that you could explain it to someone else, or reproduce the triangle in a sketch. Focus on its color: the depth, the shade, the gradient of its color. Focus on its shape, the position of triangle points on the wall. Focus on its size, by running your physical eyes along the edge of the mental projection. This, being the most limited element, is the easiest to focus on when attention wanders.

Notice: (1) There are only three elements in a simple, visual impression—color, shape (the features), and size. (2) When you focus on any one of the three elements, the triangle becomes stabilized, and the wall recedes from awareness. So, to tune out input coming through the phy-sical eyes, it is useful to deliberately focus on the color, shape, and size of the inner-eye projection. Rest, no input. Close all three eyes.

Keep your physical eyes closed. Project the green triangle inside your head. Go blank. Project it again. Go blank again. Do this until you get the idea of being able to choose a mental focal point, and produce it inside the third eye at will.

Notice: (1) With your eyes closed, the discrimination between the visualized green triangle and other input that is coming from inside yourself becomes much more obvious. (2) You can deliberately move your mental focus from sector to sector of this internal input. The usual sectors consist of: the triangle itself; the awareness of the room that sits in front of your closed eyes; your own body dimensions, especially the front of your face; your own judging or doubting thoughts about the accuracy or importance of visualizing green triangles; memories about times that you have attempted mental work before; plans about what visualization might lead to; and fantasies arising from the self. (3) When you are concentrating on one sector of internal input, the other sectors recede from awareness, just as the wall receded when you focused on the projected triangle.

Move your mental focus between the sectors of internal input. The usual sectors are: body dimensions; residue of the room in front of your closed eyes; judging or doubting thoughts; memories, plans, fantasies. Last of all to be recognized are the sectors of concentration consisting of the front of your face, and what has been called "the Watcher" in meditation.

Notice: (1) The last discrimination is usually made between the green triangle and "the watcher." This is the sector of inner input that is experienced as "Somebody is watching a green triangle." It is the last sector of possible intrusion of personal thoughts into a visualization. (2) By deliberately rotating mental focus between the sectors of input, you find that they become more recognizable when they intrude, and easier to move away from when you redirect concentration to the triangle, by concentrating on its color, shape, and size.

EXERCISE TO STRENGTHEN INTERNAL IMAGES

The expectation in strengthening something is that you isolate it, and keep practicing its function until it is strong. This would be like strengthening a muscle; you would isolate the biceps, and pump that muscle until it increases in lifting power and endurance. It is very diffi-

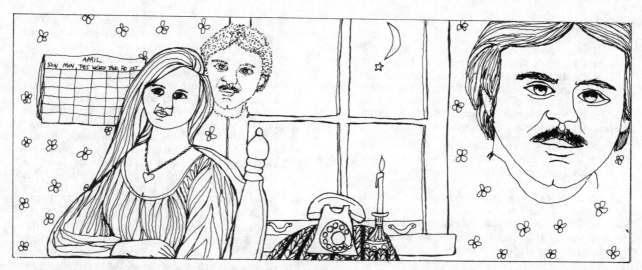

Pick a friend at a distance, that you want to contact. Visualize the friend's face, and move your concentration between the shape, the size, and the color.

cult to strengthen the intensity and endurance of mental images by forcing your attention to stay glued on a green triangle, and isolating it by willing other input to stay out of your mind. This would be like the old exercise "don't think of an elephant," wherein much of the available mental focus is concentrated on keeping elephants out—blocking intrusions, rather than on strengthening the triangle. To reduce blocking of intruding input and forcing of attention to a single point, you must direct attention to the triangle, by letting it become so beautiful that you want to look at it for a long time. The strength is in the beauty, for the mind is willing to concentrate on something beautiful for a long time.

Visualize the green triangle inside the third eye. Deliberately rotate your attention between the three elements of the triangle. The color: focus on the tone of green, the shading, the surface patina—anything of green that is interesting enough, beautiful enough to draw attention to the color of the triangle. *The shape:* focus on the position of points and lines, isoceles, equilateral. *The size:* run your focus along each line.

Pick a friend, at a distance, that you want to contact. Visualize the friend's face, and move your concentration between the three elements of the pictogram. The face has a fantastic surface for engaging attention. The colors of a complexion are endlessly shaded and textured. The bony structure has infinite combinations of shape to gaze at. Size can be variable.

Notice: (1) Although you are working from a memory face, the imagination is already filling in the gaps between pieces of memory. Clearly,

the eyes could be a different color than what appears to you, and the hairline shaped in a different way. (2) Your focus on the distant friend deepens as you allow imagination to play out against the image.

Visualize the face of the friend. Let the brain move, without thinking, to a pictogram that represents that friend.

Notice: (1) The brain moves easily from a literal memory to an abstraction of that memory. (2) The concentration is still locked to the absent friend when you move to the mandala, so long as your own thoughts have not intervened, or your concentration moved to another point.

The most critical part of a reading is that the pictogram, the triangle of the absent friend, be seen as absolutely neutral, beautiful but neutral, and that no intruding input be present when this neutral surface is questioned. When it is neutral, and no thought is present, let the triangle show you the emotion that your friend is experiencing at that exact moment.

This is a situation of see/think, in that the triangle will initiate visual changes in the absence of your own thoughts. The thinking part of the brain, for once, assumes the unusual role of putting an interpretation on the visualization, after it has already gone by. It is interesting how a simple triangle can be known in the imagination as excited or depressed, or witty, or shy. Yet the thoughts will attribute meaning to any impression that is held inside the mind's eye.

Notice: The potential of see/think can be extended to highly complex diagrams of distant targets.

TRANSCRIPT OF A PSYCHIC READING

This section from a transcript illustrates the kind of highly personal patterns of thought and behavior that become available information when images are free to carry a question from its antecedents in the past, into its future, and into its place of relation to the other categories of the client's life. I chose it because it shows a clear mental pattern, and because the client asked some questions about the mechanics of reading.

Patricia J.
Bolinas, California
March 1978

Pat: I am in therapy, and I have a lot of fears. I want to understand more about these fears, and to get rid of them.

Helen: My first reaction is that I am in a danger zone. My body is afraid, and my thought wants to go to other people, to ask them what I am being afraid of, where the danger is located. The first set of impressions comes from the past; it has to do with a repeating scene between your parents. She stays close to you, and he moves in and out—eventually he stays out. Now there remains in your mother a scanning, like a watchtower light, that is always out there, into the adult world, scanning for what he might do. Her body is with you, and the statement is, "I'm here, with you," but the concentration of her mind is "out there," preoccupied with some danger point that she does not report. So there is an odd feeling of her being physically present, but located elsewhere in her emotions. The child is scared at not being included in where the woman's thought goes, and it's also exciting: "I could go there too; and if I could be the target of the situation that she's visualizing, then I've got her. Her thought would be pinned on me," And that's where your mind went, it traveled into her danger zone and shared it with her.

Your mother defends herself with an idea of the undefended gate. Her thought goes to the undefended gate. That represents the sector of your life together where outside trouble might creep in. The sector that runs smoothly is defended; consequently, no thought has to go there, it doesn't hold her attention. Thought goes to the possibility of what might happen at the unsmooth gate, the sector that has problems.

In the present, there is an uneasy carryover of the early pattern. In presenting yourself in any new situation, there is a feeling of safety, of going to be included, if you can manage to present yourself in the position of the endangered outsider. I see the old thought of the mother, scanning like a searchlight, around for where the enemy plane is zeroing in. If she spots the plane, and you have managed to be the target of the plane, then "Ah! My child is being threatened." She tracks the plane, and gives it full attention, which includes yourself. So, as an adult, there is an underlying pattern in your thinking, that you will be ignored in situations that are peaceful to yourself, and be sought after, be valuable in, situations where you happen to be standing in the undefended gate, vulnerable to the attack of whatever the situation most fears. This pattern of thought underlies all the different categories of your life—your love of people, your health, the progress of your career. That when any situation becomes profitable to the self, easygoing, there is a great uneasiness that the attention will turn away from you, that the rug is going to slip, that the attention of the situation will turn to whatever menaced all of you from the outside. So your thought then turns to the possibilities of danger, and how to engage that danger, although the situation that you occupy may be 90 per cent free of outside interference. The thought automatically locates at the undefended gate, so that it fills your mind, and seems to be real and present. Your automatic, mistaken idea is that the others too, the beloveds, are also thinking along the lines of possible threat, or that they are so tuned out or insensitive that they cannot see it standing there.

Pat: How does this affect my marriage?

Helen: What's his name?

Pat: Seth J.

Helen: I see that if you walk into a room full of men that you have never met before, and if there are men there who look overtly charismatic, very in the world—they may have a good profession, a well-put-together life—that you don't notice them. You are not looking because they don't carry a sense of inclusion, according to your pattern. What you're looking for is, "What's he afraid of?" Okay, you can see this, even in somebody who has a very good cover. Now, in this room, you will be very sensitive to, be drawn to, the one out of many who is preoccupied with some point of nervousness, a fear of his own. You would feel comfortable with that man; you could walk over and have a conversation, a relationship. We could sit here and enumerate dozens of relationships that follow that pattern. Now, Pat, if a man is really well put together, doesn't have a big fear, or doesn't want to let on, it will seem to him that you bring it out of him, that he is only aware of being afraid around you.

Pat: I'm the witch.

Helen: Yes, they will say, "I feel crazier around you than I feel around anybody. Why is it that I'm thinking about the one thing in the world that scares me to death, when I'm around you."

Pat: Seth says that to me all the time, that I upset people and then he has to patch them up again.

Helen: From another point of view, if a real fear situation develops for Seth, he can easily draw you into it, and pass it over to you for handling. Inadvertently, people will use you for their own causes. The signal that you put out is that you are willing to listen to a bad situation.

When I focus on the marriage, I get your man, your husband, and the man that he is afraid of: big, tough, a Hell's Angel man. From the inside perspective, you follow your pattern, and flirt with the motorcycler, the danger. Several ideas converge in your mind here, illogically, but according to the pattern, that you will make the marriage firm by drawing off the danger. This has a line of action to the past, where, if you become the victim of your Dad's anger, then you won Mom hands down, because that's where her thought always goes anyway. So there are fantasies of being hurt by somebody: not maimed really, just pushed around, feelings hurt, used, or put upon. In these fantasies, you have the idea that you sacrifice yourself for your friends. You didn't want it to happen to them; so you drew attack, humiliation, onto yourself. Very fascinating, because, from the outside, you are the one who flirted with the hated danger, sat on the cycle. You are the wick by which heat can travel into a situation. Being fascinated by what others fear, you try to help them, and bind them to you. In this process, you become the means by which danger can enter your marriage. Seth is appealing to you to stay away from trouble.

Pat: What does he look like?

Helen: Physically? I have no idea.

Pat: But you saw us together.

Helen: No. I got a diagram that describes your interaction. He could have come in as a stick figure, as a stereotype. He could come as a diagram of pinpoints, the movements of which give me the message of your marriage interaction. The importance is the guidance, the message. Do you think that way? Was the description accurate?

Pat: Yes.

Helen: Good. Then it's useful. Also, I know that you are attached to flirting with danger too, but I doubt if you act it out on the back of a Harley-Davidson. Your message came in a symbol that reads to me.

Pat: How do I stop it? I want that marriage to be good, I want it to work, but it's been a constant crisis.

Helen: You don't need a psychic for that question.

The traditions have clear advice, both the version of mental tradition that we are used to—psychotherapy— and the spiritual traditions that contain methods that you can use to intervene in your own thoughts. You will only act on situations that appear in your thinking. I'm not making light of your situation when I say that the future of it rests on the elements that are prominent in the repeating pattern of thought. You will pick out those elements in any situation. They will attract your attention, and fill your mind, so that they seem to be the only reality present for you to act on. Learn to focus your mind, so that you can keep your thoughts concentrated on the stable elements in the marriage, without panicking and automatically switching on the thought of danger from the outside. Learn to recognize the moment when your thought locks onto danger, and intervene, so that you can circumvent your inevitable action toward the point of danger that seems real to you. I know that it sounds like these patterns are tangible things, solid, like pieces of furniture that you have to move around. But you can choose where to place your thought. This is not avoidism. If real danger comes, you would be the first to know. This is working to move your thought toward what you have established as the objective situation, rather than letting the pattern automatically turn to the elements of a situation that it habitually seeks.

SUGGESTIONS FOR FURTHER READING

Robert Ornstein, ed., *The Nature of Human Consciousness.* W. H. Freeman, 1973.

Putoff and Targ, *The Papers on Remote Viewing.* Available through Stanford Research Institute.

Joseph Goldstein, *The Experience of Insight.* Unity Press, 1976.

Helen Palmer, M.A., Ph.D., is in private practice as a psychic counselor, working mainly with people who are developing their own paths by means of therapy and the techniques of meditation.

She is a clinical psychologist whose clairvoyance developed unexpectedly nine years ago during the practice of self-hypnosis to deal with a long emotional crisis. Since that time her intuition has stabilized and expanded, so that her way of working with people has moved from that of psychologist to that of psychic.

She has taught psychic work at numerous California centers, including Esalen, U.C. Berkeley Extension, the California School for Professional Psychology, and Antioch West.

Currently she continues a private practice, and leads private groups in the development of intuition.

Flower Essences:
Catalysts for Transformation and Health
Richard Katz

The Bach flower remedies use the subtle energy of 38 different wildflowers to activate positivity in areas of emotional blockage. When we increase our mental and emotional well-being, the physical body has a better chance of staying healthy. In this article, Richard Katz discusses this wonderfully simple and gentle method of self-healing.

"There is no true healing unless there is a change in outlook, peace of mind, and inner happiness."

Dr. Edward Bach

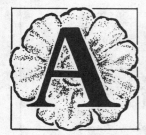

Any sensitive soul who has made friends with forest and field knows how nature heals and uplifts the human spirit. The spontaneous harmony and varied forms of life satisfy our longing to feel unity with the cosmic order, to overcome the painful illusion of the isolated ego.

Flowers, particularly, are our healers and teachers, expressing the unique personality of each plant species in beautiful form, color, and fragrance. They are the universality of the divine source expressed in radiant individuality, and without the fear, doubt, anger, and confusion that separates us humans from our true selves.

Dr. Edward Bach of England (1886–1936) was one who knew the healing power of nature and the needs of people to reconnect with their inner natures. He was a visionary healer who deeply understood the inner nature of health and dis-ease. Dr. Bach expressed his vision in *Heal Thyself*, written in 1931.

"Disease is in essence the result of conflict between the Soul and the Mind, and will never be eradicated except by spiritual and mental effort. Such efforts, if properly made with understanding . . . can cure and prevent disease by removing those basic factors which are its primary cause. No effort directed to the body alone can do more than superficially repair damage, and in this, there is no cure, since the cause is still operative, and may at any moment again demonstrate its presence in another form. . . .

"Let it be briefly stated that disease, though apparently so cruel, is in itself beneficial and for our own good, and if rightly interpreted, will guide us to our essential faults. . . . Suffering is a corrective to point out a lesson which by other means we have failed to grasp, and never can it be eradicated until that lesson is learnt."[1]

According to Bach, one major lesson we are to learn from dis-ease is that we need to harmonize our personality with our soul, or higher self. The word

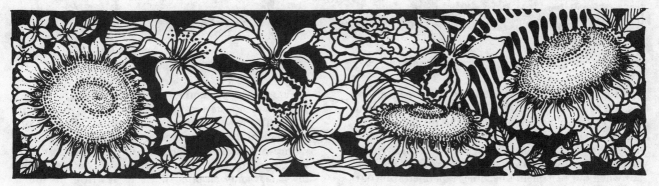

Flowers, particularly, are our healers and teachers—expressing the personality of each plant species in beautiful form, color, and fragrance.

The Lessons of Bach Flower Essences
Richard Katz

Agrimony—inner peace, honest cheerfulness.
Aspen—fearlessness, openness to experience.
Beech—acceptance, tolerance, understanding differences.
Centaury—inner strength, inner direction.
Cerato—trusting inner guidance.
Cherry Plum—courage and balance under extreme stress.
Chestnut Bud—observation, learning life's lessons.
Chicory—selflessness, appropriate giving and receiving.
Clematis—grounding, presence, manifesting inspiration.
Crab Apple—inner and outer cleansing, harmony, proportion.
Elm—self-assured confidence.
Gentian—perseverance, confidence despite setbacks.
Gorse—faith, hope.
Heather—listening to and caring for others.
Holly—compassion, universal love (heart center).
Honeysuckle—present-centeredness, letting go of the past.
Hornbeam—confidence of energy and ability, involvement.

Impatiens—patience, understanding, acceptance.
Larch—self-confidence, creative expression (throat center).
Mimulus—courage, confidence, understanding, faith.
Mustard—joy, serenity, peace of mind.
Oak—brave perseverance, strength.
Olive—revitalization, renewed interest in life.
Pine—self-acceptance, accepting mistakes as lessons.
Red Chestnut—sending calm, healing thoughts to others.
Rock Rose—self-transcending courage.
Rock Water—flexibility, spontaneity, self-nurturing.
Scleranthus—decisiveness, stability.
Star of Bethlehem—healing of trauma and shock.
Sweet Chestnut—prayerful faith, even in dark times.
Vervain—moderation, relaxation, openness.
Vine—sensitive leadership, respecting others.
Walnut—freedom from limiting influences.
Water Violet—involvement, service, humility.
White Chestnut—quietness and clarity of mind.
Wild Oat—clarity in life directions, vocation.
Wild Rose—enthusiastic interest in life.
Willow—releasing blame, accepting responsibility.
Rescue Remedy (Star of Bethlehem, Rock Rose, Impatiens, Cherry Plum, Clematis)—centering, grounding during extreme stress or emergency.

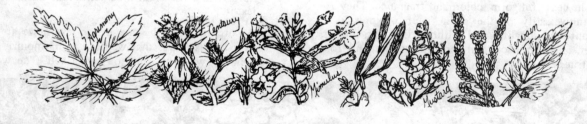

"personality" comes from the Latin "persona," meaning "to sound through," and referring to a mask worn in a dramatic play. Personality is the mask our spiritual self wears—the roles it plays in acting out our life drama. It can serve us well, because it is the vehicle through which we actively express our inner qualities, but when our personality becomes separated from our inner being, we become cut off from life's purpose and the source of our vitality. Thus inwardly split, we are subject to limiting thoughts, feelings, and the physical manifestations of dis-ease.

Bach's own life is an inspirational example of attunement to life's purpose. His dedication to the service of healing sustained him through the most trying circumstances. Even the threat of death early in his career only inspired Bach to reaffirm his life's work, and in the process to restore his health completely.

Although successful in both allopathic and homeopathic medicine, Bach disregarded fame and convention. Following inner guidance, he left his London practice in 1930 to seek the source of health in the simplicity of nature, in her healing flowers. Highly sensitive, Bach selected those flowers whose vibrations brought balance and harmony to the mind and emotions. He prepared the essences by floating the blossoms in a bowl of water in the sunshine, or by lightly boiling them. Using brandy as a natural preservative, he diluted the essences twice, for stock and individual usage. The standard dosage was four drops, four times daily.

Bach prepared 38 different essences, each responding to a particular personality imbalance, awakening the "dormant" inner quality needed to replace it. This work required much strength of purpose, because Bach often experienced the various states of imbalance and disharmony before finding the needed flower. It was only after he felt he had completed his work, in 1936, that he released his spirit from its physical form.

The lessons of Bach's life are contained in the flower essences he left us. For example, the *Wild Oat* essence helps open us to the realization of life direction and purpose; *Larch* helps free our self-expression and creativity from the fear of failure; and *Walnut* helps us steer clear of the influence of dominant personalities, ideas, and past patterns, in order to remain true to inner guidance.

The *Holly* essence represents another of the major lessons of dis-ease: the need to reconnect with the unity of life, to experience ourselves as emanations from one divine source. It vibrates our heart center with the awareness of universal compassionate love.

According to Bach, the illusion of separation is the root of our suffering and of the many ills of our world. When we feel separated from our higher self, from the unity of all life, we create attitudes of fear, greed, envy, hatred, and confusion. Limited thoughts and expectations can become self-fulfilling prophecies, as when the fear of dis-ease produces an actual illness. Yet the tremendous power of the mind can also create healing, as Dr. Bach recognized when he wrote, "The greatest gift that you can give to others is to be happy and hopeful yourself; then you draw them up out of their despondency."

Dr. Bach observed, as have many others, that people's beliefs and behavior form repetitive and predictable patterns—very definite personality types which he found to be keys to his flower-essence system. These personality types represent crystalizations of thought, feeling, and action into fixated patterns which may once have been appropriate (e.g., in early childhood), but now severely limit the healthy flow of life.

Such fixated personality patterns have physical consequences, as modern studies of psychosomatic and stress-related dis-ease have shown. Personality types that create chronic patterns of mental and emotional imbalance create tendencies toward chronic dis-ease, such as cardiovascular disease[2] and cancer.[3]

How can we change these limiting patterns? The first step is *awareness* of the patterns and of the need to change. This means taking *responsibility* (without blame or guilt) for having created our present state of health, and realizing our power to create change. (The *Willow* essence can help with this lesson.)

Flower essences can stimulate a painful awareness of disharmony, particularly if we have been previously numb to its existence. For example, many people have adjusted to fear and worry as everyday constants, and are barely aware of their existence. As they begin taking the *Mimulus* essence, they develop a new attitude toward life experiences, welcoming them as challenges and opportunities for growth. Once they have tasted this new awareness, the habitual anxiety and resistance to life experiences is felt as a painful contrast. It then becomes clear that the attitude, not the experience, is the problem.

The pain accompanying this new awareness of restrictive attitudes can be called a "healing crisis," for it is the beginning of the break-up of long standing emotional/mental patterns, and not merely a worsening of condition. Although it may take some time, and it may require creative efforts along with the flower essences, the release from the bondage of conditioned behavior is an invaluable step along the road to health.

After awareness, the next step is transformation. (Some people are ready to go directly into transformation, without need of a "healing crisis.") In the case of *Mimulus,* fear and worry often begin falling away naturally, as the qualities of faith and inner courage grow stronger and stronger, nourished and guided by the *Mimulus* essence taken four times a day. The flower essence does not eliminate the feeling of fear, as would a tranquilizing drug, but helps liberate the energy needed for creative, healthy growth, which is currently bound up in excessive fear.

Flower essences, then, are not really "remedies" in the conventional sense of something external which can supply something we lack, or manipulate our condition into a particular state. Limitations and illness are treated not as enemies to be conquered, but rather as misdirections of life energy to be gently guided back to the source of our life flow. Dr. Bach summarized the transformational effects of the flowers when he wrote:

> "The action of these remedies is to raise our vibrations and open up our channels for the reception of the Spiritual Self, to flood our natures with the particular virtue we need, and wash from us the fault that is causing the harm. They are able, like beautiful music or any glorious uplifting thing which gives us inspiration, to raise our very natures, and bring us nearer to our souls, and by that very act to bring us peace and relieve our sufferings. They cure, not by attacking the disease, but by flooding our bodies with the beautiful vibrations of our Higher Nature, in the presence of which, disease melts away as snow in the sunshine."[4]

Flower essences are thus *health catalysts* which can energize our own health process without unduly interfering in its natural flow. We need this catalytic assistance when we get stuck in the inertia of habit, the fear of change, and the depletion of vitality that comes with living unbalanced lives.

When choosing flower essences for our individual use, one to three essences will usually suffice. These will represent the key priorities for unlocking our healthful energies at a given time. (Using too many at once tends to confuse the process.) Since we often don't see ourselves clearly, it is frequently helpful to have a friend or experienced practitioner help select the essences and stimulate our self-awareness. Radiesthesia (pendulum analysis) and other tools for heightening intuitive awareness (e.g., the *I Ching*) can help us tune in to more hidden life patterns. Using affirmation statements with flower essences can enhance their effectiveness (e.g., "I accept myself," with *Pine*).

New flower essences are usually given as our emotional patterns change. Flower essences can also be used with more immediate moods and mental states to help us regain balance. (For example, *Gentian* or *Mustard* can be used for depression, *Elm* or *Larch* for self-doubt.) The "rescue remedy" combination has been used for grounding and centering during physical and emotional trauma and emergencies. With such short-term use, dosage is frequent, but only for as long as needed.

The use of flowers for health is more in the spirit of traditional herbal medicine, with its attunement of human beings, nature, and spirit, than of modern chemical pharmacology. Bach would often refer to himself as an herbalist. The flower essences are used in such minute dilution that any direct chemical effect is negligible. Rather, they work by vibrational resonance, much like the sound waves of inspirational music, or the light waves of great art.

Modern physics and ancient mystical tradition argue that we live in a world of vibrations. The holographic paradigm of brain researcher Karl Pribram and physicist David Bohm postulates that physical "reality" is but a projection of patterns of frequencies of nonphysical energy, which is interpreted by our consciousness as our physical experience. Flower essences are thus an exquisite vehicle for transforming our reality by projecting harmonious vibratory patterns to be assimilated by our fields of consciousness.[5]

By resonating with the healthful vibrations of the flower essences, we can experience the blossoming of our inner essences. We ourselves can become health catalysts for the reconciliation of our human world with nature and spirit.

NOTES

1. Edward Bach, *Heal Thyself* (C. W. Daniel, 1931, 1973), pp. 6 and 8.
2. M. Friedman, and R. H. Rosenman, *Type A Behavior and Your Heart* (Knopf, 1974).
3. O. C. Simonton, and S. Matthews-Simonton, "Belief Systems and Management of Emotional Aspects of Malignancy," *Journal of Transpersonal Psychology,* 7, no. 1 (1975): 29–48.
4. Phillip Chancellor, *The Handbook of the Bach Flower Remedies* (Keats, 1980).
5. Marilyn Ferguson, "Karl Pribram's Changing Reality," *Re-vision,* 1, no. 3–4 (Summer/Fall, 1978). See also the article by her in this section.

SUGGESTIONS FOR FURTHER READING

Edward Bach, *The Twelve Healers and Other Remedies,* C. W. Daniels, 1933, 1979.

Nora Weeks, *The Medical Discoveries of Edward Bach, Physician.* C. W. Daniels, 1940, 1976; Keats, 1980.

Flower Essence Quarterly, Published by the Flower Essence Society, Box 586, Nevada City, CA 95959.

Bach Flower Essence Stock Bottles, a newsletter, and replies to written correspondence are available from:

The Dr. Bach Centre, Mt. Vernon, Sotwell, Wallingford, Oxon 0X10 0PZ, England.

For information on American flower essences, local practitioners, and the latest research on flower essences, write the Flower Essence Society, P.O. Box 586, Nevada City, CA 95959; (916) 265-0163.

Richard Katz is a counselor and teacher who brings to his work in flower essences more than a decade of experience in ways of natural health and psychological and spiritual growth. He is currently researching essences of California flowers, and is founder-director of the Flower Essence Society and Editor of the Flower Essence Quarterly.

The Planetarization of Consciousness, Will, and Activity

Dane Rudhyar

This visionary article describes a monumental shift in consciousness, inaugurating a new era of understanding. It involves the emergence of the planetary self. Each of us has the potential to perceive ourselves as integral aspects of a larger being; unique just as each cell is unique to the body, yet organically related to the whole. This is perhaps the ultimate meaning of holism.

Reshaping our sense of individualism is not an easy task; it requires our concerted efforts. We must release old concepts in order to embrace a new paradigm. Dane Rudhyar offers us valuable keys for merging with the current evolutionary trend.

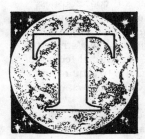

The absolutely logical thing, but the thing that hardly anybody really likes to believe, is that a human is part of humankind, which is part of the Earth, which is part of the solar system, and the galaxy, and so on. There is no reason *not* to think that the Earth is an organism and we are part of it; that we are cells in the body of that great organism, the Earth.

If we understand this, we are compelled sooner or later to realize that we can never deal completely satisfactorily with any situation if we look only from the point of view of the individual person. A person is a larger whole to all the cells in his or her body, but is also just one of the millions of components of the larger, greater whole which, from a practical point of view, I would call the planet Earth. But although our planet Earth is an organism, it is not merely a *physical* organism. In its totality it includes the material sphere, the biosphere (the sphere of life), what Teilhard de Chardin called the noösphere, and perhaps a pneumosphere (a spiritual sphere). In fact, according

This article is adapted from material that first appeared in *An Integral View* (Spring/Summer 1979), and is reprinted here by permission of the author.

to an ancient idea, the aura of the Earth, as it were, extends through what was called the *sublunar world,* which ends at the orbit of the moon. (So actually our astronauts never left the Earth when they landed on the moon, because this marks merely the periphery of our aura.)

If we take this attitude, the next logical step is to begin to realize that humankind as a whole has a certain *function* to perform within the organism of the Earth. I have often stated that we can think of humankind as the cerebrum (or nervous system) of the entire Earth, and that our function is to transform or translate all the activities of the Earth into consciousness. That is to say, our function (or *dharma*) is to bring to a state of consciousness any and all types of activities taking place within the total being of the planet. This is, of course, what our nervous system and our brain do, or can do, in terms of the activities of our body. I should add that we now know that a great yogi is able to understand and to control life processes taking place within all the cells and particles of the body; so perhaps the collective mind of humanity eventually may be able to understand and control all the processes occurring throughout the entire planet.

Next, there are two basic factors to consider if we want to understand fully what is historically occurring on this Earth and in humankind at any moment. The evolution of nature on the Earth is the first factor with which to deal. According to ancient doctrines, this evolution is cyclical, periodical; it passes through various phases. Humankind also evolves with it, and every human being is caught up in the tide of evolution, of humankind as a whole. We now know historically that the great migrations of races, the movements of people from one place to another, were produced by the drying up of whole regions. For instance, the drying up of the Gobi desert at one time sent the Huns and Mongols upon India and Europe; the Sahara desert was once a very fertile region; and who knows what is going to happen to California?

This evolutionary picture deals with nature, then, and therefore affects the development of any culture. We are bound to our culture; we imbibe it from our moment of birth, and we are molded by it. We are molded by our language, and anybody who speaks several languages well knows that you cannot express yourself in one language the same way as you do in another. We are completely dominated by cultural development. What is happening to our culture as a whole transcends completely what happens to the individual, whether or not one's idea of consciousness is expanding. This does not mean that the individual is not important. But we have to give up the idea that the individual comes first in society.

Many teachers tell us that society is a collection of individuals; but *this is not so*. We are born as members of a society; we are not born as individuals. Even the sense of "I" develops slowly in babyhood. We are born at a certain place and time as a certain expression of mankind for a certain purpose. If we believe that the Earth as a whole and the cosmos as a whole are living organisms (in the sense of an organized system of interdependent activities), then there is a purpose for every human being. That purpose is to focus at a certain time and place something which is an answer to the need of that time and space where the person is born and develops.

Two factors must always be considered. First, we must consider changes within the evolutionary pattern of the globe and changes in the culture of which we are a part. Then, we have to deal with our own changes as individuals who, if we want to become true individuals, have to emerge—to sever our attachment to the culture to which we were born and in which we were raised.

No one is an individual until he or she has definitely, actually, emerged from his or her culture; for so long as we take for granted all the paradigms within our society, we are not individuals; we are merely specimens of our culture, with only superficial modifications of type and temperament. These superficialities of character do not really constitute what we should call our true self, our essential individuality. We haven't reached that sense, that uniqueness, the truth of our being—our *dharma*—our essential potential of being. It is the task of our being to actualize this potential; but we cannot actualize it unless we are first relatively free of what we have accepted unquestioningly, unless we assess the value of all the things which have been imparted to us from the time of our birth.

Unfortunately, we have developed in our Western world, and particularly in America, a culture which is completely based upon individualism, and not only on individualism but on the *personal* aspect of the individual. I came to America in 1916 when I was 21, and

it was amazing to realize the degree to which, in this new world, everything was "personal." And it has become increasingly so. Everybody wants to do his or her own thing, as a person; not really as an "individual," but as a person who has had a certain type of training, type of body, and capacity to act. Our collective mentality presents us with difficult problems. We have first to understand what we really are as human beings who are parts of humanity and who are involved in the vast cyclic development of the whole planet. How can we gain such an understanding?

The basic purpose of occult groups is to make known a process of individual transformation, usually called "the Path," or the way of discipleship and initiation. This path takes into consideration the cosmological and metaphysical evolution of the universe, but it is focused rigorously upon the accelerated development of individual human beings and the step-by-step expansion of their consciousness, *plus* a repolarization of their relationships to other human beings and to society in general. This occult path deals with a process of radical transformation of the human being: a total and, in a sense, irrevocable transformation, during which the center of consciousness is gradually transferred from one plane of being to a higher one that is *more inclusive,* that encompasses more and more. What is basic on the Path is the transcending of what today is our normal feeling of being "I myself." The individual has to acquire a new "frame of reference" for all he or she knows, feels, or responds to.

This is a very difficult process! What it implies, first of all, is a change of "images." The first condition for that change of images is to have a conscious realization of the meaning of what has happened within the last century or so. This alone can enable us to clearly understand the nature of the old images and symbols on which our culture was based, images which are now obsolete. We can, of course, become fascinated by other cultures and their mystical or religious imagery. We may join a Sufi, Buddhist, Vedantist, or Zen group. But these images are also old; the cultures are, in most cases, slowly dying out. What is more important is to understand the basic principles on which our culture, and whatever culture we are interested in, has operated, and to further realize what today, at this particular point of human evolution, is possible.

The word *consciousness* has been used and abused for the last fifteen years. What has usually been said does not make the meaning of the word clear. The Hindu speaks of a sea of consciousness as being the essential reality, but a consciousness without anything

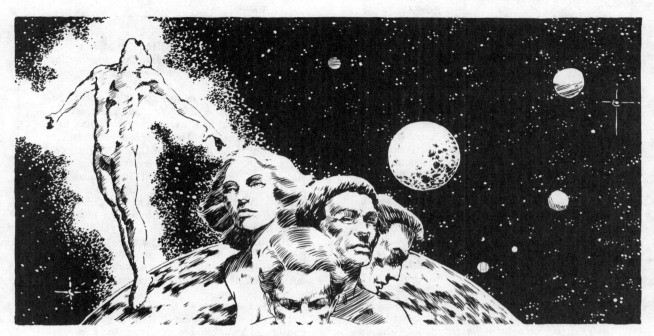

The thing that hardly anybody likes to believe is that a human is part of humankind, which is part of the Earth, which is part of the solar system, and the galaxy, and so on.

to be conscious of certainly has nothing to do with what we call consciousness in the Western world. The usual translation of the Sanskrit word *chit* as "consciousness" is probably not at all accurate, and this is true of many philosophical Sanskrit words.

From my point of view, what is essential in existence is *activity.* What we primarily and undeniably experience and know are activity and change. The trouble with so many of our systems of philosophy is that they are the philosophy of grown-up people who have already developed a certain kind of mentality based on their experiences, their problems, and their conflicts. Out of these the philosopher builds some kind of theory which to him best explains what life and his personal reactions to it have meant to him, what seems most important, crucial, or spiritually comforting at the time. Yet, one should really start from the beginning, from the experience of the baby and the little child. The experience of change, the experience of activity, is the only thing that is absolutely evident. The child is not born as an individual conscious being. Yet the child's organism reacts instinctively to an immense variety of internal and external changes. Animals do the same thing. But the difference between a human being and an animal or a plant is that plants and animals only react to those

ever-changing impressions, and a person has the capacity not only to react to them, but to *respond* to them.

There is a great difference between a reaction and a response. A conscious response implies the presence of a center, aware of the different activities occurring within the field of its existence, and of the relationship between these activities. *What we call "unconscious" is what cannot be experienced by or related to the center of the field.* Something is there in the field, but it cannot be related to the center. Therefore, it is unconscious. Thus, consciousness implies a center. And it also implies an awareness by that center of the activities of which it is the centralizing focus. The essential point is that, although animals merely act and react, human beings can respond and change their responses. They can also respond in a way which is *not* according to the essential truth of their being. An animal always reacts in the way that is right for its life situation; a person can respond in a way which is not natural, which is not true to his own being. Humans are the only living creatures who can be what they are not, and by being what they are not, to consciously learn, after various crises and tragedies, what they truly are. That is the meaning of the concept glorified by some sects (particularly among old

(Text continued on p. 202)

Immortality of the Soul
Ram Dass

The universe is composed of one "stuff"—call it shakti, call it prana, call it consciousness, call it love, call it God, call it the Spirit made manifest—whatever you will, it is *one* stuff. But within this one homogeneous stuff exist patternings, or separate entities. You could think of the whole in the same way as you think of a DNA code: a set of predisposing factors affects how each individual pattern relates to all the rest. For convenience, let's call this pattern a soul.

Let's start at the point where a soul is "separate" from the rest, and has a unique set of predisposing characteristics. In the Hindu literature, these are characterized in terms of the proportion of three forces: the forces toward light; the forces of fire, or heat, or action; and inert force. Manifestation, or the need to incarnate—or reincarnate—is determined by the disequilibrium or imbalance among these three forces, for anything but perfect balance reflects some form of attachment, or uniqueness, or "specialness." These, then, are the seed conditions for an incarnation.

The soul goes on from birth, to birth, to birth. Each lifetime is a set of experiences which the soul passes through, and which affect its karmic predicament. A soul that is unconscious of its predicament, that is, a young soul with this disequilibrium of forces, makes its choices mainly in such a way that it increases its own personal security, gratification, and power. Choices made this way tend to increase karmic disequilibrium; that is, such choices "add" karma. If you do something that goes against the flow—for example, an act of violence, greed, or lust, out of attachment—you add to your own karmic predicament, or *negative* karma.

This article first appeared in *Alternatives Magazine* and is reprinted by permission of the Hanuman Foundation.

That is, you affect the balance in such a way that later these seeds will manifest once again, in ways that will be connected with your own suffering.

It must be kept in mind that it works the opposite way as well. If you act again out of personal desire and perform good acts, but goodness in the "righteous" sense, which is not necessarily in harmony with the flow, you create *positive* karma. That positive karma will also *force* incarnation. You may incarnate among the heavenly hosts, among angels or *devas*, or you may stay 500 years in great feelings of well-being and contentment and pleasure. Then that, too, will be over, and you'll go on with your work. Such may be the fruits of the karma you create by your righteousness. Thus both positive and negative acts which are done out of personal desire accrue karma.

Once you begin to awaken to this predicament, you understand that the wheel of birth and death will continue as long as your karma continues. Your choices then start to be in tune with the flow. Choices made in harmony with the will of God create no new karma, for they do not come out of personal desire. An awakening being may be in a state in which her or his acts do not produce new karma; they work out past karma. Unconscious beings constantly create new karma, making their journey longer and longer. An old soul who has awakened so that he is not creating new karma exists in form to work off old karma, life after life. He ultimately arrives at a point where his karma is used up.

Someone once asked the Buddha, whose karma was used up, "Where will you go after you die?" His answer: "Where is the fire after the fuel is used up? Answer: it isn't." This is the ending of the Samsaric wheel of birth and death. Now, there is a choice for an individual at this point. Such an individual *may* continue to manifest in a totally dharmic way, no longer out of personal karma, but by identification with collective karma. There are beings, like Christ, who come to Earth or to another plane

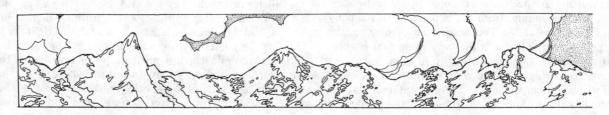

not because of their own personal need to work out karma, but in order to be an instrument for the working out of others' karma. These are not separate individuals in the same sense that you and I are. More precisely, they are instruments of the will of God. They have no personal karma.

Many realized beings have themselves finished with karma while their bodies continue to exist because of karma, or the inertia, of their own. For example, Ramana Maharishi, when asked whether he would heal his body, which was suffering from cancer, answered, "No, this body has served its purpose." His devotees cried and pleaded with him not to leave them. He answered with some surprise, "But don't be silly, where could I go? It's just that I have finished with this body." The body was working out its own karma; the cancer was the karma of that body. Ramana Maharishi didn't have cancer. His body had cancer. Ramana Maharishi was free to use that vehicle or leave it.

As you become more conscious, you become an appreciator of your own karmic predicament. You honor your karma, good or bad. Your point or objective is the cessation of suffering, and the cessation of suffering comes from the cessation of clinging. Clinging is another word for karma. When you become free, then you are part of the totality of the universe. But though you are part of the One, and no longer have unique karma, you are still a separate entity— this is a paradox of the One and the many. At that point, your will and God's will are in perfect harmony; then you *are* God, yet you are still separate!

For any one life to be meaningful, ultimately you must have the perspective of the Akashic record, the record of all incarnations. Buddha, it is described, looked back at one point and in a moment's time—since higher consciousness is not linear—saw his last 99,000 incarnations. It's important to have a time perspective about this dance of life, for we tend to get lost in the intricacies of life experiences.

A story that I like to recount because of the perspective it gives, concerns the duration of our incarnation. The image that is presented, again within the Buddhist tradition, is the image of the mountain which is six miles wide, six miles long, and six miles high. Every hundred years a bird flies over the mountain with a silk scarf in its beak and runs the scarf over the top of the mountain as it flies past. The length of time it takes that silk scarf to wear away the mountain gives some sense of the duration of time in which you have been experiencing the cycle of birth and death and birth and death. Each lifetime, within that perspective, is like a blink of an eye. Like tiny insects that are born in the morning and die in the evening, so it is with our lives. We are born in the morning and die in the evening, again and again. Each time we are born, for the experiences to truly work, we get "lost" in the incarnation. It is this attachment—or entrapment—that creates or works out our karma.

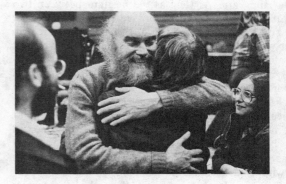

Ram Dass, author of Be Here Now *and other books, is a widely followed spiritual teacher. He is a founder of the Hanuman Foundation, an organization dedicated to furthering spiritual well-being in the society.*

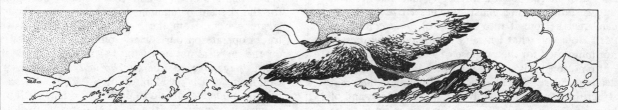

(continued from p. 199)

Gnostics or in tzarist Russia) as the doctrine of "salvation through sin." If people sin hard enough, they may become so disgusted that they begin to understand what they are. One may become a saint by means of a process of violent psychic reversal or conversion.

An objective understanding of the individuality of a human being is most important today, because one of the deepest challenges mankind faces, especially in America, is a revaluation of the meaning of "being an individual." We have to give up as obsolete the concept of the rugged individual of the frontier days. This *image* of the aggressively independent and unrelated individual, with its basic possessiveness, greed, and ambition for success, regardless of what happens to other individuals, is still inherent in the human psyche today. As long as this image is basic in the human psyche, there can be no essential transformation of the individual.

After human beings realize that what is essential for them is to try to learn what is their truth of being, their *dharma,* the thing they are born for, they may eventually reach a stage of consciousness wherein they no longer have any choice, because they can be only what they are. As long as we hesitate between two courses of action, we are not yet fully what we are; we still have the possibility of being what we are not. But when we come to the point where what we are is so absolutely ingrained in our consciousness, our feeling, and our will that we cannot act otherwise; then we have become more than a person, we have become an Entity, that is to say, an *operative principle* in the universe. We are fulfilling our function in terms of the need of mankind and of the Earth at the time and the place where we were born. We have become that function. We have become a truth in action, in terms of what is possible for human beings.

That is, at least in one sense, the end of the process of human metamorphosis. By following the path of initiation, step by step, we detach ourselves from our culture, from all the possessiveness and aggressiveness of the biosphere. And let us not forget that the biosphere is, after all, a world where the basic law of life is "eat or be eaten." It is not a very nice place to live, but we human beings must start here. Eventually we can emerge from it into a realm of *mind consciousness.* However, what I mean by *mind consciousness* is not mind used for the purpose of survival or satisfying our emotions; it is a mind for which it is natural to be dealing with the great laws and principles, the great structural forces of the universe, of our planet, and of humanity as a whole. To develop that mind is to be truly human. The individual becomes fully what he or she was meant to be from the beginning of the world. One has overcome the downward pull of material entropy. One expresses a particular *quality* of being, an aspect of divine nature.

If a great many people could reach this state of existence, not only the condition of society, but even the whole biosphere would be transformed. Yet it should be rather obvious that if one had to wait for every one of the several billions of persons living on the Earth to reach this state, the Earth and humanity would never be totally transformed. The Earth as a whole has its own rhythm of evolution. The Earth and humanity evolve according to cosmic rhythms; individuals according to their own patterns. The two react upon one another. If, at a crucial time of the Earth's evolution, there were not numerous individuals who had reached that condition in consciousness, the collective evolution of mankind would be delayed by the inertia of institutions, by the failure of human beings as individuals to perform their duty and their *dharma.* This could imply some kind of planetary tragedy.

Many people today know of the vow of the Bodhisattvas who renounce Nirvana until *every sentient being* on Earth has reached that condition. Unless there were an evolution of *nature as a whole,* and not an evolution of only individual persons, it would be most unconceivable that all sentient beings would ever reach the condition of Nirvana, because in our world a tremendous force of inertia exists. Such an inertia can only be overcome by a transformative process operating on the planet as a whole. We do act and think within this planetary whole; but we can only operate within limited fields of action if we act *only* as individuals. Just as the cells of our body will not transform themselves until our greater being experiences a radical change of consciousness which can actually transfigure these body cells, so the greater whole, Earth, must be active upon its lesser wholes, human beings, in order for us to develop and become focal points for the action of that greater whole.

To become such a focal point is to act as an avatar. An avatar is a person who has so transformed his individual being that he is able to become a focal point for the descent of planetary forces operating from a greater whole, from the planet or the galaxy. These forces operate on our society, our culture, as well as on the physical nature of the Earth; but at a certain point they have to operate *through* a personage, a God-man, a "Divine Manifestation." Thus, if we are fully to understand, and to positively orient ourselves to what is occurring in the world at this time of global crisis, we need to consider two movements: a descent of the greater whole polarizing the ascent of individuals open to larger horizons of reality.

Unfortunately, most people in the consciousness movement look at the New Age as something emerging, going up, up, and beyond. They are seemingly unable to picture also a movement coming down from the greater whole, reaching down to us, the smaller wholes. Individuals who are no longer imprisoned in the fortified castles of their egos and their cultural traditions can become attuned to this descent. It does not matter too much whether one calls it evolution, God's will, or the impact of a spiritual hierarchy. What matters is one's ability and willingness to believe in its reality and power and to become identified with it.

In other words, we are facing today a situation requiring of the true pioneers of a new and future civilization that they open their minds to more than what the consciousness movement usually implies. They should see through and reach beyond what very often turns out to be a kind of spiritual narcissism, in which one becomes almost completely involved in one's own betterment, one's own evolution and transformation. Transformation, yes; but for what? In terms of what?

Human consciousness and human activity—collective as well as individual—moves from a smaller frame of reference to a larger one. The smaller deals with an approach to reality and a variety of experiences which are basically physical, emotional, mental, cultural. But when the truly planetary field is reached and properly understood, man will realize that this field no longer deals primarily or exclusively with physical matter, because the real Earth and humanity in their widest aspect transcend physicality; and every liberated individual is a functioning part of a vast planetary wholeness that is inherently a spiritual entity.

To realize that these are facts of human existence is today of great importance, because recently we have been too much involved in ourselves and in developing our personal potential and our individual consciousness, without any greater frame of reference than ourselves. One cannot develop satisfactorily in such a way. All the talk about love, and fanciful ideals actually mean very little unless one is able to feel and constantly experience the "presence" of the greater whole. Whatever we do should be in terms of that larger frame of reference, not in terms of ourselves and our progress. We can become fascinated by all sorts of techniques, each one guaranteed to develop a special path to higher consciousness, but where does this lead humanity?

In the past all such practices were done in terms of religion, thus in terms of the purely transcendent kind of formulations of an ideal of power, love, and perfection. People worship a personal God or hierarchies of gods, or great personages and masters. Many words; many images! The reality behind them is that we are all part of the larger unit our planet constitutes. Now we are at last able to realize that these gods and superhuman, superphysical beings symbolize or embody functions of the etheric body, or mind-body, or spiritual body of the Earth. There is, in fact, only one planetary mind, the mind of humanity-as-a-whole. Our minds are not individual minds. They are like radios; we tune into the planetary mind. Sometimes the radio-mind is full of static; sometimes the connection is very clear and what we hear is inspiring. We may be able to improve our radio, and succeed in getting more communication over greater distance. But it is the one mind with which we get in touch. Man actually does not create anything. Man responds, man interprets, and man understands.

Without such understanding, most of our efforts at self-development and personal happiness lead to spiritual miscarriages. One has to have a wider, clearly perceived, deeply felt frame of reference; one has to feel, think, and act according to it. Vague feelings, an imprecise, diffuse sense of floating in the rarefied air of eagerly believed-to-be mystical experiences, are not enough. We may speak of having reached cosmic consciousness, but what of it? The question is what you can do, here and now; what your *dharma* is. Fulfill it by facing your karma and by courageously, persistently going *through* it toward freedom and peace.

In terms of the new movement of consciousness and human potential, what happened in the '60s was very valuable, and indeed quite wonderful. It was necessary because we had to try to break away from many cultural hang-ups, from the lure of success and power, from the rat race of big business, and all the things typical of the American scene. This had to be done even if it meant only escaping, moving out without purpose, blindly reacting to the past. But now we have to do something else; we have to begin to build. We have to act and to try to find what we are here *for*. And this means thinking, building a clear, vibrant, creative understanding, which requires courage, determination, perseverance, and self-discipline. May we all find within ourselves the needed source of power, the love that blesses all sincere efforts, the peace that *is* understanding!

SUGGESTIONS FOR FURTHER READING

Dane Rudhyar, *The Planetarization of Consciousness.* A.S.I. Publishers, 2nd ed., 1977.

_____, *Beyond Individualism: The Psychology of Transformation.* Quest Books, 1979.

_____, *Culture, Crisis, and Creativity.* Quest Books, 1977.

_____, *We Can Begin Again Together.* Seed Center, 1974.

_____, *Occult Preparations for a New Age.* Quest Books, 1975.

Dane Rudhyar is a Promethean philosopher and creative personality who, for more than sixty years, has attempted to transform the character of the assumptions and patterns of thinking that structure our way of life and our Western culture. He is the author of more than a thousand articles and some 35 books. He is perhaps most well known for his pioneering reformulation of astrology in philosophical and psychological terms. In an age of specialization and compartmentalization, Rudhyar stands out as a man of many achievements—in music and the arts, literature and poetry, and, most recently, in formulating a new approach to a psychology of transformation. Rudhyar has been inspired by an integral philosophy and by his dedication to promoting a new, global organization of a transformed humanity.

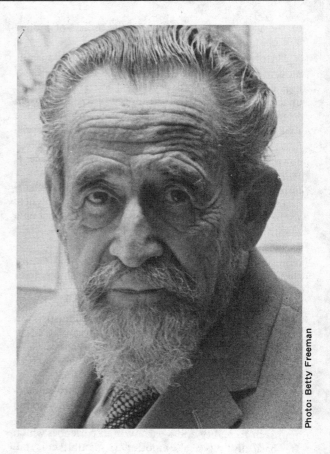

Photo: Betty Freeman

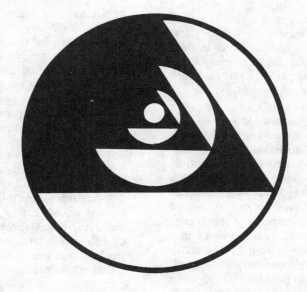

Surrender, Healing, and Divine Grace
Aerin Land

The work of Sri Aurobindo and The Mother is considered to be among the most visionary literature to emerge in the last century. Their combined writings truly presage a new age of consciousness.

Sri Aurobindo was educated in England and became a Greek scholar before discovering his native culture of India. He later immersed himself in the study of Eastern religion and thought, and moved to Pondicherry, India, where he settled down to a life of teaching and writing with a small group of disciples. Sri Aurobindo became one of India's greatest thinkers, leaving behind a wealth of spiritual wisdom in his prolific writings.

The Mother, of French origin, received her name because of her devotion to the Divine Feminine Principle, which she embodied in her life. She met Sri Aurobindo in 1920, and they remained together for the next thirty years, as complementary aspects of one soul essence.

The blending of East and West in the teachings of Sri Aurobindo and The Mother offers the Western reader a unique opportunity to grasp mystical understandings of the East in a form accessible to Western thought.

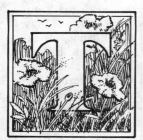 he writings of Sri Aurobindo and The Mother have clarified and widened my own experience as a spiritual healer. I am in no way trying to promote a religion, or the idea that anyone should blindly follow them, for this is not my purpose, and even more, not theirs. I hope, instead, to present them as the gifted visionaries they were; they left behind a wealth of information and guidance on the future of evolution. One of the aspects of their work I find most attractive is their work on the transformation of matter, something I have always felt was the basis of the manifestation of a New Age. What I want to describe is an actual process of healing: the basis of spiritual healing and the basis of physical transformation. What I hope to present is a message central to their work, central to my own experience, and central to all of us who aspire to be instruments of the transformation which will bring about a New Age.

True healing is a process of opening ourselves to divine grace by means of surrender—creating a greater wideness in our being for the descent of spirit. Most illness is a result of resistance in our physical, vital, or mental natures to the guidance of our soul. When we are able to surrender, when we become quiet and still within, an opening is created in us for divine grace to transform us. As matter, our physical nature is the most resistant to transformation, to realizing its divine nature. Life on Earth is ultimately an evolutionary process of spiritualizing matter and materializing spirit, of enlightening the physical nature. The transformation of the physical begins in the body, by an increased receptivity to divine grace and the accompaying movement, or "force" of spirit.

Why this concern with the body and the physical plane in the work of spiritual healing and transformation? In *The Supramental Manifestation Upon Earth,* Sri Aurobindo wrote,

"If our seeking is for a total perfection of the being, the physical part of it cannot be left aside; for the body is the material basis, . . . the instrument which we have to use. A total perfection is the ultimate aim which we set before us, for our ideal is the Divine Life which we wish to create here, the Life of Spirit fulfilled on earth, life accomplishing its own spiritual transformation even here on earth in the conditions of a material universe. . . . A Divine Life in a material world implies necessarily a union of the two ends of existence, the spiritual summit and the material base. The Soul with the basis of its life in matter ascends to the heights of the Spirit but does not cast away its base; it joins the heights and the depths together. The Spirit descends into matter and the material world with all its glories and powers, and with them fills and transforms life in the material world so it becomes more and more divine. The transformation is not a change into something

205

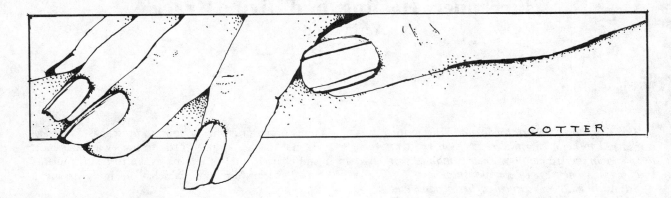

In the laying on of hands, what is created often is a peace in which one who is sick may dissolve the resistance that was causing the illness.

purely subtle and spiritual to which matter is in its nature repugnant and by which it is felt as an obstacle or shackle binding the Spirit; it takes up matter as a form of the Spirit, though now a form that conceals and turns it into a revealing instrument."[1]

In many religious teachings the body is the very impediment that keeps us from God. In Sri Aurobindo and The Mother's path of integral yoga, all aspects of consciousness are to be embraced and transformed. In this lies the wholeness we seek. On Earth, it is when our visions are finally made manifest in life that we feel the most complete, when we are not having to deny, repress, or escape one aspect of consciousness in order to experience another. It is the self within that craves expression in every aspect of who we are, even the most material, so that all may be brought into greater truth, perfection, and beauty. In this opening between spirit and matter lies the miracle of healing, for miracles are accomplished by means of the descent of forces of a higher plane of consciousness into those below. With grace all disharmony and illness are brought into a greater light, and whatever obstructed our self-expression is cast away. This is the basis of spiritual healing. Grace comes to us by sincere surrender—the offering up of whatever we are and whatever comes to us—to the divine. In healing, if we become silent within, that which has been causing us pain and suffering can be transformed.

When we speak of surrender we must differentiate it from the idea of release. In certain psychological therapies, for instance, the tears, screaming, and other forms of release may or may not signal a breakthrough, a surrendered state. Release may be a means that helps a person learn to surrender, but it is not an end in itself. A person can go on releasing for years while focusing on the debris of the mind. The important point is whether or not the person continues to fight for his or her own higher consciousness. There may be many dramatic releases happening outwardly, although inwardly there has been little progress.

With surrender, a deep peace will ultimately follow. It is only when we are able to become still with whatever bothered us (about ourselves or others), to widen and include what has happened as a part of our experience, and then move on, that we have broken through. This is the real surrender—when the "contagion" has lost its charge and no longer takes us away from who we are. In the laying on of hands, for example, what is created often is a peace in which one who is sick may dissolve the resistance that was causing the illness. After receiving a spiritual healing, the one who is healed is usually quiet and filled with inner joy, a melting into the divine. This is a state of surrender.

Surrender is generally a hard concept for Westerners to understand. It is seen as a weakness, or as giving up one's free will. But before rendering a verdict, we must take a closer look and ask ourselves the question, to what do we ultimately surrender? The Mother offers clarity on this point:

"By surrender we mean . . . a spontaneous self-giving, a giving of all your self to the Divine, to a greater consciousness of which you are part. Surrender will not diminish, but increase you; it will not lessen, or weaken, or destroy your personality, it will fortify and aggrandize it. Surrender means a free, total giving with all the delights of giving; there is no sense of sacrifice in it. If you have the slightest feeling you are making a sacrifice, then it is no longer a surrender. . . . Most people seem to look upon surrender as an abdication of the personality, but that is a grievous error. For the individual is meant to manifest one aspect of the Divine Consciousness, and the expression of its characteristic nature is what creates his personality; then, by taking the right attitude towards the Divine, this personality is purified of all the influences of the lower nature which diminish and distort it and it becomes more strongly personal, more itself, more complete."[2]

It is a great realization to see that the soul has a personality, that God has a personality uniquely expressed in each of us. The reality of this truth is evident in the personalities of inspired spiritual teachers. Each of them has realized union with the divine by some form of surrender, but for each the expression of this union is slightly different. One's gift may be to touch another's soul with song; another is able to provide great clarity for the mind; another embodies the Divine Mother and heals all who are open to her energy; another is strongly disciplined; another lives simply and bears the gift of humor; and so on. This surrender is not a surrender into some grey world where all of our dreams, visions, creativity, and unique expression are given up, but a surrender in which all that we are is permeated more deeply and thoroughly by the divine. That within us which was previously veiled in obscurity and ignorance is brought into light.

This surrender is a dynamic movement of identification with the divine, rather than a passive "giving up." Surrender in relation to healing is the state in which we are able to be quiet and still inside with whatever adversely affects us. We are no longer identified with our resistance and the resulting pain. By means of surrender, negative vibrations may be rejected before they ever enter our being, and what results is a dynamic identification with the health, peace, and joy of the divine consciousness. We see that we can be inwardly still, while outwardly active and effective. With surrender we are brought closer to our soul, which becomes our center.

As we come into greater contact with the soul, we are taught the real value of discrimination. This is a crucial point. Surrender does not mean accepting the

Alone In the Woods
Armand Ian Brint

The sharp smell of pine
marked the only
passage of time;
spun its evergreen
history
beneath the sun.

I asked,
"What in the world
    am I doing here?"
There was no answer
except,
a bluejay laughed—
somewhere.
I looked up—
without warning,
the wilderness conformed
to my palm
like a stone snatched
from the bottom of a childhood stream.
Everything fit
without seams.

I stood beneath the trees,
a million miles from
the normal chaos of leaves and
enormity of sky,
until
only a pebble,
the memory of a bird
and the obliteration
of my original question
remained.

invitation of any and all vibrations that come our way, but rather to be able to see what is true and right for us. With surrender there is the protection of grace; it is the divine which moves us. We refuse to parley with that which will do us harm. We know what to trust, what to have faith in; we know what is of divine consciousness because our soul is touched.

It seems that one thing that holds us back from surrender is a fear of being taken advantage of, of losing ourselves in a manifestation of falsehood. We live in a time when dubious organizations, in the name of spirituality, boast large followings. Yet surrender is not necessarily dependent on any external form, such as "religious" organization or person. The experience may be a spontaneous self-giving, an opening in ourselves to descent of spirit. It is also possible that one may recognize the divine in another, and a surrender takes place before words are even exchanged. The key to discrimination always is to be in touch with the divine within, and to commune with that part of another. In a perfecting soul there is little difference between the outer personality and the divine within. It is knowing the divine in ourselves that allows us to be profoundly open to healing relationships. Learning to surrender requires great trust and faith in the guidance of our soul. Then, if we are being manipulated or controlled, if something is pulling us away from who we are, we will know it.

As we surrender our resistance we become receptive; a greater opening to divine grace is created in us. Grace can be seen as the constant availability of the help and mercy of God. In spiritual healing, a manifestation of grace is the descent of spirit into matter. It is through this descent of spirit, through grace, that a healing transformation is possible. In order for this to occur we need to develop a greater receptivity in all our being, including a receptivity in the body itself. The body, the physical world, is infused with light when we surrender our resistance and become receptive to grace.

> "The first condition (for receptivity in the body) is to remain as quiet as possible. You may have noticed that in the different parts of your being, when something comes and you do not receive it, it produces a stiffening—something hardens in the vital, in the mind or in the body. There is a clenching and this tension hurts."[3]

> "The Grace is always with you; all help is constantly given; so all depends on the receptivity and openness of your being. The more you are unified and receptive, the quicker [the transformation] will go."[4]

In spiritual healing, when we have felt ourselves being healed or are healing another, we may experience a rush of energy flowing into us. This descent is usually first felt as an intense, almost solid feeling of peace and stillness which pours forth and settles into us from above. It is important to note that the descent, as a manifestation of grace, is available to us through our receptivity. If we are in any way trying to "pull" it to us, we may draw in something else entirely. The descent of spirit, for the purpose of healing, is generally attracted by gentleness and simplicity. Sincerity and faith will let the grace act in its highest form. When we are touched by the descent of spirit, everything inside us is quieted. We become deeply appreciative of all we've been given and of all

we are. We remember grace; we remember self. Our body is made alive and responsive to a higher calling. Within this awareness, we see that the body and all matter may be "light," yet simultaneously exist in the physical. The paradox vanishes and we realize that the divine body can be a reality on Earth.

> "When you arrive at the work of the transformation of the body, when some cells of the body are more ready than others, more refined, subtle, and plastic, begin to feel concretely the presence of the Divine Grace, the Divine Will, the Divine Power, the knowledge which is not intellectual, but knowledge by identity, when you feel this even in the cells of your body, then the experience is so total, imperative, so living, concrete, tangible, real that all the rest appears as a vain dream . . . thus one can say that it is only when the circle will be created, when the two extremities will touch, when the highest will manifest in the most material, that the experience will be totally decisive. . . . It would seem that one never truly understands until one understands with one's body."[5]

The transformation of the physical by making our highest spiritual visions manifest on Earth is the ultimate purpose of this terrestrial evolution. If heaven is truly to be on Earth, then we must bring the peace, power, and love which we experience on an inner plane into our outer life. When we do this, we realize that all we create that is beautiful, and all that we appreciate as being beautiful, raises the vibration level of Earth. The Mother said beauty itself is a path to the divine, and beauty and love are ultimately the outcome of our transformation. When we are touched by love and beauty we remember who we are. We begin not only to heal others, but to heal everything around us. As we surrender and let the divine act through us, all we do and all we are begins to express the beauty that is our soul. We actively participate in the creation of a new age and the life divine on Earth.

> "The Perfect Consciousness accepted to be merged and absorbed into the unconsciousness of matter, so that consciousness might be awakened in the depths of its obscurity and little by little a Divine Power might use in it and make the whole of this manifested universe a highest expression of the Divine Consciousness and the Divine Love. . . . For this world of matter is the point of concentration of all worlds; it is the place where all the worlds will have to manifest. At present it is disharmonious and obscure; but that is only an accident, a false start. One day it will become beautiful, rhythmic, full of light; for that is the consumation for which it was made."[6]

NOTES

1. Sri Aurobindo, *The Supramental Manifestation upon Earth* (Sri Aurobindo Ashram Trust, 1973), pp. 6–7.
2. Sri Aurobindo and The Mother, *On Surrender and Grace* (S.A.A.T., 1970), pp. 16–17.
3. *Ibid., On Physical Education* (S.A.A.T., 1967), p. 122.
4. Huta, *White Roses,* Parts I–III (Sri Aurobindo Memorial Fund Society, 1973), p. 178.
5. Sri Aurobindo and The Mother, *On Physical Education,* pp. 91–92.
6. *Ibid., Conversations* (S.A.A.T., 1973), pp. 79 and 114.

SUGGESTIONS FOR FURTHER READING

Satprem, *Sri Aurobindo, or, The Adventure of Consciousness.* Harper and Row, 1968.

For more information on the writings and ongoing work of Sri Aurobindo and The Mother, write to the Sri Aurobindo Ashram, Pondicherry, India.

Aerin Land has been interested in the teachings of Sri Aurobindo and The Mother since first reading Sri Aurobindo, or, The Adventure of Consciousness. *He is a minister of the Gentle Brothers and Sisters, where Sri Aurobindo and The Mother's teachings form part of the basis for instruction in psychic development and the growth of consciousness. Aerin also offers classes through the Berkeley Holistic Health Center in the use of Tarot as keys for insight into life.*

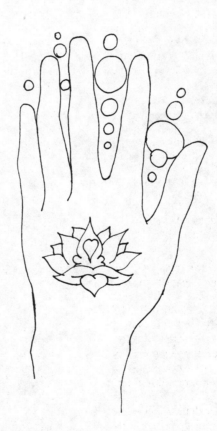

Section IV:
Relationships
The Family, Intimacy, Sexuality, Aging

"Let love develop inside your heart. The purer the heart becomes, the more love will come out; and one day you and love will become one."

Baba Hari Dass

"Let there be spaces in your togetherness,
And let the winds of the heavens dance between you. . . .
For the pillars of the temple stand apart,
And the oak tree and the cypress grow not in each other's shadow."

Kahlil Gibran

"If you love a person, you love him or her in their stark reality, and refuse to shut your eyes to their defects and errors. For to do that is to shut your eyes to their need."

John McMurray

"If I wish anything for my sons, it is that they should have the courage of women, who in their private and public lives are taking greater and greater risks, both psychic and physical, in the evolution of a new vision. This new kind of 'being man' can help to bring a true equality to love between the sexes, and create a new freedom of sharing."

Adrienne Rich

"Children have an uncanny ability to get inside our unconscious selves and know what we're feeling and thinking without a word being said. Children are beautiful teachers."

Gerald Jampolsky

"We are a new breed of old people. We are the elders, the experienced ones. I believe that the wisdom and experience of old people, linked with the new knowledge and energy of the young, can be the basis for valuable analysis, social redesign, and improvement."

Maggie Kuhn

Introduction
RELATIONSHIPS: The Family,
Intimacy, Sexuality, Aging

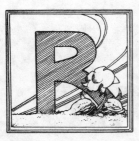

elationship is the fabric that weaves together our universe. Affinity to what we like, or what we need, is the attractive quality of relationship. People, animals, plants, thoughts, actions, and dreams meet in the crucible of relationship.

Nothing exists outside of relationship. We are interdependent and interpenetrating beings. As we become cognizant of the delicate intricacy of our lives, we see who we are, and what we seek for fulfillment. Choices in relationship express our inner nature. Our family, friends, lovers, community, job, and environment all exist in relation to us, and we to them. Especially important is the quality of the relationship that we have with our self, or many sub-selves, that define us from the inside.

Relationship provides a mirror to reflect back to us what we value. The articles we have collected for this section on relationship highlight the universal human joy and struggle of sharing intimacy. An overriding theme is "relax, trust yourself, and let love flow in a natural way." We have presented positive images with direct personal messages. Let them support you in building strong relationships that take you where you want to go. For generations, we have looked outside ourselves for support and validation. Today, out of sheer necessity, we are reclaiming the wealth of love that resides within, for our self-nurturance. As we contact the place of being within the human form, we suddenly become free to acknowledge and celebrate the innate beauty of others.

Possibly no area of our life is as sensitive and vulnerable as our sexuality. Great pain has accumulated because of the misuse of sexual energy. We can learn to address and minister to our wounds, and facilitate healing in this area. We have included teaching on the very explicit aspects of making love, complemented with a highly inspirational piece on the holistic nature of sexuality. Insights into children's sexuality and the gay experience are shared to give a full picture of human sexual response.

Family health is also highlighted. Caring is centered in the home. Our culture seems to have lost sight of this truth. Basic holistic practices bring a family into harmony. Living well together, sharing responsibility, being in touch not just mentally, but physically, emotionally, and spiritually, keeps the family connected.

Our elders have been incredibly victimized by the superficial values of the modern world; so we present here holistic perspectives on aging. The powerful guidance and love that older people can offer are waiting for acknowledgment. We need elders to help restore wholeness to our society.

The topic of embracing death and disease concludes our discussion of relationships. In the passing of a loved one, we are confronted with our own deep attachments, our own fear of death. Everyone involved can grow from being real and united in this transition.

Relationship is our teacher. We see our patterns project outward, again and again. From infancy until old age, we are perpetually growing. No matter how often we take new partners, and watch ourselves change in appearance, the essential part of us remains the same. This being, unique to each of us, relentlessly seeks to express itself, saying, "Accept and love me for who I truly am."

Relationships Survey

How well does each statement describe your patterns
of thought and action?

1. I have a variety of satisfying relationships.
2. I freely give and receive love and support.
3. I feel comfortable in expressing my sexual needs and desires.
4. I enjoy touching and sharing physical, emotional, and spiritual contact with others.
5. I am comfortable with the masculine and the feminine parts of myself.
6. I have meaningful relationships with people of all ages, including children and elders.
7. I am in harmony with, and share affection with, members of my family.
8. I am willing and able to respond to the needs of my friends and family in health or during illness.
9. I take enough time to be alone and nurture myself.
10. I have a positive self-image, which I express freely in relationships.
11. I am accepting of nonorthodox forms of relationship, i.e., homosexuality, bisexuality, celibacy, extended families.
12. I have worked out the resentments from unsatisfying experiences with family and lovers.
13. I have learned to live with separation and death of loved ones.
14. I am open to important new relationships.

The Care and Feeding of an Intimate Relationship
Philip Manfield, Ph.D.

We humans are social animals. We invest much of our time and energy in relationships. We look outward to partners to share our adventures and reflect back to us the qualities we love and hate.

Dr. Manfield discusses the dynamic that attracts people to one another. He follows relationships through the initial phase of exhilaration and high expectations to the stressful period that arises when communication breaks down. Practical suggestions for handling upset and rebuilding a relationship are offered. The "fair fighting" ritual of George Bach is presented to help struggling couples resolve dissatisfaction and alienation, and to refocus on their original intention for merging.

Featured with this article is "Healing The Heart," by Dajawn Breaux. In opening to an unconditional expression of love, our hearts can release the longing, sorrow, and blame that we so often call a "broken heart."

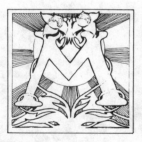

ost people would like to have an intimate and committed relationship with another person. As we can see from recent divorce statistics, however, most attempts at intimacy are short-lived. I believe that a primary cause for this apparent failure is a widespread lack of information. People seem to assume that intimacy grows naturally, all by itself; that it need not be cultivated. I would rather think of intimacy as I would any other growing thing: the better it is cared for, the more beautifully it grows.

To obtain information about the care and feeding of an intimate relationship, let us look at how an untended relationship develops, and where it can run into difficulties. We first learn about relationships as children; we learn by interacting with and observing those around us. In particular, we learn an enormous amount from our parents. We develop judg-

mental attitudes, rules about how things "should" be. By the time we are ready to form our own intimate relationships, we have a pretty firm idea about how relationships should and should not be. We have an image of how a man is supposed to behave and how a woman is supposed to behave. So, when we go out into the world seeking a partner, we usually try to act the part of our idealized man or woman; and we seek, in part, someone who will also conform to our idealized image.

CHOOSING PARTNERS

The idea that opposites attract appears to be true. In choosing a partner, we tend to be attracted to someone who possesses a quality that we lack. A flighty person tends to be attracted to someone who is down to earth and practical. A serious, intellectual type is often attracted to a vivacious and bubbly person. We are attracted to people who can add something to our lives, something in which we ourselves are weak or altogether lacking. Whether consciously or not, we wish this new person to teach us, to show us how to enrich our lives.

In varying combinations, all people are both practical and impulsive. Their minds and their bodies complement and balance each other. Thus, when we find ourselves viscerally attracted to someone whose qualities are different from ours, we may also notice our minds evaluating whether this match would be a practical one. We observe the image that the other person is presenting, and we evaluate whether this person will be able to take care of our needs. If a woman is nurturing to those around her, her prospective partner may comment to himself that this woman would make a good mother. Or perhaps the woman is fairly aggressive, and the man, lacking in aggressiveness, thinks to himself that she might give him the little push he needs in order to be more aggressive himself. The man, on the other hand, may present the image of someone who is solid and reliable, and would make a good provider; or he may present the image of someone who is very gentle and not to be feared.

So, for a combination of emotional and practical reasons, two people form a partnership. During the outset of the partnership, all goes according to their expectations. Suppose, for instance, that John and Sue have each presented to the other a gentle, cheerful image, which both found to be a welcome relief from their memories of their parents, who were always fighting. Though some irritations and dissatisfactions do arise between John and Sue, these are small and easily overlooked.

THE BEGINNING OF CONFLICT

As long as the irritations and differences between John and Sue are small, there will be no real problem; but over time, years perhaps, substantial differences and irritations are bound to arise. These will present a problem. John knows that part of Sue's attraction to him has been his gentleness, a quality she has commented on many times. If he shows the anger that he is feeling, how will she respond? Will she still want to be with him? Sue has similar concerns. When John wanted to watch football on television, and she wanted to watch a play, it was easy for her to avoid a conflict by simply giving him his way. But now that differences are arising over more substantial issues, like how to discipline the children, she feels too strongly to simply give in. She wonders, however, if John will think her willful and aggressive, and become displeased with her.

In addition to these problems, another type of problem arises. Sue was originally attracted by John's great generosity. Her parents had always been ungiving, and so it felt special for her to be the recipient of John's generosity. Now, it is upsetting her to see how John squanders much of their precious resources on gifts. Similarly, John was originally attracted by Sue's playfulness. He was a hardworking, serious person, and he found it uplifting for him to be around Sue's playfulness. Now, in the midst of his career struggles, he is irritated by Sue's constant requests that he take time away from his work to have fun with her.

BUILDUP OF STRESS

Stress is created as partners strive to fulfill their childhood fantasies of "the good life." Since "the good life" is a symbol, an oversimplified representation of happiness, it is frustratingly elusive, and usually unsatisfying if finally attained. Additional stress is created as parents, children, and careers compete with the marital relationship for attention and

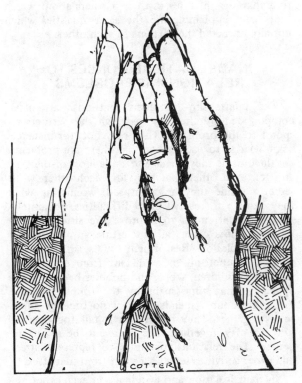

The forces which initially bring a couple together remain active throughout their relationship.

time. There doesn't seem to be enough of anything or anyone to go around. Partners often neglect their own personal needs. In their struggles to cope, the partners put increasing emphasis on performance, and they become more needful of each other's assistance. Concern about performance leads partners to be critical of each other's different styles; each wants the other to do things "right." Each may blame the other for unsuccessful coping behavior. The message of "I'm right, you're wrong" replaces the appreciation of each other's differences that the partners once shared.

Thus, the forces that initially bring a couple together remain an active force throughout their relationship. The images that people initially present to each other become restrictions on spontaneous behavior. Behavior that is inconsistent with the images that were originally attractive can represent a danger to the stability of the relationship, and is thus often avoided. Qualities in one partner that the other originally thought refreshingly different can, in times of stress, be seen as irritating obstructions. Nine out of ten couples that come to me for marriage counseling find that the qualities in their partners about which they are complaining are the same qualities which initially attracted the partners to each other.

INADEQUATE RESPONSES TO RELATIONSHIP PROBLEMS

The relationship problems that arise are often compounded by the way in which the partners respond to the problems. They may not, for instance, acknowledge to each other that there are problems. On the outside they manage to smile most of the time and tell each other that they love each other, while secretly inside they are confused, wondering what they can do to resolve their difficulties. Separately, they make attempts to improve the situation, but these attempts often fail and create an even greater sense of isolation. Resentment builds, and the partners feel more and more distant from each other. Activities, children, work, and hobbies become more appealing than time spent by the couple together. Soon the couple spends little or no time by themselves together. They forget how to talk together and how to play together. They cease to be sexual together. The relationship comes to represent stress, and other activities serve as a relief from that stress.

In their isolation and avoidance of each other, the partners rely more and more heavily on indirect means of communications. Rather than say, "I don't want to spend our money on a new car this year," one might say, "Don't you think a new car is a little extravagant for us right now," or, "You might as well forget going away for a vacation this year." Rather than say, "I'm feeling distant and irritated with you, and I don't want to make love with you tonight," one might say, "I feel tired, and I have a headache; so not tonight." If one partner wants a particular appliance or tool replaced with a newer model, that partner might complain often about the appliance or tool until the other partner gives in and suggests buying a new one. These indirect communications bring further distance to the relationship.

SELFISHNESS: SATISFYING WANTS AND NEEDS

How people get their wants met in a relationship is very important. In some relationships, it is considered selfish for one partner to ask the other partner for something directly. The unselfish way to get needs met in those relationships is to hint at what those wants or needs are; if the partner does not

want to respond, he or she can pretend not to notice the hint. This process avoids the unpleasant situation in which one partner is asking for something, and the other partner is saying, "No." The fantasy in these relationships is that if people really loved each other, they would be selfless in their attempt to fill all their partners' needs and make their partners happy.

These relationships usually run into problems. Hints are often not clear enough to express a real need, and many needs go unfilled as each partner tries to guess whether a hint was ignored or just not received. Many times I have heard people express to their partners in a shocked tone, "You didn't know I wanted that all these years? I thought you just didn't care enough to do it for me." The person most able to take care of me is me, and if I expend my energies trying to take care of my partner, leaving my needs to be taken care of by her, it is likely that we will both end up dissatisfied. No one can make another person happy. People can only make themselves happy and share their happiness with others. If my partner is always trying to please me, I will have trouble knowing whether the wants that she is expressing are actually her wants, or whether they are a reflection of what she thinks I want. The process of guessing what is in the other person's head is easily avoided by direct communications.

Before entering a relationship, one looks after one's self. There is no shame in satisfying one's own needs when one is unattached; this is not considered to be selfish. One is very much involved in one's own individual life. Entering a relationship is no reason to give that up. It makes no sense to me that a person should have fewer needs satisfied after entering a relationship than before. Why would a person want to give up growing after entering a relationship? One chooses a partner partly because of his or her differentness from one's self. One hopes to learn and grow with this partner. If a person's image of a relationship leaves no room for this process of individual growth, then it is time to reexamine what he or she has learned and accepted about relationships.

REBUILDING THE RELATIONSHIP

To understand the process of rebuilding a relationship, let us go back and look at the original weaknesses that brought about the current difficulties. The partners each felt compelled to maintain the image that had originally attracted the other partner. As the partners changed, they grew further and further from those images, until they could no longer bear to maintain the images. When they began to behave in ways inconsistent with those images, their partners reacted with feeling of resentment and betrayal. In addition, with the mounting stresses of family and career came a growing emphasis on practical needs, and a gradual loss of appreciation of differences between partners. Resentment grew, and with it isolation. Each partner tried separately to find his or her own solutions, but failed and felt more isolated. The emphasis in the partners' lives turned more and more from enjoying to coping. Time together became often unpleasant and reasons were found for avoiding contact. Partners who found it hard to ask directly for what they wanted turned more and more to manipulation and indirect communications.

ACKNOWLDEGE THE PROBLEMS

I believe that a first step in rebuilding a troubled relationship is to acknowledge both the problems that exist in the relationship and the feelings each person has about the situation. This is often difficult and painful to do. It cannot be done if the partners attempt to protect each other from the painful truth. Most often, the truth is less painful than the catastrophic fantasies that people create when trying to guess "the horrible truth." They wonder what truth could be so bad that they must be protected from it.

To tell the truth requires a confidence in one's partner's ability to take care of himself or herself. To be able to tell one's partner what one wants or needs, one must be able to rely on the partner to also tell the truth, which includes saying "no" when the request is for more than he or she is willing to give. The partner must be relied upon to refuse, rather than to acquiesce and begrudge cooperating with the request. Two people who are beginning to tell each other the truth about what they think and feel have already taken a big step toward turning a faltering relationship around.

WORK IT OUT TOGETHER

Once the problems have been identified, both partners must actively participate in addressing the problems *together*. Until the problems have been described out loud, this combined participation would be impossible. Problems are most effectively dealt with if treated as relationship problems, rather than as problems of one partner or the other. If my behavior upsets my partner, then we have a problem. She has a problem because she is experiencing an upset, and I have a problem because what I am doing is upsetting to her and interferes with our feeling close.

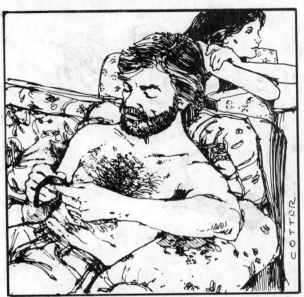

Problems are often compounded by how partners respond to each other. They forget how to talk together and how to play together.

It is unrealistic for only one partner to attempt to solve a major relationship problem. This would be like trying to take a family photograph of one's own family. There will always be someone missing from the picture. If partners doubt each other's willingness to be cooperative, then they will need to ask whether or not each partner has the other's best interests at heart. A spirit of cooperation is necessary for partners to be able to work their problems out together.

MAKE TIME FOR THE RELATIONSHIP

A second step is to recall the origins of the relationship, and focus on the original purpose of being together. This purpose usually has to do with adventuring, having fun together, feeling loving, and feeling loved. In this light, the recent emphasis on coping and functioning can be seen in perspective and cease to have such great significance. Partners can again appreciate and enjoy each other's differences. It is important that partners who have busied themselves and kept distant from each other now create time to be alone together. Doing so may require a special effort. Couples may need to set aside periods of time in which neither partner will have prior commitments to children, work, or anything else. Children can learn that parents periodically need this undisturbed time together; parents must learn to make their needs clear to children. This alone-time can be

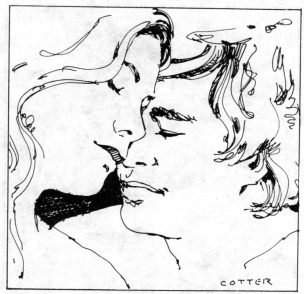

The first step in rebuilding a troubled relationship is to acknowledge the problems in the relationship and the feelings of each partner.

spent being sensual together, talking, walking, or doing any of the many things that felt good when the relationship was young.

EMOTIONS IN RELATIONSHIPS

The purpose of business is usually to produce a product; so it is most important at work that people function well. The purpose of home, if one were to think of home as having a purpose, would probably be to be happy, and happiness has less to do with producing a product or functioning. Happiness is a feeling, and it has a lot to do with emotional contact and intimacy.

Emotions need not make sense. They have their roots in the body, rather than the mind, and they don't require a reason to exist. A common mistake that people make is to insist that their feelings and the feelings of those around them be justifiable. This is like demanding a justification for a cough or a sneeze.

Requiring a justification for feelings causes them to be bottled up inside people, rather than expressed: if a person does not understand a feeling, he or she will then not feel free to express it. Most often, feelings are subtly felt before they are actually understood. For example, people might find themselves secretly resisting doing something because they have an irrational sense of misgiving about doing it, and they feel a need for a logical explanation before they will express their misgivings. The result is usually

frustration for everyone involved. If the misgivings finally become understood and explained, the question asked is usually, "Well, why didn't you tell me that sooner?" And the answer is, "I didn't know that's what I was feeling." This kind of situation can be avoided if partners encourage each other to occasionally be somewhat irrational, and to express feelings for which there is no apparent reason.

I find it helpful, in understanding how feelings work, to think of an analogy between a person's feelings and a reservoir. The reservoir has inlets and outlets. This analogy works equally well for anger or sadness, but, for the purposes of explanation, let us take anger as the example. Here the "inlets" are a person's upsets. For example, one of your inlets might be an upset that you have when you are driving your car and another car cuts you off. An outlet might be yelling: leaning your head out the window, and letting the other driver know what you think of him or her. Here, the anger is not stored in your reservoir very long. It begins entering the reservoir when your car is cut off, and it is let out, in spades, when you yell out the window.

Take the case of Joe. An inlet for him is an upset when his boss reprimands him. He chooses to store the anger generated in him by that upset rather than risk losing his job. He spends the rest of his day with his anger reservoir at a high level. The situation is aggravated as he thinks during the day of how his boss treated him, and his reservoir fills even more.

One can think of the inlets as the reasons for the feelings, but once the reservoir has been filled, it is irrelevant what the inlets were; all the anger is mixed together indistinguishably, and what is needed is to lower the level in the reservoir before it bursts. Driving home in rush-hour traffic yields Joe some welcome relief: "What the hell does he think he's doing?" "When are they going to finish that f---ing road work?" But these outlets are not enough, and when Joe arrives home, he is still brimful of anger. Fortunately, at home, he finds that the phone bill isn't paid yet, and that his son's roller skates have been left on the front lawn. He finally has an opportunity to unload all that anger he has been carrying around all day. "Why isn't the phone bill paid yet?" he snaps at his wife, and at his son, "And I thought I told you to put your skates away when you've finished playing with them. How many times have I told you . . ." If Joe thinks he needs reasons for his feelings, then he will have to find an excuse whenever he needs to explode.

Some people don't ever let their feelings out. They keep themselves under control at all times, and main-

Healing the Heart
Dajawn Breaux

"As I sat cross-legged, staring out across the ocean and the ever-darkening sky, I clearly perceived myself as a lighthouse. My crossed legs and lower torso were the foundation and tower of the lighthouse, and my neck and head were the roof of the structure. My chest was the glass-walled lens through which my heart was generating light and pure energy outward in all directions. There I sat with my upper torso beaming out feelings of warmth and passion.

"I can't explain what I felt like as this image continued to hold me, but I knew these feelings of love were not attached to any one person or thing or any one place. Rather they seemed to be nonspecific and nonparticular feelings of goodness and happiness that I was offering to everyone and everything. It didn't matter to me at that time whether or not I got anything back for my love. I was pleased just to be a channel through which it could flow."

Ken Dychtwald, *Bodymind*

Though it may not have been as dramatic as Ken Dychtwald's, most of us have had some sort of inspiring experience while alone in the grandeur and beauty of nature, an experience that transported us beyond the little world of our personal concerns, and instilled in us a sense of awe, great peace, and good feeling. These experiences are the best examples that I can think of to express the nature of the feelings in the heart and the essence of love. Because of a lack of love in our childhood and our struggle to get it from someone else in romantic relationships, most of us have a distorted ideal of what love is and how to have it in our lives. I would like to share with you what I have learned about love and how we can fill our lives with it.

Love is an inherent power associated with the heart region that produces pleasant and exhilarating feelings. There is a corresponding sense of fulfillment and good will; the world appears to be perfect, in harmony, lacking nothing. Love is a mystical experience, mystical because it opens us to a perspective beyond our alienated relationship to the world. We experience the integrity of the universe. We become an integral part of its wholeness.

The heart is the center, the axis upon which creation unfolds. To be in that center is to be in love. Most of us, however, live halfheartedly; this precious essence of our being, so vulnerable and deep, is closed off, hidden, protected. We have built a big wall so that nothing can get in and hurt this most vital part of ourselves. We want to feel safe, but we are miserable. Not only have we protected ourselves from the pain, we have shut out the beauty and joy of life.

As love flows from within, it pushes on the barriers that we have constructed to defend ourselves from our fears and insecurities. Allowing this force to push aside these walls of our separate identities creates a crack in our world view. It is a giant and terrifying step to venture forth naked, trusting in and surrendering to the inner knowing that, at the heart of everything, there is love.

Let's take a closer look at some of the misconceptions that prevent us from taking that big step. In the beginning we were born with a brand-new heart, perfectly capable of loving. (Even if there are influences and patterns carried over from previous incarnations, we have a somewhat fresh chance in every life.) Most of our parents have had no experience with real love; they were love-deprived. Our open expression of our need for love served as a ever-present mirror to them of their own unfulfilled needs. All too often they reacted in defense and resentment to the pain within themselves. Out of frustration they blamed themselves and us for the responsibility that love demanded of them. In many ways they punished themselves and us unknowingly. In these reactions and confusion, there was no love; we became love-deprived.

Out of this mixture of pain and frustration, guilt and sense of duty, they attempted to control love. We had to learn tricks to get it, and actually we hardly ever got the real thing, only myriad substitutes. If we did what they wanted us to, we got a pat on the head and a cookie. If we bothered them when we weren't supposed to, or didn't behave in the prescribed manner, we were rejected, and made to feel unworthy of love and their approval. We were taught that love was conditional. Our parents possessed it and could give it or take it away, depending on a long list of rules.

(continued on p. 222)

(continued from p. 221)

The world our parents grew up in and the world that we live in now is not a world of love. The collective ego of humanity has not taken that giant step. We all have learned to adjust and protect ourselves from the indifference and alienating aspects of the social structure. Our need to feel and express the more sensitive and loving parts of ourselves has been repressed. Behind the walls of our defenses is anger. Deeper still is our belief, charged with fear, that we are somehow inadequate and unworthy, that we will never know love. Our hearts, like a starved lion, hunger for love. We feel that love is so scarce that when we find some, we must jump on it, devour it. Thus the next pitfall, our misconceptions about romantic love.

I'm sure that the word love conjures up for most of us images of Hollywood romance. We grew up believing that some day Mr. or Miss Perfect would come along, and we would magically fall in love. They would give us the love we always wanted, make us happy, and fill up the lonely emptiness of our lives. But for some reason, everytime we "fall in love," it never works out the way it's supposed to. Our expectations are never completely met. We are disillusioned, and feel hurt and wronged.

In romantic love, our capactiy to feel love is perverted by our misconceptions and our history of unmet needs. We don't unconditionally see and love another person. We fall in love with an illusion created by our own state of deprivation and expectations. We are therefore mostly concerned with how our lover can fulfill our needs and dreams. In *The Art of Loving*, Erich Fromm said, "The active character of love can be described by stating that love is primarily giving. . . . The person whose character has not developed beyond the stage of receptive, exploitive, or hoarding orientation, experiences the act of giving, but only in exchange for receiving. Giving without receiving is for him being cheated." This is one of the biggest obstacles to expression of our love in a rich and healthy relationship.

A mature relationship to love is progressively realized as we dissolve our resentments and sorrow for our unloved past. These old emotion complexes blind us to love. We need to learn how to grow up emotionally, to take care of the needs that went unmet in childhood. To begin with, we need to remember how to love ourselves, to return to the innocence of our infancy. To feel love, to give and receive it fully, we must feel truly worthy of it. Our greatest challenge here lies in developing deeper and deeper levels of honesty by acknowledging and sharing our feelings and thoughts.

Inner honesty means trusting that we are naturally lovable when we are being ourselves. If we hide and do not share our inner self, then we are acting as if we are separate, covering something up that we believe will cause someone to reject us.

Next, we need to realize that no one can give us love. It doesn't come from anyone or anything "out there." It is an inherent power and state of being that we can meet and share in, but it cannot be given back and forth like a commodity. Love is within. It is at all times present. We need to open our hearts to the infinite reservoir of love and goodness within. Thus others will feel safer and more readily open their hearts around us.

"Love is being totally open, vulnerable. It is dangerous. You become insecure. We cannot ask how to love; we cannot ask how to surrender. It happens! Love happens, surrender happens. Love and surrender are deeply one.

"But what is it? And if we cannot know how to surrender, at least we can know how we are maintaining ourselves from surrendering, how we are resisting surrendering. That can be known and is helpful: How is it that you have not surrendered yet? What is your technique of non-surrendering? If you have not fallen in love yet, then the real problem is not how to love. The real problem is to dig deep to find out how you have lived without love, what is your trick, what is your technique, what is your defense structure, how have you lived without love?"

Bhagwan Rajneesh, *The Book of the Secrets*

The answer to these questions will require more than an intellectual effort. It will have to be lived through. We must allow ourselves to be transformed through it. This is dangerous because we will not remain the same. We cannot control it. Much of who we thought we were will fall away. To know love, we must be in love.

To live wholeheartedly, this is the secret of life.

SUGGESTIONS FOR FURTHER READING

Betty Bethards, *Sex and Psychic Energy*. Inner Light Foundation, 1977.

Erich Fromm, *The Art of Loving*. Bantam, 1963.

Liz Greene, *Relating*. Weiser, 1978.

Ken Keyes, Jr., *The Conscious Person's Guide to Relationships*. Living Love Publications, 1979.

Bhagwan Rajneesh, *The Book of the Secrets*. Harper and Row, 1974.

Dajawn Breaux has pursued an eclectic study of psychotherapy methods and holistic modalities. He resides in Santa Cruz, where he practices Psyche-Postural Integration, a form of deep emotional and body work. He also does psychic readings and healing, and teaches classes in how to develop and use these skills within a transpersonal approach to counseling. Dajawn is presently writing a book called The Seven Chakras and the Art of Psychotherapy, Meditation, and Healing.

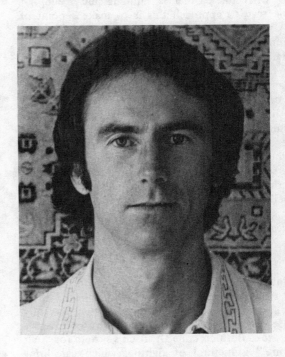

tain a steady tone of voice. In terms of the reservoir analogy, they deny themselves use of all their natural direct outlets. As a result, their reservoirs don't drain. They may be afraid to open any of the outlets for fear that all their stored-up feelings will come bursting out uncontrollably. They may be afraid of possibly hurting someone; so they don't let any out. With the inlets open, and the outlets closed, the reservoir fills. When it remains at dangerously full for a long time, the body instinctively finds an indirect outlet for the feelings. A "well-behaved" youth may break out in a heavy case of acne or other skin irritations. A "good-natured" mother of three may become severely depressed. A "smooth" businessman may develop an ulcer, or take to drinking heavily to "relieve his tension." A "nice young man" may experience frequent headaches. One way or another, the anger finds an outlet.

HANDLING FEELINGS AND UPSETS

Using the reservoir analogy, I find that the possibilities for handling feelings boil down to (a) developing safe outlets, (b) keeping inlets closed, or (c) finding a way to eliminate inlets altogether. Examples of a safe outlet for anger might be watching a spectator sport and shouting at the referee; playing an active sport; screaming in one's car with the windows rolled up; or getting involved in some sort of physical labor. Keeping inlets closed is accomplished by knowing what situations cause upsets and avoiding them, or by confronting upset situations as they arise. For example, if you have a slight upset about your boss reprimanding you in a certain manner, you might attempt to tell him in a direct, unemotional way about your upset. For major upsets, it may be difficult to stay unemotional. You might also attempt to perform at work in a way that is not likely to draw you into conflict with the boss; or you might change jobs.

I have noticed something about communicating upsets. Progress stops with the word, "you." As soon as I begin telling someone else about his or her part in my upset, he or she stops listening and begins thinking about what to say to prove his or her "innocence"; and an argument ensures.

From the foregoing, we can see that a third step in rebuilding a relationship is for both partners to learn to share their thoughts and feelings with each other every day. They need to avoid assuming that they know what the partner is thinking and feeling. A simple way to approach this is to make a point of using sentences that begin with the word "I," and avoiding sentences containing the word "you."

Marriage counselors often suggest structured exercises for couples to try in order to improve their communication skills. This structured communication can be valuable, by circumventing or inhibiting "old habits," automatic response patterns that have become unproductive, and by allowing people to explore new possibilities. In one exercise, a couple sits together in a quiet place. Taking turns, they each say three sentences to the other. The first sentence begins with the words, "I think"; the second with the words, "I feel"; and the third with the words, "I want." This exercise can make it easier for the partners to communicate their own thoughts, feelings, and wants.

CONFLICT RESOLUTION

Finally, the partners must express and let go of their stored-up resentments, and must learn to resolve conflicts. I recommend either of two books by Dr. George Bach, *The Intimate Enemy* or *Creative Aggression*. Both describe Dr. Bach's system for "Fair Fighting," a method of fighting which can bring couples closer together. The method consists of a collection of structured fighting "rituals," ways in which anger and discontent can be expressed in a safe, constructive manner. My wife, Janet, and I have used this system for many years and find it to be very valuable.

The basic idea behind "Fair Fighting" is that in an intimate relationship there is no such thing as a win/lose situation. When it appears that one partner has won, and the other has lost, the victory is temporary at best. Sometime soon the loser "gets back." This may take the form of "guilting" the winner, being late, forgetting to do something for the winner, withdrawing, being sexually unresponsive, becoming physically abusive, or any of many other possibilities. Ultimately, both partners lose. "Fair Fighting" is intended to make it possible for both partners to win.

There are two reasons why people fight, according to Bach. One is to blow off steam, and the other is to cause something to change. When someone is blowing off steam, he is usually in no condition to be negotiating a sensible change. Bach designed separate fight rituals for blowing off steam and for causing change. It is the responsibility of the person who is dissatisfied to declare whether he or she is interested in irrationally blowing off steam or in rationally fighting for change. Both processes are important, and they don't productively mix. If John is irrationally angry and also wants a rational change, Bach would advise him first to discharge his anger, and then, when he has cooled off, to talk about change. During the first process, Sue can simply hear John's anger without responding, knowing that John is only expressing his hostile feelings, and not demanding any change from her. When he asks for her to change, in another ritual, she will need to respond with her side of the matter.

Another payoff to "Fair Fighting" is that the stronger member of the couple doesn't have to hold back and protect the weaker member from the full force of his or her wrath. There is always a built-in handicapping in the rituals. Rituals are safe; nobody gets destroyed. When on participates in a ritual, one can give it his or her all.

The "Fair Fighting" rituals are carefully structured to avoid needless escalation of hostilities. As a part of the structure, both parties must agree to participate before a ritual can begin, keeping in mind that it is in both parties' interest that the aggression be released in a harmless way. Each ritual has a time limit, usually two or three minutes. There are rituals for different situations: there is one to be used when both people are angry, another to be used when only one person is angry. At the end of every fight ritual, there is a physical bonding, like a hug, a kiss, or a handshake, depending on how the partners are feeling toward each other at the time. The bonding is an expression of the caring spirit in which the fighting has been done. Then there is a twenty-minute cooling-off period during which the subject of the anger is not discussed. This prevents the back-and-forth exchanges that so often add fuel to an already hot fire.

Even if a relationship is in a state of crisis, there is often hope for solving the relationship problems. At such a time, when the relationship's survival is threatened, the partners have less to lose; they may feel freer to take risks and experiment with some new patterns of relating. It is during crises that I have seen people make the most dramatically constructive changes in their lives.

The suggestions given here for building or rebuilding a relationship will, I hope, point out some new directions for partners who are wanting a more intimate relationship, or who are sincerely attempting to reconnect with each other after having grown apart. More important than any outside guidance that such a couple might receive, I believe, will be their own individual commitments to each other to work together in solving the problems in their relationship. Just as we must sometimes work through difficult times in our individual lives, we must also work through difficult times in our relationships before we can again feel close.

SUGGESTIONS FOR FURTHER READING

George Bach and Herb Goldberg, *Creative Aggression*. Avon Books, 1974.

George Bach and Peter Wyden, *The Intimate Enemy*. Avon Books, 1970.

Virginia Satir, *Conjoint Family Therapy*. Science and Behavior Books, 1967.

_____, *Peoplemaking*. Science and Behavior Books, 1972.

Everette Shostrum, *Man the Manipulator*. Abingdon Press, 1967.

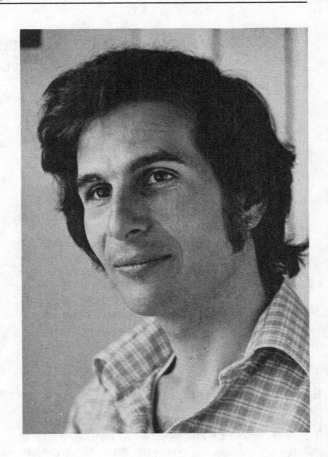

Philip Manfield, Ph.D., is a marriage and family counselor in private practice. He has offices in Oakland and Walnut Creek, California. His primary professional interest has been to help individuals and couples to build intimate and satisfying relationships. In addition to his clinical practice, he and his wife, Janet, also a marriage and family counselor, lead frequent relationship-enrichment workshops for couples. Dr. Manfield also teaches at Vista College in Berkeley, and conducts research in interpersonal relationship dynamics.

The Nature of Sexuality
Layna Verin

Sex is not the exclusive playground of the young and the beautiful. We all love it, need it, and deserve it, throughout our lives. More than intercourse, sexuality is the primal world from which we emerge and which we reenter in our intimate moments.

This moving article by Ms. Verin taps the pulse of sexual urgency that celebrates the very nature of our being. Her appreciation of sexual expression awakens feelings of wonder, awe and joy. What a relief from the commercial stereotypes that glut the media and pollute the image of sex in our hearts and minds!

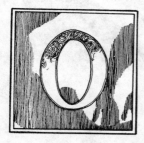ur sexuality is the deepest and most primal impulse, we possess. Repressed, it drains our vital energies and weakens all our faculties of mind and body. Fulfilled, it becomes a great creative and regenerative force. Sexual liberation does not lie in mastering techniques which see our bodies as pleasure mechanisms, but in the realization that our bodies are holy and that sexual relationships are a sharing of the divine energy that animates the universe.

"Divine am I inside and out, and I make holy whatever I touch or am touch'd from."
    Walt Whitman

Sexuality. How many millions of words have been written on the subject? How many tomes on erogenous zones, timing, positions, location and duration of caresses, on the use of hand, tongue, and genitals, and, above all, on the newest of status symbols: the orgasm.

True, much of this has been liberating. We are a puritanical people, and need to be untaught the fears and prudery that have been imposed on us. Unfortun-ately, the teaching has been more instructional than enlightening. Like childbirth, medical care, and education, our sexuality has fallen victim to the pervasive mechanization that distorts and debases the most fundamental aspects of our lives and of our human nature.

MEANING AND FUNCTION OF SEXUALITY

In the beginning was procreation. Procreation and fecundity. The primary urge of life is to be: to pursue its existence and to reproduce itself. Nature, in its limitless inventiveness, evolved from the most simple methods of cell division a separation into sexes. One of these is so fashioned that it enters into and fertilizes the other, which then nourishes and protects the newly conceived life within its body, preparing it for the moment of emergence. Thus variation in heredity is assured, and a more complex order of life realized. To ensure that mating occurs, nature created, in both the male and the female of all species, an irresistible impulse toward union.

Nature did not indulge in this creative fantasy to provide *Homo sapiens* with more and bigger thrills. The thrill is an intrinsic aspect of the sexuality. Sexuality is something far more profound than an instrument of pleasure. The glow in your eyes, the texture of your skin and hair, the warmth or humor of your smile, the timbre of your voice, the grace with which you move, these are all sexual. Sex is the essence of the life force, and you as a sexual being are an instrument of the life force.

Sex is an exchange of energies, an exchange of aspects of ourselves, imprinting ourselves on the body and soul of another human being, changing and being changed. Sex is the realization of self through loss of self. I become you and you become me in my arms.

When there is mutual surrender, some essence of the lover enters all the cells of the body, the nervous system, and the brain. There is an enhancement of individuality by the sharing and surrender of individuality.

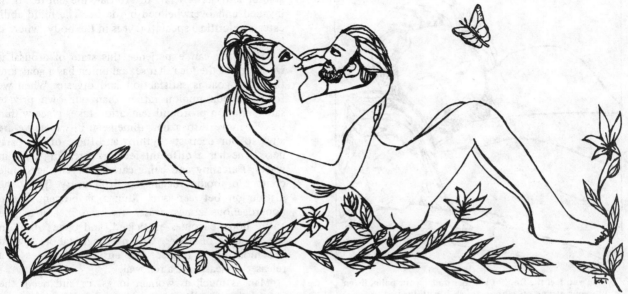

Sex is an exchange of energies, changing and being changed—the realization of self through loss of self. I become you and you become me in my arms.

THE MECHANIZATION OF SEXUALITY: AMBIVALENCE AND ALIENATION

Sexual intercourse that is failed communion—that is, mechanical excitation, mechanical friction, and mechanical come—is one of the fatalities of our civilization, one of its most tragic results, if not *the* most tragic. Wilhelm Reich believed that all our other tragedies stem from it. He hoped to transform the world on the foundation of sexual surrender.

To the degree that one is loveless, one inflicts lovelessness on everything and everyone with whom one is in contact. It is perhaps the sum of these acts of lovelessness striking against one another, jarring one another, and setting in motion further currents of lovelessness that makes our lives go so awry. In losing contact with our sexual selves, we have lost more than we know.

There is an almost schizophrenic ambivalence in our prevailing attitudes toward sexuality. Though sex is used as an instrument of power and domination, an expression of ego, a mechanism for relieving tension, a means of a "high," underlying all this is the hope that the sexual act will accomplish miracles, will release us from our feelings of alienation, and make us real to ourselves. There is a deep longing for the regenerating communion of true sexual passion.

THE QUESTION OF TECHNIQUE

Our exaggerated concern with technique, with sex as sensation, with orgasm as a goal perpetuates the split in ourselves, carries us away from sexual fulfillment. It is not technique we need; rather, we need to be at home in our bodies, to possess our bodies. We need not technique, but an openness to experience, a feeling of genuine appreciation and love toward our partner. Technique, as we understand and use it, is the intrusion of mind where mind is a hindrance.

In more primitive, less repressed societies than ours, young people at puberty are taught ways to pleasure and satisfy each other. These are learned as an accompaniment to the uninhibited flow of sexual energy, not as a substitute for it; as art, not technology; as the art of enhancing joy. Technique imposed upon inhibition remains mechanical; but freedom from the mechanical is what we all crave.

VARIATION AND DIVERSITY

What even the best of the sex manuals ignore is that no two human beings are alike, and that nowhere is our essential diversity more unmistakably expressed than in our sexuality. There is tremendous variation

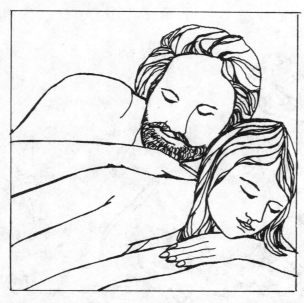

When you feel the flesh of another under your palm, listen to its murmuring pulsations, touch it with love.

in temperament and sexual drive. What thrills one person might bore another. Not everyone enjoys the sensuous delights of lengthy prelude. Not everyone needs or desires prolonged union. There are people who experience orgasm almost at a touch. There are others in whom the flame of passion does not so easily consume itself. What may be surfeit for one may be far from enough for another.

The exigency of desire also differs from situation to situation and from mood to mood. There are moods in which lovers take joy in caressing each other the whole night long without orgasmic consummation—and others when even the flinging off of clothes seems an interminable delay.

Desire may ebb and flow. It is only our fears that prevent this ebbing and flowing. An erection need not be sustained without interruption: It can sigh, subside, and reassert itself. It's true that the penis has a life of its own, humorously and sometime inconveniently. He's a whimsical and ironical fellow, raising his head at inappropriate moments and abasing himself when he longs to strut. But such whimsy is no life-and-death matter: anxiety is its own punishment.

EXCITEMENT AND AROUSAL: ORGASM

Because of our anxiety, because of ignorance or impatience, we do not give ourselves time to be. We confuse excitement and arousal. Excitement is usually genital and superficial. In arousal, the entire self is invaded and overwhelmed by desire. The mind abdicates as a critical spectator: it is in the body, where it belongs.

All of us can experience this state of arousal if we let go of the idea that sexual union has a goal, and that this goal is satisfaction and orgasm. When we focus on communion rather than our own private satisfaction, a profound relaxation takes place within us. We move into a new dimension in which we are alive to our deepest rhythms and those of our partner. Time has a different feeling, spreading itself in waves. Caressing and being caressed, even the simple contact of bodies begins to thrill every fiber. The distinction between such things as erogenous and nonerogenous zones ceases to have meaning. The entire body becomes eroticized, and opens itself to the flooding of desire. One no longer labors toward the moment of release: the entire experience is a release, a release and a renewal.

Man as much as woman longs for and needs the union that results when there is deeper arousal than simply erection and tumescent ache. Man, no less than women, is cheated by its absence. Passion in a man kindles a woman. Passion in a woman kindles a man. It is the body's complete sensual-sensuous abandonment to feeling.

I have known sensitive, ardent, and physical women who did not experience full orgasim for more than a year after marriage though they were deeply in love. When the orgasm came, it came in its own time and unexpectedly. With complete trust came the capacity for complete surrender.

There is much about orgasm that we do not know. And what is usually defined as orgasm is only one kind of orgasm, and not the deepest nor the most profound. There are orgasms that are explosive and shattering, orgasms that are light and laughing, orgasms that are an unhurried and tranquil dissolution. There are orgasms in the clitoris, in the vagina, in the uterus, in the entire body. Orgasm takes place everywhere.

ALIENATION

Unfortunately, the split in ourselves, the split that tells us that we have a body and that we have a mind, rather than that we *are* a bodymind, the split that separates us from the Earth and all living things, and that alienates us from each other—that split also dominates the sexual relationship. Man is alienated from and fearful of woman, the indispensable vehicle of his completion. Woman, though closer to the tides of life by virtue of her menstruation and child-bearing, is fearful of and alienated from the vehicle of her completion and of her fecundation.

It is because of this fear that promiscuity is elevated to a mode of sexual fulfillment. When the thrill is conceived of as merely genital, the more bodies one encounters, the more thrills one will experience.

Hidden behind all the frenetic activity is the heart's cry for the warmth of another human being, the longing for the trusting, passionate embrace in which flesh and soul are inseparable.

> "Sex is the greatest pleasure, the highest ecstasy, the supreme form of giving and receiving. . . . It has in itself everything."
>
> A. S. Neill

Love without lust and lust without love are equally unfulfilling. Love-lust, there is the beauty. If men and women did not feel lust, there would soon be neither men nor women. Not lust, but cold, indifferent, hostile copulation is our enemy. It is the use to which the lust—the desire—is put that makes all the difference. It is the way in which it is expressed, the quality of the union to which it leads, that make it a depressing exercise in futility or an affirmation of life.

THE QUESTION OF AGE

Neither age nor programmed concepts of beauty determine the boundaries of desire. Sexuality is not exclusively the province of the young and nubile, as our culture would have us believe. Desire, in later years, may be less insistent and demanding, but it may also be more serene, more appreciative of nuances and tenderness. What the body loses in elasticity and vigor, it gains in wisdom. The idea that there is something ungainly and obscene in sexual relationship between those who have passed the menopause is a relic of our thoughtless assumption that aging and senility are synonymous.

I had the good fortune to know a woman who fell madly in love when she was in her middle seventies. She was fat; her legs were somewhat bowed, her thighs loose and fleshy. Wrinkled and pudgy, she seemed the antithesis of what we associate with sexuality.

One day her lover, a man a few years younger than she, walked in while I was in her apartment. I watched in awe as her bosom began to rise and fall in the most passionate rhythm. A flush that began at her temples spread over her neck and suffused her breasts. Her skin glowed. Her aged hands gestured with grace and vitality. Her voice took on resonance

---

The Oldest Feeling
Summer Brenner

it is the oldest feeling in the world to me
walking on the beach along the ocean
holding onto the arm of someone I love
this

is the oldest feeling in the world to me
the feeling I've been doing this forever
and ever and ever and ever
putting

my foot next to another's in the sand
walking next to that one
arm folded into arm

the sense of journey
the constant voyage
that changes as little as a breaker over a
    particular rock
arm and arm in a corridor of the oldest feeling
    in the world to me

the beach might as well be outer space
and our short walk a flight through eternity

---

and trembled. At that moment she was Aphrodite, and to see the transformation was an experience I shall never forget.

Old as they were, the years that these two spent together were the most beautiful of both their lives.

SEX AS ADORATION

At its highest and most profound level, sex is adoration: adoration of life in the form of woman or man. This level is accessible to those who are imbued with a sense of the sacredness of their bodies and of their union.

For others who would like to make such a union possible for themselves, but to whom it still seems strange and mystical, a ritual exists which may help them to the self-surrender they seek. This ritual is one of the techniques of the Eastern teaching known as Tantra, a teaching in which sexuality as adoration holds a supreme place.

The lovers prepare themselves carefully, bathing and anointing themselves. Incense, candlelight, and beautiful surroundings create an atmosphere conducive to a meditative union. The lovers sit facing each other, the woman on the thighs of the man, with her legs twined around him. Though joined sexually, they remain motionless, deeply attuned to one another, and such rhythmic pulsations as occur, occur within the body, in a state of outer stillness. The senses are focused on an awareness of oneness, the blending of separate energies into one stream. Whether what happens is or is not orgasm is unimportant; there is union at the deepest level, a sense of exaltation and peace.

When a man and woman are able to surrender themselves fully to each other, such a ritual is unnecessary. It may be desirable for its own sake, because of its aesthetic beauty, but the quality of adoration does not depend on it. The body is not a lesser thing and the soul a greater. The body that houses the soul is the soul. Our divinity is in our bodies, in every fiber of our being. Our sexual juices are no less divine than the creative impulses of our minds and hearts.

FULFILLMENT

Each satisfying sexual encounter shared in lovingness is a rebirth. We shed invisible layers of silt, apathy, resentment, and suppressed fury, and in their place appears a vibrant interest in and tolerance of others. Everything appears in an easier and friendlier light. We feel weightless and buoyant.

Our moistures refresh each other like rain on the Earth, and the heat of our passion pours like sunlight into every pore, into every atom of every cell. As the Earth opens to the rain and the sun, so we open to life.

The child in us is reawakened. Our ears hear sounds to which, a day ago, they were oblivious. Our touch becomes more sensitive and delicate, our eyes aware of a radiance that emanates from and surrounds all living things.

The fulfillment of our senses delivers us from our broodings and discontents into the now, into the excitement and challenge of the ever-present moment. It fills the body and soul with joy, fostering in us impulses of candor and generosity, opening in us unknown springs of creativity.

In full measure our sexuality returns to us what we have given of ourselves, unlocking the mature forces of body, mind, and spirit, unifying them and making us whole.

A LAST WORD

When you feel under your palm the flesh of another, touch it with love. Let your hands listen to the murmuring pulsations under the skin, to the wandering blood, muscles, the fibers, each speaking their own language and asking:

"Oh, press deeper, deeper, softer, more gently. Hold, lift, place yourself here and here. Stroke and caress. Move the flesh slowly down, down, immeasurable distances and let it slowly return, whispering, revealing the secret of where the knots of terror are hidden and letting them be smoothed away . . . "

Secret upon secret, the body murmuring and asking and thanking and revealing, unloosing itself to flow like a stream, like a tide, like a wind.

This essay is not theoretical. I write from my own heterosexual experience. But what I say can be true of any relationship, woman to woman and man to man, as well. The most ardent description of a sexual encounter I remember reading in the past few years was written by a lesbian, Violette Leduc, in La Batarde. And the most naked, lucid, and courageous discussions of sexuality I have heard in the same period have been those broadcast by the Gay Men's Collective on Berkeley's Pacifica radio station, KPFA.

SUGGESTIONS FOR FURTHER READING

Erich Fromm, *The Art of Loving*. Harper and Row, 1956; Bantam, 1963.

Anaïs Nin, *Diaries*. Vol. 1 through 7. Harcourt Brace Jovanovich, 1966-1980.

Nancy Phelan and Michael Volin, *Sex and Yoga*. Harper and Row, 1967.

Wilhelm Reich, *The Function of the Orgasm*. Noonday Press, 1971.

Walt Whitman, *Leaves of Grass*. There are many available editions.

Realizing Sexual Potential
Joan Spiegel, L.M.F.C.C.

Sexual education is a welcome addition to a holistic understanding of self and relationship. The insightful observations Ms. Spiegel shares here are ones that she has found to be helpful for people working on sexual problems. She discusses the mechanics of sex with the attitude of personalizing and sensitizing a couple's communication. In this way, they can mutually share satisfaction in lovemaking.

In letting go of inhibitions, and exploring intimacy in a playful and relaxed way, we are less likely to be self-critical and goal-oriented. We learn about sex through practice. Enjoy your lessons!

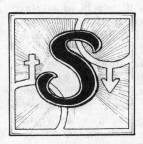 exuality is a natural expression of who we are. To realize our sexual potential is to be in touch with our bodies and our sensations, so that they can be an instrument of satisfaction of our needs. It is to feel all right about our bodies as an expression of us. We want to feel a real connection and rapport within ourselves and with partners. Communicating clearly and freely is an essential aspect of sexuality. Saying "no" when we mean "no" is what makes saying "yes" really meaningful.

We will examine what helps and hinders us in realizing our sexual potential. This paper is written for people of all sexual preferences. There are common elements of sexuality that we all experience and can learn from, to more fully enjoy our sexual experience.

PLAY AND SURRENDER

During sexual activity, people are most vulnerable. When we are feeling vulnerable, we would like to know that it is safe to be without defenses, to be lost in an experience. Fully participating in sexual activity is allowing ourselves to take all the time in the world to build up the excitement necessary for a physically satisfying experience. Teasing and touching and flirt-ing, playing and laughing, flowing in the moment, letting our bodies dictate the next move, giving up the idea that sex is a "performance" and that there is a "right" way to be—this is a reachable goal.

Begin to explore. Touch and stroke in different ways just for the sake of the experience itself. Play! Be outside of objective time. For a man, let it be all right *not* to have an erection all the time. For a woman, let it be okay not to please her partner at every moment. Shed some of the armor that we all carry around with us throughout our daily lives.

To create this kind of experience, we need to let go and give up expectations of what *should* happen. We don't need to plan the sequence of each movement. After all, sex can't be fun and be work at the same time.

TRUST

Full participation involves trust in ourselves, our bodies, and our partners. It is being comfortable in a state of vulnerability and openness. For this, we need to know that our bodies can function well in sexual activity. We need to trust that we can allow ourselves to act spontaneously and still be whole. In fact, letting go and exposing ourselves gives our partner the permission to do the same.

Trusting also means allowing our bodies to experience new sensations. Sometimes higher levels of sexual excitement than we are used to can seem frightening or uncomfortable. Just letting it be there and taking deep breaths is often all that is necessary to become more used to sensations and thus extending the range of our experience.

RESPONSIBILITY

Another aspect of full participation is being willing to take responsibility for ourselves in a sexual experience. No one can give anyone else an orgasm. The most important sex organ of all is the brain. The way we perceive how we are being touched is what causes our response. For instance, if our partner touches us exactly the same way with the same softness, gentleness, and slowness on two separate

231

occasions, but on one occasion we are in the right mood and are eagerly anticipating his touch, and on the other occasion our mind is not on the touch at all, we will have two very different subjective experiences. In that sense, our sexual pleasure is our own responsibility.

If one partner remains uninvolved and expects the other partner to provide him or her with sexual pleasure, that is not taking responsibility for one's own pleasure. Taking a turn at being passive is not what I mean by being uninvolved. In fact, taking turns at giving and receiving sometimes works out better than both partners stimulating each other continuously. When taking turns, the partner who is receiving can pay full attention to his or her own sensations and not be distracted by giving and receiving at the same time. Receiving pleasure is taking a very active part in the sexual experience. Not taking responsibility is saying or implying to our partner, "You do it to me!"

The partner giving pleasure can stay tuned into the other's signals, both verbal and nonverbal. Sometimes we get carried away with a form of stimulation that has worked in the past with our partner and miss the fact that her or she is dissatisfied this time. Asking our partner for feedback is one way to find out if what we are doing is pleasing. We can also notice the movements and facial expressions of our partner as clues.

CONDITIONS

A colleague of mine, Bernie Zilbergeld, talks about how everyone has conditions for good sex. Each person cites certain circumstances under which sex is comfortable and satisfying. Many male clients I see mention that one of their prime conditions for good, satisfying, non-anxiety-producing sex is knowing that their partner really wants to be with them, cares about them, and is as involved as they are in the experience. To have a partner as involved in his or her own sexuality as we are is one assurance that it is safe to let go, that we won't be laughed at.

Another condition many men have is that there be other options besides intercourse. When a man knows that oral and manual play is acceptable and satisfying to his partner, and that his not getting an erection would not be a disaster, he is more likely to get one.

Some men have conditions about the amount of time available and privacy. If the experience has to be rushed and there is someone in the next room, they have more difficulty getting an erection. This is

not surprising. Conditions such as lack of time or privacy create anxiety, which is just the opposite of the emotional state needed for relaxation and enjoyment, erection and ejaculation.

Most men need to know that they do not have to act on each surge of sexual energy just because it is present. They need to have the conditions present where they can say, "Yes, I would like to very much, but the circumstances do not allow anything sexual. Perhaps we could just let ourselves experience the feelings and be close to each other." This attitude would give both partners permission to experience new feelings that might be even richer than purely sexual ones.

Another condition some men and women have is that only after they have known their partner for some time and feel a degree of intimacy, do they feel safe and comfortable achieving penetration. One client informed me that he was fine once he got to know the woman he was dating, but if he tried to have intercourse on the first date, or even the second he had difficulty in getting an erection. One solution to this dilemma is to create a situation in which it is not convenient to go to bed on the first few dates, perhaps a date for coffee, or for lunch instead of a late-night dinner.

We women, too, have our conditions for good sex. When sex does not go well for us, it is usually because we have not honored them. Many times, when we are with a male partner, we allow penetration too soon. Many of us have experienced occasions when we are more turned on by manual or oral stimulation, because physiologically that is where most of our nerve endings are; and when we are penetrated, the high level of excitement seems to subside without our reaching an orgasm. When this occurs, many women think there is something wrong with them. There is nothing wrong. The fact is that there are very few nerve endings deep inside the vagina; so we tend to feel less during intercourse itself. It is the other, outer stimulation which is more likely to bring us to orgasm. When we allow penetration too soon, we cheat ourselves of our full potential experience.

BREATHING

One key to realizing our sexual potential is to focus on our breathing. Usually during increased sexual excitement, we naturally start to breath harder and faster. In order to focus, we can deliberately start to breath deeply earlier in the experience than we would otherwise. We can deliberately take deep breaths; and as we let them out, focus on the part of the body that is being stimulated: lips, ears, breasts, or genitals. This very active participation in receiving serves to increase the sensation in the area of the body being stimulated.

When actively giving pleasure, we can also use our breathing to facilitate the experience. We can watch our partner's breathing and coordinate ours with hers or his. This helps us know a little better what our partner might be experiencing, and helps us adjust our rate of stimulation to the rate of breathing.

One exercise I sometimes give my clients to show them what I mean by this is called "Spoon Breathing." The partners lie on their sides next to each other, and the one in back holds the other in the spoon or semi-fetal position, front to back. The one behind can then sense the other's breathing from the movements of his or her back. As the rhythm is sensed, it can then be duplicated. Very nice feelings of closeness and comfort usually accompany this exercise.

SELF-DISCOVERY

One of the best tools we have to discover our sexual potential is self-stimulation: masturbation. Masturbation was once thought to be an evil practice that resulted in a variety of maladies. Today we know that it not only is the best tranquilizer (with no side effects) available, but also provides a storehouse of information about our bodies. And it is the best way to train our bodies to respond sexually.

Men and women can use the masturbation experience to discover how their bodies respond to different kinds of stimulation. Many men in our culture have been taught to shut down their bodily sensations and just focus on their genitals. Sometimes the men clients I see are resistant to stroking their whole bodies. Somehow it seems "feminine" to some of them. But what is defined as masculine and feminine, we are learning, has limited our experience as human beings. When men allow themselves to open up and let their whole bodies become erogenous, they report that their orgasms become more of a total body experience instead of being solely genitally centered.

When men experiment with an exploration of their genitals, they discover the many different sensations they experience from different areas. These can help make sexual experience more enjoyable, by providing many different options for activities that had not before been thought of. Besides intercourse, other kinds of touches can be very stimulat-

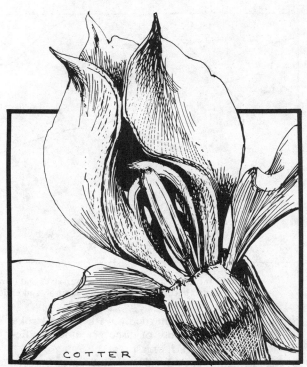

We want to feel a real connection and rapport with our partners and within ourselves. Communicating clearly and freely is an essential aspect of sexuality.

ing, and it is by masturbation with the focus on discovery that these can be found.

Women may never have touched or looked at their genitals before doing this exercise. Many women have said to me that they regard their genitals as ugly, or as looking like open wounds. I might show them pictures of different \women's genitals and point out how they are all different, just as our faces are all different. And I might point out that female genitals resemble opening flowers, if they would only look carefully. When we women begin to demystify the unknown that is our genitals by becoming familiar with them, we can then own them as part of us and be more in control of our own sexuality.

One way we might set up a discovery experience would be to create a relaxing atmosphere just for ourselves, to pretend that we are our own very special lover and to set the scene for our encounter with ourselves. We need to set aside a block of time that is ours alone, where we will not be interrupted. We might have a glass of wine, a soft comfortable place to recline onto, soft music playing in the background. We could take a bath or do some yoga to relax before

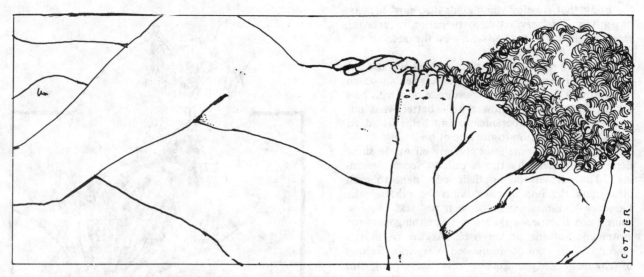

Practice, intuition, and sensitivity to ourselves and our partners are the fundamentals which enable positive sexual experience to become a comfortable, natural, and enduring part of us.

beginning. And then unhurriedly we begin to stroke our body for the purpose of discovery, not specifically to turn on and reach orgasm.

Just stroking our body all over to discover the sensation on different skin surfaces using different pressures is a great sensitizer. When I give this assignment to a client, I want to know very specifically what was discovered. Is the way her outer thigh feels the same as the inner thigh? How much pressure is satisfying, how little? Do different parts of the body feel different when being stroked with different rhythms?

What we are trying to do is help the body remember that all of it is an errogenous zone. Our whole body is responsive to sensation to some degree. Touching the whole body will help to reawaken it, will help to let us know that we are totally alive and that sex is not simply a genital experience.

Then I will have the client go on to genital stroking, again for the purpose of discovery. I will ask her to use a lubricant—not vaseline—and experiment with different strokes on different parts of her genitals using different pressures and speeds. I will ask her to take her time and explore leisurely, so that she can find out exactly how her genitals like to be touched.

Some women report that touching the clitoris directly is painful; so they prefer more generalized stroking on their genitals. Some women say the lighter the touch, the more stimulating to them. Others say just the opposite, that they like the touching to be fairly firm. There is no way a woman can find out what kinds of touching she likes without exploring for herself.

Some men start experiencing new sensations in different part of their bodies that they had never been aware of before. They may also discover new sensitive areas in their genitals that respond to different kinds of touches than they've tried before.

This kind of exploration helps the body experience higher levels of arousal and pleasure from very specific touches. When we know what these touches are, we can then show our partners how we specifically like to be touched, and we are then more likely to have more satisfying sexual experiences. There are two conditions that are absolutely necessary for increased excitement and orgasm to occur: muscle tension (myotonia) and vasocongestion, engorgement of the genitals with blood. When a person is uninvolved during sex, there is no tensing of the muscles. When muscles are not involved, there is no way for sexual excitement to increase and a satisfying orgasm to occur.

Some people notice that as sexual excitement naturally increases, the muscles of the legs tend to tense. Toes may curl. We may find that we want to grab with our hands. We may grimace and tense our face. This is all natural and part of increasing excitement that leads to orgasm. Some women may feel that it isn't "ladylike" for all this muscle tension to occur, and may consciously try to stop the natural movements. It is this self-consciousness which inhibits sexuality.

There is no way to will an orgasm. An orgasm is simply the release of the muscular tension and vaso-congestion through rhythmical muscle contractions, at eight-tenths of a second. Think of it as a sneeze of the genitals. A natural sneeze is just watching, waiting, letting the congestion build up till it lets go without any conscious pushing for it on our part. There is no way to push for a sneeze. In fact, if we try to control it, it feels worse. It is the same with orgasms. They come when they are ready. Our only job is to assist in the mounting tensions.

There is a difference between muscular tension and relaxation. It seems like a paradox to say both that one must be relaxed in order to enjoy sex and that one must have muscular tension. One can be *emotionally* relaxed and eager for the experience while at the same time tensing the muscles.

Men usually have not had as much difficulty engaging the muscles as women have. Men in our culture are trained to use their muscles as a matter of course, and getting sweaty is simply added evidence of masculinity. Also, when men are on top, as in the missionary position, there is strain on arm muscles and tensing all down their bodies, which contributes to sexual excitement. But the other side of the coin, for men, is that this position may tend to cause them to ejaculate before they really want to.

SOUNDS, SMELLS, AND JUICES

I once had a client say to me, "Sex would be all right if there were no sounds, smells, and wetness!" If it were all neat and clean, deodorized, sanitized, prepackaged with a nice neat ribbon, like our society pretends life is, then sex would have been OK for this client. Well, it isn't; and no matter how hard we try, life isn't that way either.

As we are stimulated and get sexually excited, we tend to make sounds. Some people spontaneously say words. Some people say "Don't" or "Stop," but that is just the opposite of what we really want. When we find ourselves wanting to say things while we are making love, we have a number of choices: either to hold back the sounds and thus cut off some of the experience; or to let the sounds emerge. I knew of one woman who was having orgasms and reaching high levels of excitement, but she told me the orgasms seem to get stuck in her throat. She then told me she was very careful not to make any sounds, because the walls of her bedroom were thin, and she was afraid her children would awaken. She was also embarrassed making weird sounds in front of her husband. I asked her to deliberately make sounds while

masturbating during the day when her children weren't home, as practice; and then to talk to her husband about what it would be like for him if she allowed herself to make sounds. He admitted it might be strange at first, but he was willing to try. They also decided to make love in the living room—away from the sleeping children—for added privacy. By her last report, she no longer felt her orgasms were stuck, and she was finding that her husband felt freer to be louder when making love also.

Semen has a characteristic odor, which is quite natural. The vagina too has its own odors, which are also quite natural. If the body is kept clean, these odors need not be bad or unpleasant. I've heard many women say that they do not want their partner to perform oral sex on them, even though they enjoy it, because they are afraid they smell bad.

Perhaps what we need to do is become friends with our body odors and tastes. Do you men actually know what your semen tastes like? Do you women know what your vagina juices taste like? It may be time to find out. It may be time to smell our underpants as we take them off to see what it really is. It may actually be a turn-on. No perfumes or coverups, just our natural clean odor. When it is less of a mystery to us, then we may not be so reluctant to allow our lovers to experience us in that way also.

Our natural juices, too, can be part of the turn-on of sex. As we women get more excited, our vaginas sweat. These juices lubricate the vagina to facilitate intercourse. I've never heard of a man who thought that his female partner was too wet. And women who truly enjoy sex relish the semen of their male partners. The mingling of the juices after intercourse can be just as much of a turn-on as the act itself. Of course, afterward we may want to wipe up the juices or else we have to decide who gets to sleep on the wet spot—which is also part of sexuality.

Sex can be fun if we allow it to be. We do not have to be stuck in our old patterns if they do not satisfy us. How we participate in sex is definitely a learned experience. We learn by practice and intuition, and by sensitivity to ourselves and our partners. In this way, sex can become a part of who we are in a comfortable, natural, and enduring way.

Of course, we do have to take the initiative to break out of old patterns and experiment with new ones. That is the most important step. Our own subjective experiences are the most important indicator of what pleases us and what doesn't; and they, too, may change. We all have to go at our own pace to find new discoveries and new ways of increasing our sexual potential.

SUGGESTIONS FOR FURTHER READING

Lonnie Garfield Barbach, *For Yourself: The Fulfillment of Female Sexuality*. Doubleday, 1975.

Shere Hite, *The Hite Report: A Nationwide Study of Female Sexuality*. Macmillan, 1976.

William H. Masters and Virginia E. Johnson, *The Pleasure Bond*. Bantam, 1976.

Sondra Ray, *I Deserve Love*. Les Femmes, 1976.

Bernie Zilbergeld, *Male Sexuality*. Bantam, 1978.

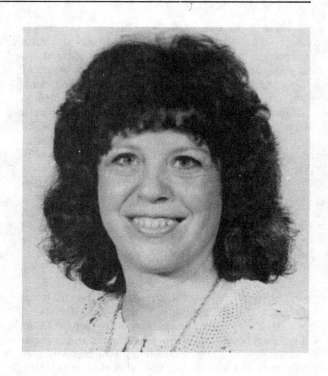

Joan Spiegel is a licensed Marriage, Family and Child Counselor, and is certified by the American Association of Sex Educators, Counselors, and Therapists as a sex educator and sex therapist. She is co-director of the Human Sexuality Education and Counseling Center in San Jose, and is on the Associate Staff of the Human Sexuality Program, University of California Medical Center in San Francisco. She has been involved in the study of human consciousness for many years, and is doing work in the field of sex and consciousness.

She has a private practice in San Jose.

Coming Out: The Emergence of Gay Identity

William Reiner, Ph.D.

Gay feelings have a life of their own, states Dr. Reiner. They are a viable position on the spectrum of human sexuality and loving. "GAY IS GOOD," echo millions of women and men around the world. A large, but heretofore invisible minority is "coming out," and claiming its right to exist in society.

The homophobic (fear of homosexuality) attitude of non-gay people is an issue we all face. Homosexuality is neither the corruption nor the aberration that our culture has believed it to be. Rather, it is an inner-directed calling that guides one to find meaning in loving members of like gender. Moralizing and minority oppression do not mitigate the emergence of gay identity.

Featured with this article is "Redefining Sexuality: Toward a Marriage of the Self," by Ruth Falk, a feminist writer and activist. She shares her experience of loving women, and of discovering the beauty, strength, and wisdom of being a part of the Women's Movement. She speaks of the androgynous (male/female) nature she has found in herself by learning to be alone and loving herself.

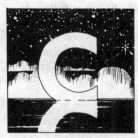

oming out of the proverbial closet to claim one's identity as a gay person is a major step toward self-affirmation. It requires inner strength to risk possible rejection from family, friends, or work associates. There are both real and imagined dangers to personal survival in this move toward authentic self-disclosure. Through trial and error, the emerging gay person learns when the time for sharing some or all of his or her gay feelings is right. Stepping into the sunlight of personal affirmation can also be exhilarating. As a gay therapist, I've learned to appreciate that "coming out" is a metaphor which describes a never-ending process of personal growth and evolution. Permission to be oneself comes from within, and is a source of personal power and strength for everyone.

Most gay people go through transitional phases of growth as they develop their individual gay identities. Most gay people become aware that they are sexually attracted to people of the same gender by the time they reach adolescence. The awakening of gay feelings for some, however, does not occur until the twenties, the thirties, the forties, or even later. Early gay feelings sometimes fade from awareness, because they are too threatening to be acknowledged; they surface eventually because they are an essential part of one's being.

Regardless of when the awareness begins, the emerging gay person will usually, consciously or unconsciously, initiate a rite of passage toward self-acceptance and maturity. The stages of growth for most gay people appear to follow somewhat similar patterns, though certainly each individual's experience is uniquely his or her own. Dr. Don Clark, in his book *Living Gay*, presents a model for understanding the transitions and life stages of gay people. I have used this model to describe four phases of growth that, I feel, illustrate some of the most common experiences of this immensely personal evolution.

BEGINNING AWARENESS

I remember, with a clarity undiminished by the passage of time, the object of my first fleeting sexual infatuation. He was somewhat older than I (he was 25, I was eight). Cupid struck at a crowded poolside one summer. Love at first sight. A gentle, outgoing young man sparked the first glimpse of what erotic attraction for other men would be like for me later. I had never before experienced the warm sensation that rose up from my belly and spread over me in vibrant waves. The intensity of my excitement over him pushed an alarm button from deep inside. All my heterosexual programming told me that my feelings were wrong. I felt alone. Those first stirrings of sexual arousal I knew had to be my secret.

The beginning awareness of homoerotic feelings for most of us is tinged with some fear and confusion. The natural attraction for people of the same gender

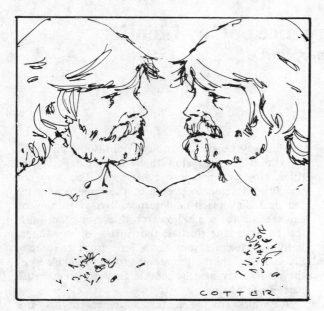

A natural attraction for people of the same gender is undeniable. Sexual feelings toward people of the same sex touch us to the core.

is undeniable. It signals awareness that one is different from other people, and, in that differentness, alone. Other people around us are not acknowledging gay feelings; there seem to be no visible models for men loving men or women loving women. An undercurrent of fear and scorn is all that is immediately detectable in people's response to identified homosexuals. It is clear that gay feelings and thoughts should be kept underground. Survival, especially for gay children and adolescents, seems to hinge on keeping an essential part of one's identity inside. Feelings in general become suspect; expression of them might lead to the expression of the deeper, more forbidding ones. There is often a tactical retreat from anything or anyone who might trigger one's sexual responsiveness. The vital life force is kept in temporary hibernation.

SELF-ACKNOWLEDGEMENT

The passage of time and the sweet ebb and flow of maturing sexual and emotional attachments to others brings the spring thaw. Early awakenings of sexual feeling come into sharper focus. There may be experiments with lovemaking or homoerotic play with peers or identified gay people. Undeniable sexual attractions for people of the same sex touch us to the core.

There is a growing acknowledgment of gay feelings and a willingness to explore their meaning. Questions seek answers. What does it mean to be gay? Are there other gay people like me? What will my life be like if I'm gay? Should I keep that part of me secret? What will happen to me if I don't raise a family? Is there something really wrong with me? Can I change and become heterosexual?

One's senses become attuned to subtle innuendos from others about their thoughts and feelings on homosexual love. Antennae are primed to detect other kindred gay spirits as yet unrecognized. Oppression is often keenly felt, as family members and friends carry on the heterosexual tradition of ridiculing gay people by thoughtless forms of humor.

A solitary trip to the library to search out one's origins usually leads to dreary reference books which chronicle the history of modern-day psychiatric witchhunts of gay people. Homosexuality is interpreted in many ways:

1. A form of arrested psychosexual development.

2. A mortal sin, a crime against nature, a theme which leads many gay people to the priesthood or to the spawning of the "best little boy or girl in the world" syndrome.

3. A form of perversion and a training rite for child molesters (although child molestation is a decidedly heterosexual phenomenon, by all the facts and figures).

4. A mental condition which a few noted psychiatrists and psychologists have "cured" by such extreme remedies as electro-shock to the genitals to punish homoerotic arousal.

5. A "deviation" involving insatiable sexual appetites and promiscuity. "Promiscuous," of course, is a term we use to describe someone who is more sexual that we are.

6. And so forth.

These harsh myths and stereotypes lose much of their inhibiting power when subjected to the slightest amount of soul-searching and personal examination of real people's lives. The questions open the mind to new possibilities, once the pretense and dogma about the "one true path" of heterosexuality is revealed. Gay feelings have a life of their own, and are just another position on the spectrum of human sexuality and loving. Mental-health professionals clearly cannot change a breast man into a leg man with any certainty, much less bridge the terrain of sexual preference. Gay sensibility, that elusive quality of humor, wit, style, and outrageous mockery of social convention so often attributed to "flamboyant" gays, is cultivated from the outside.

COMING OF AGE: ADOLESCENCE

Acknowledgement of one's gayness leads to action: the pursuit of sex and love. Initial forays into the gay world are a mixture of excitement, disappointment, fulfillment, heartache, adventure, and all else that befalls us poor mortals in the formative stages of adolescence. Typically, it's a time for learning about other gay people, and exploring sexuality. The release of bottled-up sexual energy is intoxicating; the reality of sexual pleasure more often than not meets one's fantasies. There is frequently a strong urge to have it all now, to make up for lost time.

Someone who comes out during adult years, after establishing strong roots with family, business, and community, may need to make up for a denied gay adolescence. Family and friends are convinced the person's gone mad, staying out till all hours, getting into romantic entanglements that are totally out of character with his or her established image. Eventually, however, life becomes more settled. One feels more secure within a more clearly defined gay portrait. Close friendships with other gay people become anchors to be used when needed to deal with the turbulent waters of the voyage ahead.

ADULTHOOD

Individual identity is carved from one's unique life experience. Adulthood for the developing gay person comes with the knowledge gained during adolescence. An evolving sense of mastery and power stems from an understanding and appreciation of one's gayness and the struggle for authenticity in a world fearful of its own richness and diversity.

The challenge of creating a lifestyle and relationships is met. One learns to be comfortable with those parts of oneself that make up the "public person" and those that make up the "private person." Coming out does not necessarily mean sharing your personal sexual life with everyone indiscriminately. Sharing one's gayness with others can be an invitation to intimacy and trust.

Usually the accumulated anger and rage that most of us gay people feel toward those who have been oppressors has found some measure of release. There is a sense of balance from knowing that life is worth living in spite of homophobic roadblocks that get in the way. Love relationships deepen. The capacity to love oneself is reflected in the bonds that are formed.

The old sexual bugaboos have, for the most part, been retired to the refuse pile, where they rightly belong. Homophobic myths about oneself and other gay people have largely been debunked, although sex-negative conditioning runs deep. The challenge of identifying the traces of our ancestral sexual fears and conditioned attitudes can be experienced as an invitation to grow. A cultivated sense of the outrageous sharpens the eye of the hunter. Illusion and heterosexual pretense become a tired old drag that no one wants to wear. Dogma and fear do not die easily; the struggle belongs to us all.

SUGGESTIONS FOR FINDING GAY RESOURCES

1. Most universities have a Gay People's Union that can put one in touch with local gay organizations and resources.

2. Most large cities have a Gay Community Center or gay activists' organizations.

3. Gay newspapers and magazines list clubs, organizations, and other resources. The national gay newspaper, *The Advocate,* 1730 So. Amphlett Blvd., San Mateo, CA 94402, provides comprehensive coverage of events, activities, and resources for gay people nationwide.

4. The National Gay Task Force, Room 506, 80 Fifth Avenue, New York, NY 10011 (telephone 212-741-1010), may be contacted for information about resources in your area.

5. The Task Force on Gay Liberation of the American Library Association maintains a carefully compiled bibliography of books, articles, pamphlets, and films that support a positive view of gayness. Their bibliography may be obtained by writing to them at Box 2383, Philadelphia, PA 19103.

6. *GAIA'S GUIDE* is an international guide to gay organizations, community centers, stores, bars, etc.

(Text continued on p. 242)

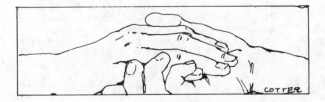

Redefining Sexuality:
Toward a Marriage of the Self
Ruth Falk

We need to develop new words for sexuality. Our language has developed out of a linear perspective in which everything has been segmented. People are called either heterosexual, bisexual, homosexual, or lesbian. We are many selves, and flow in and out of these dimensions. Why try to fit our total being into a box that may fit only one aspect of us? Although most people express their sexuality by loving the opposite sex, that does not mean they never have had loving and sexual feelings for the same sex.

It would be healthful for all of us to define ourselves as people from our inside, from our feelings, not by outside definitions into which we must force ourselves to fit. In that way all our parts can emerge freely.

I prefer not to label myself, and I think in terms of over-all sexuality. I feel everyone is born with the potential to love both women and men. If society did not say we had to choose, most people would let themselves experience loving and sexual feelings for both sexes.

WOMEN LOVING

After years of relating to men sexually, I allowed myself to explore my loving feelings for other women. This has been an important transformation for me. Relating to women has unquestionably brought me closer to myself. Today I feel more powerful, and have a deeper sense of love and respect for myself and for other women. The permission to love other women in the emerging women's movement has been very exciting and freeing. We have gained and continue to discover a new sense of ourselves. We have created our own culture, our own community, our own religion, our own ethos and set of values, our own spirituality, which many call Womenspirit. What has emerged out of our movement are very powerful women (both physically, mentally, and spiritually strong) with a reverence and respect for everything living, a recognition of the cyclical nature of the world, and a posture toward the world of *allowing* everything to unfold rather than trying to *control,* which has been the dominant mode for centuries.

As we each participate in the world, we bring with us our women's culture, our celebration of the emergence of the feminine. With our strengths and new perspectives, we will be a healing force in this country.

INTIMACY

The relationships we are evolving in loving other women have been exciting. I have gotten a clearer understanding of myself. Because we don't follow traditional sex roles when we relate, there is a freshness, a newness about experiencing same-sex relations. Each of us is striving to experience all our different selves and to take full responsibility for who we are in the relationships. A new type and understanding of intimacy is evolving.

In the women-to-women relationships in which I have been involved and know about, two strong individuals come together and share intimacy. We are not looking for our other "half." One partner isn't expected to be the breadwinner and the other the nurturer. We experience taking turns in all variations of these roles. Each of us learns how to receive and how to give.

In sharing roles and exploring all our different parts, we are evolving toward an androgyny of the self. Receptive, soft, open, compassionate, passive, feeling: these qualities are traditionally labeled *Female* in this society. Aggressive, strong, hard, driving, objective are labeled *Male.* Exploring androgyny, I am learning to integrate these different parts of my total self. I am fuller and stronger in expressing my active and receptive sides, and admire and appreciate this wholeness and freedom in others.

One of the keys that I have learned in intimate relationships with women is the importance of keeping my own space and of the time I need to be alone.

Sections of this piece have been excerpted from *Women Loving: A Journey Toward Becoming an Independent Woman* (Random House, 1975), and *High Adventures: Ace of Wands,* a visionary work on the celebration of the reemergence of the Feminine Principle in this culture (to be published soon), and are reprinted here by permission of the author. To obtain a copy of *Women Loving,* send $8.35 postpaid to WOMYN, P.O. Box 7083H, Berkeley, CA 94707.

SPACE WITH ANOTHER PERSON

"We close the doors
between us
for reasons of warmth."
Diane Fabric

When you like someone a great deal, it is difficult to keep your boundaries, your own space. I have found when I am intimate with someone, it is especially difficult for me to take the space I need for myself, to be alone or to do my work. When I love someone, I like to be with them often. But I have learned that if I don't take the time I need to be with myself, I lose my center, and the relationship and I begin to suffer.

I told an old friend from back east about this concept. She said it is still hard for her not to take her lover's need to be alone as a rejection of her. This is something we all need to work on.

At one time in my life, having a man and a relationship was more important that taking care of myself. I felt that relationships came first, my work and myself second. Most men are often still caught up in traditional sex roles, and are very demanding of a woman's time. In my experience, women are more supportive of each other's needs.

THE PLEASURE OF BEING ALONE

We hear very little about the pleasure of being alone with oneself. When I was younger, I was so afraid of being alone that I thought of it mostly in negative terms: loneliness, isolation, no lover. The image of a woman alone conjures up thoughts of a woman without a man: a "single woman." For me, exploring other meanings of being alone has been very enriching and nourishing.

"What's wrong with that girl? She's eating dinner alone!" When I was in my early 20s, I would feel very ugly inside if I were eating dinner alone in a public place, wondering what people were thinking of me. I remember one time going out with the "nice Jewish Boy of My Life" for dinner, and seeing a lady at another table, eating dinner alone, on a Saturday night. How sad and pitiful she looked to me. What was really sad and pitiful was my relationship to this man. I would have been better off eating dinner alone than being in that painful relationship.

My friend who encouraged me to spend more time alone said that she could never imagine me taking long, hot baths and relaxing. I had no sense that being alone would help me be closer to myself. Constantly going out to meet other people was doing me no good. As I began to spend time being closer to myself, I began to realize that my essential love—that primary lover I had been searching for—had to be me.

One of the first things I did alone was to take a vacation. For the first time I experienced the excitement and comfort with myself that I usually relied on from a best friend. This time I had no interest in, nor felt any pressure to be with, other people. The sheer delight of being alone after a full day of sun, sound, wind, and foam rolling upon foam. A cool breeze through my room. A hot shower. Walking through my room nude; cool cream; and then cool sheets. Reading, high-beamed ceiling with shingles interlaced. How can you do all that with someone in your room? You can, but it's just not the same.

I have discovered that there are two different levels of nurturing. One level is the nurturing I need to comfort and protect myself when I am in pain. The other is the nurturing I do or receive to pleasure myself. I do not want to be doing good things for myself only as rewards or as comfort when I am in pain. I want pleasuring myself to be a part of my everyday life.

MARRIAGE OF THE SELF: FUTURE VISIONS

From my frantic search for Mr. Right to my experience of women loving, I now see an evolution toward a marriage of the self. I fantasize often about intimacy, about sexuality, and about the form of our relationships. As we go deeper into ourselves, in a sense we are reclaiming our childhood, ourselves as children . . . we become our original selves. Now that I love myself, loneliness and solitude have taken on new meaning for me. I am my primary lover. I experience the "mother within." I look to the future with hope and excitement as I imagine hundreds of women and men taking vows to the self: to nurture ourselves, to be responsible for our own lives, to experience all our parts and sides. We have become individuals with roots in ourselves, and we live our lives as a journey.

(continued on p. 242)

(continued from p. 241)

As time goes on, people will continue to form intimate relationships, but the focus need not be confined to the couple. A community of strong, powerful individuals, moving fluidly between being friends and lovers, is develop-

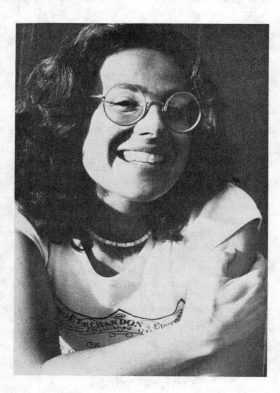

ing, where affection and love are shared amongst equals. Many of us envision a tribe of kindred souls that will span the country. When we love ourselves in our totality, we will feel deep love for many.

Author Ruth Falk lives in Berkeley, California. Her pioneer book Women Loving *(Random House) explores feelings at such a deep level that thousands of women and men have said that the book was a turning point in their lives. Her movie/novel* High Adventures: Ace of Wands *is a visionary book celebrating the re-emergence of the Feminine Principle in this culture. She is currently producing the feature film* High Adventures *based on this novel.*

Falk, who sees creativity as a channel for self-growth and transformation, consults on writing and creativity in the Bay Area. She has served as consultant to several institutions in-

Falk, who sees creativity as a channel for self-growth and transformation, consults on writing and creativity in the Bay Area. She has served as consultant to several institutions involved with social-action programs. Falk received her Masters from Harvard in Education and Social Policy. She was Consultant, Section on Youth and Student Affairs, at the National Institute of Mental Health for six and one-half years and was responsible for funding such youth projects as runaway houses, free clinics, hotlines, and women's centers. She is author of numerous professional papers on prevention, mental health, and transformation.

(continued from p. 239)

SUGGESTIONS FOR FURTHER READING

Dennis Altman, *Homosexual Oppression and Liberation*. Outerbridge and Dienstfrey, 1971.

Betty Berzon, *Positively Gay*. Celestial Arts, 1979.

Rita Mae Brown, *Rubyfruit Jungle*. Daughters, 1973.

Don Clark, Ph.D., *Living Gay*. Celestial Arts, 1979.

_____, *Loving Someone Gay*. Celestial Arts, 1976.

Christopher Isherwood, *A Single Man*. Avon, 1978.

Jonathan Katz, *Gay American History: Lesbians and Gay Men in the U.S.A.* Crowell, 1976.

Paul Monette, *Taking Care of Mrs. Carroll*. Avon, 1979.

Sappho, *Sappho: A New Translation*. Trans. by Mary Barnard. University of California Press, 1958.

Charles Silverstein, *A Family Matter: A Parent's Guide to Homosexuality*. McGraw-Hill, 1977.

C. A. Tripp, Ph.D., *The Homosexual Matrix*. McGraw-Hill, 1975.

Ginny Vida, *Our Right to Love: A Lesbian Resource Book*. Prentice-Hall, 1978.

Patricia Nell Warren, *The Front Runner*. Bantam, 1975.

Edmund White, *States of Desire*. Dutton, 1980.

William Reiner, Ph.D., is a psychologist and consultant in private practice in San Francisco and Marin. He has worked extensively with gay people, and on gay-related issues as a therapist to individuals, couples, families, and groups.

Teaching Our Children About Sex
Anne Bernstein, Ph.D.

Dr. Bernstein casts a clear light on how we do and should school our children in the facts of life. We teach our children about sex from the first moment they enter the world by the way we touch and care for them, by the way we allow pleasure in the sensuality of intimate contact.

As children grow older, the example that parents give, in how they conduct themselves with family members, close friends and lovers, creates a far deeper impression than any verbal instruction. In growing up, children learn that their sexual explorations may not be appreciated in certain situations. Parents and children can establish guidelines that meet their mutual needs, and thus avoid embarrassment and hurt feelings. In essence, parents and children teach one another about the joy and responsibility of expressing sexual energy.

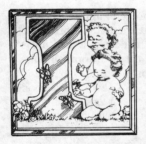
'm going to do a better job talking to my kids about sex than my parents did with me" is a frequent vow in today's households, but a difficult one to put into practice. Even without saying a word about sex, though, we speak volumes by the example of our lives. Children learn by observation; they are acute receivers of nonverbal messages. For them, as for us, actions speak louder than words.

Sometimes we actually teach what we want to teach. Often, we do not. For instance, parents who tell a child that it is all right to masturbate, but do so with voices flat and controlled, are giving a double message. Their words say one thing, but their intonation says that on a deeper level they believe just the opposite. Children then are left with ideas and feelings about sex that they can neither question nor explain.

BABIES AND SEX EDUCATION

Teaching about sexuality begins at birth. The touching and handling and caressing that loving parents provide teach infants to relate warmly to others, whereas touch deprivation leads to emotional and physical problems. From their parents, children learn either "I am a lovable person whom others will care for," or "I am unlovable and must protect myself from caring too much for anyone."

To like oneself one must like one's body. How others respond to one's body is an important part of how we feel about ourselves. Spoken and unspoken messages set the tone for who and what can be touched, and for the conditions under which children can see, show, or ask questions about bodies. Is it okay to touch Mother? Father? Her breasts? His penis? Until the child is how old? Can he still look after he can't touch? And how will he be stopped when the line is drawn? The way parents touch children, as well as family and cultural attitudes toward nudity and modesty, bodily pleasure, or physiological development, all affect a child's sexual development, leading to positive or negative attitudes toward the body.

Toilet training provides an important arena for transmitting attitudes about body parts and processes. The young child values his waste products as part of his body. If he is made to feel that his bowel movement or urine is bad, he may internalize these attitudes, and start to feel that he himself is bad. Dr. Warren Gadpaille, in *Cycles of Sex*, decries calling the sex organs by "nursery or babytalk words which, in their initial application, refer to excretory functions," because they foster "the association between sexuality and dirtiness." Similarly, Selma Fraiberg points out that children who discover that the genitals, which give them pleasure, disgust their parents will often feel that their genitals are bad, that their feelings are wrong, and that they are unworthy as people.

"I ENJOY BEING A GIRL (OR BOY)"

Feeling good about being a girl or a boy is another important source of self-esteem. To like the fact of one's own sex, one must feel good about one's genitals. It is hard for a child to feel good about himself if his parents would have preferred him to have been put together differently.

In learning about sex differences, children learn both facts and values. But until they see evidence to the contrary, both sexes assume that everybody is "just like me." Seeing the body of a naked child of the other sex will stimulate questions about why there's a difference. Boys may ask, "Where's her penis?" or "Why doesn't she have one, too?" From girls, the questions may be "What is that?" or "What happened to mine?"

Unless complicated by negative attitudes toward the little girl's sexuality, penis envy is common but harmless. Teaching more about other sex differences is often useful when children first begin to ask questions about genitals, so that each sex is defined by what it has rather than what it lacks. Both sexes need to understand that they are specially designed, "on purpose," to be different so that they can make babies together when they are grown up.

Masturbation is one way that children explore their bodies' potential for pleasure. Although most children do masturbate, some 40 per cent of their parents think that it's "not all right" for them to do so, according to a study reported in *Family Life and Sexual Learning*. There is, however, considerable evidence that masturbation is a sign of healthy normality.

As early as 1905, Freud wrote that the sexual instinct is aroused by maternal affection as well as by direct excitation of the genitals. Later research supported this connection. Child-development researcher René Spitz, M.D., who observed infants throughout the first year of life, found that babies who received virtually no nurturance did not masturbate, even though they received all the usual stimulation involved in ordinary diapering and bathing. Those whose mothers had personal problems that hindered the quality of the care they offered showed some self-stimulation, but no genital masturbation. The babies given the best maternal care all began to masturbate by their first birthdays. The study concludes that infantile sexuality develops spontaneously with quality nurturance, clearly demonstrating that it is both normal and healthy (Gadpaille, p. 62).

This does not mean that parents cannot or should not put limits on their children's masturbation or

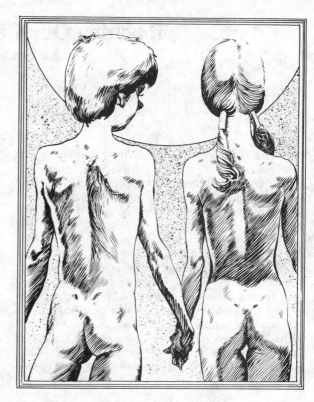

Until they see evidence to the contrary, children of both sexes assume that everybody is "just like me."

other sexual activity. Preschool children, even toddlers, have already learned that there are appropriate times and places for many of their activities: eating is done at the table, sleeping in the bedroom, elimination in the toilet. Masturbation need not be treated differently. A parent may say: "I know it feels good to play with your penis (or clitoris or vagina), and it's okay, but it makes me uncomfortable when you do it here in the kitchen where I have to work. I would feel much better if you would go to another room, where you can have privacy." This parent acknowledges that the child's good feeling is appropriate and respected, but also takes care of his or her own discomfort, without leading the child to confuse the parent's needs with his or her own.

WHAT ABOUT FAMILY NUDITY?

Parents' attitudes toward their own bodies have an important impact on their children's sexuality. If parents hide their bodies and are embarrassed upon being discovered unclothed, children will learn that there is something shameful about the human body.

Casual and unaffected parental nudity conveys the message that parents are "at home" in their bodies.

Parental nudity is sometimes thought to be over-stimulating to children. I think it is the attitude of the adults—how they feel when they are undressed—and not the nudity itself that can be distressing.

Seductiveness, not nudity, is what overstimulates children. Parents can be seductive without being nude and nude without being seductive. A look at other cultures shows us that nudity is not necessarily damaging to children. It is the emotional messages the parent is broadcasting, not how many clothes he or she is wearing, that influence how children will feel. If parents are self-conscious about being undressed, they will transmit anxiety and doubt rather than comfortable self-assurance. If this is the case, parents can quietly request privacy, avoiding a show of distress.

"UPROAR" DURING THE TEEN YEARS

Puberty is a critical time for youngsters' evolving sense of themselves as sexual beings. Parents' responses to the physical changes in their children go a long way in shaping their sexual self-esteem. Often criticism of the child's sexual development is veiled in comments about clothing and makeup, rules for getting home, and choice of acceptable companions. A father who feels aroused by his adolescent daughter's womanhood may react with anxiety and denial. In so doing, though, he may lead his daughter to blame herself for the change in him, which she sees as rejection. She is left feeling that she has done something wrong by becoming sexual.

Children need to know that sex includes emotional intimacy as well as sexual intercourse and making babies. By watching their parents' marriage, they learn how sexual intimates relate. Is the love between a woman and a man mutually supportive, caring, tender, responsive, and responsible? Or is it exploitative, critical, barren, and debasing? What they see at home as children will influence their expectations of what is possible for them when they become sexually active adults.

In our culture, experts agree that openness does not include making love in front of the children. Witnessing adult sex can be both overstimulating and evocative of scary misconceptions. Of course, children sometimes wander into their parents' bedroom at inopportune times. These occasions are best handled without panic or guilt about wounded young psyches.

Telling the child you want to be left alone and will be available in a short time is usually sufficient for the time being. Later you can explain what you were doing and ask if the child has any questions. Hearing you speak of the love and pleasure of sex will help counteract any impression of violence. Clear, simple, and forthright answers to questions can give children the information they seek without compromising your own intimacy and comfort or overstimulating the children.

WHAT PARENTS NEED TO KNOW

Clearly, we cannot avoid communicating about sex to children. The way we relate to one another and how we talk about sexual differences, reproduction, and relationships form a part of their sex education. How then can we guide them in their efforts to integrate their sexuality into their lives as whole people when this is a task very much in progress for most of us? In order to help the children we love, we must first explore our own feelings about sexuality and become comfortable with them. To be clear with children, we must first be clear with ourselves, recognizing our abilities and limits, and acknowledging our true values.

There will be mistakes. But mistakes can be remedied. Elizabeth Canfield, a prominent sex-education counselor at the University of California at Los

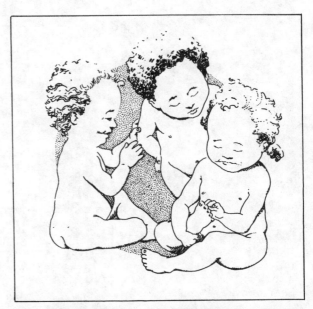

Teaching about sexuality begins at birth. To like oneself one must like one's body.

Angeles, suggests: "It's a marvelous experience to walk up to a child and be able to say: 'You know, I've done some more thinking about our discussion the other day, and I've decided what I said didn't make sense, so let's talk some more.' A child (or friend, neighbor, student, employee, lover) will be so delighted with this admission . . . that a whole new world of communication will have opened up!"

By keeping the communication channels open about sex, parents who establish themselves early in their children's lives as receptive in dealing with sexuality will find that when their children have questions or worries to be cleared up, they will turn to their parents.

For information does not equal permission. Socially inappropriate behavior is more often the result of ignorance than of knowledge. None of us, child or adult, does everything we know to be possible. Nor do we want to. But when we know the score, we can choose which tune to sing, fitting the song to the scene and to characters with whom we share the platform.

SUGGESTIONS FOR FURTHER READING

Anne C. Bernstein, Ph.D., *Flight of the Stork.* Delacorte, 1978; Dell, 1980.

Stephanie Waxman, *Growing Up Feeling Good: A Child's Introduction to Sexuality.* Panjandrum, 1979.

Warren Gadpaille, *Cycles of Sex.* Scribner's, 1975.

Sol Gordon, *Let's Make Sex a Household Word: A Guide for Parents and Children.* John Day, 1975.

Wardell Pomeroy, *Your Child and Sex: A Guide for Parents.* Dell, 1975.

Anne Bernstein, Ph.D., is a California-based family therapist and the author of The Flight of the Stork, *a book about how to discuss sex and birth with children.*

The Role of the Family in Holistic Health
Casi Kushel, L.M.F.C.C.

We all experience some kind of family most of our lives; it can be anything from the traditional nuclear family to a chosen family, selected for support and shared values. Whatever the form taken, the family can be a tremendous source of nurturing and stability. It gives us each a base of support and encouragement from which to build our lives. Unfortunately, we often take our families for granted or neglect the interrelatedness necessary to maintain a healthy family atmosphere. Ms. Kushel suggests some exercises which may increase awareness and understanding between family members. Taking the time to do these simple exercises together will greatly add to your appreciation of each other.

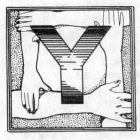

our family . . . what do you think and feel when these words flicker across your mind? Your Mom? Sunday dinner? Raised voices? Your grandmother's house? Perhaps you have begun a family of your own, and the first image that comes to you is the day your son was born? Or the nasty fight that heralded the beginning of the end of your marriage?

Are you living with your family of origin, the one into which you were born? Do you and your spouse live together? Perhaps you share your life with a chosen family selected for support and shared values. Children? Grandparents? Living with someone? We all experience some kind of family most of our lives. We all live in a social network. Yet when we think of our health and well-being, the one thing we rarely consider is our family, the people with whom we live and interact daily.

How do we look at the family in this new age of holistic living? What should it do? What can we expect from it, and how do we keep it healthy? To begin with, the family is a system in which everyone is affected by and affects everyone else constantly.

"Healthy systems produce individuals who both are autonomous and have a sense of belonging or identification with the family and the world around them. These healthy, functional families are able to communicate clearly and congruently. They encourage independence and provide loving support for their young. They are consistent with discipline and encourage appropriate responsibility. Most importantly, they allow for individual differences and are willing to make appropriate changes in family rules as children grow and circumstances change. Often these healthy families share spiritual or political values, and are involved with their community" (Peper and Kushel, 1979).

We all hope to have a fair share of our emotional and psychological needs met in our families. When we experience ourselves as valued, loved, and nurtured, we glow with energy and health. Often, however, our family life does not provide this feeling of well-being. We fight, misunderstand, feel bored, blame, swallow our feelings for fear of hurting or being left, or do not even find time for our families.

FAMILY CHECKLIST

We are often unaware of how well our support systems serve us. Here is a checklist of some of the important components in family interaction. Sit quietly and mull them over for yourself. Give careful consideration to your experience of your family. These should be relevant no matter what size or shape your family is.

COMMUNICATION

Does your family communicate well? Clearly and congruently? Do you feel really listened to? Are you interested in what the people you live with have to say? Do you share feelings, or just chitchat? Are there words that are never said, topics never mentioned? Can you ask for clarification if you do not understand? Does it sometimes feel like someone says something with their words, but his or her body says something else? Does one member of the family tend to talk for everyone else?

FEELINGS

Are a full rainbow of feelings expressed and encouraged? Are children allowed to express anger? Is it okay for Dad to cry? Is joy applauded or hushed with guilt? Can some one person's anger dominate everyone else's activity? What happens when you say "No"?

PLANNING

Can the family plan something from start to finish and put it in to operation? Are leadership roles assumed? Who is in charge? Who makes decisions? Are the parents willing to be responsible but respectful of other's expertise?

AUTONOMY

Is your family flexible enough to accept differences in its members? Is there privacy? Can a person be alone and not cause hurt feelings? Are independent activities supported? Is each person's uniqueness appreciated and nurtured?

INTIMACY

Are the parents an intimate couple? Do they go out alone? Support each other emotionally? Make love? Share the responsibilities of the house lovingly? Do they model health in their habits?

TOUCHING

Does your family touch? Do people hug? Is it permissible to ask to be held?

RULES

Are the rules in the family explicit? Do you have unspoken rules, like "No one may ever criticize Dad," or "If something's wrong, it's probably John's fault"? If no one says exactly not to do something, is it all right to do it?

CONFLICTS

Are conflicts resolved or just avoided? Do some issues persist unresolved for years?

Now share this checklist with your family. Talk about it. Is there anything about your family that you would like to change? This may lead to another family issue which you discover as you interact. How does your family deal with change? Who usually initiates it? Is it always the same person? Does the idea of discussing a change you might want to suggest excite you or make you feel anxious? If it makes you feel anxious, consider getting some professional support for positive change for your family.

FAMILY THERAPY

There is a whole new field of behavioral medicine developing now. Supported by the trend to holistic health, this discipline looks at how people's behavior affects their health, teaches new skills, and encourages self-responsibility for wellness. Just as you would demand from your health professional that she treat "the whole person," insist that you be seen in your social context.

A growing part of this new field is family therapy. Family therapists treat the structure of the family, alter the relationships of family members, teach communication skills, foster age-appropriate behavior, and create space for individual growth in a supportive environment.

Families most often come in for therapy when the couple is experiencing serious enough difficulties to consider divorce, or a teenaged member has been busted, or one of the kids is "acting crazy" and the family wants him fixed. People often have family therapy suggested to them if their child is having continued trouble in school or has been labeled a schizophrenic, or if a member has a disease or some other handicap that affects the functioning of the whole family.

All these are excellent reasons to see a family therapist. But they are not the only good reasons. If you answered any of the questions above in a way that made you feel uncomfortable or dissatisfied, consider bringing in your family for a checkup. Therapy can be a place to learn new skills, and to create support for families going through transitions or coping with major life changes.

It is also a setting in which to consider our most important life options. Should we marry? What kind of a couple contract reflects our ideals? Is this a good time to have a child? How do we organize our family for a new member? How do we anticipate our children's leaving home? What plans would improve our retirement? How do we prepare for death?

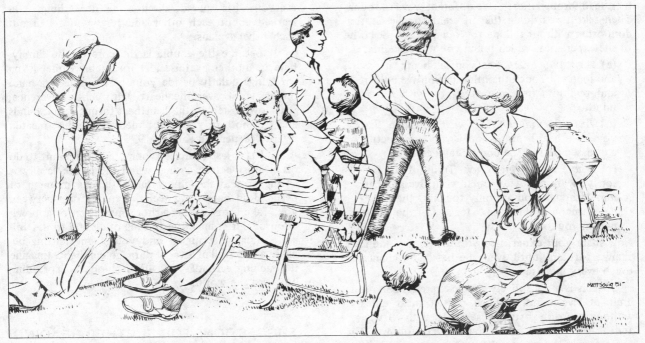

Your family is a core ingredient of your environment, a system in which everyone is affected by and affects everyone else constantly.

FAMILY EXERCISES

Aside from working with a professional, you can share many valuable experiences with your family at home. Here are ten exercises that you can do yourselves and that will promote clearer communication, encourage intimacy, and give you each an opportunity to learn some new things about yourself and the people you share your life with.

1. Pass out a sheet of paper to each member of the family. Have everyone make a column for each family member, and write the person's name at the top of it. Under each name, write three things that you think that family member thinks about YOU. Take turns reading your answers and discussing them. Did you know he thought you thought *that*?

2. This exercise is sometimes called *Appreciations and Resentments* (Bach and Wyden, 1970). It is best in pairs. Choose a partner. Arrange yourselves so that you are sitting facing each other. One partner begins by offering three things which he or she resents about the partner. The partner must listen without responding until the first partner is finished, and then may say, "Thank you for sharing that," or "I understand." No more. The first partner then continues with a list of three things he or she appreciates about

the partner, and the procedure is repeated. Then the two reverse roles. The exercise is repeated until each member of the family has had the opportunity to "resent and appreciate" everyone else.

3. For this exercise, you will need a very large piece of drawing paper. Each member is given a different-colored crayon. The family is to cooperatively draw a picture. This is to be done in silence, with no previous instructions or directions. Each member's work will be identifiable by their color. Everyone find a place around the paper which is placed at a table or on the floor. Now begin. Work for five minutes. Now look. Who has the most color on the page? Who has the least? Did anyone get left out? Is it a picture of something or a lot of individual pictures? Was there a silent leader? Did everyone look to one person for direction? Discuss everyone's feeling. Prepare to try again. Turn the paper over, and begin another work of art. Leave room for everyone; encourage the shy one. Change leaders. Now how does that feel?

4. This is a touching exercise. Touch is an extension of our emotions and thought. This is an opportunity to practice and get feedback on how well your touch expresses your feelings. Choose a partner, and

then read through these three different ways to touch. Then take turns doing the different touches in random order without talking to your partner. See if he or she experiences which touch you were sending.

(a) *A grasping touch.* Feel yourself being "needy and lonely." Touch the other person's shoulder, and pull him or her toward you with this in mind.

(b) *Experimental-clinical touch.* Imagine that you are a health professional who is inspecting a diseased part of the body. Stay detached.

(c) *Whole and loving touch.* Think of the person you are about to touch with love and caring. Although you are only touching the shoulder, remember this is an extension of the whole person you love.

Now share your experience with the family, and then change partners, until everyone has had a chance to touch everyone else.

5. This is a deceptively simple exercise. Set a time limit of five minutes. Each person must quickly, without censoring, start a sentence with "I want," and finish it with any thought that follows. The other family members follow each other quickly in sequence, not pausing to think or respond to the others' wants, or even to try to make sense. Keep this up, rapid fire, one right after the other, for the full five minutes. Are you surprised by what you said? Did you learn anything new about your family? Were you able to listen to others' "I wants" without judging them or feeling responsible? Share your feelings about what you learned with the others.

6. This one is for the couple only. Each partner writes on a piece of paper five things that most impressed them when they first met. Then write one line which begins "I chose you because," and finish it with the reason you chose this person over all the other possible mates. Then share your lists and discuss how you feel about those five qualities now. Finish by sharing your last sentences.

7. Again you will need a piece of paper for everyone in the family. Have everyone write down three rules that everyone in the family knows are true. Then write down three more rules that you think are true, but no one has ever said out loud. Discuss the first set until everyone agrees that these are really family rules. Now discuss the second set. Does everyone agree on this set of rules? Are there any rules you would like to change? Discuss this.

8. Each member of the family takes a five-minute turn, telling the family "What I would do if I just found out that I had only one month to live." When everyone has shared, discuss the new things you learned about each other and how you felt about each other's plans.

9. Because the couple is the core of the family, here is another exercise just for them. While sitting (or lying) quietly beside your partner, place a hand on his chest over the heart. With gentle reverence, with love, listen to the heartbeat through your hands and feel both of you surrounded with and permeated by love (Peper and Kushel, 1979).

10. This last exercise is one you might want to do often. Just before eating, while the entire family is sitting around the dinner table, share a moment of peace. Join hands and feel the energy pass between you. Take turns leading a short invocation of appreciation of our connection to each other and to the universe. Imagine yourself and your family sitting beneath a waterfall of love, of pure, golden light. Imagine it touching each of you, uniting you and spreading out over the world.

SUGGESTIONS FOR FURTHER READING

G. R. Bach and P. Wyden, *The Intimate Enemy: How to Fight Fair in Love and Marriage.* Avon, 1970.

Ravi Dass, and Aparna, *The Marriage and Family Book: A Spiritual Guide.* Schocken, 1978.

R. D. Laing, *Knots.* Vintage, 1970.

Shirley Gehrke Luthman and Martin Kirchenbaum, *The Dynamic Family.* Science and Behavior Books, 1974.

Salvador Minuchin, *Families and Family Therapy.* Harvard University Press, 1974.

E. Peper and C. Kushel, "An Holistic Merger of Biofeedback and Family Therapy," *The American Theosophist,* 67, no. 5 (1970), pp. 158-168.

Virginia Satir, *Conjoint Family Therapy.* Science and Behavior Books, 1967.

Casi Kushel, Co-Director of the Biofeedback and Family Therapy Institute, Berkeley, is a licensed Marriage, Family, and Child Counselor. Her speciality is family therapy. She is on the faculty of the California Graduate School of Marital and Family Therapy, Marin, and has been an associate staff member at the University of California Medical Center in the Human Sexuality Program, San Francisco. Her private practice is in Berkeley, California. Currently she is engaged in research on psychic healing and its application to developing a holistic model of psychotherapy.

"Who Put the Geraniums in the Water Pitcher?": Direct Care of the Bedridden Family Member

Alta Picchi Kelly, M.S.W., M.P.H., Ph.D.

Taking care of a loved one who is ill can be an intimate and rewarding experience. It can also be frustrating and trying. The health of any one family member always affects that of the entire family. When a family member is ill and requires care, there usually must be a readjustment and shift of responsibilities throughout the household. The extra responsibilities can, at times, cause resentments. This article talks about the challenges involved with "home nursing," and presents some useful suggestions on how to make the whole experience a healing one for all concerned.

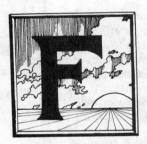

Few experiences can have the emotional impact of being awakened in the middle of the night by a crying child, who, you discover, as you stumble from your bed, has vomited on her bed and is as hot to touch as fire. Or of the phone call from a friend telling you that your husband is coming home from a ski trip with a broken leg. Or of the day when your mother's doctor meets you in the hospital corridor, and says, "Well, there is really nothing more we can do for her here. You may as well take her home."

As you pick yourself up from the floor, wondering "Why me?" and "How am I going to cope?" and "What do I do first?" you begin to enter the world of accidental and unskilled at-home nursing.

Every family at one time or another faces the problem of caring for someone who is sick or injured. It is a common but stress-filled experience for all families and most adults. Today, with the increased expense of health care for long-term illnesses or injuries, and with the increase in the size of our aged population, we have become aware that we need to learn again how to take care of a family member at home.

Caring for a family member at home can be a rewarding and growing experience for the family, or it can be a difficult strain. Forethought and planning in family health management can ease a stressful situation. The techniques and information from holistic health, when integrated with traditional skills of at-home nursing, add a new dimension to caring for the sick and assisting them in their own inner healing.

But whether it's the 24-hour bug or your mother's final illness, forethought is something that will make handling the at-home nursing situation much easier. For years the American Red Cross has offered classes in home nursing. Their textbooks offer fundamental information on basic skills and are a good reference for bedside nursing. Any person who has the *desire* and the fundamental knowledge to work with an incapacitated person at home can be responsible for most of the bedside care.

Holistic Home-Style Nursing is a new field in family health. There are basic ideas associated with the new practice. Holistic Home-Style Nursing assists in the patient's inner healing and well-being by:

- giving physical care and support;
- working as a team member with the person who is ill, the family, and the medical community;
- recognizing that the patient is aware of and controls his own body processes at some level, and is acting upon the body's feedback messages;
- accepting feelings as part of health;
- recognizing that home-style nursing is helping, not rescuing;
- rewarding health, not illness;
- supporting open and effective communication between yourself, the patient, and meaningful others.

KEY CRITERIA FOR NURSING SKILLS

There are several at-home nursing skills that can be observed in caring for any sick person at home.

251

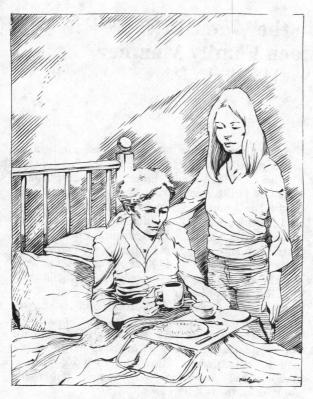

Sickness is a crisis in anyone's life, affecting the person's self-concept and body, as well as the family environment.

SAFETY

This essential factor applies to the ill person, the at-home nurse, and the family. Safety is very important in prevention of disease, and is the major criterion for deciding how to handle and dispose of soiled articles, discharges from throat and nose, and body wastes. Washing hands after each contact is the key to preventing the spread of disease.

COMFORT

Comfort for the ill person and the core person are important. Comfort means less stress and strain for both. A clean, dry, well-made bed and supporting pillows placed at the proper height for good bedside nursing is essential to necessary rest and sleep, and will create less wear and tear on the home-style nurse. Comfort that fosters self-help and self-care is important for rehabilitation and recovery. The ill person should share in preparing this environment, as much as he or she can.

ECONOMY

Careful thought should be given to deciding what is the best and most efficient use of energy, time, money, and equipment. Planning uses of household items, and of shared responsibility with family members, will save money and materials, and make the best use of energy.

EFFECTIVENESS

Any system should be tested for its usefulness. Questions asked about ways of providing care should be: "Does it work?" "Is it safe for the ill person and me?" "Does this way foster a team approach to care?" "Will it save time, money, and equipment?"

When illness occurs in a family, adjustments and living arrangements usually have to be made to fit the new situation. All family members should be involved in planning the distribution of household and work tasks. Good common sense, good judgment, and open communication are an essential part of the holistic ways of home nursing.

THE SICK ROLE

Sickness is a crisis in anyone's life. Once illness is noticeable in the body, it has an effect on the person's self-concept and, as stated previously, also affects the social and family environment of that sick person. People respond to illness in a variety of ways. One person may see himself as being martyred; another might see herself as having a privileged status, and act this out in demanding behavior. The self-concept influences the person's response to any treatment regimen.

Talcott Parsons has characterized the sick role as having rights and duties. The rights are the freedom from blame and from normal roles and task obligations. The duties, which put limits on that freedom, are to do everything possible to recover and, when necessary, to seek technically competent help.

Since our society recognizes this sick role and the facts of illness, and bases its treatment on this role behavior, persons who are ill have been rewarded for conforming to the role, and those who deviate from accepted behavior have been punished. The result has been a tendency to rob the sick person of his or her status as a human being. People have been treated as good or bad patients according to how passive they are in interacting with the medical community. Health institutions and medical practitioners would like to have obedience, dependence, and gratitude. This traditional mixture of charity and discipline is a practiced technique for removing initiative from people, who in this way become less trouble for the caretakers.

In contrast, when the basic ideas of holistic health are used in at-home nursing, the sick person is able to exercise greater initiative and to maintain more of a sense of wholeness and self.

FAMILIES

The family working together can overcome difficulties in caring for one of its members who is sick. Balancing the support needed to promote wellness with the discipline required in any regimen of treatment can be a challenge, for the whole family is affected when one member is ill. A simple illness can affect people by changing their relationships, roles, responsibilities, and functions within the family. Illness can create a substantial amount of stress. The techniques of stress reduction and open communication can be of great use, not only for the sick person but for family members of all ages.

OPEN COMMUNICATIONS

Holistic health has come to accept as its own the idea that open communication between people and especially between loved ones is important in improving and maintaining health. In the pioneer work done by Simonton and Matthews-Simonton, the importance of open communication in the recovery of cancer patients was amply exhibited. Their work on the family support system and those working with cancer patients can be translated into home-style health-care practice.

ACCEPTING FEELINGS

Issues of families and health (especially ill health) always arouse a variety of feelings, and the greater the degree of illness, the more feelings come up. Sometimes the feelings that come to the surface seem inappropriate. Some family members may be able to express such feelings, and others may repress them. If you're doing most of the bedside at-home nursing, it will be a great help to you and the bedfast person to accept the fact that people have feelings and emotions and that not all of them seem "acceptable." There really are no appropriate, inappropriate, mature, or immature feelings about illness. It doesn't help you or anyone else to tell yourself that you should or shouldn't feel such a feeling or think such a thought. Your first step is to accept that you do have these feelings—so does everyone else, from

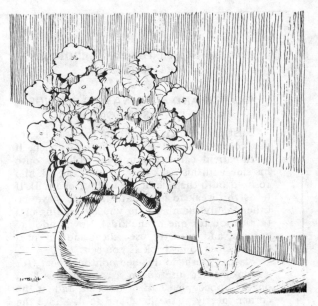

granddad to baby. The next step is to recognize that the whole family needs love, tolerance, and acceptance, and to begin to develop open, supportive communication. Begin with yourself.

Communication that is effective, open, and supportive encourages the expression of feelings, both your own and those of others. It's listening and responding to others while maintaining integrity. It is supporting the person who is ill, and encouraging responsibility and participation without babying or rescuing. It means rewarding health by encouraging the effort of self-care, commenting when the person is looking better. It means spending time as a family or individual with the person who is bedfast, in activities unrelated to the illness. And it means continuing to support and communicate with the person who is ill when he or she gains better health.

HOLISTIC HEALTH TECHNIQUES THAT CAN BE USED IN ACCIDENTAL AND UNSKILLED HOME-STYLE NURSING

Many different techniques of healing can be brought to bear on returning a person to wellness. The value of some of these techniques is immediately apparent, and these can be integrated into the care of the patient. Let us consider some of these.

Holistic nutrition is based on the concept that food is natural medicine if it is fresh, wholesome, and alive. Feeding is always a part of caring for someone who is ill. Holistic nutrition can easily be integrated in natural and normal stages into at-home nursing.

Home-Style Nursing Techniques
Alta Picchi Kelly

A QUICK AND EASY WAY TO CHANGE A BED WITH SOMEONE IN IT

First get your fresh bedding ready (I like to use colored sheets) and within easy reach. If your patient can still grip a bit, roll him onto his side with his back toward you, and ask him to hold onto the side of the bed (or bed rail). If he is too weak to hold onto the side, have another family member help you by holding him (a nice job for one of the kids). Now, undo the corners, and push the used sheet and any padding as close to his back as you can.

Place a fresh double-bed contour sheet (for a twin-size bed; use queen size for double bed) on the unoccupied half of the bed, and fit the corners neatly at the head and foot. Shove the fresh sheet and clean padding up against the ones being removed. Now roll your patient over onto the clean side, and ask him to hold on again. Go to the other side of the bed, and slip off the soiled bedding. Pull the clean sheet and padding across the bed under him, check to see that all bedding is smooth, and tuck corners of sheet at head and foot. Ease your patient back onto a nice, clean bed. Replace top sheet and blankets, and you're all set.

THE BED BATH

There really isn't much to giving a bed bath. All you need is a wash basin, washcloths, mild soap, lotion, bath powder, plenty of towels, and fresh nightwear. To give a bed bath, you simply start at the top and work your way down, washing and rinsing as you go. Be skimpy in applying lotion; use it only on areas like the shins, where the skin looks dry. Too much lotion will make the skin tender and more susceptible to bed sores. It's a good idea to give a bed bath just before you change the sheets, so that you don't have to be careful about soiling the sheets.

TOILET FACILITIES

This is an ever-present problem if your patient is bedridden. If she can use a bedpan, very good; keep the pan clean and near the bed. When it is needed, have her flex her knees; place the bedpan at the side of the bed, with the open end toward the foot. At a signal, with your hand at the small of the back, you lift as she lifts her hips, and with the other hand you slip the bedpan under her. If she is able to sit up, support her back. Have toilet tissue available. Then leave the room to give her some privacy unless she is too ill to remain alone. When she is finished, return, clean her if necessary, and remove the pan promptly. Have hand-cleaning facilities available for her. Take the pan to the bathroom, empty and clean it, and return it to the room for next use. (A human note: *warm* a cold bedpan before placing it under the patient, by heating it with warm water.)

DIVERSIONS

People who are sick need peace and quiet to recover, but they also need to feel that they are part of the family, not isolated and left out. Some people like visitors, and some don't. Some folks like friends and family to visit and share their life with them. Sometimes the best

---

The use of *herbs* as healing agents is known and practiced throughout the world. Herbs are easily available, but careful use is required in the sick room. Herbs, like some pharmaceutical medicines, can have unusual side effects when used together with some medications; so always check with your herbalist or medical practitioner before using any herbs for teas or in other ways.

Breath, a key of life, is used in sick-room care by both the ill person and the at-home nurse to reduce stress and pain, and to promote feelings of calmness and peacefulness.

Massage has always been a part of sick-room care. It has been used to reduce stress, stimulate blood circulation, and prevent bed sores. *Reflexology,* or massage of the feet, increases circulation and assists the body in stimulating sluggish organs and nerve endings. *Shiatsu* can often relieve pain and discomfort of advanced illness. It is the application of a slow, deep finger pressure along the acupuncture meridians. It can be used effectively within the normal process of massage.

Autogenic Training and other forms of autosuggestion, to relax the mind and create a focus on well-

thing about a visit is when the person leaves. Children and animals needn't be kept out of the life of someone who is bedridden or ill. They can bring comfort and diversions to a sick friend or relative.

If your patient is bedridden for any length of time, he may enjoy having pictures of his friend, awards he has won, plaques that honor or amuse him, a favorite poster or print.

Television, radio, tapes, and records help pass away time in bed, as do books, papers, and magazines. Being read to can be a rewarding, shared activity.

Often churches will bring home communion to the sick and bedridden. Some folks enjoy keeping a link to their church.

Eating is fun for some folks, and if his digestion is all right, treats of food during the day can help break up long hours in bed.

Having the bed near a window that has activity outside it provides another source of entertainment.

THE PATIENT IS RECOVERING, BUT THE NURSE IS FALLING APART

Supernurse, there isn't such a person. On days when nothing goes right, when all you do is clean up messes of various kinds, when you feel like hiding in the broom closet, indulge yourself. Martyrdom went out 1,400 years ago. If at all possible, find someone to do bed-sitting for as many hours as you can afford, and take this time for rest and relaxation. Hire someone to come in to do once-a-week housecleaning. If anyone offers to give you a hand, *believe* them; let them help out. Share your burdens. Take care of yourself. Dress better than you ever have. Get out to the hairdresser for a good cut. Keep your weight near normal. Practice stress reduction with yourself and family. Take family outings and enjoy your time away from home. Don't spend a lot of time with activities that make you aware of feeling trapped and unhappy. See yourself as a person with style, insight, a unique person, living well.

ness and healing is new to the practice of health. It has been found successful in helping to reverse some serious diseases and illnesses.

The healing aspects of *meditation* are well-known in Eastern thought. More recently, in the West, we have found that there needs to be a correct posture and type of meditation for specific human conditions, but use of meditation by both the at-home nurse and the ill person and the family can relieve tension and stress.

These are just a few of the techniques and practices that can be used in at-home nursing. Doubtlessly, home nursing and holistic health will merge together and develop a new way to practice health care.

SUGGESTIONS FOR FURTHER READING

Berkeley Holistic Health Center, *Holistic Health Handbook*. And/Or Press, 1978.

Ruth M. French, *The Dynamics of Health Care*. McGraw-Hill, 1968.

Mary Kate House, "Home-Style Nursing," *Journal of the American Medical Association*, vol. 240, no. 22, (Nov. 24, 1978).

Richard Jackson, *Holistic Massage*. Sterling, 1980.

Talcott Parsons, "Definitions of Health and Illness in Light of American Values and Social Structure," in E.G. Jaco, ed., *Patients, Physicians, and Illness*. (Free Press, 1959), pp. 165-187.

Kenneth R. Pelletier, *Mind As Healer, Mind As Slayer*. Delta, 1977.

The Revolutionary Health Committee of Hunan Province, *The Barefoot Doctor's Manual*. Cloudburst Press, 1977.

Martin E. P. Seligman, *Helplessness*. W. H. Freeman, 1975.

O. Carl Simonton, M.D., Stephanie Matthews-Simonton, and James Creighton, *Getting Well Again*. Tarcher, 1978.

Alta Picchi Kelly received the B.A. in Social Welfare from California State University, San Francisco, in 1968, and the M.S.W. from California State University, Sacramento, in 1970. She received the Master of Public Health degree from the University of California, Berkeley, in 1973, with a specialization in Maternal and Child Health. She received the Ph.D. in Psychology from Paideia University, Berkeley, California, in 1979. She is currently a member of the faculty and staff of Paideia University, and is maintaining a private practice as a marriage and family counselor in the San Francisco Bay Area. She is co-editor of the recent book The New Healers: Healing the Whole Person *(And/Or Press, 1980).*

Liberating Aging: An Interview with Maggie Kuhn
Ken Dychtwald, Ph.D.

Maggie Kuhn is one of the great leaders and spokes-persons of our time. At the age of 73, this slight, fragile-looking woman is making a unique contribution to the liberation of aging in America.

Banding together with a small group of like-minded friends, she cofounded the Gray Panthers, which in ten years has become a coalition of more than 10,000 people of all ages who are committed to an activist approach to social change. To date, she has written two books and numerous monographs on various aspects of aging, health care, work, older women, and religion.

Maggie Kuhn is an inspiring example of what a dynamic and positive influence our elders, given proper respect and support, can have on our pursuit of wholeness.

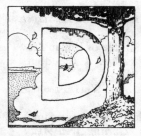

ychtwald: Do you have any special feelings about being an elder at this particular time in history?

Kuhn: This is indeed a New Age—an age of liberation and self-determination. I'm glad to have reached seniority at this time. I feel free to speak out and act in ways that I was not able to when I was younger. I'm 73 years old, and I haven't dyed my hair and I can't afford a face lift. I enjoy my wrinkles and regard them as badges of distinction—I've worked hard for them!

I guess that when I think about it, there are three things in particular that I like about getting old. First, you can speak your mind, as I certainly try to do—but you have to do your homework first; otherwise you'll quickly be dismissed as a doddering old fool. The second thing I have liked about getting old is that I have successfully outlived a great deal of my opposition: many of the people who were my detractors

before are not around anymore! And then the third thing that I've especially liked about getting old is that it's really kind of a miracle to be able to tap into the incredible energy of the young, while making use of the knowledge and experience that comes after living a long, full life. Having the power and energy of these two worlds is an enormously vitalizing and inspiring experience.

I think of age as a great universalizing force. It's the one thing that we all have in common. It doesn't begin when you collect your social security benefits. Aging begins with the moment of birth, and it ends only when life itself has ended. Life is a continuum: only we—in our stupidity and blindness—have chopped it up into little pieces, and kept all those little pieces separate. I feel that the goal of successful aging is to keep on growing and learning and becoming a mature, responsible adult.

Dychtwald: Do you think that most people view aging in this positive fashion?

Kuhn: Sadly, most people don't yet view aging in this way, and too many of my older peers are unhappy with their predicament. We must be proud of our age. We can be proud of our history and our experience. We can be proud of our survivorship and our capacity to cope with change. We're *not* wrinkled babies—although there are lots of people and programs that have purported to serve us, but instead treat us like wrinkled babies, powerless and dependent. Our goal should be responsible adulthood. We're the elders of the tribe, and the elders are charged with the tribe's survival and well-being!

Dychtwald: Many elders seem to feel that they are the victims of stereotyping and negative cultural images of aging. Would you agree?

Kuhn: Yes, absolutely! And in many cases, we elders are just as responsible for creating and sustaining these beliefs. To my mind, there are several myths that are the most debilitating in their effect on elders.

First, there is the myth that stereotypes old age as a disastrous disease which nobody wants to admit having, but which affects us all. Old age is not a disease—it is strength and survivorship, triumph over all kinds of vicissitudes and disappointments, trials and illnesses. In addition, the "diseases of aging" have for too long been confused with the normal developmental processes of aging. Many of my peers suffer from preventable, reversible illnesses simply chalked up to "old age." The medical establishment, with its overemphasis on sickness and disease treatment, has refused to take geriatric medicine seriously; either that, or it does not think that geriatrics is "exciting" enough. For example, with the omission of geriatric medicine and gerontology in most medical schools, young doctors are poorly equipped to diagnose many physiological conditions which can lead to irreversible mental impairment. In this way, aging as a disease becomes a sad, self-fulfilling prophecy. Nearly 50 per cent of the patients now in nursing homes need not be there! Geriatrics is not a fad or a pacifier for us older folks. It is the hope of our future bodies and selves.

Another myth is that old age is mindless: you know, you can't learn anything more after thirty, and then after fifty it's just a question of time before senility sets in.

Dychtwald: Do you feel that this senility is real, or is it just a form of cultural suggestion?

Kuhn: I think that a lot of so-called senility is not irreversible. It is induced by frustration and despair, because old people have no place, really, no status. Also, old people are often so heavily medicated that they seem senile. And other forms of brain disease are due to gross neglect by an insensitive medical profession, which frequently fails to diagnose and treat older people caringly and appropriately.

Old age is not mindless! I recently saw some statistics from a study at Harvard, where a group of men at the age of 71, who had been tested over a period of twelve years, scored at least 15 points higher in the I.Q. average than they did in the beginning. Not a bad sample! Psychological studies have shown that there is no limit to learning.

Another wrong and cruel myth is that old age is sexless—that in one's old age human sexuality withers and declines, and one's interest in being loved and having love fades away. I can tell you that it's not that way. Sex need not wither. In fact, it may take a whole new turn. Indeed, it ought to be flourishing right up to rigor mortis!

Old age can even be a time for a great deal of fresh sexual exploration. A growing number of us old women are involved sexually, in varying degrees of

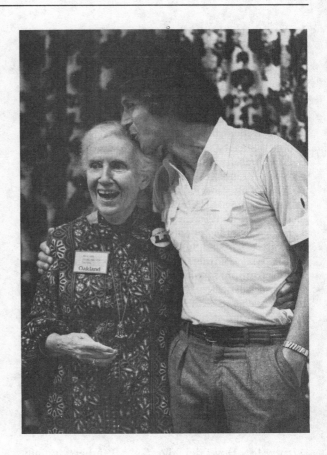

intimacy, with men who are younger than us. What is known about such relationships? Old age can certainly be a time for sexual and sensual pleasure and discovery.

A fourth myth is that old age is useless. This myth comes because our technological society scrap-piles old people as it does automobiles. We elders have all kinds of skills and knowledge, and I submit that if we got our heads together, there wouldn't be a single problem that could not be solved. Mandatory retirement is a perfect example of this type of agism. It results in and perpetuates the image that old people are useless and unproductive and at best only capable of rest and play. It creates artificial barriers between age groups and violates the older workers' right to choose and to exercise control over their work life. It forces many to live on reduced and fixed income. If older people could choose to remain workers in the mainstream of society, then they might realize more fully their ability to control their own lives while usefully influencing the direction of society.

A fifth negative myth that prevails in our culture is that old age is powerless. But if you really look at the demography of the United States and Canada, there is enormous power in our numbers. In the United States, there are about 24 million people over the age of 65, making up about 11 per cent of the population. By the year 2010—or even sooner, according to present trends—the percentage of older people may double. Society's response to these demographic shifts will profoundly affect people of all ages and human conditions.

What some describe as the "plight of the elderly" will not appreciably improve without basic change in society, including an active and intelligent involvement of our older population. Most of my life is now committed to tackling these issues through the work of the Gray Panthers. The Gray Panthers are a national coalition of old, young, and middle-aged activists and advocates working to expose agism's destructive web and to challenge all forms of age discrimination in our society. The Gray Panthers have become an outspoken national movement which emphasizes the relationship between personal growth and self-development to the pursuit of larger goals, such as self-determination and liberation from stereotyping. As a coalition of old and young people working together for change in the larger public interest, we also demonstrate interactional lifestyles and actions which counter agism in all its oppressive forms.

Dychtwald: How did the Gray Panthers initially form?

Kuhn: The Gray Panthers began in 1970 when six of us, friends forced to retire from national religious and social service organizations, decided to pool our efforts and to help one another use our new freedom responsibly. Our initial personal reactions to compulsory retirement were anger, shock, and a sense of loss—loss of friends, status, income, and purpose in living. We had seen the lives of once vigorous colleagues trivialized and wasted in retirement periods. The course of action we determined for ourselves was to use our knowledge and experience, our network of contacts and relationships, and our ample free time to work for broad-based social change.

The Gray Panther movement now includes people of all ages, working in more than seventy active networks across the country. Our social thinking and strategy are openly pluralistic, and there is a great deal of exhilaration and vitality in our diversity. The people who make up the Gray Panthers have committed themselves to the creation of a society in which self-actualization and human values receive the highest priority. With our various networks and task forces, we Gray Panthers have been monitoring social problems and critiquing social policies, with an underlying concern for social justice.

Dychtwald: How do you see the Gray Panthers as being different from the many other so-called senior citizens' programs in existence?

Kuhn: First, let me say that "senior citizens" is a euphemisim which we reject as insulting and demeaning. I prefer to be called by my name, or, if not, I'd like to be identified as an "old person" or an "elder," for this is what I am.

I suppose that at present our movement has three characteristics which distinguish it from other groups of elders. First, in many ways, we are a relatively radical group, since we are an age-integrated action-coalition working for *change*—not just adjustment or accommodation to the exisiting order. Second, we are very much concerned about all forms of injustice and oppression, including unjust treatment of citizens because of their age. And third, we are experimenting with new, flexible structures and with multiple leadership, in the belief that human relationships are more important than bureaucratic hierarchies: our network doesn't depend on a lot of machinery to keep it running.

Dychtwald: In what kinds of activities have the Gray Panthers been involved?

Kuhn: In the past eight years, we have undertaken a wide range of tasks and programs. In the beginning of our coalition, we focused a great deal of energy around nursing-home reform and elderly consumer affairs. We've staged demonstrations at meetings of the American Medical Association and the National Gerontological Society, and I've testified before the House and Senate on aging, health, welfare, media, mandatory retirement, and a variety of other topics. In the last few years, since the Gray Panthers have grown considerably, we've been able to expand our efforts to include task forces to monitor the operation of courts, banks, insurance companies, and municipal agencies, such as planning commissions and zoning boards. Another area that we are examining involves the way older people are depicted on radio and television and in advertising. Through our "Media Watch" we target programs that make older people look useless and helpless. As more people of all ages become sensitive to the problems and possibilities that surround aging, we'll become more able to launch a large-scale effort to improve the conditions for living and aging in America.

As political activists, we believe that if we are truly to liberate ourselves from the oppressive age stereotypes that society imposes upon us—at all ages—we must involve ourselves in social action. And effective strategies for social change invariably require knowledge of the past and present state of the issue, as well as knowledge, in most cases, of power, politics, and economics. Our thesis, then, is that action and mutual education are interlocked, and that knowledge becomes power only when it is informed and informs our action.

Dychtwald: Can you give an example of the way in which the Gray Panthers work to affect social change?

Kuhn: A simple yet clear example occurred recently with respect to public transportation. Everyone knows that the lack of public transportation is a national disgrace and a major cause of the social isolation of many old people. But it often requires pointing out the obvious to make younger people recognize that many elderly citizens are completely dependent on public transport.

In Philadelphia, where I live, and where public transportation is less than adequately available, a coalition of groups of older people took stock of their need for safe, economical transport, and pressed for reduced fares for riders over 65 and for rescheduled bus routes. Hard data about declining ridership and increased fares and costs were secured by research teams, who also studied what other communities were doing with dial-a-ride serivces and free rides in non-rush hours. When the board of the Transportation Authority met, older residents packed the meeting and demanded consideration of their request for reduced fares. Mass media covered the meeting, and spokespeople argued their case with hard facts based on inventories of human needs, dollars and cents, and ridership tables. A carefully reasoned argument won the day!

Older Philadelphians have, in the past year, demonstrated their approval by greatly increasing their use of buses and trolleys. Thus, by example, they helped restore public confidence in a transportation system that had been operating ineffectively, and simultaneously demonstrated their ability to affect and improve public systems for the elderly.

Dychtwald: What is particularly exciting about you and about the Gray Panthers is your willingness not only to examine and speak out on significant social and political issues, but also to explore and experiment with new lifestyles and ways of being. Do you find the role of "lifestyle explorer" a difficult one to assume so late in life?

Kuhn: In many ways, it's always difficult to try new things and take risks, but in our old age we become more free to innovate: we're free to burst out of our wrinkled skins and be creative. Of course, it takes some planning to do this, and a great deal of support and confidence. It also takes examples, but if we allow ourselves to look, we see that history presents us with countless examples of alive and creative older people.

In fact, I take this possibility one step further, since I feel that old people have a particular responsibility in our society to develop, test, and try on for size new roles. As elders, we should see ourselves as being responsive to the needs and questionings of our younger friends and family. When we are kept apart from those who will live on after us, we deprive ourselves, and we also deprive the young; our society is correspondingly weaker because we have not lived together. Without interacting as we were intended to do, young and old rarely communicate, share experiences, or give each other mutual support. There is so much that we all could be doing with and for each other! There is absolutely no excuse for any of us to give up and retreat into our own private worlds because of our age.

Dychtwald: I suppose that in many ways you are the best example of your philosophy and attitudes regrading the potentials inherent in the aging process. Here you are, at the age of 73, a national celebrity who has been instrumental in affecting a great deal of social and political change. When you were young, did you envision that this would be in store for you in later years?

Kuhn: To tell you the truth, I really can't believe that it's all happening. All of my life I was primarily involved in groups and group activities, and so never was one for celebrity or personal acclaim. It's all so exciting! Often it's quite frightening, too: now that I am in this position, more than ever I need support, friendship, love, criticism, and assistance. My life has become so challenging that I feel more alive now than I ever did. It's just terrific!

I feel particularly inspired by the realization that aging is a transitional phase, rather than a phasing out. Instead of retiring from life, I am pleased and excited to be able to recycle and redirect my goals. I continue to realize that old age is a time of great fulfillment—personal fulfillment—when all the loose ends of life can be gathered together.

For further information about the Gray Panthers, write: Gray Panthers, 3700 Chestnut St., Philadelphia, PA 19104.

SUGGESTIONS FOR FURTHER READING

Simone de Beauvoir, *The Coming of Age.* Warner, 1973.

Robert Butler, *Why Survive? Being Old in America.* Harper and Row, 1975.

Alex Comfort, *A Good Age.* Crown, 1976.

Maggie Kuhn, *Maggie Kuhn on Aging.* Westminster Press, 1977.

Gay Luce, *Your Second Life.* Seymour Lawrence/ Delacorte, 1979.

For biographical information on Dr. Dychtwald, see his Bodymind *article in Section II.*

SAGE
Adelaide Kendall

SAGE is a Bay Area community organization ad-dressing itself to the special needs and talents of those over 60 years of age. Our culture has not been kind to its retired citizens. Instead of being appreciated for their experience and wisdom, they have been cut off from family life and looked on as an unwanted burden.

SAGE is reversing this trend by creating commun-ity programs, where self-responsibility, intimacy, and positive imaging are valued and practiced, and which are tailor-made to suit the energy of the over-60 population. Relaxation, exercise, massage, breathing, and autogenics provide structures of growth with which to lessen the grip of social alienation and the fear of death.

Training is offered for people working in core groups at the SAGE center, or for those who work in institutional situations. An emphasis on caring and sharing is communicated to all community workers and creates an enthusiasm which is contagiously healthy. SAGE is a model program which will un-doubtedly be an inspiration for senior citizens to evaluate their own centers of re-creation throughout this country and the world.

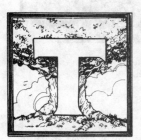

he words for which "SAGE" stands—Senior Actualization and Growth Explorations—are the cornerstones of its philo-sophy. Contrary to the atti-tude that growing old means marking time on the fringes of existence, SAGE's view is that the later years of life can be a period of discover-ing ways to self-fulfillment and of exerting control over one's life.

The foundation of this process is the establishment of human bonds. Society tends to cut adrift its older members, who, just as when they were younger, have needs of belonging and well-being. But meeting these needs becomes difficult because of changes in income and standard of living, physical decline, and the feel-ing of being considered worth less.

SAGE has programs for relatively healthy people over sixty who can travel to its premises, as well as for people who are less independent or who live in institutions. The participants learn basic skills and techniques geared to the individual that are practiced within groups as well as alone. Self-approval replaces group competition, and the pleasure generated by individual gains sparks the formation of an enthu-siastic, caring group.

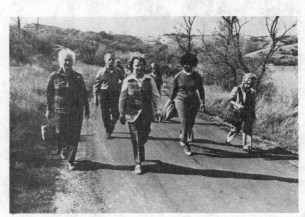

The SAGE spirit is not a mystery revealed to a select few—it is an outlook fostered by a belief that people can grow at all ages.

Without denying the physical problems of aging, the SAGE approach suggests that some of these prob-lems may be diminished by appropriate planning of activities that coordinate mind and body. The meth-ods below are described as they are used with relative-ly healthy, independent participants in "core" groups. However, the staff has adapted these methods for the program in institutional settings.

RELAXATION

The SAGE process begins with relaxation, a state that eludes many because they do not know how to reach it. Tension caused by fear and worry accompanies growing older, and sometimes tension patterns from earlier years persist. Also, long periods of lack of exercise result in reduced oxygen intake. Relaxation helps relieve tension and makes oxygen available.

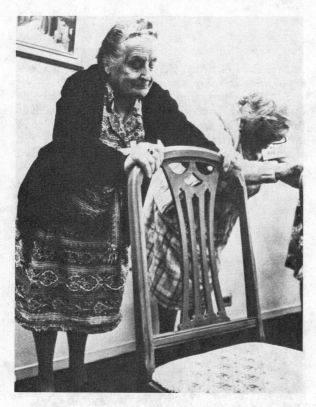

Various exercises promote easier motions in sitting, getting up, and walking.

ROLL BREATHING

Roll breathing is a beginning step toward relaxation. The term originates from the wavelike motion created when the breather, lying on his or her back, inhales so that the diaphragm first expands fully. The chest fills with air, and as the air is exhaled, a forceful audible sound is encouraged. Thus, the breather absorbs a maximum amount of oxygen; relaxes the muscles of the chest, diaphragm, and lower abdomen; and increases the blood flow.

This is a safe and effective means of correcting habits that result from shallow breathing. Gradual increases in oxygen intake appear to be beneficial to older people, and some report breathing exercises to be more refreshing than a nap.

PROGRESSIVE RELAXATION

This procedure involves alternately tensing and relaxing all the body muscle groups. In doing so, one learns to distinguish tension from other body sensations and to lessen muscle tension consciously when it arises.

AUTOGENIC TRAINING

Developed in Europe and adapted by Dr. Wolfgang Luthe, this method consists of phrases that the learner repeats to himself or herself in such a way that the mind and body relax. Relaxation eases tension that often contributes to high blood pressure and insomnia.

MASSAGE

Massage is used to revitalize the body, soothe muscular tensions, restore body tone, and build a supportive emotional atmosphere. Participants begin by massaging their own facial muscles and neck. Later they massage each other's hands and feet.

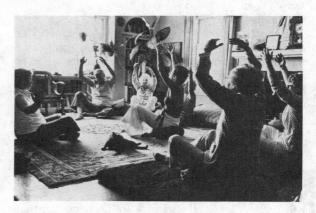

Several exercises coordinate breathing and movement to improve respiration and circulation.

PHYSICAL EXERCISE

Various kinds of exercise promote easier motions in sitting, getting up, and walking. Several exercises coordinate breathing and body movement to improve respiration and circulation. Emphasis is not on mastering techniques or straining, but on moving at a personal pace without stress. The criterion is what one's own body feels. It is important to pay attention to the fact that most participants have had little exercise and thus are unready for a vigorous program.

Slow, graceful limbering of seldom-used muscles increases body tone and improves balance.

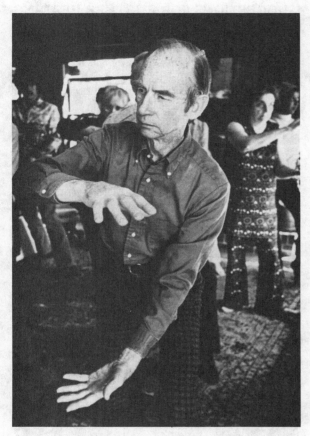

The slow, graceful movements of T'ai Chi help to limber muscles and increase balance.

SENSORY AWARENESS

Deep relaxation is the stepping-stone for sensory awareness and guided imagery. Several methods are used by leaders to help the participants visualize in the mind's eye experiences and images that are unique. From this process comes a greater understanding of oneself and an awareness of the control that individuals have over their physical and mental well-being.

This is only a brief summary of a few selected activities. Music and art enrich the program, and new ideas are tried to maintain the excitement of discovery. A significant aspect of the program is the opportunity for discussion. At first hesitant to talk about their hopes, fears, failures, and successes, the groups gradually emerge from their reserve. They disclose their deepest concerns. And within the intimate SAGE atmosphere, they can even discuss death and dying. Slowly barriers disappear and the sense of community strengthens.

In fact, the "sense" of community has transformed into a "SAGE Community," set up by core graduates of four groups. It evolved from a desire to continue the caring, learning, and sharing they experienced in "official" groups. It is significant that this community was formed and is sustained by its members, independent of staff. Currently they meet once a week on the SAGE premises.

One of the principal differences between the core program and the institutional program is that the process within the institutions is less easily defined. Many people in institutions are over the age of eighty. Often they have been lonely longer, have felt less stimulation, have been less mobile, and are more likely to suspect that death is close at hand than most of the core-group members. Because of indifference

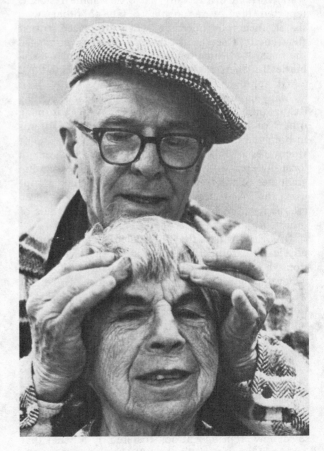

Massage helps to soothe tension and build a supportive emotional atmosphere.

or neglect, these residents succumb to feeling helpless. Coaxing them to use their minds and their muscles requires a special approach. The program is brought to the institutions, and many members have to be awakened to its possibilities. Even so, there are some residents who cannot participate at all.

The program has had a profound effect in the four institutions that SAGE serves in the Bay Area. So strong has been the sense of isolation among residents that they often did not know each other's names. With the SAGE staff they began to be more aware of life around themselves and of submerged feelings waiting to be tapped. Warmed by patient encouragement of the SAGE staff, residents have talked in ways almost forgotten. As a result, they speak of greater intimacy and increasing communication among themselves.

The program has caused a second look at the environment and at opportunities that the personnel who work in institutions can offer. Some residents reported they were unable to talk to others who shared their rooms because beds were placed so that they couldn't see each other. Employees rearranged the beds. And some employees, seeing happier possibilities for their charges, are willing to try a modified SAGE approach on their own.

Many inquiries come to SAGE for help in modeling its program. SAGE has several ways of informing others of its work. These include training of interns in both the institutional and core programs, rental of videotapes of SAGE in action, workshops, classes in local colleges, and nationwide presentations. Several graduates of the training programs are leading groups using the SAGE process. And a few graduates of core groups have become leaders and assistant leaders of other core groups.

SAGE recognizes the importance of an appropriate physical environment, not only for those in institutions, but for those still living independently. SAGE is developing plans for a center for older people that will accommodate their special needs in terms of location, transportation, mobility, safety, ventilation, temperature, dexterity, lighting, acoustics, and functions. Included are nursing and medical facilities. The hope is that the plans will get to the drawing boards, and that money will be found for construction. The belief is that such a center will be not merely a good physical plant but also an environment that engenders deep friendships.

The SAGE spirit is not a mystery revealed to a select few. It is an outlook fostered by a belief that people can grow at all ages. With exposure the spirit can be contagious. Isn't it time to risk catching this spirit?

SUGGESTIONS FOR FURTHER READING

H. A. De Vries, *Vigor Regained.* Prentice-Hall, 1974.

K. Dychtwald, *Bodymind.* Pantheon, 1977.

M. Feldenkrais, *Awareness Through Movement.* Harper and Row, 1972.

B. Geba, *Breathe Away Your Tension.* Random House/Bookworks, 1972.

_____, *Vitality Training for Older Adults.* Random House/Bookworks, 1972.

E. Kübler-Ross, *On Death and Dying.* Macmillan, 1969.

H. Selye, *Stress Without Distress.* Lippincott, 1976.

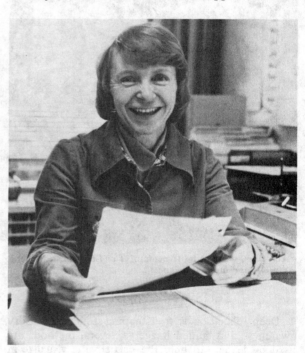

Adelaide Kendall's Bachelor's and Master's degrees in the fields of psychology and education led her to explore the fascinating world of the very young. As a result she helped develop and worked in experimental programs for "normal," emotionally disturbed, educationally handicapped, and mildly and severely retarded children. The relationship between physical health and emotional health in all age groups has always intrigued her. Now, as a SAGE staff member, she is especially aware of needs and hopes in the later stages of life.

On Embracing Death and Disease
Glenna Gerard

Disease can act as the catalyst for profound changes in our consciousness. Ms. Gerard shares with us her view of disease as a learning experience. In the light of her father's disease process, she has come to realize that disease is a powerful force in our evolution, frequently catapulting us into expansions and transformations of ourselves and our worlds.

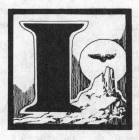 once suffered a crush fracture of a major bone in my foot. The orthopedic surgeon who attended my foot viewed the fracture as a "disease" to be treated in a specific manner. I, however, experienced the fracture not as a disease, but as a reality which had come into my life to teach me about an aspect of myself which was not in balance and needed attention. For me the entire experience was health-giving. Obviously, whether the fracture was a health-process or a disease-process was a question relative to the doctor's individual perspective and mine, which were quite different. Of course, when confronted with the doctor's model, I could have changed my belief structure and considered myself "diseased." Yet that would still have been my own choice: ultimately it is always I, and not someone else, who am personally responsible for the definition of myself as healthy or diseased.

Each of us possesses the power to define our own health, because no matter what the circumstances, we may always choose the manner in which we relate to them. This power of choice resides in every person, at every moment of his/her life.

When an aspect of my life—be it physical, emotional, mental, or spiritual—engenders discomfort, and *I choose* to assume the position of helpless victim, I automatically cast myself into unhappiness. Joy goes out of my life, and is replaced by discomfort, resentment, anger. These states of feeling are reactions to the disease process, reactions consistent with the perspective I have chosen. But consider: what law obliged me to choose that particular vision? None, of course. At every point in the process, I have the option of changing my perspective, At any time I can decide to enter a relationship with the disease which integrates it into my life, without anger and without resentment.

I have made this choice, for the integration, not the rejection, of disease. This decision has transformed my vision of myself and of those around me. I now understand that disease is one of the most powerful forces for change in the individual. The attempt to integrate the disease process demands that one seek to understand and appreciate its function within the totality of one's life. To fulfill this demand one must first achieve a high degree of detachment; one must disidentify from the disease process. Without making this move, one is virtually helpless against a myriad of negative feelings about oneself when seeking to answer the question: "Why is this disease present?" It is only too easy to see the disease as a negative judgment on oneself, and when one is prey to such feelings, it is impossible to see the situation clearly. Only upon abandoning all judgment and becoming an "objective witness," relative to one's life and to the disease process, can one attain clarity and understanding, infused with compassion.

It is this shift into the "witness" state of consciousness that provides the first powerful experience of transformation: you begin to see your entire life in a new light. You find that you need no longer be involved in the pain and suffering which resulted from labeling certain aspects of your life as negative, and from identifying yourself with these aspects. You become able to view your life with a detachment which allows you to appreciate the contributions of all its elements to its totality.

Since disease may motivate such a radical shift in consciousness, and the consequent transformations in one's life, it must be considered a powerful force for change.

TERMINAL DISEASES

Terminal diseases, i.e., those which normally lead to death, are likely to demand an even more far-reaching transformation: one in which the individual is required literally to die to his old way of life, and to be reborn into a new, more expanded, vision of reality. In fact, this transformation is often precisely the purpose of a terminal disease process: the purpose is a death. Whether the disease leads to death in a symbolic sense—the death of old patterns in one's life and the opening of one's vision onto new horizons—or to physiological death, *the process is intrinsically the same.*

We have begun to hear about individuals whose terminal diseases, such as cancer, have motivated a transformation which, in relation to their previous way of life, is essentially equivalent to death. Sometimes the transformation is actually followed by the resolution of the disease. In other words, the purpose for which the disease entered the patient's life has been fulfilled: he has released whatever aspect of his life gave the disease meaning and, with that, it has dissolved.

In other cases, terminal disease may present itself to take a person through his physiological death in a particular way. Here the transformational process centers on resolving the fear of death. The individual is asked to see death not as *the end,* but as one more transforming experience. Anyone who can meet his death with an awareness, and an appreciation, of the learning that it holds for him is indeed a transformed human being, compared to the individual for whom death is a fearful occurrence to be avoided at all costs.

Further, these transformations into which a person may be catapulted by illness are not limited to the individual in whom the process manifests physiologically, but extend beyond him to encompass all those who are involved with him. The changes in these others are often as great in magnitude as those in the sufferer himself. This truth has become very real for me during the past three years as I have watched my own evolution through the experience of my father's disease.

A PERSONAL EVOLUTION

In 1974 my father was diagnosed as having a form of cancer known as Hodgkin's Desease, which originates in the lymph glands and then extends itself to other areas of the body. I remember my mute shock when I learned of the diagnosis, then my frantic attempts to convince my father that he should undergo treatment. Hodgkin's is one form of cancer in which conventional medical treatment has been quite successful in extending the life of the individual, and I wanted my father to live as long as possible. My father, on the other end of the telephone line, was telling me that he did not wish to face the disease in this manner, and was confident that the only thing to do was to rest into his faith in Christ's love. (My father is a minister and a very religious man.) I found myself using every subtle trick I had ever learned to sway his decision. In the middle of my argument, a little voice within me suddenly said, "What is it you are really concerned about? Is it what will happen to him if he must face his death, or is it what might happen to *you* if *you* must face his death?"

As the realization that I was really afraid for myself began to crystallize, doors creaked open which I had closed many years before, and the closeted contents poured forth. Questions stampeded into my consciousness, demanding answers. "Why are you afraid of your father's death? Why do you feel that it is your responsbility to save him? Why do you need to play a part in his decision about which path he will take? Why does the fact that he is going to come up and spend four days with you terrify you to the point of suggesting that your brother come along?"

As I rummaged through my consciousness, trying to bring some clarity to this tumult that had ripped my view of our relationship up by the roots, I began to get glimpses of how that relationship had been formed, and of the multitude of patterns in my own life that had been constructed on the very same foundation.

It was not until my father's cancer had permeated my own reality that I began to examine deeply such things as: the way that fear lurked in the corners of my intimate relationships with men, and molded my actions; my propensity for constructing impersonal relationships in order to avoid accepting people on an intimate level; my need to be in control, not only of my own emotions, but of other people's as well; my beliefs about the strength of aggressive actions and the weakness inherent in a receptive position; and last, but certainly not least, my fear of my own death.

Immediately I realized how incomplete it was to think of the disease process as my father's alone, for its effect on me was shatteringly profound; I understood that it was mine as well. In fact, I am beginning to see that for one person to resolve a disease process, all persons in any way affected by the disease must resolve the issue for themselves as well. Only when they have done so can they provide a clear and loving environment which supports the "diseased" person and facilitates the work he/she has to do.

We are all interlocking spheres of energy, emotion, and thought, parts that make up a whole greater than our sum, and the harmony within each of us is essential to that of the whole.[1]

Dealing with the issues brought to the surface by the penetration of my father's disease process into my being—attempting to find my own vision of myself among the crosshatchings of the reactive patterns involved—has been, and continues to be, a major work in my life. It is not easy work for me, nor has it been easy for my father. His disease has been a most difficult gift to learn to accept and truly to appreciate. There has been much pain, but it is the cleansing sort of pain that accompanies the clearing of a garden, overrun with weeds, in preparation for the birth of a new crop. As the process continues to evolve, I find more and more of myself; my strength and my trust in an all-encompassing order, filled with compassion and joy, which reaches beyond the boundaries of my perception, continues to grow.

With deep personal conviction I can now state that disease may frequently catapult us into an expansion and transformation of our view of ourselves and of the world, and may thus become a powerful force in our evolution. I further believe that insofar as we can appreciate and use the learning opportunities that disease presents to us, to that same degree we can integrate our multidimensional reality into a growing whole, which reflects the joy inherent in living.

I now know that the way in which a disease process affects me depends entirely upon the relationship I have established to what is going on in my being. If I have an appreciative, loving relationship with all aspects of myself, if I have integrated them into a whole within which I am joyful, and if I radiate that joy, then I am healthy in the face of any disease. If I have accepted the disease process as part of my reality, and am able to appreciate the nature of what is going on within my body—and what it signifies in

the evolution of my life—then I am healthy. I am healthy because I am whole, because I have not attempted to cut off any part of me, to reject a portion of my reality. Rather I have tried to integrate all the aspects of which I am conscious into a whole which is in harmony and which reflects the joy inherent in all of life, including death.

For me, the words *whole* and *healthy* are synonymous, and the words *holistic health* are an obvious combination. I cannot imagine health which is not holistic, health which does not involve the whole, for health is the harmony of the whole, and disease is a statement of its fragmentation and disharmony.

It is not the technique that a practitioner uses—whether acupuncture, herbology, or chemotherapy—that enables him to foster health in any given individual. The deciding element is the nature of the interaction between "patient" and "healer." Does the healer embody and communicate a state of consciousness which comprehends the totality of the person he is dealing with? Is the patient ready to receive and appreciate an expanded vision of himself relative to the disease process? The answers to these two questions will determine the degree to which health is fostered in *any* interaction.

Such is my vision of health and disease. I have chosen it because it brings light into corners of my life which were previously dark, because it fosters the expansion of my consciousness to encompass new dimensions of my being, and because within it I perceive the key to a worldview in which all of life, in its myriad forms, is appreciated and celebrated. Each one of us is a multitude, seeking, through a process of evolution, to become one. Disease is only one dimension through which we are propelled toward the health and harmony of unity.

Glenna Gerard is deeply involved in the exploration of transformational states of consciousness, in particular those that can be reached by maintaining a focus of unconditional love and acceptance of one's own beingness. She works with other people, both individually by means of bodywork and collectively by using group energy to heighten and accelerate the exploration. Glenna has also worked as a technical specialist in the field of medical diagnostics and as a writer of biomedical educational material.

---

[1] This last thought takes us into the realm where disease is perceived as a force for change in the evolution of man as a collective being.

Section V:
Society/Environment
Work and Education, Community,
Social and Planetary Consciousness

"In numberless animal societies, the struggle between separate individuals for the means of existence disappears; struggle is replaced by cooperation."

Charles Darwin

"I will show . . . that Nature has set no limit to the perfecting of the human faculties, that the perfectability of man, henceforth independent of any power that might wish to arrest it, has no other limit than the duration of the globe on which Nature has placed us."

Benjamin Franklin

"Our highest endeavor must be to develop free human beings who are able of themselves to impart purpose and direction to their lives."

Rudolph Steiner

"Let us put out minds together and see what kind of life we can make for our children."

Sitting Bull

"Economic growth is like any other kind; it can be good or bad. Is physical growth a good thing? Yes, of course. When my children grow, I am very pleased. But if I should suddenly start to grow again, it would be a disaster. So I'm not saying that economic growth is always bad. What I'm saying is that we must stop pretending that such growth is always good."

E.F. Schumacher

"What man is there over whose mind a bright spring morning does not exercise a magic influence?"

Charles Dickens

Introduction
SOCIETY/ENVIRONMENT: Community, Career, Social and Planetary Consciousness

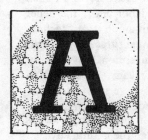generation ago Teilhard de Chardin cited forces at work in the world that would eventually draw mankind into an awareness "that they are inseparably joined elements of a converging Whole." More and more we are perceiving that society, as a collection of individuals, is largely a reflection of their health. The cumulative impact of the society (social networks, economics, political climate, cultural values, etc.) also influences personal health. A link exists between the society and the individual, a continual feedback loop, simultaneously affecting the health of each. The environment, another major determinant of health (providing the food we eat, the air we breathe, the energy we consume, etc.) is also directly affected by individual and societal priorities. Simply put, there are three great tiers of life intimately bound one to another. Health results from the balanced activity of all three. Therefore, to effect wholeness, we must act responsibly as a member of each.

Clearly we have reached an impasse in the life of our society. New revelations from the fields of science and human potential have had a tremendous impact on our lives. And for better or worse, the relative calm of days gone by has given way to the exigencies of the present and the future. Our lifestyle has changed so much in the last few decades that our so-called advanced technology is strained to keep pace, and the social institutions initially designed to insure our welfare now often stand as impediments to it. We are a restless people, attempting to preserve some of the old, and incorporate the meaningful new, while resisting the temptation to succumb entirely to the automaton existence of freeways and fast-food counters.

The dizziness of life has for too long set us adrift on imponderable seas. Our fundamental sense of "fitting in" is all but an abstraction, and the small comforts of home and family, those things that nourish us most, teeter on the edge of extinction. In short, we find ourselves dislodged from community and the social structures that so profoundly influence our lives. When you add this to our increasing estrangement from nature, our very survival comes into serious question.

Dire as this picture may seem it is not without hope. It is the unseen nature of crisis to exert an opposite force toward resolution. In that resolution lies the seeds for new growth. Gathering stormclouds inevitably produce rain, and after the rain the sky regains its clarity. The storm may have caused great damage or only minor discomfort. So too, we have a choice either to add to the mounting chaos, or in our own small way to relieve some of the pressure by taking a different route from the majority. Many pursuits helpful in achieving this alternative course are offered in this section.

We have not attempted to cover all areas pertinent to society or the environment. Rather, we have chosen from what we consider to be salient areas. The articles here are meant to illustrate certain progressive schools of thought, but do not constitute a complete blueprint for the future.

We begin this section with an overview of where we have been and the course we may take, as a society, in the future. Professor Harman's article sets the tone for the rest of the section. From this starting point, we jump to education, one of the basic obligations of a society, and also one of the most important factors in shaping the attitudes of its members. After education comes pursuit of a career. Here we apply some of the lessons of the consciousness movement in creating a livelihood which is both rewarding and a constructive contribution to society.

Any discussion of a society would not be complete without a look at its economic values. It seems easy to single out culprits responsible for our current col-

271

lective plight, but excessive consumption does seem to figure prominently in the rise of these troubled times. The production ethic permeates our national character and its ruling motto, "Bigger is Better," threatens to implode upon our environment, economy, and individual sense of well-being. To the extent that we have each placed excessive material gain above the common good, we have contributed to the power and malevolence of this force. The following, related articles discuss the skills necessary to interact in a group when interpersonal and business considerations take on equal values, and the concept of "right livelihood."

We turn next to the arena of politics, but not in its usual sense. Here we speak to the politics of personhood. The power hidden within our own unique beauty can change society and even the planet. It is this individual discovery that leads inevitably back to the healing of our environment.

Our look at societal transformation is completed by a revolutionary examination of the meaning of communities. We are, beyond a shadow of a doubt, social creatures, and yet the reasons that bring us together may in fact only increase our separation. This article brings a new vision of wholeness to our ancient urge to live and work together.

We turn our attention next to the health of the environment, beginning with the very personal environment of the home. Here is an example of how an energy-efficient, integral home can operate. From the province of the home we move to the creation of the urban environment. Most of us live in cities, and life amidst the noise and pollution often seems a mixed blessing. In fact, many people labor under the belief that cities must suffer a certain amount of "technological malaise" in order to qualify as a city. This article dispells those misconceptions by clearly illustrating that we have the means (right now) to design urban centers which preserve the benefits of city life within an ecologically sound environment.

One of the chief liabilities of modern-day cities is their nearly total segregation from the natural environment. For this reason we have included some material which deals specifically with recontacting the healing quality of nature.

In the midst of our presentation on healthy environment we must call attention to what is potentially the most glaring threat to the accomplishment of this goal; namely, nuclear fission. If we are to heal ourselves and the earth, our energy demands must be brought into balance with the fragile ecologic needs of our internal and external environment. This, too, is holistic health.

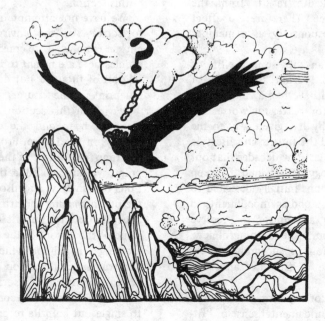

Society/Environment Survey
How well does each statement describe your patterns
of thought and action?

1. My work brings me a sense of satisfaction and a feeling of accomplishment.
2. I feel better away from work than while there.
3. I can create a fulfilling occupation for myself.
4. I feel economically exploited.
5. Money is vulgar.
6. I have to justify my expenditures.
7. My work takes priorities over my relationships.
8. I see a positive side to the obvious confusion and upheaval in our society.
9. I am politically apathetic.
10. I feel a sense of nurturing and belonging in my community.
11. My child's school is supportive of his or her individual needs and talents.
12. I would like to see businesses and communities decentralized and scaled down to meet personal needs.
13. I consider cutting down my energy consumption a hardship.
14. I consider myself ecologically active.
15. I am concerned about the impact of high technology on the environment.
16. I am excited about the possibilities of natural alternative energy sources.
17. I am not aware of any pollution in my immediate environment.
18. I feel dependent upon my automobile.
19. I feel my personal health is affected by the health of the planet.
20. I feel a real kinship with nature.

Prospects for the Future:
Metamorphosis Through Metanoia
Willis W. Harman, Ph.D.

In this lucid presentation, Professor Willis Harman outlines some of the basic factors and assumptions responsible for the long-term modernization of society. By examining paradoxes within these assumptions, recent countertrends, and emerging paradigms, he comes to the conclusion that a massive restructuring of society is not only imminent, but may already be underway.

Although Professor Harman is acutely aware of the growth pains accompanying this "trend shift," his words inspire hope for a benevolent future.

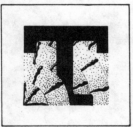

he task of interpreting the present and anticipating the future is aided if some appropriate interpretive concept can be found. Seeking this is somewhat analogous to identifying the Industrial Revolution at the time Watt invented the steam engine.

Understanding that both surface events and deeper institutional change are shaped by much more slowly varying long-term trends, we are led to examine characteristics of the long-term modernization trend that started eight or ten centuries ago in Western Europe and eventually affected all the world. This trend began with the secularization of values at the end of the Middle Ages, and played itself out through the development of modern science, capitalism, the Industrial Revolution, democracy wedded to material progress, the modern technological explosion based on applied science, and incorporation of an ever-increasing fraction of human activity in the mainstream economy.

In the last two decades we have become increasingly aware of the problems of success—of the dilemmas

of highly industrialized society. These dilemmas appear to be intrinsic to advanced stages of industrialization and modernization, and thus to basic characteristics of the trend itself. They have led to growing resistance to all aspects of the long-term modernization trend and an emerging vision of a different future. This resistance is manifested in a host of social movements, intentional communities, and voluntary associations which may be likened to the "imaginal cells" in the pupal stage of metamorphosis. These cells proliferate (whilst other larval tissue is degenerating) and prefigure the adult insect which will eventually emerge. Similarly, the social movements and experiments may expand to bring about a "transindustrial" society, whose defining characteristics can already be discerned.

Most basic of these defining characteristics is the dominant vision of reality. Societal metamorphosis is predicated on a still more fundamental change, namely, transformation of the basic premises upon which modern industrial society ultimately rests. This belief-system transformation is appropriately denoted by the Greek word for religious conversion, *metanoia*, a "fundamental change of mind." Metanoia starts with individuals and small groups, but ultimately expands to become the transformation of the belief systems of whole cultures.

An interpretive framework such as this one is not *true* or *false;* rather, it is useful or not useful. It can be tested by seeing whether further events, through the next year or two, substantiate its fitness and its usefulness. It suggests that the important political dimension of the future is not Left versus Right, but continued modernization and material growth, contrasted with movement toward a "New Age" society with a radically different social paradigm. The framework further implies that the most critical issue before us is how well we handle the transition period.

NOTES ON THE EMERGING WORLD VIEW

The French historian F. Braudel, in his introduction to *The Mediterranean and the Mediterranean World in the Age of Philip II,* explains why he found

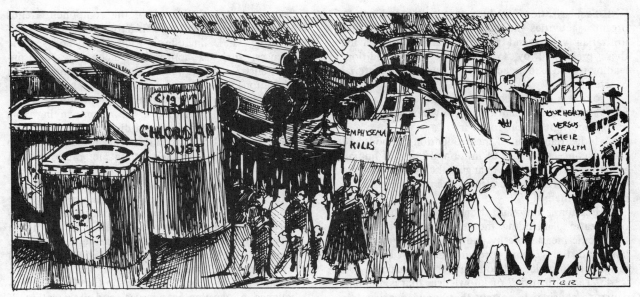

In the last two decades we have become increasingly aware of the problems of success—of the dilemmas of highly-industrialized society. These dilemmas appear to be intrinsic to advanced stages of industrialization and have led to growing resistance to all aspects of the long-term modernization trend and an emerging vision of a different future.

it necessary to write three separate histories of this place and time. One is a history of events—accessions to power, revolutions, treaties, laws, wars. As he says, "We must learn to distrust this history," because of the deceptive apparent relationships between actions and events. In this common form of history, actions appear to cause events, rather than both being manifestations of a deeper flow. Thus Braudel writes a second history, of institutions and institutional change. But this too fails to deal with all the forces present; so a third history is needed, of those enduring factors and patterns—climate, demography, basic cultural characteristics—which change only very slowly during the centuries, but which nonetheless shape the more rapidly varying changes.

At this deep level of the societal structure, every society forms around some basic paradigm, some tacitly assumed set of fundamental beliefs about man, society, the universe, and the source of authority. Very rarely in history has this basic world view gone through rapid and fundamental change. Lewis Mumford, in his *Transformations of Man*, estimates less than half a dozen such transformations in the entire history of Western civilization, the last one being the ending of the Middle Ages. He reminds us how dramatic was the value shift involved: "All but one of the seven deadly sins, sloth, was transformed into a positive virtue. Greed, avarice, envy, gluttony, luxury, and pride were the driving forces of the new economy." In the realm of beliefs, the shift from the medieval perception of a cosmos alive in every portion to the post-seventeenth-century scientific view, of regular phenomena in a "dead" universe devoid of mental or spiritual properties, was equally dramatic. All institutions in society were intimately involved in these changes, both being shaped by the evolving world view and also helping to shape it.

We have seen, particularly in the last two decades, evidences that the long-term trends of modernization, including evolution of both world view and institutions, may be turning in a new direction. There is some reason to think that this could happen with what in historical terms is extraordinary rapidity, and that we may be living through a period of great wrenching, during which it will be particularly important to understand what is going on, and to develop the ability to ride with the transformational currents.

THE LONG-TERM MULTIFOLD MODERNIZATION TREND

The centuries-old multifold modernization trend which started in Western Europe some eight or ten centuries ago has since spread to affect practically all the peoples of the globe. It involves a number of component trends, of which the most fundamental started with a shift in basic cultural beliefs and values:

1. Secularization of values, that is, the tendency to organize activities rationally around impersonal and utilitarian values and patterns, rather than having these prescribed by social and religious tradition; leading to and associated with the concept of material progress.

From this root belief-system change stem a number of other component trends, of which some of the most important are the following.

2. Industrialization of the production of goods and services, and eventually of more and more of human activities, in the process changing the quality of those goods and services, and also of the work involved in producing them.

3. Economic rationalization of social behavior and organization, including the tendency for all things to become measurable by and purchaseable with dollars, and the growing predominance of economic rationality in social and political decision making.

4. "Technification" of knowledge, that is, the tendency to consider important that knowledge which is useful in generating manipulative technology, and to downplay claims that there can be an important body of knowledge about wholesome human values and goals, personal growth and development, and spiritual aspirations.

5. Increasing per capita impact on the physical environment and per capita use of resources.

6. Increasing centralization, bigness.

7. Specialization, impersonalization of roles.

This fundamental multicomponent trend is inherent in the institutions of modern industrialized society; its perserverance is implicitly assumed in most projections of the future. Yet there is impressive evidence that a trend-change is not only possible but may be well underway. This evidence of the plausibility of incipient transformation is of four kinds:

1. *Social movements* which amount, in the aggregate, to a broad countertrend force, and which include a vision of a different future than the modernization trend would lead toward.

2. *Basic contradictions* in modern society which create pressure for restructuring.

3. *Historic indicators* of approaching revolutionary change being presently visible.

4. *Basic premises* underlying the form of modern society showing signs of undergoing fundamental change.

SOCIAL MOVEMENTS

Since the early 1960s numerous social movements have become visible which can be interpreted as pro-

tests against one or more of the component trends identified above, and as affirmations of a "New Age" society. These include a wide variety of specific focuses, such as appropriate technology, environmentalist, conservationist, holistic health, person liberation, feminist, technology assessment, voluntary simplicity, human potential, "new transcendentalism," and numerous others. The accompanying table shows how these various and diverse movements can be interpreted as a countertrend force tending to deflect society from continuing along the path of further "modernization."

We are speaking here about industrialized societies, but a counterpart to the countertrend movement is to be found in the Third World in the form of a "liberatory development" movement offering an alternative to economic development in the sense of striving to become like Western (or Communist) industrialized societies. "Liberatory" development would place the emphasis on human liberation and well-being, self-reliance of developing peoples, and preservation of cultural values, rather than on strictly economic goals and mindless adoption of Western technology.

BASIC CONTRADICTIONS

Behind these social movements are some very real contradictions faced by modern industrialized societies. As examples, consider the following five assumptions that tend to be taken for granted, but lead to questionable conclusions.

1. Fulfillment comes from the consumption of scarce resources. This assumption is woven through the structure of materialistic modern society; it underlies the standard economic indicators, the concept of economic growth, the idea of planned obsolescence. The dominant institution in modern society is the economy, and the performance of the economy is judged on the consumption of goods and services, all of which use up scarce resources and exude polluting waste. Hedonistic consumption, once a vice, is now promoted; frugality, until recently a virtue, is now bad for the economy. Yet the entropic handwriting on the wall is clear: frugal we must become. The consumption ethic leads inexorably to global competition and conflict of increasing proportions.

2. Employment is a byproduct of economic production. Thus as industrialized societies face limits to the amount of production, while pressures continue to increase labor productivity, meaningful work becomes a scarce commodity. But modern society also rightly considers employment (i.e., satisfying social roles) for its citizens to be essential to their well-

being. Employment in this sense is the individual's primary relationship to society, through which (s)he makes a personal contribution and receives affirmation in return, and in the process builds essential self-esteem. The assumption that employment (jobs) is a mere byproduct of economic production is in contradiction to this concern.

3. It is not practicable to ask the rich of the world to significantly decrease their material standard of living to redistribute to the poor. Yet they clearly cannot afford not to. World distribution of food, income, and wealth is far more uneven than is the distribution in any single country, even those with the most notoriously unjust political orders. Yet there seems to be no workable proposal to correct this situation. Instead, economic and demographic forces conspire to cause the maldistribution to grow steadily worse. The rich "North" partakes of a feast that the world's limited resources cannot sustain, while the teeming populations of the impoverished "South" remain trapped by poverty, illiteracy, and high birth rates in a remorseless cycle of deprivation, and the threat of ultimate "wars of redistribution" grows ever more imminent.

4. Technology will solve social problems. Economic and technological growth have brought abundance and problem-solving capabilities, and have liberated humankind in numerous ways. Yet in recent years technology has contributed to new kinds of scarcity (e.g., of fresh air and water, of waste-absorbing capacity of the environment); it has proven to be in some measure problem-generating; the institutions which house it are accused of being enslaving. New and alarming democracy-threatening aspects have begun to surface. For example, the possibility of major dependence on nuclear power poses grave threats to civil rights and liberties, such as the mandatory psychiatric examinations proposed to insure the mental stability of persons having access to dangerous nuclear fuels and waste. More fundamentally, the very momentum of economic and technological growth leads toward the automatic making of far-reaching social decisions (e.g., the growth imperative, "autonomous technology"), in effect bypassing the political process.

5. Science will produce the knowledge we need. Modern society has developed science and technology that enable it to accomplish feats which other societies could only dream about. Yet it is clearly confused in matters of guiding values and ultimate goals. The deepest value commitments and the ultimate goals of all societies that ever existed have come from the profound inner experiences of some group of

Long-term Modernization Trend and Countertrend Components

Trend	Countertrend
BASIC	
Secularization	"New transcendentalism"; quest for meanings
Industrialization	Reaction against "industrialization" of education, health care, agriculture, etc.
Economic rationalization	Reaction against dominance of economic rationality over ethics, social rationality, human values
"Technification" of knowledge	Search for knowledge of human values and goals
DERIVATIVE	
Technological, economic, and material growth	"Limits-to-growth" arguments; proposed change in qualitative nature of growth emphasis
Increasing use of inanimate energy sources	Energy conservation; "conserver society" movements
Increasing institutionalization of innovation	Challenge to "technological imperative"; technology assessment movement
Increasing bigness of technology, centralization	"Small is beautiful"; appropriate technology; decentralization movements
Urbanization	Reruralization movement
Increasing impact on environment	Environmentalist movements, rise of ecological ethic
Increasing power of weapons	Nuclear disarmament movement
Movement toward a single world economy	Small-country self-determination movements, demands for reshaping the international order
Increasing specialization, influence of technical elite	Politization of scientific and technical decisions, with public participation; "defrocking" of the experts
Tendency for ties binding individual to institutions to become impersonal	New emphasis on community, family values, human relationships, human potential movement, person-liberation
Acquisitive materialism as the mainspring	Voluntary simplicity movements

people—religious leaders, prophets, mystics, poet-philosophers, or in some visionary cultures the majority of the adult population. Some form of systematic knowledge of the world of inner experience, publicly validated and widely disseminated, would seem to be among the knowledge most needed to guide society in its crucial choices. Yet modern society's official knowledge system—science—tends to assume *a priori* that these experiences will in the end be explained (or explained away) as epiphenomena from a perishable brain, and has steadfastly excluded these phenomena from its field of study. The prevailing view in the culture is that such systematization of, and consensus on, inner wisdom is impracticable.

Paradigm Upheaval
Peter Schwartz

What's going on is morphogenetic. Morphogenesis is the process of the change of form (it's like, for example, how the galaxies evolved out of the chaos, or how one wave gives way to the next wave in the ocean, and so on); it's how forms evolve. But it's not a process which works very linearly. Instead, it's an accretion of a whole bunch of changes into a new order.

In the midst of all that's going on now, there are a whole bunch of threads that give cause for optimism, on the one hand, and for pessimism, on the other.

I think the women's revolution is probably the most positive force in the world today—that is, if the world really is changing that way. The kind of values or state of mind that has traditionally been associated with the feminine are precisely the kind of perceptual structures that are necessary to understand and to nurture the change that's in process, so that it comes out better rather than worse.

What I see happening in the women's movement is this. I think that the women who thought for a long time they had to behave like men to be successful in the world are now discovering that, because of the victories of the ones who first had to behave like men to carve

out a place, they can both be successful and be women in their own terms. And that's a fundamental pervasive change which will have a long-lasting effect on society for the good.

The women's movement, the current religious revival, and the microelectronics information movement are fostering new ways of thinking about society.

Another strong force is the religious revival that's going on. Now, that has both its up side and its down side. The up side is that people are really reflecting on the meaning of their lives, and discovering the values of deeper sources, focusing on the significant, not the trivial. On the other hand, I'm worried about some of the potential negative consequences of religious movements, such as highly organized religious movements, which tend to be highly authoritarian. Probably more evil has been done in this world in the name of religious belief than anything else. And that worries me, because in times of trouble like the ones I think we are facing, it's relatively easy to look for the kinds of answers that those kinds of religions offer. Still, the deeper part that is motivating this re-

HISTORIC INDICATORS

A third kind of evidence comes from sociological studies of past periods of revolutionary change in various societies. These studies indicate that typically there are precursors of such fundamental transformations, in certain social indicators which rise some years prior to the revolutionary change period and subsequently decline. These indicators include alienation from the institutions of society; rate of mental illness; rate of violent crime; rate of social disruption and use of police to put down dissension; tolerance of hedonistic behavior, particularly sexual; religious cultism; and economic inflation. All these indicators have risen since the mid-Sixties.

CHANGE IN BASIC PREMISES

A fourth kind of evidence is particularly significant in that it emphasizes how fundamental a change is taking place. This is the evidence pointing to change in some of the most basic, tacitly assumed premises in modern industrialized culture. New developments in biofeedback training, psychic research, and consciousness research indicate that a number of the implicit premises underlying modern positivistic science are challenged by the most recent findings of science itself.

Both in the culture at large, and in fringe areas in the scientific community, the dominant science-technology paradigm is being challenged in a funda-

ligious revival—as opposed to the form that it is taking—I see as a very positive force.

A third force that I see at work is microelectronics. Despite the dislocations that are likely to result from the development of small-scale electronics, it represents an important positive direction, if only because the existing civilization—the high-tech world that many people don't like very much—is simply not going to go away. And if it did go away, that would be a very unhappy process. So part of our task is to help nurture it in good directions.

The difference here, from almost all other sorts of high tech, is that microelectronics are cheap and broadly distributed, so that the great power there is made accessible at the lowest level of society. The individual now has direct access to this new power.

The women's and religious movements, the information movement that microelectronics makes possible, all go hand in hand to foster a new way of thinking about society, a set of tools to control and guide our lives, and a deeper reflection on values and beliefs. So that whole pattern of transformation I see as very positive.

Over-all, I think we are undergoing a shift in our basic belief structures. We're in the process of changing our fundamental beliefs about how reality is organized and what it means to be human.

I think that the most important thing for the individual to keep in mind is the old Buddhist maxim, "Do no harm." To do the least harm you can, live as well as you can.

What's worth doing? It seems to me the answer is almost everything that helps, whether it is at the national level, or in the neighborhood, or in the family, or with your children, or in your classroom. Every level where we bring more good into the world, we help, and at every level where we bring more harm into the world, we hurt. And it doesn't really matter whether we simply work in our own homes and classrooms and shops. I think an exaggerated importance is attributed to the higher levels, and I don't think there is any truth to it. It doesn't really matter what level we work at.

SUGGESTIONS FOR FURTHER READING

Irene Claremont DeCastillejo, *Knowing Woman: A Feminine Psychology*, Harper and Row, 1973.

Erich Jantsch and Conrad H. Waddington, eds. *Evolution and Consciousness: Human Systems in Transition.* Addison-Wesley, 1976.

Erich Neumann, *Depth Psychology and a New Ethic,* trans. by Eugene Rolf. Harper and Row, 1973.

James A. Ogilvy, *Many-Dimensional Man.* Harper and Row, 1979.

Peter Schwartz is Director of the Strategic Environment Center at SRI International, formerly Stanford Research Institute, where he carries out studies on the future for government and corporations. He is a former President of the Portola Institute, and currently a Director of the Smith-Hawken Tool Co., an importer of fine English garden tools.

mental sense. Survey data indicates a significant cultural shift in the direction of more interest in spiritual and psychic matters, particularly among the better educated. The challenge amounts to a reconsideration of the outmoded "warfare between science and religion" (presumably won long ago by science, hands down). The growing suspicion is that traditional religion and conventional science alike are both partial and flawed, and due to be superseded by a more unified view of reality.

In fact this development has been progressing for some time. Once-taboo areas of science—notably sleep and dreams, creativity, hypnosis, unconscious processes, psychosomatic theories of illness—have become legitimated. Psychic phenomena such as "remote viewing," precognition, and psychokinesis are being explored with renewed interest. Altered states of consciousness related to those traditionally known by such terms as meditation, contemplation, and "graces of interior prayer," are being tentatively explored via biofeedback training and other routes.

The implications of these recent research findings in these areas are paradigm-shaking, indeed. Some representative examples are as follows.

1. Unconscious knowing is far more extensive than ordinarily assumed, and includes not only the sorts of knowledge of "involuntary" bodily processes brought to light by biofeedback, but also unconscious knowledge of the various realms of psychic phenomena.

2. Because of the preponderance of the unconscious in our mental processes, there are previously unsuspected powers associated with beliefs, images, suggestions, etc.

3. Mind is ultimately dominant over biological processes (rather than being some sort of epiphenomenon deriving from them).

4. Mind is extended in time and space (as evidenced by such phenomena as "remote viewing" and precognition).

5. Minds are joined, in ways other than the usually assumed physical mechanisms of communication.

6. Mind is ultimately predominant over the physical world, as evidenced by psychokinetic phenomena.

7. Thus the arguments by which an earlier generation of scientists had declared the fundamental tenets of religion to be illusion turn out themselves to be invalid.

8. Hence we are led to revised views of the possibility of knowing meaning in life, of transcendent goals for the individual and society, of the significance of "losing one's mind," of birth and death.

THE POSSIBILITY OF A "NEW" SCIENCE

As physicists have learned to reconcile once-contradictory wave and particle pictures of elemental physical stuff, so we today are learning to reconcile inner and outer perceptions of reality, and physical and spiritual aspects of human experience. This is no mere theoretical argument by the academics. All about us are signs of involvement of ordinary people —pursuing spiritual disciplines, adopting holistic approaches to their own health care, becoming interested in questions of death and dying, investigating the paranormal. The culture is no longer so sure that fundamental concepts of religion and spirituality are outmoded by the impressive explanatory powers of positivistic science; no longer so sure that psychic phenomena (seemingly contradictory to materialistic science) are explained away as deception, error, and fraud; no longer so sure that the search for a universal moral order is fruitless.

In simplest terms, the historical development of modern science, because of its being an integral part of the long-term multifold modernization trend, took on a particular bias. Although *all* of our experience is "subjective" in the most basic sense, science undertook to study exhaustively only that portion which is our subjective experiencing of the data of our physical senses—meanwhile ignoring if not disparaging that part of our subjective experience which has to do with nonsensory, intuitive knowing. Initially this amounted to a sort of "division of labor" *vis a vis* the church. However, the methods of science became extremely powerful in generating technologies for manipulating the physical universe. As a consequence, their prestige led to an overshadowing of the inquiries of the humanities and religions into matters of value and meaning. Knowledge that could generate new technologies became that knowledge deemed of most worth, and the whole of science took on the prediction-and-control values of technology-focused knowledge.

This rise of materialistic science has been one of the most remarkable evolutionary leaps in the history of man. Its essence embodies a remarkable proposition, namely, that objective knowledge should not be based on religious or traditional authority, nor be the guarded property of an elite priesthood, but should be empirically based and publicly verifiable, open and free to all. It required, and obtained, consensus on the rules of validation. Thus we do not have (in general) Russian chemistry versus American chemistry, or Hindu astronomy versus Christian astronomy. Around the globe there is only science, the best set of conceptual models and empirical relationships yet available, continuously tested in public by agreed-upon procedures.

Now we are approaching a similar development in the other half of human experience, wherein the rest of subjective experience becomes subject also to the same sort of open, free, publicly validated search for empirical truth. This new, noetic* science would eliminate the apparent contradiction between the experiential understanding of Hindu, Moslem, and Christian. For the first time in history we see emerging a growing, progressively funded body of empirically established experience about man's inner life, particularly about the perennial wisdom of the great religious traditions and gnostic groups. For the first time, there is hope that this knowledge can become not a secret repeatedly lost in dogmatization and institutionalization, or degenerating into manifold varieties of cultism and occultism, but the living heritage of all mankind.

---

*The root of the word "noetic" is the same as for the words gnosis, diagnosis, agnostic, and knowledge; it refers to intuitive knowing. William James used the term in *The Varieties of Religious Experience* in defining mysticism.

SUGGESTIONS FOR FURTHER READING

Fernand Braudel, *The Mediterranean and the Mediterranean World in the Age of Philip II.* Harper and Row, 1972.

Willis Harman, *An Incomplete Guide to the Future.* W. W. Norton, 1979.

Ronald Higgins, *The Seventh Enemy: The Human Factor in the Global Crisis.* McGraw Hill, 1978.

Lewis Mumford, *The Transformations of Man.* Harper and Brothers, 1956.

Mark Satin, *New Age Politics.* Dell, 1979.

L. Stavrianos, *The Promise of the Coming Dark Age.* W. H. Freeman, 1976.

Willis W. Harman is Associate Director of the Center for the Study of Social Policy, SRI International; Professor of Engineering-Economic Systems, Stanford Universiity; and President of the Institute of Noetic Sciences. His academic background was in electrical engineering and physics; however, he was one of the pioneers in humanistic psychology, and his 1969 paper, "The New Copernican Revolution," reprinted many times, is far better known than any of his engineering accomplishments. He has been a "futurist" for 13 years, and several years ago summarized what he had learned in a small book, An Incomplete Guide to the Future.

Toward a Rationale and Model for Basic Education
Hobart F. Thomas, Ph.D.

There are certain fundamental qualities of character which are necessary for the development of happy, secure, and successful human beings. If our basic educational system does not contribute to the building of these qualities, it is then building on a weak foundation. It is easy to teach tangible facts and figures. Self-awareness, self-expression, noncompetitiveness, and an awareness of contributing to a greater whole need also be gently but clearly cultivated. Each person has his or her own set of talents and strengths, which we must make room in our schools to encourage. The following article speaks of a model for education now in practice at Sonoma State College in California. The focus is on the discovery of one's inner directions and talents, and learning how to live one's life accordingly. This seems like a simple idea, but until recently it has been overlooked in the rush for more superficial means of satisfaction and success.

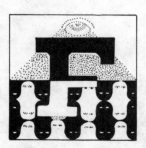

or many years I have believed that the development of "character" deserves priority in education. I would argue that once a person has arrived at a certain stage of maturity, the rest of the education process is, relatively speaking, smooth sailing. If, on the other hand, we do not try to cultivate certain fundamental qualities of character, we are likely to be wasting time in superficialities.

I would suggest that character, for the purpose of this discussion, is composed of the following attributes: (1) self-awareness; (2) mastery of suitable means of self-expression; (3) engagement in activity which is congruent with one's own nature; (4) the ability and willingness to assume personal responsibility for one's life; and (5) an awareness that one is part of a larger totality and a sense of responsibility to that totality.

SELF-AWARENESS

This concept refers to knowledge of one's unique personal qualities, a sense of who one is, including one's needs, aspirations, and values. I find Schumacher's comment about the centering process to be helpful in clarifying this concept:

"All human activity is a striving after something thought of as good. 'Good for whom?' Good for the striving person. So, unless that person has sorted out and coordinated his manifold urges, impulses, and desires, his strivings are likely to be confused, contradictory, self-defeating, and highly destructive. The 'center' obviously is the place where he has to create for himself an orderly system of ideas about himself and the world, which can regulate the direction of his various strivings."[1]

The charge is to find out something about our own nature, what we want out of life, and then to attempt to live in accordance with our own system of values. This is a reasonably fair description of a self-directed person. The antithesis is one whose life orientation consists largely of following someone else's orders.

In our present culture, and perhaps in most cultures, finding out about one's own nature is not given much attention in educational institutions. For the most part in the Western world, such investigation has been the province of the psychoanalyst, who usually gets to the person long after the educational system has finished with him. Yet there is a model provided for us by certain primitive cultures, among them the American Indians, in the practice called the Vision Quest, in which the young person spends long periods fasting in the wilderness until he or she receives some sense of inner direction, perhaps in the form of a vision, perhaps in some other form. This procedure was given a central place in each person's education and received cultural support. Years of experience in the fields of psychotherapy and education have made me want to devise some model suitable for our culture which might similarly enhance self-understanding.

In order to delve deeply within oneself, relatively unstructured time and space are needed. Yet the traditional education model, based largely on informational input, the acquiring of skills, and the demand to conform to externally imposed standards, is the very antithesis of those models generally devised for bringing about self-understanding. Faced with this conflict, one is tempted to forgo the possibility of synthesis and simply choose one way or the other. Indeed, the reconciliation of two such contradictory approaches is a big order. One might well ask whether this is not demanding too much of the educator. Do we not have a right to assume a certain degree of maturity on the part of our students? Is it not sufficient for us merely to teach our field of expertise and to require of our students only the mastery of this specific area? Perhaps so. I wonder, however, if there is a place within our educational institutions for the consideration of more fundamental issues. In order to do so, we must develop procedures which tap deeper layers of the self, those oft-neglected hidden regions which contain the secrets so vital to our completion as human beings.

SELF-EXPRESSION

Various forms of self-expression seem to come naturally to the young child; yet soon the child learns to relinquish his or her unique ways as a price for obtaining social approval. Picasso speaks precisely to this point when he admonishes that instead of trying to teach children how to paint, we should learn from them. Creative thinking in any field relies on the acceptance and expression of nonrational processes, such as dream fragments, fantasy, and imagination. Consider Jerome Bruner's remarks about the conditions of creativity: "My advice, in the midst of the seriousness, is to keep an eye out for the tinker shuffle, the flying of kites, and kindred sources of amusement."[2] Yet, these processes are all too vulnerable to the requirements for socialization. Almost by definition socialization means "growing up," putting away childish things. All too often this results in a denial of those very qualities which give meaning to human experience. Charles Darwin in his autobiography poignantly describes his loss of delight in art and music while he was heavily concentrating on the rational side:

"My mind seems to have become a kind of machine for grinding general laws out of large collections of facts, but why this should have caused the atrophy of that part of the brain alone, on which the higher tastes depend, I cannot conceive . . . . The loss of these tastes is a loss of happiness, and may possibly be injurious to the intellect, and more probably to the moral character, by enfeebling the emotional part of our nature."[3]

The development of creativity in adults calls for a rediscovery of the childlike, expressive qualities of the individual. The modes differ for each person. For one, musical expression seems to come naturally; for another, bodily movement, such as dance or athletic activity; for others, it may be painting, sculpture, woodworking, mechanical work, or drama, poetry, etc. The form of expression matters little.

Daniel Rhodes speaks of art as leaving traces of one's life, and expands the concept of self-expression to include more than typical art forms:

"Making 'art' is impossible. All one can do is leave traces of one's life. This cannot take preconceived forms . . . . The trail, if it is truly a mark of honest expression, will be uniquely valuable; it will objectify the inner life and furnish guidelines into the still unknown . . . . Expression has to do with our total selves, our identity, and it takes many forms besides those we call art. A whistled tune, a gesture, the shape one gives to an old pair of shoes. It is search, awareness, projection. Perhaps what we honor with the name of art are those projections of selfhood which we feel to be completely honest. If art forms *inhibit* the search, they must be discarded or transformed. If the trail one leaves in work and living becomes confused, obscured, or contradictory, never mind. That may be a sign of truth, and is to be preferred to easier, neater configurations. The outward forms of painting and sculpture give no assured avenues toward the genuine or the valuable. They exist only as possible vehicles among many others."[4]

In addition to his emphasis on the authenticity of expression, Rhodes calls our attention to another aspect of the creative process, namely, the acceptance and valuing of work which is "confused, obscured, or contradictory." Here is another illustration of something which conflicts with traditional pedagogical practices. Generally speaking, school is a place where one is expected to learn how to get the right answers, not a place to act "confused, obscured, or contradictory." How can institutions of learning maintain standards of excellence, but at the same time encourage students to be free enough to make mistakes and fail? Typical class structures do not allow for

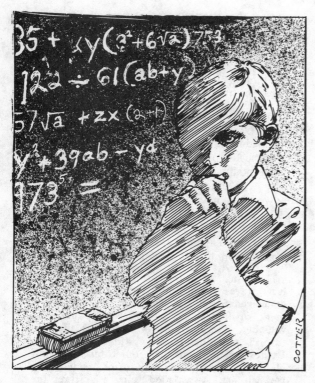

Traditional class structures do not allow students the freedom to experiment with different modes of self expression.

such individual experimentation. Are there other models which might provide for a more thorough exploration of personal modes of expression? If so, then what kind of standards need be employed?

CONGRUENT ACTIVITY

George Bernard Shaw commented once that "labor is doing what we must; leisure is doing what we like." Therefore, the wise person is one who learns the art of spending a large portion of life in leisure: doing what he or she wants to do. Hans Selye in his studies of stress cites examples of successful people in many fields who meet this criterion. The list, a long one, includes such diverse figures as G. B. Shaw, Pablo Picasso, Winston Churchill, Albert Schweitzer, Henry Ford, Pablo Casals, and Bertrand Russell.[5] "Leisure" thus defined does not refer to a lack of activity, but rather to full engagement in something one enjoys doing. Selye sums it up by saying that since work is a basic need of man, the question is not whether to work, but what kind of work is play.

Again we are confronted with a paradox. Those who have made the greatest contributions in all fields seem to be those who have learned how to play. And the attitude of play takes us back again to the child. Playful activity is that which is engaged in just for its own sake. It is not "good for something." It *is* its own purpose.

Traditional curricula, with the possible exception of recess, do not include playful activity. Is there a place for such education in the models that now exist? Is it possible within our educational institutions to develop individuals who have learned how to connect their work and play so that they can live deeply satisfying lives? If people like Selye are right, such individuals are also likely to contribute the most to society.

ASSUMING PERSONAL RESPONSIBILITY

For several years I have been observing students in situations in which they must assume responsibility for what they learn and organize their learnings into a personally constructed system of values and style of life. The cultivation of this attribute of self-responsibility hinges largely on the creation of an environment in which most of the impediments to making personal choices are removed. Under such circumstances it is not so much a question of what the person in charge *does* as what he or she *does not do*. In most life situations, the individual is oriented toward meeting externally imposed requirements. The attitude thus engendered is primarily one of "What is expected of me?" An extreme example is a totalitarian regime in which one merely follows orders. If, on the other hand, no one tells the individual what to do or, even more important, if whoever is perceived as being in charge clearly expects the person to do what he or she most deeply wants to do, a profound shift in orientation ensues. Such a shift is usually accompanied by much inner turmoil, and if it is to "take," there must be great commitment by all concerned. The gravest temptation for all is to avoid the pain of change by lapsing into familiar modes of behavior. The student is tempted to avoid the awful responsibility of free choice by searching for some external authority who will do the choosing. The educator is tempted to short-circuit the process out of a fear that somehow the individual is not capable of assuming this responsibility and will make a mess of things. Indeed, the creative process—in this case, the creation of a self—is more often than not an unpredictable and messy affair. Students undergoing

(Text continued on p. 288)

Education in the New Age

Jack Canfield and Paula Klimek

"I hear and I forget, I see and I remember, I do and I understand."

Old Chinese proverb

In a growing number of classrooms throughout the world, education is beginning to move into a new dimension. More and more teachers are exposing children to ways of contacting their inner wisdom and their higher selves. The beauty, depth, and quality of the responses to these new approaches is a source of constant amazement and inspiration.

The essence of education in the New Age is one of holism and synthesis. True education means providing an environment in which the student's self-regulated learning process can unfold naturally. The word *education* comes from the Latin word *educare*, "to lead out from within." What teachers are now interested in leading out from within is the expression of the self—the highest qualities of the individual student's unique soul.

Holistic education is, of course, more a perspective than a collection of methods: it views the student as being engaged in an integral process of unfoldment under the direction of his or her higher self. This process is perceived as taking place in a universe that is also constantly evolving: each of us is seen as an important part of the larger planetary and universal evolution of consciousness.

The following activities are now being used in more and more classrooms across the country. They are given here as examples of the many creative possibilities in working and living with children.

There are certainly many more creative and exciting ways to work with developing the physical self in school than the traditional gym period. Perhaps not every student will tune into each way presented, but with enough options students can find what George Leonard would call their "ultimate athlete," or their highest and best physical self. Here are a few of the approaches now being used in classrooms.

NEW GAMES

New Games were originated in the early 1970s by Stewart Brand (producer of the *Whole Earth Catalog*), George Leonard (author of *Education and Ecstasy*), and a host of others dedicated to new forms of play stressing cooperation, trust, and fun rather than competition, stress, and winning. Originally developed for large outdoor festivals, New Games have begun to be increasingly used in classrooms for teaching cooperation, for relaxing tension, for releasing stored-up energy, and for creating a learning environment based on fun. We have observed that when students discover they will not be criticized or excluded, their whole attitude toward the use of their bodies changes. They become more involved and less self-conscious.

The games, explained and illustrated in *The New Games Book,* include Hug Tag, Prui, Ooh-Ahh, Hagoo, Stand Up, the Lap Game, and 53 others. Almost all are suitable for classroom and playground use. For example, Hug Tag follows the same rules as classical tag, but with one major exception: the only time a player is safe is when he/she is hugging another player. The rules are adaptable: players might decide, for example, that only three people hugging are safe.

These games involve a lot of physical touching in a nonsexual way, which is a basic need we all have.

Children of all ages love physical exercises and seem to be particularly fascinated with yoga: they move easily into all sorts of contortions. In addition to being enjoyable, yoga exercises help children to relax their muscles and develop their balance; they stimulate the circulation and restore energy. We have also noted dramatic changes in so-called "hyperactive" children; they become better able to concentrate.

If you put out a call to parents and friends in your local community, you'll probably find that there are many people involved in dance and movement who would love to work with you and your kids. Basically, any area of physical growth that excites adults can be done with children. The spontaneity and freshness they evoke always bring a new sense of aliveness to the classroom.

(continued on p. 286)

(continued from p. 285)

THE MARTIAL ARTS

We recently sponsored a workshop by Victor Miller and Terry Dobsen, co-authors of *Giving In to Get Your Way,* a book on aikido and conflict resolution. They have discovered that one of the most profound teaching tools is the physical metaphor—having the student experience the conflict in his or her body by movement or improvisation. A few moves from aikido can easily illustrate the concept of the difference between resisting and flowing with what is happening. Tai Chi, Kung Fu, Judo, and Karate all contain similar lessons on such themes as blending, concentration, awareness, and trusting one's body. This is the best way we've found to get the individual attention of the more difficult students.

SENSE OF SELF

Learning to love oneself, to accept all the parts and subpersonalities, all of one's feelings, images, thoughts, and sensations, is one of the most important tasks of the personality's development. One can only bring the quality of love into the world if one has it grounded within one's self.

There are three general areas which are essential to developing a positive self-concept: a sense of belonging, a sense of competence, and a sense of worthwhileness. Gerald Weinstein, a professor in the Humanistic Education Center at the University of Massachusetts, refers to these qualities as "connectedness, power, and identity."

An important aspect of developing positive self-concept is hearing positive things about yourself from significant others. One activity we use again and again is the "strength bombardment." Each student is the target for two minutes. The rest of the class tells the target person things they like about him or her. Another student records all the statements, and later gives this list to the target student. We suggest the following guidelines to the students. The target person may not talk during the process (this avoids his or her discounting the feedback). The students are asked to make eye contact with the person to whom they are talking, and we ask them to begin statements with "I like——" or "I appreciate——," rather than "You are——." (The first is a personal reaction; the second is likely to be judgmental.) The response is incredible. People generally are not aware of the positive aspects of themselves which others perceive.

CIRCLES

The magic circle and circle-time programs consist of the teacher sitting in a close circle with eight to ten students and engaging in a series of discussions that are sequenced developmentally to increase their self-awareness, self-confidence, and effectiveness with others. Another major outcome of circle work is phenomenal progress in the students' ability to truly listen to one another and to respond in an authentic, caring, affirming, and nonjudgmental manner.

Each day there is a selected topic for discussion, such as:

my favorite thing to do alone;
something I wish I could have;
a fear I have to overcome;
something I do well;
something about me I don't understand;
a time I really used self-control;
a hard decision I'll have to face;
a time I felt put down.

CHANTING

Children are naturally rhythmic, and chanting fits well into the classroom. Chanting can be used as meditation, for focusing the group energy, and for evoking the qualities of peace, love, joy, and unity. When the whole class creates a unified vibration through sound, there is a tremendous uplifting effect. An example of a chant that works particularly well with children is:

Happiness runs in a circular motion.
Life is like a little boat upon the sea.
Everyone is a part of everything anyway.
You can have it all if you let yourself be.

MEDITATION/CENTERING

Centering can also be extended into work with meditation in the classroom. (Advice: if you're teaching in a public school, don't call it meditation, call it "centering." Every school wants children to be relaxed, attentive, and creative, and that's what they will get.) The first difficulty is to get kids to close their eyes and to validate this need for inner space.

A wonderful way to do this, we have found, is to use the tools the media are providing. An example might be to ask, "What's this thing called the Force in *Star Wars?* How does Luke communicate with it? How does it help him?" The next question is, "Well, would you like to have this kind of experience?" (The answer is always an overwhelming "Yes!") "Well, we can try this and see what happens. There are some ground rules you will need to follow." At this point the kids are more than ready. The media has done a lot of the work for us. Consequently, they quickly learn such benefits as being fully present before a test, solving their problems through contact with their own inner wisdom, and learning to relax. We were amazed to find out how tense kids really are and how grateful they are to learn how to work in this way. Some said:

"I've learned to be more calm and to understand other people's feelings better."

"I've learned I have lots of light."

"I am as calm as the sea."

"I am the silence of the forest."

"I will say what I feel with love in my heart."

These children of the New Age are incredibly conscious and will teach us an incredible amount—if we truly open to them. They will create new developmental models. By working in the transpersonal dimensions we find a window into the new. The only requirement is to provide a space and an environment where these beautiful young spirits can open up and allow their wisdom to be seen.

KEEPING UP

The following publications cover the latest developments in New Age education.

National Holistic Education Network Newsletter (P. O. Box 1233, Del Mar, CA 92014) is published several times a year by Anastas Harris, who began the network. The Network also sponsors an annual conference on holistic health and holistic education and publishes the *Journal of Holistic Education.* Membership is $10.00 per year. Write for more info.

Journal of Humanistic Education and *Celebrations: The Newsletter of the Association for Humanistic Education* are both published by the Association for Humanistic Education, P.O. Box 1345, Carrollton, GA 30117. Membership is $15.00 per year. They also sponsor an annual conference and several regional conferences on humanistic education.

The Association for Humanistic Psychology (325 Ninth St., San Francisco, CA 94103) and

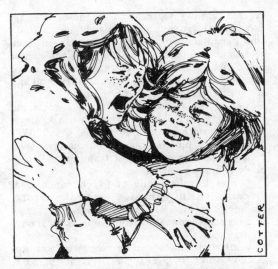

In the game of Hug Tag, the only time a player is safe is when hugging another player.

the Association for Transpersonal Psychology (P. O. Box 3049, Stanford, CA 94305) both have education networks and many active members who are teachers. Both organizations have journals, newsletters, and annual and regional conferences. We recommend membership in both.

Synthesis (830 Woodside Rd., Redwood City, CA 94061) presents articles on psychology and education based upon and aligned with the theory and practice of psychosynthesis. Subscriptions are $8.00 per year.

For further recommendations, consult *A Guide to Resources in Humanistic and Transpersonal Education* by Jack Canfield (available for $5.50 from the National Humanistic Education Center, 110 Spring St., Saratoga Springs, NY 12866). This guide contains annotated references to more than 500 resources, including books, curricula, classroom exercises, tapes, films, curriculum development projects, newsletters and journals, growth centers, consulting organizations, and professional associations with a special interest in the areas of humanistic and transpersonal education.

FURTHER TRAINING

Several groups and organizations have recently emerged that conduct both professional

(continued on p. 288)

(continued from p. 287)

teacher-training workshops in these new approaches and workshops designed to facilitate the personal growth and expansion of consciousness of teachers as people. Each center has a slightly different orientation and focus; so we suggest you write for brochures from all and see which ones strike a harmonious chord.

Center for Humanistic and Transpersonal Psychology and Education (Johnston College, University of Redlands, Redlands, CA 92373) conducts an undergraduate and master's level program in humanistic and transpersonal psychology and education.

Center for the Study of Psychoeducational Processes (Ritter Annex, Temple University, Philadelphia, PA 19122) offers degree programs in humanistic education and sponsors an annual conference.

Confluent Education Development and Research Center (P. O. Box 30138, Santa Barbara, CA 93105) is a comprehensive confluent education center which sponsors workshops, provides consultants, publishes the *Confluent Education Journal,* and disseminates confluent curriculum materials.

Development and Research in Confluent Education (Department of Education, University of California, Santa Barbara, CA 93106) is developing curriculum and training teachers in the area of confluent education. Their aim is to integrate the knowledge and activities of the human potential movement with the traditional classroom curriculum, thus creating a more total or holistic learning situation.

The Hill Center for Psychosynthesis in Education (Old Walpole Rd., Walpole, NH 03608) offers an intensive year-long training program for education using the holistic approach of psychosynthesis to enable teachers, and their students, to actively cooperate with their own natural processes of growth.

Human Development Training Institute (7574 University Ave., La Mesa, CA 92031) publishes materials and conducts workshops on the Human Development Program, designed to develop children's self-awareness, self-confidence, and human relationships.

Institute for Wholistic Education (Box 299, Star Route, Muir Beach, CA 94965) conducts professional training workshops for educators and mental-health professionals, consults with school systems, and publishes books and tapes in wholistic education.

Interface/Beacon College M.A. Program in Holistic Education (230 Central St., Newton, MA 02166) offers professional training, an M.A. degree program, and workshops in the areas of holistic education, counseling, and health. Write for a brochure.

Mandala (P. O. Box 796, Amherst, MA 01002) is a newly formed educational consulting and publishing group which offers pre- and in-service training courses in humanistic education, circletime, communications skills, etc.; it

(continued from p. 284)

this process are not often likely to enhance their mentors' chances for tenure and promotion!

The preliminary research we have been doing for the last seven years seems to indicate that rather profound character changes do occur in many persons committed to this approach. Our experience also indicates that, once a person is operating from a personal center, he or she is then more highly motivated to pursue cognitive areas of learning which relate to this center.

The following excerpt from an interview with a graduate of the School of Expressive Arts illustrates one person's progress during a two-year period:

"During the first semester of the College, a lot of people were running around playing school. We set up lots of classes and groups, and soon, I think, I was able to see through all that as a substitute for learning what was more personal and important. One thing that meant a lot to me that first year, though, was gaining a feeling of self-worth. I learned how to be with people and how to be alone. I got acquainted with my rhythms in this respect.

"In the second year, I was able to put into effect what I'd learned in the first. I got an old house and began fixing it up into a home. I learned how to work with wood, build furniture, sew, make clothes. I also had time to get into reading more. I got interested in Indian history, psychology, novels. I was able to find courses and other resources connected with these interests. This place weaned me from needing others, and helped me realize that in the final analysis all you have is yourself. I learned to take initiative for what I wanted. I

also publishes books of activities and a series of yearbooks in humanistic and transpersonal education.

National Humanistic Education Center (110 Spring St., Saratoga Springs, NY 12866) conducts seminars in humanistic education and makes available books and reprints of many articles in the area of humanistic education.

New Games Foundation (P. O. Box 7901, San Francisco, CA 94120) publishes a newsletter and a list of New Games Training Workshops across the country.

NEXTEP Fellowship Program (Southern Illinois University, Edwardsville, IL 62025) offers degree programs in humanizing classroom learning environments; theirs is one of the most comprehensive efforts in the field.

Philadelphia Center for Humanistic Education (8504 Germantown Ave., Philadelphia, PA 19119) conducts teacher-training workshops and distributes humanistic education books and articles.

SUGGESTIONS FOR FURTHER READING

New Games Foundation, *The New Games Book.* Doubleday, 1976.

Jack Canfield, *The Inner Classroom: Teaching with Guided Fantasy.* Prentice-Hall, 1981.

———, *Teaching Students to Love Themselves.* Prentice-Hall, 1981.

Jack Canfield and Harold Wells, *One Hundred Ways to Enhance Self-Concept in the Classroom.* Prentice-Hall, 1976.

Deborah Rozman, *Meditating with Children.* University of the Trees Press, 1975.

Matt Weinstein and Joel Goodman, *Playfair.* Impact, 1980.

Jack Canfield, M.Ed., is past director of the New England Center and the Center for Whole Being, and is currently Director of the Institute for Wholistic Education in Muir Beach, California. He is a skilled trainer in gestalt therapy, transpersonal psychology, and humanistic/ wholistic education. He is also past president of the Association of Humanistic Education.

Paula Klimek, M.A.T., is a holistic education consultant, counselor, and writer. She is the major facilitator of the M.A. program for educators, counselors, and health educators at the Interface Foundation in Newton, Massachusetts. She is the former Director and founder of the Human Development project, a Title III grant in wholistic education in Rhode Island. She is a consultant to numerous schools and has been a member of two university faculties.

learned to get what I wanted out of required courses and still make As. I feel that I'm just beginning my education, which will go on for the rest of my life. I'm ready to leave now and go out into the world."

That is just one example of what we have discovered to be a relatively consistent pattern in students committed to this program. The pattern is basically holistic rather than fragmented in nature. In it the individual has the opportunity to search deeply within, to discover something of who she is, to learn what she needs in order to survive. The mastery of these skills is accompanied by feelings of self-worth, an attitude of self-reliance, and a sense of personal direction. The development of these basic attributes of character and the ability to cope with the process of living allows for the emergence of intellectual and aesthetic interests. Education for this person, as she indicates, is now likely to be a lifelong process.

RESPONSIBILITY TO A LARGER WHOLE

Complementary to the development of individuality and self-reliance is the awareness of one's relationship to something more than oneself. Such a relationship can be experienced with immediate family, friends, community, various social, cultural, political or religious groups, or all of humanity, and in the more sensitive among us can include a reverence for all life and a sense of oneness with the cosmos. The expansion of the concept of self to include more than the individual ego can occur spontaneously in meditation or in interaction with others where communication is based on open, honest dialogue, and where manipulation and exploitation are minimal.

(Text continued on p. 292)

Meditation for Children
Stephanie Herzog

Imagine you are walking into a typical classroom full of energetic children. You notice their energy is scattered: some are doing schoolwork; others are busy discussing last night's TV shows; two children are throwing erasers at each other; five hands are raised, waiting for the teacher; and seven others are gathered around the teacher, all trying to talk at the same time.

Now imagine walking into another classroom. As you enter the room, you immediately feel a sense of calm. You notice that the children are engaged in many different activities: some are reading in a corner, others are doing math, a few are listening to a story. They all seem absorbed in what they are doing, and there is a pleasant vibration of harmony. The children's faces are friendly and bright. Several children come up and ask your name; they lead you over to the table they are working at to show you the books they are writing. The teacher is sitting with a small group, teaching a language lesson, looking totally relaxed and comfortable. The teacher and the children flow easily in and out of one another's worlds. This classroom is very different from the norm: it feels as if the children's and the teacher's awareness have been opened to new ways of seeing.

I am convinced that such children can exist in our schools. Last October my classroom was transformed from the typical one to the new type described. I started using meditation, and a wonderful thing began to happen: the students' self-direction increased so much that I seldom had to discipline—a caring, loving atmosphere evolved almost like magic. Other professionals, including a state evaluation team, visited my classroom, and were amazed by the level of creative thinking and care exhibited by the students.

I first heard about using meditation with children at a district "inservice"—a day when lecturers come to speak to teachers about new, innovative ways of teaching. Dr. Deborah Roz-man, author of *Meditating with Children*, spoke about using meditation in the classroom. She discussed the way concentration and the imagination are developed by meditation and how a sense of community in the classroom is created. This helps children find an inner calm and centeredness which become special tools with which to face the trials of growing up.

I decided to try it the very next day. I was a little nervous at first about leading the children through a meditation. I wasn't sure how they would respond. I was also a bit nervous about how the parents might react when the children described to them what we did. But I gathered the children into a circle around me, and told them we were going to do an exercise that would give them more energy for their work and help them concentrate better. I had them close their eyes and relax all their body parts, breathe quietly five times, and concentrate for a while on a star between their eyes while imagining having a good day and doing the very best they could on all their work. After the exercise I had them tense their bodies, to bring themselves back, and open their eyes. The children sat very quietly for a few minutes. Then I asked them to go to their activity centers and start their work as usual. And to my surprise, they did.

Now, on any normal morning some children will not go straight to work. Instead, they will meander around or visit with a friend until I remind them. But immediately following the centering exercise, all of them went quietly to work and were fully absorbed until noon. Usually after a few hours the children begin to get restless and have trouble concentrating. But this morning was different; for the first time the children were deeply focused and stayed zeroed in on what they were doing. The results proved to be consistent. Each morning we did the same routine and the children went quietly to work. They were usually able to stay centered and tuned into my directions for three hours. I began to enjoy teaching in a way I never had before and found myself looking forward to coming to class. Generally, teachers expect a hectic day. But now the children radiated a peaceful energy that flowed into me; I would start to radiate a peaceful feeling from my being in turn, and it would all multiply.

At first, when leading the whole group, I realized you cannot keep your eyes closed all the time; there will always be the few who may disturb. You have to keep your feelers out, making sure this child isn't going to get up and wander around or that child isn't going to make faces at So-and-so. All of a sudden you may hear giggles because this kid is teasing that kid. With regular practice the children gradually get used to the daily exercise and a close watch isn't necessary; they go right into it.

Before I started using the centering exercises, I maintained the type of discipline where the children suffered natural consequences if they disobeyed one of the rules in the classroom. For instance, if children kept shouting out at me and would not allow me to speak to the group, the consequence would be to have them pick up litter around the yard at recess time. About a week after I started using centering, I realized I wasn't having anyone pick up papers anymore.

Before I used meditation, I found that whenever I was speaking, some children would not be listening. As all parents and teachers well know, it is always a struggle to get everyone listening at the same time. After I started using meditation, I began to notice that all of the children were quiet the whole time I was speaking; they were so attentive, their eyes would be right on me. I began talking more to their inner beings—it kind of flowed naturally. I began to relate more from the feelings in my heart, something that's usually hard to do in a classroom. I felt as if they were actually hearing me from deep inside.

After such wonderful results, I decided to meditate on my own every morning right before the children come to school. I go into my classroom, keep the lights off, and lock the door. I do several yoga exercises, then I close my eyes and relax all body parts. I imagine that a golden waterfall of love is flowing down from high in the cosmos through the top of my head and down into my heart, then out from my heart to everywhere in the classroom. I imagine breathing in love and breathing out love. As I do this exercise, I get a warm feeling in my heart which gives me an inner strength that lasts through the whole morning.

I find it very valuable to meditate before I lead the children through a centering activity. In fact, to the extent that I allow myself to become uncentered, anxious, or scattered, the children begin to become anxious and noisy

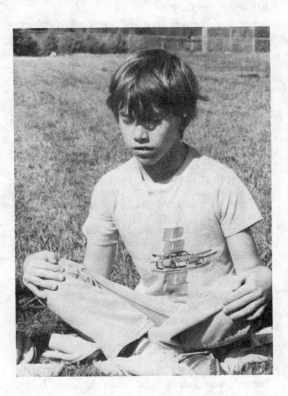

too. They pick up my energy and send it back like a mirror. I then become more uncentered, and it snowballs. Now I try to stay calm and centered all day.

A few mornings, some children came early to school and were waiting outside my door when I arrived. I invited these children to come in and center with me. These were the best meditations! I felt a special closeness between their beings and my being.

After using meditation about one month, I started to notice other changes. The boys and girls were beginning to play together more. In the mornings before school a large group of boys and girls began to congregate on the playground and they would have discussions. Usually children just wander around by themselves in the morning, a few boys playing over here and a few girls over there—definitely not together. When I saw boys and girls together in a circle, talking, I thought, "Wow, what's happening? They are really beginning to see each other in a different way." I feel this happened because the children were tuning into their

(continued on p. 292)

(continued from p. 291)

inner worlds every day and some of the blocks that children have—such as the attitude, "I'm not going to have anything to do with that person"—began to disappear. It all happened spontaneously, in a way they weren't even aware of. They began to have more feeling for one another; so they just naturally began to relate more.

I had a student named Sharon who at the beginning of the year didn't have much self-confidence. It really showed in her body language, in the way she walked. Her face was not happy. There was pain in her face and much uncomfortableness. Her eyes were not opened all the way. She had trouble getting along with other students, and constantly felt she wasn't doing a good job in reading and math. Actually she had much ability; it was her attitude that was defeating her. No matter what encouragement and positive strokes I gave her, she continued to feel badly about herself, school, and life in general.

After we began the centering activities and through the rest of the year, I began to notice a real change in Sharon. She began to be able to stay with her work, concentrate on it, and feel good about it. Academically, she progressed very nicely. She began to have pride in herself, and her whole face changed. It be-

came fuller and brighter. Her eyes became sparkly and opened up. She began to walk much straighter, with a bounce of confidence, and she began to play with other children well. I feel this all happened to Sharon because she changed inside. She no longer needed confirmation from outside, from myself or others in the classroom. She found an inner center where she felt good about herself.

Meditation is a wonderful tool for increasing a child's use of the right hemisphere of the brain. The exercises automatically increase awareness, creativity, intuition, and imagination. Meditation requires no timely preparation as do most academic subjects. It's effortless effort. The meditations using the expansion of the imagination have been most successful. The children love them—and simply shine with energy and quiet excitement afterwards. I lead the children through guided fantasy journeys, such as the balloon meditation (see box), right after lunch every day. When a child practices using his or her imagination consciously, it's a lesson in self-mastery. Learning to control the imagination brings a developed consciousness that can aid creative problem-solving.

You can begin using meditation at home and in the classroom any time. It is best to talk about it with the children a few days before

(continued from p. 289)

In an educational setting, one can foster a sense of responsibility beyond the self by valuing each person's experience and cultivating the ability to make it articulate. It is not enough merely to work in isolation. Being in school includes an obligation not only to learn for oneself, but also to contribute one's learnings to the pool of human knowledge and understanding. In the School of Expressive Arts, this principle of challenging the individual to engage fully in what he or she deems most important and to share it with others in a variety of ways has resulted in a rather unique community, rich in energy and resources. In order to make use of such a learning community effectively, one must risk opening up to knowing and being known to others. Those who have learned how to take this risk are likely to experience a total, continuing process of education which deals with the very process of living itself. One student described it as, "Here I can't come to school and leave myself at home."

In these circumstances the community itself, an organic, dynamic pool of human resources, becomes the primary medium for education, with each member being at one time a teacher, at another a learner. Most important, the price of membership is not the loss of individuality but its celebration.

NOTES

[1]E. F. Schumacher, *Small is Beautiful* (Harper and Row, 1973), p. 95.

[2]J. Bruner, *Knowing: Essays for Left Hand* (Harvard University Press, 1965), p. 18.

[3]C. Darwin, *Autobiography* (Collins, 1958).

[4]Daniel Rhodes, "Erosion II," *Ceramics Monthly.* 20:27 (Fall, 1972), p. 27.

[5]Hans Selye, *Stress Without Distress* (Lippincot, 1974).

you are going to start, to prepare them for what is coming. One teacher I know had the chidren discuss energy and becoming aware of energies in ourselves as a preparation to beginning. You may wish to tell them you will be starting a new program which you will be using until the end of the year. Repetition and regularity are the most important factors. Describe what the exercises will be, and how they will be using their imaginations and opening their hearts. This isn't just ordinary fantasy games; it is a scientific method of holistic living, relaxing body tensions, breathing to get in touch with feelings and release them, concentration to focus the mind, and imagination to expand the awareness and probe hidden potential.

SUGGESTIONS FOR FURTHER READING

Christopher Hills, *Nuclear Evolution: Discovery of the Rainbow Body.* University of the Trees Press, 1977.

————, *The Rise of the Phoenix: Universal Government by Nature's Laws.* Common Ownership Press, 1979.

Christopher Hills and Deborah Rozman, *Exploring Inner Space: Awareness Games For All Ages.* University of the Trees Press, 1978.

Deborah Rozman, *Meditating With Children.* University of the Trees Press, 1975.

————, *Meditation for Children.* Celestial Arts Press, 1976.

Stephanie Herzog received her B.A. (cum laude) from the College of Notre Dame (Belmont, Calif.), where she was elected a life member of Kappa Gamma Pi, the National Scholastic and Activity Honor Society of Catholic Women's Colleges. She also earned her California Standard Life Elementary Credential through the College of Notre Dame. Stephanie has been instrumental in introducing new methods of teaching reading, meditation, and awareness activities in the classrooms of the Scotts Valley Elementary School District in California and has helped lead many "Meditation With Children" seminars since joining the University of the Trees Community (Boulder Creek, California) in 1977. She is currently teaching at University Community School, a newly opened wholistic elementary school in Ben Lomond, California, and is writing a book describing her three years of experience teaching meditation and awareness activities in the public schools, an accomplishment supported by local school superintendents.

Hobart F. Thomas is Professor of Psychology at Sonoma State University, California. He received his Ph.D. from Stanford University in 1951. In addition to a practice in clinical psychology, he has served as consultant to a wide variety of organizations. For many years he has been involved with the task of developing holistic educational models in public institutions. He and his wife have three grown children, and currently live in Santa Rosa, California.

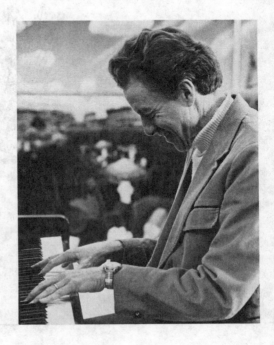

A Guided Fantasy
Deborah Rozman

Start by having the children sit with their backs straight, cross-legged and eyes closed, no one touching. Slowly tense and relax each body part, beginning with the toes, left foot, right foot, etc., up to the top of the head. Then say:

Breathe in slowly through your nose, keeping your mouth closed as I count to 5. Now hold to 5 (count 1-5). Now breathe out through your nose very slowly (count 1-5). (Repeat this five times with the children.) Now, keeping your eyes closed, look inside your forehead to the spot right between your two eyebrows and stare at that spot. That spot is one of the doors into the center of your being ... Now concentrate on that spot by putting everything you feel or think right there and see if you can feel a deep peace, deeper than when you sleep at night ... (pause) ... stay there with it, be still ... (pause ... if the children are ready, go on; otherwise bring them back at this point and repeat daily for a while) ... Feel a balloon inside that center. Now we are going to blow up our balloons. But these balloons are very special. They never burst, they just keep expanding and expanding and expanding. Feel your balloon expand. Now, blow it up in your mind a little bigger, and bigger, and bigger ... (pause) ... Feel it getting so big that it is bigger than your head and is expanding everywhere ... Feel it bigger than this room, feel it bigger than the city, bigger than the country, bigger than the oceans, bigger than the whole world ... (long pause) ... Now blow it up once more so that it is bigger than the whole universe and all the stars and the planets and the sun are inside your balloon too, and imagine that every idea and every thought and every feeling is inside the balloon ... (pause ... at the right time, depending on age of the children, bring them back, slowly) ... Now, letting the energy out of the balloon, coming back into the world, back into the room, back into the center ... Let's tense the body, take a deep breath, and open the eyes.

Excerpted from *Meditating With Children*, by Deborah Rozman (University of the Trees Press, Boulder Creek, CA).

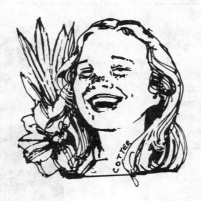

Creating Your Dream Career
Lynne Whiteley Novy

For many people, work is what you do to get money to buy things. But what if we could have our dreams come true? What if we could spend our time exactly as we want to? Very few of us would really want to spend our 16 or so waking hours a day under a palm tree. Knowing what we want to do enables us to do it. In this article Lynn Whiteley Novy presents information and exercises to help us create our dream career.

"In the process of growing up, many people lose their sense of magic, joy, and playfulness. They become part of the practical, logical, sensible world that is determined, predictable, and finite. They become adults and abandon the world of magic and dreams. They "fit in," earn a living, and make do with what they have. They have accepted the belief that life is hard, that people can't have what they want, and that you need to settle for what you get in life.

"You can argue for your limitations or you can be magical and powerful enough to make your dreams real. The choice is yours."

Cherie Carter-Scott

"You are
never given a wish
without also being given the
power to make it true.
You may
have to work for it,
however."

Richard Bach,
Illusions

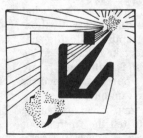 ife, for most people, is about fitting in. It starts with finding your place in the family— the oldest, the youngest, the kid in the middle, or the problem child, the model child, the only child—and then doing whatever it takes to get Mom and Dad's attention for performing the role. It goes on in school, figuring out the right an-swers to give teachers to get decent grades to get out of school so some university will let you in. And when you get into university, you pick a major, a slot to slide into at 18 that's supposed to lead to a career success at 40. Never mind that after slogging through law school you discover, before age 30, that you don't like spending your days doing what lawyers do.

"Fitting in" is the cornerstone of The Great American Myth that there is some *way* to be and some *thing* to do so that at some *time* in the future you'll have it made and life will be wonderful. Some people spend their whole lives in search of The Thing To Do That Will Make Life Turn Out.

In the search, we look to parents, teachers, counselors, wives, husbands, friends, and experts for advice. And they willingly narrow the field. Mom and Dad warn you to be practical in this time of economic crisis. The Bureau of Labor Statistics lists the fastest-growing employment fields in *The Occupational Outlook Handbook,* so you can fit into what's going to be hot in the next ten years. Employment counselors, in doom-filled tones, explain that the job market is tight, that MBAs are a dime a dozen, that more taxi drivers have PhDs than not, that teaching is flooded, and that you'd be lucky to land a job as a steno-typist or computer programmer. Almost everyone tells you to steer clear of the glamour fields— publishing is too competitive, fashion is too cut-throat, photography is too insecure.

In the good old days it was easy to find The Thing To Do. It was obvious. You just did what Dad did. Or you did what Mom did. Then, as now, most people fit themselves into a life's work based on possibilities, availabilities, other people's opinions and fears. Most never stop to ask, "Hey, wait a minute! How do I want to spend my days? What do I want?"

Looking inside yourself for the answer to the question, "What do I want to do with my life?" is the specialty of Motivation Management Service, Inc. (MMS), a San Francisco corporation dedicated to helping people discover their dreams and making them happen.

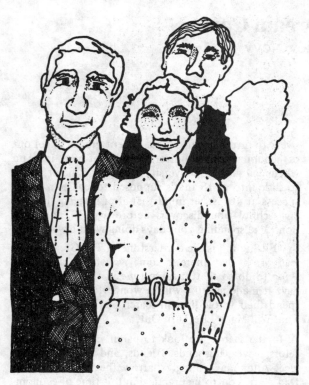

The myth of "fitting in" is that there is a particular *way* to be and *thing* to do that will make life turn out well.

The MMS approach is not about fitting in. It's about discovering within yourself the elements, or substance, of what turns you on in life and creating out of those things the form in which you will do it. You choose your career based not on an outer-centered reality—what the world says is available to you given what you look like, what you know or what your current skills are—but based on an inner-centered reality, doing those things that resonate to your inner self.

Founded in 1974 by Cherie Carter-Scott, MMS has two basic premises: people have inside them a beautiful and powerful place that knows what they want, trusts their choices, and loves themselves and others; and people can have their lives be exactly the way they want them to be. The discovery of "that place that knows" happens in a consulting process developed by Cherie out of her personal quest for what to do with her life. It's different from most consulting in that MMS consultants do not give advice or opinions. Instead, they ask questions that encourage people to look inside themselves to see what, in substance, they truly want, rather than what they *think*

they can have or what they're willing to accept. They then help the person put together a plan to realize what he or she wants.

SUBSTANCE vs. FORM

Usually when people are looking for what they want to do with their lives, they think in terms of a specific kind of career or job that already exists. They immediately want to know the *form:* will it be doctor, lawyer, beggarman, thief? At MMS people are invited to look for substance first without figuring out the form.

Before she started MMS, Cherie discovered that she loved being with people, and she liked asking questions without having to know all the answers or be an expert. She liked being around people who were willing to take risks, and she liked to see people inspired and excited about their innermost dreams. She also knew that whatever she did, she wanted to have fun and she wanted to be totally herself, however weird others might think her. This was the substance of what she wanted. If she had tried to attach an existing career form to this list, possibly MMS would never have been born. As it happened, Cherie began with consulting people and then developed workshops for people to break through the things about themselves that hold them back from having their lives the way they want them. Cherie's life's work has evolved into a philosophy that inspires people to rehabilitate their natural sense of inner knowing, so that they can make choices based on the true path of their being (inner-centered reality) rather than on the scattered voices of their mind telling them what they *should* do for the approval of others (outer-centered reality). To listen to your own inner voice and absolutely love yourself enough to trust your own choices against all odds and authority is so opposite to the way most people live that Cherie calls people who live their lives this way The New Species.

"Dreamers are always ridiculed and criticized by people who have accepted that they can't have what they want," Cherie says. "You can agree with those people and lead an acceptable, appropriate life that no one can criticize, or you can take risks and go beyond what is comfortable. To stick with what is safe and acceptable is to sacrifice your dream, to deny that feeling inside that makes you unique."

Each of us knows what we want if we are willing to look and if we are willing to tell the truth about what we hear from that little inner voice. It's risky to tell the truth about what we want because most of us don't believe we can have it. Our minds give us a thousand reasons why what we want won't work, isn't the right thing, is stupid, isn't viable, can't happen, and is impossible and impractical. What takes guts is trusting yourself enough to say what you want out loud and back yourself up by doing whatever it takes to make your dream real. You have to be willing to truly allow yourself to have what turns you on.

"The people who make a difference in this world are the people who go after their dreams," Cherie says. "They are the people who are willing to look inside, see what they want and move mountains to make it happen. They are willing to take risks and to be powerful enough to cause their dreams to become realities."

GETTING CLEAR

At MMS, consulting sessions allow people to look inside themselves and say what they want without judging it as right or wrong, good or bad, possible or not. The consultant directs the person and keeps him focused when it gets uncomfortable or seems hopeless and all he wants to do is say "I don't know," and escape to a hot fudge sundae or a cigarette.

The following exercises are ones that you can do by yourself with paper and pen. Be aware that in these processes you will be hearing from two different parts of yourself. The part you are looking for—the being—is the little voice that knows what things resonate to you, what things are fun, exciting, adventurous, meaningful for you. This part is most often felt coming from the center of your body; it's the part people refer to when they say, "I had a gut sense" about something. The other part—the mind—is usually a louder, more active voice in your head that tells you all the reasons you can't do or be or have what your being says you want. Sometimes the things your mind tells you sound like they are being said by someone else. Indeed, they often are things your Mom or Dad told you, information your teachers gave you, or warnings the government has issued.

For the purpose of these exercises, think of your mind as a tape recorder, and all those voices from the past as tapes recorded throughout your life. For the moment, suppose that you can just play those tapes, hear them, and not have to believe them or do what they say. Just let them play as you do the exercises and listen for the being's voice.

1. Make a list of all the things you love to do with your time. Travel, play tennis, make love, dance, write, talk to people, whatever. These are the things you would do if you could have it any way, if you

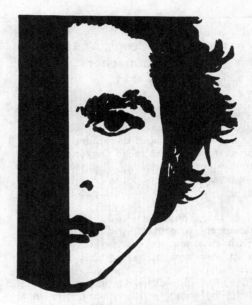

If you know you only had six months to live, how would you spend that time?

could do absolutely anything your heart desired, if money were no object, if you had no obligations. Write down whatever comes up. Just notice if your mind tells you that this is silly, if it gives you reasons why what you wrote is ridiculous or if it says that this is a waste of time. Hear what your mind says and then ask yourself again, "If I could have it any way, what would I do with my days?" You are not searching for a particular job or career field right now. You are just writing all the things you like to do, that turn you on. Keep writing until you feel the list is as complete as you can make it.

2. Shortly after you have completed the above list, the voices of your mind will probably come on like gangbusters. Take a clean sheet of paper and empty your head onto it. Write down all the doubts, fears, reasons why you can't have those things, admonitions about wasting your time, all the "shoulds" and the "what ifs." Probably one of the loudest refrains will be: "But I couldn't do just this stuff and support myself." Notice if your mind is immediately putting form to things, trying to fit your "wants" into a job category. When your mind runs out, put this paper aside and go on to the next exercise.

3. Make sure you are in a quiet place where you won't be disturbed for at least fifteen minutes. Close your eyes and center yourself. Take three deep, relaxing breaths. Now, in your mind's eye get a clear picture of yourself lying in your bed, awakening to-

Economics As If People Mattered:
E.F. Schumacher
Lorin Piper

"Human beings have both brains and hands and enjoy nothing more than being creatively and usefully productive, rendering service and acting in accordance with their moral impulses. Unfortunately, modern technology increasingly frustrates them in fulfilling all three of these very basic needs."

E. F. Schumacher

Right Livelihood is one of the eight paths to enlightenment presented by the Buddha; it is the path that concerns itself with work. The Buddhist sees work as having three purposes: to give a person a way to use and develop his faculties; to help him overcome his egocenteredness by joining with other people in a common task; and to produce the goods and services needed for existence.

Ernst Friedrich Schumacher, a student of Buddhism, was an economist whose primary concern was the quality of people's lives. As a Rhodes scholar in economics, an economic advisor to the British Control Commission in postwar Germany, and for twenty years the top economist and head of planning at the British Coal Board, he had the expertise and insight to deal effectively with economic policy. But despite his impressive credentials and a fine scientific upbringing, Schumacher was not afraid to consider spirit and conscience, moral purpose and the meaning of life as equally important for economic theory.

In 1973, his book *Small Is Beautiful: Economics As If People Mattered* was published. In it Schumacher tells us what we already know, but still need to hear: that our happiness has nothing to do with the gross national product. To concentrate only on material goods and their production and not on people is to be motivated by greed. And when we live in a world motivated by greed, everyone loses.

Schumacher's economic theory, as presented in *Small is Beautiful,* began to develop in 1955, when he was invited to Burma and other developing countries to assist their leaders in de-

All quotes and much of the information in this article come from an interview with E. F. Schumacher published in *Co-Evolution Quarterly.*

ciding what kind of help the West could give them. He soon found that really only one form of aid was available, and it required replacing the primitive tools of the developing countries with the huge machines and technologies of the west. "But," said Schumacher, "the developing nations did not have the industrial base they needed to support such technologically advanced systems, which meant that this 'answer' we were trying—indeed, are still trying—to force down their throats was no real answer at all.

Per capita income and statistics can be totally misleading when used to estimate the quality of people's lives.

To make the high technology we give them work, they need to make a tremendous investment of capital—which they do not have—in fuels and fertilizers, pesticides and spare parts, training programs and complicated machinery, almost none of which are now available in such countries. If they want these high-technology systems and equipment—and we do teach them to want them—there is only one place they can get such things: from us, and at our prices. What we are doing, you see, is offering the developing nations no real solution at all. We are merely showing them how to trade one form of bondage for another."

Schumacher became aware that what the developing countries could really use was an "intermediate technology": a technology that would tailor tools, small-scale machines, and methods of production to the needs of the countries themselves, a technology that uneducated people could understand and manage even on a village level.

In 1965 Schumacher founded the Intermediate Technology Development Group (ITDG) in London. The purpose of the organization was to "facilitate the flow of practical information about these technologies, conduct original research into new tools and methods, and in some cases take on the actual manufacture of IT equipment." One great IT story concerns the Zambian egg packer. A Zambian firm wanted a machine that made egg trays. When they approached a Western company to design it, they were given a proposal for a huge machine that would make a million trays a month. Schumacher said, "This was far beyond the needs or the resources of the Zambian packer; so we designed a miniplant that was just what the firm wanted. And our little plant was soon ordered by other Third World countries—then by the Canary Islands, Spain, Ireland, Canada, and even the United States. This and similar experiences soon taught us that the so-called 'advanced' nations frequently need as much help in scaling down their technologies as the emerging countries need in scaling theirs up."

Also while in Burma, Schumacher studied at a Buddhist school. Of this experience he said, "There, for the first time, I realized that you do not find clarity in the mind, but in the heart. And the heart will not speak to you unless you quiet yourself and liberate yourself from such masters as greed and envy. But if you can do this, you will find, in the stillness that follows, insights of wisdom that are obtainable in no other way. You will begin to see things as they really are. You will become enlightened. The Buddhists call this vipassana. Well, I don't claim to have attained vipassana, but I did come away from Burma with a different view of things. And in the beginning, as I saw my life in this new light, I was very unhappy. The things I had been doing had ceased to make sense.

"But then I realized that 'life must go on,' that I must apply my new insights to what had become my life's work. And as I struggled to do that, I gave various lectures and wrote papers. And they were compiled eventually into the book *Small Is Beautiful.*

"So I did not set out to change economic theory. I set out to find the answers to the metaphysical questions that bothered me. *Small Is Beautiful* just happened to be one of the outcomes of that very personal quest."

It was in Burma that Schumacher also discovered that per capita income and statistics can be totally misleading when used to estimate the quality of people's lives. When he went to Burma in 1955, it had an annual per capita income of $50.00. And yet he met there people who were extremely happy. They ate and dressed well, and they lived in beautiful houses suited to their climate. They had no time-saving devices, and yet they had plenty of leisure time which they enjoyed. The simple and gracious lives of the people in Burma contrasted sharply with the "more is better" theory of the West. Schumacher saw life in America and Germany as full of pressures and constant agitation. He saw England as somewhere in between, being both underdeveloped and overdeveloped, and he realized that he felt comfortable in England. This gave him an idea which he says he was tempted to release as the first Law of Economics: "The amount of real leisure a society enjoys tends to be in inverse proportion to the amount of labor-saving machinery it employs."

(continued on p. 300)

morrow morning. Get a clear picture of the setting—what nightclothes you're wearing, items that are in the room, what the light is like. You are feeling fabulous this particular morning. You know it's a beautiful day, and you can't wait for it to begin. With the rest of this process, you will take yourself on a fantasy excursion through your perfect day. This is a day you would live tomorrow if you could have your life be exactly the way you want it. Ask yourself specific questions and lead yourself on this journey moment by moment, letting yourself go wherever the fantasy takes you. The more attention you give to detail, the more deeply you can be involved in this process and the more you can take from it. The kinds of directions you might give yourself include asking yourself "What do I do then?" as you get out of bed. Watch

the answer play in the movie of your mind. Describe in detail the clothes you put on ("what would really feel good to wear this morning?"). Do you have breakfast? If so, what favorite foods do you eat? At home or in a restaurant? Follow yourself through a whole day until you return to bed at night. Try not to judge; just let the movie play and see where you go, what you do.

After the fantasy, open your eyes and write down all of the things in your perfect day that seem important to remember.

4. Take a clean sheet of paper and pretend that you have just received advance information on your life delivered through a reliable source that you trust totally. The advance information is that six months from now you will be struck by lightning. Write down

(continued from p. 299)

In *Small Is Beautiful,* in his essay on Buddhist economics, Schumacher points out the differences between Buddhist and modern economics. The modern economist is used to measuring the standard of living by the amount of annual consumption, assuming that the person who consumes more is better off than the person who consumes less. A Buddhist economist would, on the other hand, see consumption simply as a means to human well-being, and would consider the goal to be maximizing well-being while minimizing consumption. Whereas the modern economist sees work as nothing more than a necessary evil, the Buddhist sees work as a primary vehicle for forming a person's character, and Buddhism sees purification of character as the essence of civilization. Of the "more is better" theory, Schumacher has said, "Karl Marx was right 150 years ago, when he said, 'Be careful. If you build too many useful machines, you will soon have too many useless people.'"

Everything has become too complex. And, just as Marx foresaw, this complexity and sophistication has made us useless. It distracts us, puts so much strain on us, and makes us so narrowminded, so bothered, and so specialized that we no longer have time to become wise.

We have, you see, in a way, advanced into hell. We have become a society rich in means, but poor in purpose, and I do indeed think it worthwhile to change that situation. I believe that a gentler technology, a technology with a human face, could once again take control of work away from the machines and put it back into the hands of the average worker. I'm talking only of returning our society to a human scale, of putting people in charge of their destinies once more. I'm talking about overthrowing the machine in favor of the tool. As Gandhi said, we do not need mass production, but production by the masses.

Mass production is sophisticated and highly capital-intensive, and gulps down ever-increasing amounts of energy. It concentrates the people who use it into crowded cities, and is inherently violent, ecologically damaging, self-defeating in its demands on natural resources, and stultifying for the individuals who must make it work.

The intermediate technology which makes production by the masses possible is vastly superior to the primitive technology of bygone ages, but much simpler, less expensive, and less oppressive than the supertechnology which now dominates our society. One might call intermediate technology a "self-help" or a "democratic" or a "people's" technology. I call it the hope of the future.

E. F. Schumacher died in 1978. His work and words become more relevant with every passing day. As he tells us, we have two great teachers in life: nature, and the wisdom of the ages as embodied in the great religious teachings of the world. To put aside greed for the sake of the good, the true, and the beautiful is to give our lives values worth living for and worth working for.

everything that is important for you to experience, do, produce, have, accomplish between now and your final day. If you knew you only had six months, what are the things you would do, the ways you would spend your time between now and then?

5. Review what you wrote in exercises 1, 3, and 4, and underline or list on a separate sheet the items or themes that recur or seem particularly important. These are the elements—the substance—of what you want. Take each element and write out the qualities of that particular thing which make it a turn-on for you. For example, some of the turn-on qualities of tennis might be that it is fast-paced, involves competition on an individual rather than team basis, and is physically very active.

Review and hone down all your lists until you have one clear list of specific things you want to do, specific qualities that you want in your days, and specific items that are important in terms of your whole life.

6. Read your list several times. Let yourself experience being excited by the things you have written. Now, ask yourself very clearly the following question: "If I could have it any way, what would I do that I would call career?" If you get an immediate answer, a clear one that seems to come right out of your core, you'll know instantly. If you go blank, just notice that the answer is not apparent yet. If you get a Ping Pong match between your mind and your being, in which your being voice tells you an an-

swer to the question and your mind voice censors it, just notice that there is an answer you may not be ready to hear just yet. Wherever you are at this point is perfect.

Sometimes people get a clear announcement of exactly what they want to do, and then proceed to make it happen. Often people get a clear idea of the ideal elements that resonate, but they do not yet know what form it will take.

One of Cherie's early clients was sure that there was no way she could have the elements of what she wanted in a career. At 40, when surgery ended her singing career, she was terrified because she thought she did not have "marketable skills." During consulting, she saw that the three things that turned her on most were shopping for beautiful clothes, eating out at terrific restaurants, and speaking French. Although this seemed to her not a lot to work with, she agreed to trust the process and to allow for the possibility that she really could have what she wanted even though she hadn't a clue what it would look like. Her homework was to do some research, even though she didn't know what she was researching exactly, at clothing stores, restaurants, and places where French is spoken. The end result was magical. Within two weeks, she took a sales job at a fashionable clothing store. Her first week on the job, the store manager discovered that she spoke fluent French, and invited her to act as guide and translator for a famous designer who was in town from Paris. Her job was working in a fashion environment where she got to speak French while eating out at fancy restaurants.

The key is to discover what you want substantively and *know* that form will follow. The scary part is totally trusting yourself to know what you want and to continue to trust when it seems you haven't a clue how it will materialize, and everyone around you thinks you're crazy.

PUTTING TOGETHER A PLAN

Your plan can be a long-range broad sweep to your ultimate goal, or it can be a short-term plan for the next phase, or both. Whatever its scope, it must be specific and must set out clear steps for you to follow.

1. Write a statement of the end result you want from this plan. If you do not yet know the form your new career will take, your end result for this phase might be to create form from the elements that you want it to have. Write as detailed a description of what you want to have happen as you can.

2. Write an open-ended general list of all the things you can think of that you could do or must do en-

---

Work
Margaret M. Stevens

There is a story about a man who died and found himself in a beautiful place, surrounded by every conceivable comfort. A white-jacketed man came to him and said, "You may have anything you choose—any food—any pleasure—any kind of entertainment."

The man was delighted, and for days he sampled all the delicacies and experiences of which he had dreamed on earth. But one day he grew bored with all of it, and calling the attendant to him, he said "I'm tired of all this. I need something to do. What kind of work can you give me?"

"The attendant sadly shook his head and replied, "I'm sorry, sir. That's the one thing we can't do for you. There is no work here for you."

To which the man answered, "That's a fine thing. I might as well be in hell."

The attendant said softly, "Where do you think you are?"

Margaret M. Stevens,
Prosperity is God's Idea

---

route to the result. Empty your head of all the possible things, large or small, without thought about the order of them.

3. Go back and review the list. Break complicated items into small pieces, and use active verbs to state each thing to be done. Specific, clearly stated items that tell you exactly what to do to complete them get done. Things that have undefined pieces are hard to confront. For instance, "Call Jack Simon for appointment about bank loan" is likely to get action more quickly than "Investigate bank loans."

4. When your to-do list is as complete as you can make it, go through the whole list again, and put dates beside each item to show when you will have that piece done. If you think you don't know a date, just take a guess and put one down anyway.

5. If your plan is a long one, you may want to rewrite it in order of deadlines. This document is your blueprint and timeline to reach the result you have stated you want. The next step is to take the item with the nearest deadline and go do it.

GOING FOR IT

For most people, getting clear on what they want is fun and fairly easy. Putting together a plan is often uncomfortable, but it's exciting to see things taking shape. Where the going gets tough is in backing the choice, committing to it, and going for it 100 per cent. At MMS, this is called the support phase of consulting.

A natural reaction for most of us when we begin to see what we want and how we could make it real is fear. Somehow it's scary to be on the road to having what you want. There's a statement of personal power in claiming that you are going to make something important happen just because it's what you want. People around you will tell you that you can't do it—unless they are doing what they want themselves.

Find at least one person who can support you in realizing your dream, someone who believes you can do it and who wants you to have it and who won't get in your way with opinions, judgments, or advice. Tell that person exactly what you want him to do to support you. And then let him. You may want him to listen to you without judging or giving unwanted advice. You may want him to do some of the things on your plan with you. You may want him to have a copy of your timeline so that he can ask you how you're doing with meeting your deadlines.

However you set it up, you are, of course, your own best support. You must trust yourself and back your own choice against all odds. The payoff is having a dream Thing To Do that's fun for you, that's true to you, that turns you on because it's right for you. You don't have to look for a place to fit into; you *are* the place.

SUGGESTIONS FOR FURTHER READING

Richard Bach, *Illusions*. Delacorte Press, 1977.
Richard Nelson Bolles, *What Color Is Your Parachute?* Ten Speed Press, 1972.
Harry Browne, *How I Found Freedom in An Unfree World*. Macmillan, 1973.
Cherie Carter-Scott, *The New Species*. Motivation Management Service, Inc., 1978.
Tom Jackson, *Guerrilla Tactics in the Job Market*. Bantam, 1978.

Lynne Whiteley Novy, who has claimed since age six that her primary purpose in life is to do all the adventures of the world, has created several dream careers for herself. She spent eight years in New York as a travel-magazine editor, which allowed her to discover purposeful adventures throughout the world while being paid for the privilege. She is now living in San Francisco, where she is general manager of Motivation Management Service, Inc. She created her current dream career by means of the consulting sessions described in this article.

Cooperative Group Dynamics
Anne Robbins, M.A.

The mutual support of a cooperative group is a highly rewarding experience. It is also something very difficult to achieve. Learning to be effective and responsible in a group is a way of learning about being effective and responsible in the world. It is a communication skill that can immeasurably enrich our lives. One of the most precious rewards of the Berkeley Holistic Health Center has been the opportunity to share our strengths and weaknesses in a group situation and to know a group energy that is more than the sum of its parts. In this article Anne Robbins presents some guidelines that she has found valuable in her work with group process.

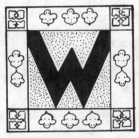 hy is it so important to learn cooperative communication in groups? This article deals with the issue of groups for two reasons. (1) Groups are inevitable. This modern, crowded Earth demands a high level of association between members of our species to exist, to procreate, to survive. These associations can be loose or tightly knit, from workers in a big business to roommates. (2) In addition, groups have become a conscious choice for many people. We have chosen groups to combat loneliness, to form ecologically and economically efficient living units, to create businesses, families, social and community change, etc. Given the close quarters of both chosen and inevitable groups, we have some choices to make about the nature and structure of our relationships.

Why do we need to learn to cooperate in these groups? Even if we choose to acknowledge our inevitable interconnectedness and to seek cooperative communication, this may not be enough to combat the alienation, intimidation, or inefficiency many of us experience in groups. We see a loneliness around us that results much more from individuals' not knowing how to relate to each other in a group than from a scarcity of people. We "can't see the forest for the trees." The special complexity of group interaction thus demands that we learn of a clear and ordered process for working in groups, one that encompasses both emotional and objective goals.

Moving toward these goals can be confusing and difficult. We're not only taking new roads in the world, but finding it necessary to build new roads inside ourselves. How do we propose to do this pioneering work? What are some of the roadblocks? What plans make for a smooth, efficient, and joyful process? In this article, I outline the steps of a planning process that have proven effective.

A. DEVELOP AGREED-UPON, CLEAR OBJECTIVES

What are we doing here together? What are we about? A clear definition of goals should be established; e.g., "We're here to support each other in solving personal problems," or "We want to get a collective backery business going." In personal problem-solving groups, members can construct simple statements of purpose to indicate to the group the work they're "contracting" to do. Begin by suggesting, "Fantasize about 100 per cent of what you want (not what you think you can get), and we'll work from there." This concept of agreed-upon, clear objectives paves the way for the work of the group.

B. ESTABLISH AGREED-UPON METHODS OF OBTAINING GOALS

How shall we proceed? How do we want responsibility delegated, decisions made? What are the standards of performance? How can members be accountable to the group? Establish clear guidelines. This is especially important in nonhierarchical groups, where the absence of structure may constitute a tyranny in itself. To keep the work joyful and efficient, people's work goals should realistically match their available time and interest.

303

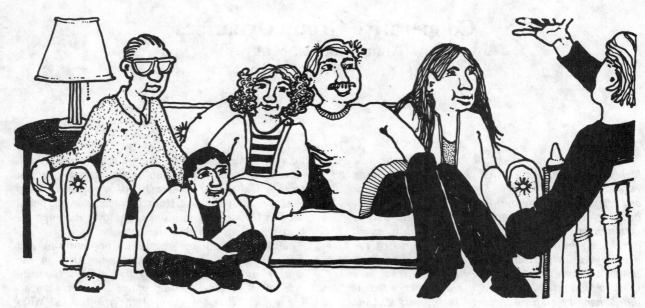

The special complexity of group interaction demands that we develop a clear and ordered process for working together that encompasses both emotional and objective goals.

Other important questions are: What are the ground rules for group process? How can we most efficiently structure meetings? Members can indicate on a sign-up sheet what (and how much time) they want on the agenda. It's also advisable to have someone (this can be a rotating function) be responsible for the cooperative management of time. She or he may also maintain an objective overview, contributing observations about group process and communication transactions. This may involve mediating a conflict, pointing out repetition, digressions, and interruptions, and in general doing what is needed to smooth out snarls in communication.

C. BE HONEST WITH EACH OTHER ABOUT CRITICISM, APPRECIATION, AND OTHER IMPORTANT FEELINGS

This is central to the group's vitality and efficiency. Agreed-upon methods, goals, and standards are effective only if they are reinforced by people's honest responses.

1. "CHECK-IN."

It's important to share feelings that detract from your presence in the group. The energy it takes to hold back a feeling can seriously diminish a member's

contribution, and the uncomfortable side effects of withheld feelings are contagious. If covered or obscured, they can be reflected and magnified to dangerous proportions, sucking in the rest of the group's energy. We really do exert profound influences on each other. It's helpful to start out meetings with a "check-in," during which each member briefly states how she or he is feeling at that moment. This combats withdrawal, connects people, and identifies the atmosphere. E.g., "I'm feeling really tired from studying all night; I may want to lay low this group." This may free other members from wondering if the person was angry at them, displeased with the group, etc.

2. STRUCTURE AN EVALUATION PERIOD AT THE END, FOR CRITICISM, SELF-CRITICISM, FEEDBACK, APPRECIATION.

Here you can pick up on anything important that may have been overlooked during the meeting. In our competitive culture, there is often great hesitancy about offering either critical or appreciative feedback. A structured evaluation helps people learn these skills and ensures that this important task gets done. Some helpful focusing questions are: How did it feel in here? What went wrong? How could it have been improved? What went right? What did I really like in this meeting?

3. SHARE FEEDBACK AND CRITICISM COOPERATIVELY.

Since we're taught to withhold and reject criticism or appreciation, love or anger, we need to cooperate to express ourselves.

a. Ask someone if they want to hear your feedback. "I feel angry; can I tell you about it?"

b. Make feedback simple and to the point. "I feel X (angry) when you do Y (interrupt me)."

c. Say what you want. "I want you to let me finish."

d. When receiving, if you don't want the feedback, make some arrangement to hear it at a later time.

e. Try to take it in rather than respond defensively. Look for the truth in it.

Because of our competitive programming, positive appreciation and strokes may be even harder to give and receive.

a. Look inside for what you like, anything from efficiency to someone's pretty blue shirt. Group work is challenging; we need and deserve appreciation.

b. State it simply and directly (not comparatively). "You look good" as opposed to "You look so much better today."

c. When receiving, many feel so undeserving that they feel compelled to discount the stroke with a "Yes, but . . ." counterstatement or a quick, embarrassed "I like you too." Don't respond; take it in.

4. ARRANGE PERIODIC LARGE BLOCKS OF TIME FOR THE GROUP'S EVALUATION OF ITSELF AS A WHOLE. DO WE LIKE OUR FORMAT? HOW DO WE FEEL ABOUT WORKING WITH EACH OTHER? HOW IS POWER DISTRIBUTED? ARE WE ACCOMPLISHING OUR GOALS?

D. EXPOSE COMPETITION

This is an important guideline to keep the group running smoothly and effectively. Competition may take many forms and have many causes, but one thing it universally thrives on is secrecy. It grows to looming proportions when unexposed, but loses its power in the daylight. Once it is exposed, the group can examine its origins and make necessary changes.

In general, it takes at least two competitors for there to be competition; the assumption is that no one person causes it. It's helpful if the two persons reveal *how* they feel "one-up" or "one-down," and what they get out of their respective roles. This cuts back on the vague unconditional quality which is necessary for the competitive stance (e.g., "I'm just a lousy speaker.")

Competition can be evoked by an overcrowded agenda, a lack of recognition for work done, withheld feelings, and unexposed disagreements. With so much emphasis on supportive collectivity, we may easily gloss over important differences. In dealing with competition, we find that in fact some of us *are* better at some things than others. Some of us do more than others. Some of us have conflicting values, and not everyone can work cooperatively and lovingly with everyone else. Working with this may mean, for example, a more-skilled member training a less-skilled, a person getting appreciation for work done, or exposing the nature and effects of our class backgrounds. In dealing with competition, the group cooperatively recognizes uniqueness and differences.

E. USE THE GROUP

The group can offer a powerful reflection of people and situations. Because group feedback is more difficult to discount than feedback received from isolated individuals, the group becomes more than the sum of its parts. Cultivate trust in the group (by means of honesty, checking out fears, asking for what you want, etc.) and use it.

In our individualistic and privatized culture, we're often denied the gift of discovering how others see us. This can be a powerful tool for self-growth. In addition, you can use the group for protection and support during conflict with another member. "How do other people see this?" This power of the group (created by other members' honest responses) can also make it safe for you to assert your wants without feeling like you're being "pushy."

Not involving the group can lead to some serious problems. One of these I call "minority rules." Here, the group bends over backward to not "gang up" on someone. Although most of the people in the group may have extreme conflicts with this individual, they keep it under their hat. As a result the whole group gets run covertly (in a backward direction). If you use the group here, it will be discovered that this is more than a series of individual differences, and action can be recommended. Sometimes, however, using the group may mean taking responsibility for calling in an agreed-upon, outside, objective mediator to deal with group "blind spots."

An Energy Circle
Margo Adair

This meditation should take five to ten minutes, and should shorten your meeting by enabling everyone to work together so effectively that it will more than pay for itself in time alone. Have someone read it, or ad lib an approximation to it, or make a tape that can be used and reused. If it's uncomfortable to hold hands, simply sit in silence with eyes closed.

1. First, undo anything around your waist that constricts your breathing. Sit so everyone can hold hands if possible. Hold hands and close your eyes.

2. Take a few moments simply to focus on your breathing, breathing with your belly, allowing your breath to find its most comfortable rhythm, as relaxed as a sleeping baby. . . . Imagine bringing in calming energy when you inhale. . . . Imagine releasing tension as you exhale, however you imagine this to occur. . . . Take a few moments to allow yourself to become fully present, in this place, at this time. . . .

3. Imagine a pool of energy around the base of your spine. Imagine it beginning to sink down into the Earth, drawn down by gravity, through the chair, the floor, all the way down through all the layers of the Earth . . . connecting to the very center of the Earth. Have this band of energy go further and further down with each exhalation of breath. Let any tensions of anything else distracting you from the tasks at hand go down into the Earth, carried by this band of energy that moves to the core of the Earth. . . . Imagine that occurring. . . .

4. Now imagine the band becoming a circuit of energy, as though you had roots drawing the calming, stabilizing energy of the Earth up into your body, up the cord, and your other tensions going down it. . . . Imagine feeling Earth energy spreading through the whole of your body, enabling you to feel the substance of which you're made, feeling very aware of your body, of your connection to the Earth . . . focused and relaxed.

5. Now become aware of the energy in the air, the energy of the sky, of the sun, . . . the moon, . . . of all the planets, the stars, the weather patterns, the energy of the air, of the sky. . . .

6. Now imagine drawing some of that energy in through the top of your head, . . . letting it tingle down through every cell of your body, . . . mixing with the Earth energy and then moving out again, either out through your feet, or out through the top of your head, or wherever you're inclined to let it go out. . . .

7. Now feel the potency of these universal energies moving through us, clearing us to be able to work together creatively. . . .

8. Feel the energy we create together . . . our collective energy; feel it moving around the circle as though it were moving into our left hands and out our right. Building momentum, powerful collective energies drawing us together, energy connecting each of us, creating a new whole . . . a collective consciousness . . . Energy we can use to create change . . .

9. Now focus on our intention of coming together today: our common purpose . . . what brings us together . . . what goals we share . . .

10. Go over the agenda in your mind. See us working through issues with ease, making clear decisions, harnessing and organizing our energies for our shared tasks. Notice how all this is happening. . . .

11. Notice how you need to be to best support the group, what interests you need to put aside, what interests you need to share. . . . Decide if you are willing to do these things. . . . See us all working together cooperatively.

12. See the meeting ending at an appropriate time. See everyone leaving, energized, feeling good about the shared work, a renewed reenergized commitment to the shared purpose. See yourselves succeeding in our overall goals. Notice what needs to happen for this to occur. . . .

13. Review your feelings and thoughts, any choices you've made, and open your eyes when you feel inclined, knowing that this energy will continue to carry us through this meeting, enabling us to fully cooperate and work together creatively. . . .

If the group would be uncomfortable with the complete exercise, you may choose to omit Paragraphs 3 through 8, and replace them with the following:

Let our silence give us the space we need to adjust ourselves to the task at hand. . . . Feel the energy we create together in this room . . . letting ourselves settle into being here together, affirming our common concerns. . . . Feel our collective power, feel what connects us, creating a greater whole of powerful energy we can use to create change.

Margo Adair is a socialist-feminist who over the last nine years has developed Applied Meditation, using the meditative state for practical problem solving. During this time she has also worked with people in halfway houses, drug treatment programs, and jails. Much of her focus has been on teaching Applied Meditation skills to activists to enable them to work more effectively to create change, and for a number of years she has also conducted forums addressing the relationship between politics and spirituality. She maintains a practice in San Francisco, conducting support groups, working indi-

vidually, and teaching. She travels around the country holding workshops and consulting. She is now writing a book on her work. Margo is a member of a collective which is currently compiling articles for publication addressing the issue of progressive politics and spirituality. For the past two and one-half years, this collective has applied the philosophy of dialectical materialism to understanding spiritual energies.

Tapes of this meditation and others addressing issues in the realm of personal problem solving and healing, community awareness, and organization development are available through:
Margo Adair
P.O. Box 11503
San Francisco, CA 94101

F. DEVELOP PROCESS SKILLS: WHAT TO WATCH FOR

Groups consist of potentially complex and powerful sets of relationships. It helps if we have our attentive antennae out during meetings to pick up on important information. Watch for the distribution, the quality, and the amount of energy in the room.

Define the feeling. Is it sleepy, heavy, exciting, lopsided, loving? Nurture the group by exposing it, and use the group by asking if others share your experience. "It seems really quiet in here; what's going on?" If you're bored, look into it. Is there something you're afraid of or something you want? Is the process off (abstract, phony, etc.)? Often it's good to expose this even if you don't have a tidy packaged explanation. The group can help you get to it. This unleashes creative potential, refocuses, revitalizes, and brings the group closer together. We are *a group,* not isolated individuals in the same room. Something is going on between us.

IN CONCLUSION

After all this, you may be feeling that this sounds like a lot of work. You're right. It's hard, because we're not supposed to cultivate powerful, loving support systems. We've been brought up to compete in secrecy. Wanting help may reflect our failure in this competitive matrix. Criticism and anger may be seen as provocative, and sharing love (especially openly in a group) as an embarassing loss of self-esteem. Ex-

posing these origins of the difficulty of working in groups helps develop strategies for change.

The dominant cultural values are internalized deep inside us, influencing our relations with ourselves and each other. Challenging these values necessitates profound transformations of ourselves and our relations. We're inventing new language. Primitive halting steps become powerful and sophisticated movements. Although we've been told differently, we're finding that it works.

SUGGESTIONS FOR FURTHER READING

Claude Steiner, "Cooperation," *Issues in Radical Therapy,* Vol. II, No. 4 (Autumn 1974).

Thomas Szasz, *The Myth of Mental Illness.* Harper and Row, 1961.

Mao Tse-Tung, "On Contradiction," in *Four Essays on Philosophy.* Peking: Foreign Language Press, 1968.

Jerome Agel, *The Radical Therapist.* Ballantine, 1972.

———, *Rough Times.* Ballantine, 1973.

Anne Robbins (M.A. in Community Psychology), member of Turning Point Radical Psychiatry Collective, has led women's and mixed problem-solving groups for more than eight years, been a mediational consultant for groups and families in trouble, and counselled individuals. She has taught classes at many schools and community centers in the Bay Area, and is the author of Combatting Powerlessness *and* Why Groups Are Better.

The Needs of the Person Are the Needs of the Planet
Theodore Roszak

We are all aware of the important contributions of the ecology movement on behalf of our suffering environment. In this article, Theodore Roszak, one of our most original social thinkers, outlines another, entirely different environmental strategy, one which may be developing on an unprecedented scale, with enough force to save the planet in the eleventh hour of her need. It is a force which originates within each of us and seeks to assert its fragile beauty even beneath the pervasive shadow of our industrialized world. It is a movement that is at once individualistic and planetary, for, as Professor Roszak so eloquently argues, "the needs of the person are the needs of the planet."

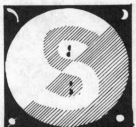 uppose the Earth is a sentient being, capable, in her own mysterious way, of intelligent adaptation and skillful maneuver for the sake of defending her life-giving mission in the universe.

If you wish, take the supposition to be no more than a convenient hypothesis, and formulate it as objectively as possible, as in the "Gaia hypothesis," which proposes that we conceive of the Earth's "living matter, the air, the oceans, the land surface [as] parts of a giant system . . . able to control temperature, the composition of the air and sea, the pH of the soil and so on, so as to be optimum for the survival of the biosphere. The system [seems] to exhibit the behavior of a single organism, even a living creature."

But if the hypothesis is convenient, why not yield to its poetry as well? For the Earth is in no way more beautifully known to us than in the ancient imagery of goddess and mother.

Further: suppose that we, in body, mind, and spirit, are subtly crafted into the fabric of the planet's

sentience as her risky experiment in self-conscious intellect.

Finally, suppose that the experiment we represent has become so dangerously infatuated with its monkey cunning, its remarkable power to subjugate and reshape, that it now jeopardizes the integrity of that global biosphere.

What, then, does the Earth do with her mischievous human children to change their lethal ways?

We might regard the sudden prominence of professional ecology as one recourse she tries. At the eleventh hour, she brings a small contingent of biologists around to the most comprehensive science of all, the systematic study of the planetary whole as the arena where culture and nature interact.

But ecology, although an indispensable expedient and one that has rallied a significant public concern, cannot rescue us on its own. It is too highly technical, too much of a specialist's approach.

The countless local pollutions that assail us each day may be irritating or ugly enough to force piecemeal adjustments here and there, now and then. But the big issues, the questions of species-wide survival and of planetary life and death that require us to rethink our culture from the ground up—the health of the atmosphere and all the seas, the vitality of the soil, the warming (or is it the cooling?) of the polar ice caps, the stability of the ozone, the future of the world food supply—these are vast imponderables for the layman to take in. Regarding such bewildering matters, the specialists might go on arguing for decades. And we may not have decades.

So—let us imagine—the Earth, in the urgency of her need, hits upon another strategy of survival, a course of wise indirection that does not at first glance look even remotely "ecological." She transforms our moral identity, working from within us to find the one motivation that is most capable of changing our bad environmental habits.

I speak of the Earth as an intentional agency, a mother striving to preserve and nurture her living variety, to emphasize that any hint of environment self-regulation which enters our ecological thought ties us to the oldest natural philosophy of our species: the worship of the Great Goddess.

We need a political ethic which is not bound to the alienated identities of individualism or collectivism. And this, I believe, is the sense of identity that the Earth brings us now as an ecological corrective: the sense of ourselves as persons, each unique, radically original, possessed of an unpredictable destiny. It is the self as Whitman sang of it in his great song: "Each of us inevitable/Each of us limitless/Each of us here as divinely as any is here . . ./I sing the songs of the glory of none, not God, sooner than I sing the songs of the glory of you./Whoever you are! Claim your own at any hazard!"

No one can say in any detail what kind of world comes of such a shameless celebration of the self. I suppose the prescription is for a Taoist anarchy, an organic commonwealth of all peoples, beings, entities, and existences. But we have no blueprints for such a future, no grand designs. Only of this much am I certain: we are at a juncture in history where personal psychology and planetary ecology—the world of nature Out There and the universe of consciousness In Here—join forces to subvert the urban-industrial dominance.

The person and the planet. Here is a connection, a political connection, which is a distinctly contemporary discovery, one that could become apparent only after our economic institutions had reached a certain critical size and complexity, a certain dizzy level of dynamism and unfeeling efficiency. Only now do we happen upon a contradiction in the social system that may be far more potent than the class contradictions to which Marx pinned his revolutionary hopes.

We are undergoing the subtle interaction which the Earth uses to protect herself from our ecocidal pressure. As the scale of industrial activity mounts, so also (at least along one important line of contemporary dissent in Western society) do our expectations of personal freedom and fulfillment. This, in turn, becomes an obstacle to the further expansion and integration of the system. So the system begins to disintegrate, a fitful process that gets registered in the news of the day as truancy in the schools, the soaring divorce rate, declining morale and rising turnover in the work force, the demise of military conscription, a growing reluctance to compete and conform, a general distrust of leaders, experts, official ideals, public institutions, . . . in brief, the spreading ethos of cynicism and recalcitrance that social theorists refer to as "the twilight of authority," "the crisis of legitimation," etc. But this disintegration is essentially creative, for, in our rising sense of personhood, we find

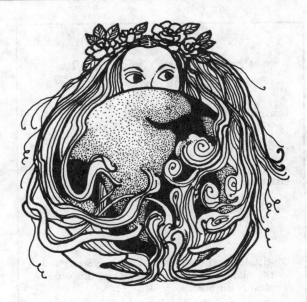

The Earth is in no way more beautifully known to us than in the ancient imagery of goddess and mother.

a peculiarly postindustrial quality of life that is wholly incompatible with the mass processing of superscale systems. In asserting the human scale, we subvert the regime of bigness. In subverting bigness, we save the planet.

Because our social thought is still torn between individualistic and collectivistic alternatives, many commentators overlook the originality and promise of such personalistic values. Think for a moment of the humanistic and human potential therapies, and of the New Age religions that have flowered so prominently in our society over the last generation. There are critics who can see nothing in these forms of deep introspection and self-discovery but a disgraceful lack of social responsibility; they are therefore quick to put these exercises down as "narcissistic," "self-indulgent," "escapist." The parajournalist Tom Wolfe sees no more in the scene than "me, me, me" and traces it all back to "groin spasms."

Like everything else that becomes widespread and popular in our society, the search for personhood can become tainted with the selfishness and acquisitiveness of bourgeois individualism. It can be vulgarized into a commodity, an entertainment, an opiate. All this is too obvious for words.

But what such quick, negative criticism ignores is the fact that, where these forms of self-discovery achieve their highest purpose (as they often do), they awaken in people a vivid awareness of their incommensurable uniqueness and provide ingenious means

Prayer for the Great Family
Gary Snyder

Gratitude to Mother Earth, sailing through
    night and day—and to her soil: rich, rare,
    and sweet
        in our minds so be it.

Gratitude to Plants, the sun-facing light-changing
    leaf and fine root-hairs; standing still through
    wind and rain; their dance is in the flowing
    spiral grain
        in our minds so be it.

Gratitude to Air, bearing the soaring Swift and
    the silent Owl at dawn. Breath of our song
    clear spirit breeze
        in our minds so be it.

Gratitude to Wild Beings, our brothers, teaching
    secrets, freedoms, and ways; who share with
    us their milk; self-complete, brave, and aware
        in our minds so be it.

Gratitude to Water: clouds, lakes, rivers,
    glaciers; holding or releasing; streaming
    through all our bodies salty seas
        in our minds so be it.

Gratitude to the Sun: blinding pulsing light
    through trunks of trees, through mists,
    warming caves where bears and snakes sleep
    —he who wakes us—
        in our minds so be it.

Gratitude to the Great Sky
    who holds billions of stars—and goes
    yet beyond that—
    beyond all powers, and thoughts
    and yet is within us—
    Grandfather Space.
    The Mind is his Wife.
        so be it.

        after a Mohawk prayer

for shaping a free identity: "doing one's own thing" in a sense that I think Socrates would have recognized as a commendable attempt at self-knowledge.

Perhaps the most impressive personalist manifestation of our day can be found in the many "liberation" movements that have emerged during the last decade in all the industrial societies: women's lib, kids' lib, gay lib, gray lib, cons' lib, mad lib, fat lib, handicapped lib. We have no sociological category for such groups with their highly selective, psychologically sophisticated forms of consciousness raising. They do not aspire to become mass movements or political parties; they are not "workers of the world" uniting into a disciplined rank and file. On the contrary, they insist on being small, autonomous, intensely intimate. For want of a better name, I have called them "situational netwroks": loose associations of our society's many victims held together by the bonds of shared suffering.

Surely no society in history has ever identified such a varied spectrum of a victimization: displaced homemakers, homosexual Native Americans, battered wives, impotent men, inorgasmic women, disabled transvestites, unwed fathers, hookers, lesbian mothers, former cancer patients, the terminally ill . . . the list goes on and on. Is there anybody who isn't a victim these days?

What is it people find in situational groupings? Yes, they find mutual aid and consolation, perhaps a means of self-defense. But most immediately they find confessional freedom, self-revelation, the healing affirmation of fellow victims. The situational group may be the one sanctuary in our big, busy, bullying world where people can come together to tell their tale, sing their song, and so find full personal recognition for all that they are as victims and (most importantly) for all that they are besides victims. In the situational networks, troubled and stigmatized souls help one another toward the self-knowledge that lies beyond shame, fear, failure, and the suffocating stereotypes of the world. The networks are a means of casting off assigned identities—"old," "gay," "female," "disabled," "addict," "ex-con"— and of asserting oneself as a surprising and delightful event in the universe.

How different all this is from the class consciousness and political agitation in which left-wing ideologies of the past specialized. Yes, here too we have an assertion of solidarity among the oppressed. But how much more refined are the varieties of suffering; how much greater the indictment of urban-industrial wrongs! Moreover, the victimized identities we deal with here are clearly seen as barriers to self-discovery that must be "worked through," redeemed, finally transcended.

"Class," we are coming to see, has never been a positive and fulfilling identity; it is, at best, a means of collective resistance, an instrument of power. But for self-discovery, power is the path, not the destination, and so cannot become an end in itself. That is why, whatever the seeming cost in immediate political effectiveness, the networks remain small, decentralized, locally autonomous, for this is the only context in which personhood can be expressed and respected.

From the viewpoint of conventional politics, situational networks are a hopeless obstacle to efficient organization; they do not produce serviceable cadres. But I think these profoundly personalistic groupings are part of a larger, unprecedented political task. Through their defiant celebration of diversity, a powerful new ethical principle enters our lives: that all people are born to be persons, and that persons come first, before all collective fictions, even those of revolutionary movements. And is this not exactly what the planet herself now requires of us? An identity that resists massification, a politics that draws us joyfully toward variety and decentralism?

It is tempting at this point to translate the person/planet connection into the familiar slogan "small is beautiful," since smallness clearly plays a central role in this transformation. But unless small means personal, unless it embraces the ethos of self-discovery, it will be no solution to our problem. This is why the search for humanly scaled institutions cannot be construed as "turning back the clock." In the past, things may have been smaller, but they were rarely personal. Rather, the institutions that governed life were stubbornly grounded in enforced identities of class, sex, age, race, caste. We do well to remember that, small as they were, the city-states of the ancient world were slave societies and fierce bastions of male, military supremacy. So, too, the sweat shops of early industrialism may have featured small-scale, "appropriate" technology, but they were instruments of brutal exploitation. For that matter, no institution is smaller than the marriage of one man and one woman; but if that marriage is built upon assigned sexual identities, it is apt to become an ugly, oppressive relationship. Whenever personhood is not respected, Sartre's dictum holds true: "Hell is other people" . . . even in a tiny room and among a few companions.

This is the missing dimension of E. F. Schumacher's economics, the main reason why he never worked out a calculus of "right size." He shrewdly perceived that small is necessary, but seemed reluc-

---

Recognition of the Mother
Gaea Laughingbird

"I will sing of the well-founded Earth, mother of all, eldest of beings. She feeds all creatures that go upon the goodly land, and all that are in the paths of the seas and all that fly: all things are fed from her store."

From a Homeric Hymn

In Tibetan Buddhism, one of the first meditation practices taught to novices is called "recognition of the Mother." It is intended to awaken deep compassion for all living things, and a sense of the sameness and equality of everything that lives. This meditation comes from the belief that each of us, because of our countless rebirths, has been the mother of every sentient thing in the world. This includes not only all human beings, but all other forms of life, insects, fish, animals, gods, ghosts, devas, plants, waters, mountains, rocks, everything that we can see or imagine.

To begin, we picture our own Mother coming toward us as we meditate. She is radiant and peaceful, totally liberated from imbalance, unhappiness, or any limitation or negativity. As we picture our own Mother in this way, and see white light radiating out of her form and all around her, we release any ill-will we may have toward her, and feel that she no longer has any space in her being for ill-will to inhabit. Just this aspect of the meditation is tremendously liberating, both practically and spiritually.

Next, we picture our other family members, our father, brothers, sisters, husband, wife, etc., and visualize them in the same way as brilliant, serene, and totally pristine. Gradually a mandala begins to form around us, composed of these people, and of the plants, animals, mountains, and other natural qualities that we allow to arise in our mind, all very light and empty, transparent yet very real. In this meditation, a katydid or a cow pie is as precious as a ruby—there is no distinction or preference between one thing and another. Even what we have regarded as obstacles and enemies—especially these, in fact—are worked with until we openly and evenly accept them as the same.

Moving into the Same Skin
Gaea Laughingbird

In the early 70s, I found myself working to save the whales. For a year, I coordinated an international project which involved a good deal of media work, correspondence, and organizational skills. Month after month, I sat typing, writing, and talking about the intelligence and greatness of whales. I had never seen a whale myself.

Near the end of my year-long project, I traveled to Japan to work for a month for the whales. It was an unpopular thing to do there, where women and foreigners are not particularly revered. At the end of the month in Tokyo, I decided to stop off for a few days in Hawaii. It was like taking a breathtaking leap from *yin* to *yang*, as the cold, wet Tokyo winter melted into the hot blues and greens and bright sun of Hawaii.

Driving along in a car, I saw the back of a whale. That instant, past so quickly, resounded in my being. I left the big island in a strange mood, feeling as if I were trying to understand something, but not knowing quite what. The tourists, the native Hawaiians, the boutique shops, the Little League all seemed opaque, somehow. I wandered from town to town rather aimlessly, keeping an eye out for what was up. Finally, I ran out of outs, and wound

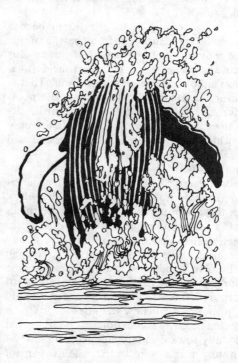

up sitting on the hot sand under the ironwood trees, praying for whales to appear. At that time, it seemed that there was nothing else in the world I wanted to do so much as that, though I had not prayed since I was young. I was not at all sure that prayers could be an-

tant to admit that it may not be sufficient. Something more needs to be added if we are to make proper use of the humanizing opportunity that small-scale operations afford us, something borrowed from beyond the realm of economic analysis. We need to infuse small, decentralized patterns of life with the distinctly contemporary insights of humanistic psychology (the work of Maslow, Laing, Rogers, Perls, May) and personalist philosophy (Mounier, Mumford, Buber, Merton), with what we have learned from the most original art and vision of the modern world.

After our long, strenuous industrial adventure, we are being summoned back along new paths to a vital reciprocity with the Earth who mothered us into our strange human vocation. In a sense that blends myth and science, fact and feeling, the Great Goddess is

indeed returning. But she returns to us by way of the deep self, out of the underworld of the troubled psyche. And her name this time is our name—yours, mine, his, hers, all our names, and for each of us the one name we have freely chosen for ourselves.

The needs of the planet are the needs of the person.

The rights of the person are the rights of the planet.

Berkeley's Theodore Roszak is the author of The Making of a Counter Culture, Where the Wasteland Ends, *and* Unfinished Animal. *His latest book,* Person/Planet: the Creative Disintegration of Industrial Society, *has recently been released by Doubleday.*

swered. My timidity made me angry with myself. Everything I had worked for during the year had been under the flag of the whale's intelligence, the whale's ability to communicate, the whale's mysterious wisdom, unfathomable songs. I sat on the sand, and worked with my various resisances. And I prayed, timidly and quietly singing without any words to the whales. Time slowed to a monotonous murmur. The breeze moved very smoothly in the ironwood trees. I looked into the ocean as into my own eyes. After some more time went by, I saw the back of a whale. I jumped up, elated, then sank down on the sand to pray in earnest, "Great whales," I said to them, "I have worked for your tribes to flourish. I come here with peace in my heart, and a wish to see you. Please gift me with the sight of your body, so that I can remember you and know you. I may never have this chance again." I felt like crying. Somehow all the years of my childhood in suburban New Jersey, all my yearning for the natural world, seemed to be unraveling around me. Far out on the ocean, a whale surfaced, spouted, and sank again into the waters. A moment later, another surfaced. Then, a great humpback whale, its white fins out to either side like open arms, rose straight up out of the water. I gasped—it was so beautiful, so slow; it touched me. It rose up to nearly its full height and, still vertical, sank grandly down again. "Oh, whale," I prayed, "please allow me one more sight of you." I had hardly

formed the thought when the whale arose once more. This time, my mind had clicked into an extraordinary focus. The whale, though far out in the ocean, seemed very close to me, perhaps twenty feet away. As it rose, its eye met mine in an ancient and wordless communion, and every detail of its being seemed to be recorded on my inner eye in a moment which is even now, years later, still precious, still fresh, still very real.

SUGGESTIONS FOR FURTHER READING

Hazel Henderson, *Creating Alternative Futures: An End to Economics*. Berkley, 1978.

Jose and Miriam Arguelles, *The Feminine: Spacious as the Sky*. Shambhala, 1977.

Dolores La Chappell, *Earth Wisdom*. Guild of Tudors Press, 1976.

Peter Berg, ed., *Reinhabiting a Separate Country: A Bioregional Anthology of Northern California*. Planet Drum Books, 1978.

Journal for the Protection of All Beings, Co-Evolution Quarterly, No. 19 (Fall 1978).

Gaea Laughingbird is vice-president of Yeshe Nyingpo, a Tibetan Buddhist center in Ashland, Oregon. She is the author of Words Themselves Are Medicine, *a book of prose and poetry about Earth, the Feminine, and inner journey. Currently she is working on a book about women spiritual teachers, and women who are working to transform the world.*

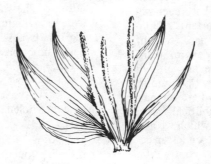

From Strategy to Wholeness:
The Meaning of Community
David Spangler

Most of us would agree that our basic sense of community is sorely lacking. The familiar social forms that once seemed so comforting now seem archaic and unresponsive to our evolving needs. What, then, about alternative systems, such as the so-called intentional communities? They certainly offer a different lifestyle (sometimes dramatically so), but are the strategies they employ fundamentally different from traditional models?

The author, David Spangler, believes they too often fall short of becoming "transformative" agents because they are (perhaps unknowingly) predicated on the same rules that underlie other, antiquated social structures. Maybe we need to ask what it means to feel whole and integral in a social/environmental setting, before we try to figure out how to get from "A" to "B." If our root concern is fundamentally changed, the community from which it springs is sure to reflect an entirely new set of rules and strategies.

This essay only hints at the future community, but the questions it raises are an essential prerequisite for establishment of any such community.

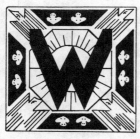 hat is the meaning of community? Not so long ago, that question would have been relatively unimportant. Community was a basic fact of life, part of the environment that formed the background for our activities. Community was where we lived, where we worked, where we married and raised families; it was the political, civic, cultural, economic, and religious life in which we and our neighbors participated to a greater or lesser degree. It was the combination of overt and subtle bonds that linked us with others in meaningful interrelationships, the functional structure of our gregariousness as a species.

This article first appeared in the *Yoga Journal* (March-April 1977), and is reprinted here by permission of the author.

In more recent years, there has been a growing sense among many, particularly within urban centers, that these bonds have been dissolving, overwhelmed by the sheer density of our anonymous togetherness. We seek our own private psychic spaces for respite and recreation; the in-depth bond-making that nurtures the community feeling withers under the pressures of depersonalized, objectified, almost mechanistic styles of work and production. Community requires time and energy; its structures include caring, communication, attention to others in creative exchange. When our time and energy become limited, our ability to nourish community is limited as well. As a consequence, we seem to be losing the experience of community.

In fact, we are all part of communities most of the time. These need not be physical places. They can be associations, sports leagues, clubs, interest groups, and the like; our families are communities, as are our marriages. The need for and the spirit of community is too entwined with the core of our human nature to be easily destroyed. It will manifest in infinite ways, in the briefest of moments, under the most trying of conditions.

What we seem to be saying when we talk about the need for a rebirth of community in our time is that, although the spirit of community is alive and well in avocational situations (clubs, interest groups, and the like), it is absent in our vocational expressions. The basic functions of society, the supplying of basic needs, material and financial, are not expressed out of a sense of over-all community; they are not interrelated and synergic, in the meaning of creating a coherent wholeness that is more than the sum of its parts.

In other words, in a small town, there is more of a feeling of how the town's institutions, like the banks, the hospitals, the food stores, the service industries, the government, the police and so on, fit together and arise together out of the wholeness of the community. People know each other; there is a sense of personhood, like an aura of connectability around the functional roles individuals assume in their daily jobs. The banker is not just a financial official; he is the fellow next door, or the volunteer fireman, or a member of a service club. He is a person. Community is not just the presence of interrelated social functions, a pattern of parts working in specialized fields making a whole system operate. It is a spirit of familiarity, a spirit of shared personhood, a spirit of the presence (and the potential) of connections and bonds beyond the functional.

In a large city, the magnitude of the social needs and the size of the institutions that must meet them obscure this extra dimension. Interchangeability becomes a virtue; efficiency and swiftness of function seem necessities because there is so much to do; the interactions of personhood only slow down the process and make interchangeability difficult (how can you interchange unique persons?). Thus, we come to see the institutions of the society (which in a small context help to define the meaning and sense of community) as faceless, impersonal, and unresponsive to our personhood. They do not communicate a sense of community but a sense of isolation, of loneliness, of being a member or a thing.

Our ability to function is only a part of our wholeness as persons. We feel a spirit of community when this reality is taken into account and we are able to participate beyond the identity of any particular fragment of our whole being. When we are treated only as functions, we become parts of a whole, not participants in a wholeness. We then lose the feeling of community because the sense of our personhood is denied or limited.

The modern quest for community, then, is a quest for our personhood and for a greater affirmation of and attention to the requirements and talents of personhood in the affairs and functioning of our society on all its levels.

To develop, organize, and run a large-scale society where the fundamental unit is the individual as person and not the individual as thing or function, and where opportunities are consciously created and maintained on all levels of social functioning for the spirit of community to manifest and to breathe, is a revolutionary (and evolutionary) task. It will require some fundamental transformations in our ways of seeing ourselves and dealing with ourselves. It will require even more fundamental transformations in our sense of how we accomplish our tasks and emply strategies of achievement. This is by no means an impossible task. On the contrary, it is as great an adventure as any that has ever confronted the human race and well within our means to achieve if the inspiration of this opportunity can call forth our pio-

neering best. Unfortunately, although many fine people and groups are responding, the strategies that are being used, particularly the strategy of the "intentional communities," more often than not work against the accomplishment of the desired new society. To understand how and why this is so, we must look at the movement toward creating new communities and the "exploration" of community.

Community is not just the presence of interrelated social functions; it is a spirit of shared connections and bonds beyond the functional.

We must also digress a moment to consider different types of change. For the sake of our discussion, I want to draw a distinction between *change* and *transformation*. Change I will define as alterations of forms or behaviors within a given system which alter the arrangement and even the structure of its contents, and may even change the outer appearance of the system, but which leave the fundamental nature of the system unaltered. On the other hand, transformation I define as a higher-order change which alters the fundamental nature of the system itself, creating a new system.

An example of this may be drawn from political circles. Many people see the ills of our society, including the loss of the sense of community, as stemming from the capitalist system; and they think that these ills could be corrected if a form of communism or socialism were instituted. Such a shift of political and economic policies, however, is only a change, not a transformation. The basic system of ownership and material possession as a criterion for evaluation of power and success remains unaltered; only the identity of the owner has shifted. A transformation takes place when ownership itself and the overvaluation placed on material production and goods are no longer considered the fundamental rules of the social system. (What may replace them is irrelevant to the example itself, although I believe the transformation would be toward a deeper understanding and practice of stewardship and custodianship, and toward person-values rather than things-values—even, in a mystical sense, learning to see the "personhood," the divine potential, of things, thus seeing things as persons rather than persons as things.)

There are often many variations of change possible within a given system; some of them appear quite radical without violating the basic fundamentals or "rules" on which the system is based. Such changes can be accomplished by forces inherent within the system. A transformation, though, changes the rules, and must be accomplished by a force from outside the system. (In short, the rules cannot change themselves.) On a human level, reason, logic, and most kinds of planning and strategy formation, can create changes, but tend to operate within a system of premises or rules. Intuition, imagination, inspiration, on the other hand, often introduce factors that are "illogical," outside the rules, and thus potentially transformative.

In spite of—or perhaps because of —our material success and technological advances, there is a great deal of dissatisfaction.

In spite of (or because of, depending on your point of view) the material success of our society, our technological and industrial advances, there is a great deal of dissatisfaction going around. Some of it results from some very real problems, such as pollution, crime, poverty, and so forth; some of it is vague, a nonspecific feeling of not finding what we thought we would amidst our successes. As a result, strategies are emerging to deal with this feeling. Since part of our dissatisfaction focuses itself on the "loss of community" in our lives, particularly amongst metropolitan dwellers, it is logical that the "strategies of discontent" should include ways of restoring this loss. Thus, we see an increasing movement during the past decade toward "intentional" communities, with every likelihood that this will become a significant social (or at least, countercultural) endeavor in the future.

The rationale for this movement is valid enough. It is not just the loss of community spirit that bedevils our large cities and organizations; it is size itself, bigness, that becomes unwieldy and wasteful of our best energies in many instances. As Dr. E. F. Schumacher rightly says, "Small is beautiful" (although there are situations where big is beautiful, too). Also, looking at ourselves as our own best resources, it is by means of our wholeness, our personhood, our ability to relate co-creatively with others, that those resources can be best and most deeply tapped for the benefit of all of us. Beyond a certain size of group interaction (at least, at the present stage of human evolution), this resource becomes lost because of forces of depersonalization already mentioned. Community as a small-scale, yet highly dynamic, human enterprise seems the answer, where the potential to work creatively may be enhanced by face-to-face relationships. There is greater opportunity for mutual nourishment to take place as a concomitant to our work, and thus a greater chance to grow and expand our capabilities.

However, at this moment, the challenge to the development of a transformed experience of community is just this rationale: that community seems an answer to certain social problems, and thus an appropriate subject to be made into a strategy. The nature of the strategy, and therefore the nature of the community, depends on the particular social problem that is focused on. If a change in political structure and functioning is desired, then the community becomes an experiment in new political forms. If economy is the focus, then the community develops around different models of finances, production, and consumption and sharing of goods. Perhaps it is a spiritual community, organized around the person or teachings of a leader, or organized to be a place where the emphasis is on inner, subjective transformation. Whatever the type, however, all these communities have in common their orientation toward a particular experiential or philosophical goal; they are strategies and means to an end. This is implied in the very term "intentional," used to describe the directed intent of a group of people to come together to achieve a purpose.

Such communities can be and often are change agents within the larger society, unless they become too isolated within their particular strategy and have goals too far removed from those of the mainstream culture. Are they transformative agencies, as well? That is more difficult to answer, since most pioneering human experiments have potentials for both change and transformation. Perhaps we could ask more specifically if these intentional communities meet the need for a rebirth of the community spirit in a way that can create the person-centered, co-creative, holistic society. Do these avowed strategic, intentional communities in fact provide a means of attainment toward such a society?

The Neighborhood
Armand Ian Brint

The neighborhood
    rattles
with reminders.
Shake it and
memories
          scatter
like
    colored
         beads.
Each is
a dazzling moment
in the
4-square-block
history
of a PEOPLE.
The beads imbed in
alleyways,   gardens,
      and
              corner
  stores,
marking a path home
through the infinite leavings.

I have already suggested that they may not. The reason lies in the fundamental nature of the transformations we must go through to co-create such a society, as reflected in this question: can a truly holistic, co-creative society, a society based on community and expressing community in the deepest sense, come into being divided into things and persons, tools and tool-users? Can it be a technocratic society in the deepest sense of that term, where technology implies the existence of that which is used as a means to an end and of that which uses it? In a co-creative society, should we not regard all that shares existence, whether it is a rock, a machine, a pool of water, a tree, a breeze, an animal, a person, a god, as a partner, a fellow person, a member of a community? Such a society may have "technologies," but in the sense of co-creative processes (the living spirit, the *deva* or angel, within the machine, within the computer, within the hammer) with whom we work, not whom we make work for us. Can we imagine or intuit such a full community of life? Can we imagine or intuit such a society, freed of this most basic

division? Surely all our other divisions against which so many modern "liberation" movements are fighting, such conditions as sexism, racism, "pollutionism," capitalism, communism, and so forth, arise from this basic separation of our world into tools and tool-users, the manipulated and the manipulators. We even define ourselves, our special human ability, as "the tool-maker and the tool-user."

Even the person-oriented community can fall into the trap of making the attainment of "personhood" the social goal.

This is not to suggest that we must stop making and using those objects and processes which we now call tools in order to experience transformation. It is to suggest that we learn to look upon such objects as partners and not just as things. We must redefine ourselves as the species that can actualize the potential of community within creation, by drawing so many aspects of creation into partnership and creativity with us, as well as by learning to enter into that partnership ourselves. Such redefinition results in a whole new perspective of our world, seeing it and all upon it as fellow persons, fellow members of community, fellow creators on many levels of potential and expression.

Do our intentional communities help us gain that perspective? Are they working to transform our sense of what community is and how far it must extend into the natural and paranatural worlds? I have found none that are doing this consistently, though some, like Findhorn with its cooperation and communication with the invisible kingdoms of nature, are attempting it. In most, and this is also partly true of Findhorn, the emphasis is not on community but on community-as-strategy, community-as-tool. New insights may be generated by such places and experiments, changes may be stimulated, but the essential system remains unchanged. *The rules of the tool-maker and tool-user remain unaltered.* There is little or no transformation.

When a community becomes a strategy, the person becomes a tool himself or herself within that community. There is a subtle difference at times between being a tool and a co-creator, between working for a common end and being "worked by" that end. Being goal-oriented is not the matter in question, but the dominance of the goal-as-value over the person-as-value. Even communities built around the idea of developing personhood can fall into this perpetuation of the system, making "personhood" as they define it a goal to which the resources of individual persons are applied. The solution is not anarchy, which, when interpreted to mean "everyone doing his or her own thing," can be destructive of personhood as well. Structure and order are not incompatible with a holistic, everything-as-person, everyone-as-partner community. The challenge is that even our idea of personhood is tied up with images of using and doing.

Space does not permit a fuller treatment of these ideas. All I wish to do here is provide a way of looking at communities and the current movement toward intentional communities in particular. To the extent that they are seen, or experienced and developed, as intentional strategies, to that extent we run the risk of perpetuating part of the basic system we wish to transform; to that extent, we may deny community even as we reach out for it.

To me, the essence of community is wholeness: the opportunity to achieve and experience wholeness and to co-create out of that consciousness a livingness that meets my needs and those of the greater whole of which I am a part. Community is the deeper reality within which I move and have my being. It is one of the names of God. Community is the gift of myself I give in endless participation with my world. It may infuse my strategies with wholeness and link them with divinity, but it is not a strategy in itself, unless it is seen as the ultimate strategy from which others come.

Community is our Alpha and Omega. It is the meaning of all we are and of all we will become. In looking upon our continued efforts to create community in our lives, we must learn to go from strategy to wholeness, that from wholeness our strategies may be born.

SUGGESTIONS FOR FURTHER READING

Gregory Bateson, *Mind and Nature.* Dutton, 1979.

Theodore Roszak, *Person/Planet.* Doubleday, 1978.

Dane Rudhyar, *Beyond Individualism.* Quest Books, 1979.

David Spangler, *Revelation: Birth of a New Age.* Lorian Press, 1979.

————, *Towards A Planetary Vision.* Findhorn, 1978.

William Irwin Thompson, *Passages About Earth.* Harper and Row, 1974.

————, *Darkness and Scattered Light.* Harper and Row, 1978.

David Spangler is a writer and philosopher/educator, primarily on New Age themes. He was a co-director of the Findhorn Foundation community in Scotland for three years, founding its educational program; upon his return to the United States in 1973, he, with others from Findhorn, founded the Lorian Association, a nonprofit educational foundation, of which he is still a director. He is a consultant to several groups and communities exploring holistic living and the New Age vision, and is currently working on his latest book, Emergence, *to be published by Seymour Lawrence/Delacorte in late 1979 or early 1980.*

The Integral Urban Home
Lee Foster

The word "integral" is defined as "composed of constituent parts making a whole." It also implies that each part is essential to the whole. This notion has been applied in a very practical way to the problem of energy consumption by a California-based nonprofit research institute.

The goal of the institute was to transform a dilapidated urban home into an energy-saving and resource-efficient environment. As you will see, their efforts have been more than successful. Each aspect of this carefully planned "integral" environment is interrelated and essential to the operation of the whole. The synergistic result is not only more energy-efficient, but personally gratifying. You become an integral participant in the environment.

The home is primarily a teaching tool, and as such provides a wonderland of commonsense, ingenious alternatives to capital-intensive, wasteful technology. There is much to learn from the Integral Urban Home if we are to turn the tide of the current energy crisis.

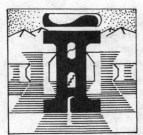

nformed people now agree that the average family's house and lifestyle, especially in the more urbanized and industrialized nations, will have to undergo fundamental changes to consume less energy and resources. But how should this be done? Where is there a model, a totally integrated example of energy- and resource-efficient living in a typical house? Suppose an average urban family of four, motivated to change their lives, but forced to live within the normal urban constraints of limited time, space, and light, asked: How can we achieve environmentally sound living? Can you show us a "different" rather than a "lower" standard of living?

This article first appeared in *The Plain Truth*, September 1978, and is reprinted here by permission of the author.

An answer is now available: The Integral Urban House, 1516 Fifth St., Berkeley, California 94710. In 1974 a California-based environmental organization, the Farallones Institute, decided to commit its resources to develop a practical working model of such a house and lifestyle. They bought and retrofitted an aging Victorian on a 6,000-square-foot lot. By thoroughly redesigning the house and grounds, they aimed to illustrate exactly what a motivated urban family could accomplish. By 1978 they had completed the prototype, which is open to the public. "A family in this house creates only 10 to 35 per cent of the environmental impact of a family in a typical American house," said Tom Javits, director of the house.

What makes the family living in this house different? In brief, they:

(1) raise all their own vegetables, most of their own fruit, plus honey;

(2) produce their own meat from chickens, eggs from chickens, and fish from a fishpond;

(3) recycle all vegetable, animal, and human wastes, calling the materials "resources";

(4) use solar energy to heat their space, water, and food;

(5) use wind energy to aerate their food-fish pond;

(6) control all insect pests with physical and biological controls rather than with poisons;

(7) reuse household water, which is recycled to the garden through a "gray water" system;

(8) generally make the best possible use of the resources available.

To learn how all this worked, I watched Tom Javits and three other house residents do their weekend chores. "Remember that when all the systems of the house are set up," said Javits, "they can be maintained in about eight hours of work per week, or two hours per person. The house shows how urban people can do this in spite of the usual comment: 'I don't have the space, the time, and the sunlight.'"

When I arrived at the house, I noticed some clues to its uniqueness even before I entered. The front "lawn" in the parking strip was alfalfa rather than the usual grass. "A square meter of alfalfa produces the feed for us to grow one pound of meat per year," said Javits.

The "sidewalks" were wood-chip rather than concrete. Several strategies were involved in this choice. The wood chips were a recycled community waste generated from tree clippings. Microorganisms in the soil could be nurtured by wood chips, but would be killed by concrete. Concrete would also compact the soil more than the chips. Rainwater could be absorbed by the wood chips rather than run off the property, creating storm-sewer problems, as happens with concrete.

When I entered the gate, I found a young lady named Joyce Liska gathering strawberries. "We grow all our vegetables and as much of our fruit as possible," she said. "The strawberries are delicious in spring and early summer, but the red leaves are also an attractive groundcover in the autumn. Most of the 'produce' from America's 16 million acres of lawn, the grass clippings, are thrown away, creating another waste-management problem."

A subtle blend of utility and aesthetics controlled the choice of all the plant materials that I saw on the property. Chrysanthemums yielded an attractive flower and a green for tea. New Zealand spinach, which is edible, served as a green groundcover.

When I entered the front door, passing under an attractive squash vine, I picked up a *Self-Guided Tour Book,* which explains the house's systems in detail. Any member of the public can visit the house weekdays, using the self-guided tour, or on Saturday afternoons, when the house residents offer guided tours. The informative book can also be ordered by mail for $2.50 (address noted earlier).

As I looked through the description of the many individual strategies used in the house and the way in which they were interrelated, they seemed to defy a celebrated mathematical axiom: the whole was greater than the sum of its parts. For example, the fish in the food-fishpond in the backyard liked to gobble up weeds tossed to them from the garden.

Besides being the director of the house and an energetic young environmentalist, Tom Javits also serves as technical adviser to the City of Berkeley's innovative program to compost its tree clippings. Javits has written several informative monographs, especially in one of his areas of expertise, chicken raising in urban areas.

As we talked, I looked out the window and noticed an odd-shaped screen contraption that looked like a triangular cage. What was that? "A fly trap that uses no poisons," Javits replied. "We put a plate of dog dung under the cage. Flies land on it. Then they fly upwards to the light, as is their nature. In the screen at the bottom of the trap are several holes, which let through the most light. The flies enter the trap, then can't get out because the holes, when viewed from above, are now dark. They buzz around for a couple of days, then die, and are fed to the chickens." So even flies are a "resource" rather than a pest at the Integral Urban House!

Later that morning I saw Joyce Liska feeding a garden snail to the chickens. Chickens are handy waste disposers, but the house residents also prize their manure as a nitrogen-rich ingredient in the compost pile.

Javits left me free to wander through the house and grounds, later returning to answer my questions.

I found Suzie Sayer in the backyard on an unusual adaptation of a bicycle, called an Energy-cycle. "I'm grinding grain," she said, "using my own legpower. Besides grinding food, this unit can be used to centrifuge honey, sharpen knives, and do several other chores. Rather than plug into a wall socket, I get exercise while doing useful work."

Everywhere in the house the idea of using sun, wind, and muscle energy rather than electricity predominated. In the backyard I saw a windmill fashioned from oil drums, called a Savonius rotor construction, pumping water for the food-fishpond, constantly aerating and filtering the water. The windmill can turn under very low wind velocities that prevail in the flatlands area where the house is located.

On the south side of the house I saw a large solar collector heating water. "We put a thousand dollars into the materials for our solar collector," said Javits. "It heats water to 160 degreees, far higher than the 120 degrees needed. In the first year of our experience, it worked to provide 95 per cent of our hot-water needs."

In winter, when the sun stays behind clouds for several days, they use a small backup electric water heater. I asked Javits how energy costs are distributed in the average American house and how this information affected planning the Integral Urban House. His best estimate is that the average all-electric house devotes 52 per cent of its energy cost to space heating, 18 per cent to water heating, and 3.5 per cent to food heating.

Consequently, much planning for the house focused on "passive" solar heating and cooling. The

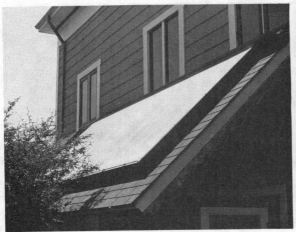

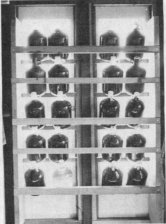

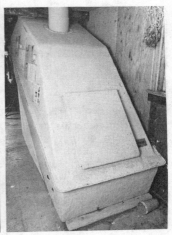

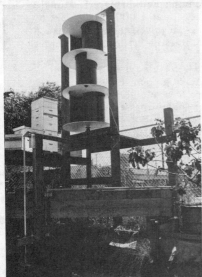

Left:
Do-it-yourself windmill made from oil drums recirculates and aerates water from fishpond. Convenient location of beehives allows fish to feed on bee carcasses that drop from hives.

Top row:
Solar panel for hot-water heating system which provided 95 percent of hot water demand during first year of operation.

Filled bottles used as passive heat collectors. Shutters on window can control amount of heat absorbed.

Swedish-made dry composting toilet produces dramatic savings in fresh-water consumption.

Bottom row:
Gray-water hoses used to recycle waste water from sinks and showers to the garden for irrigation.

Salad vegetables and herbs grow in container boxes filled with lightweight compost and drip irrigated to minimize their weight on the roof.

A greenhouse room serves as a nursery for young vegetables and opens out to heat two rooms in winter.

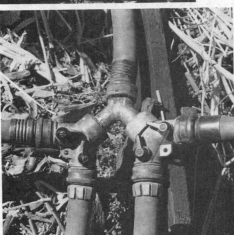

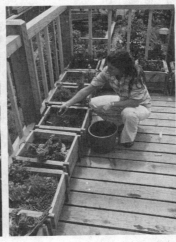

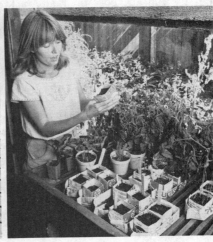

Urban Vegetable Gardening
Lee Foster

Back in 1976, I considered whether it would be possible to grow all the vegetables for my family of four on our modest-sized lot in Oakland, California. I wondered what amount of country-style food production could be achieved in the city, where I wanted to remain, where most of us are destined to live.

I had no skills at the time in vegetable gardening. Our lot is 50 by 100 feet, located on a corner, with the house centered on the land. Our chief asset is strong sun, all year round, since we are located on a hillside that faces south. Our microclimate is also frost-free.

I began slowly in 1977 with two tomato plants, plus lettuce and onions for salads. During 1977 and the first half of 1978, I devoted an hour a day to developing our land. The hard soil of our area, called Rockridge, was well-named. At a composting site near the Berkeley city dump, where all the city tree clippings were shredded and composted, I bought ample amounts of organic material to improve the structure and nutritive levels of my soil. Eventually my own composting systems managed our vegetative wastes and sustained our vegetables in their nutritional needs.

By late 1977 most of my raised beds were completed. I erected a fence to keep roaming dogs out of the 440 square feet of sunny land that I had reclaimed. That space proved sufficient, by mid-1978, to make us self-reliant for vegetables.

We east most of our food fresh, but we must store some of our warm-weather abundance for cool winter consumption. We chose freezing as our preservation strategy, despite some energy costs. With a chest-type manual-defrost freezer, the energy consumption can be minimized. The physical appearance and nutritive values of frozen produce seem more attractive to us than the results of canning and drying. I estimate that I would need about 1,000 square feet of growing space to achieve vegetable self-reliance in areas, such as Minnesota, with only a summer growing season.

By mid-78 we were enjoying the full pleasures of the vegetable garden. Each evening we ate a different fresh vegetable. Sugar peas had an appealing taste that surpassed what a supermarket could offer. Cauliflower was so succulent we ate it raw. Our lettuce had none of the pesticide residue found on most commercial produce. We developed a fondness for Oak Leaf lettuce, a tender variety you can grow, but

windows can be shuttered from the outside to keep out the sun and cool the house or keep the heat of the house from escaping at night. The shutters of some windows can be held rigid to act as reflectors, bouncing the sun's rays to containers holding liquids. The containers warm during the day and slowly radiate their heat at night. Because of such strategies, plus the complete insulation of the house, the only heat source needed in the relatively benevolent Bay Area climate is a wood-burning Jotul stove. The stove is prized for its efficiency at converting wood into heat that can be used rather than heat the escapes up the chimney. A handful of scrap lumber in the Jotul burns for a long time.

On the ground floor, a greenhouse room serves as a nursery for young vegetables and opens out to heat two downstairs rooms in winter. On the cool north side of the house, a "cool closet" in the kitchen keeps vegetables cool and aired by using convection drafts in the shade, reducing the need for refrigerator space.

Conserving water was stressed as much as saving electricity.

"Even beyond the recent concern in California about the drought," said Javits, "we have to realize that delivering a gallon of water to our houses requires energy. Our estimate is that a delivered gallon of water, after you build the dam, purify the water, and pump it to the site, costs the energy equivalent of burning a 60-watt light bulb for 10 minutes."

The amount of water used at the house is only a fraction of what the usual house consumes. "We use about 50 gallons per person per day," said Javits, "as compared with 140 gallons per day in the average house."

The figure is even more striking when you consider that the 50 gallons includes the water required to

can't buy. Our spinach came to table at its nutritive peak, rather than deteriorated by allowing days to pass between picking and eating. We grew broccoli with minimum fossil-fuel costs, using only the energy needed to import water, avoiding the heavy energy costs of conventional agriculture for petroleum-based fertilizers, farm-machinery operation, processing, and transporting the food to market and the consumer's house. We enlivened our food with our own herbs, reducing our dependence on salt. While living the joy of eating foods we had created, we also began to experience long-range economies in our food budget, which is about 17 per cent of the average American's living expense. Food costs are rising about 13 per cent per year.

Many subtle pleasures began to express themselves. The garden became a dynamic experience that changed daily. A squash plant that had just poked its head out yesterday seemed to have grown a foot today. Weather became more than a passive presence in our lives. When the chill of autumn arrived, we learned there was no point in extending the life of the bell-pepper plants. We harvested remaining peppers, then turned the ground over to cool-weather cabbage-family plants, such as brussels sprouts.

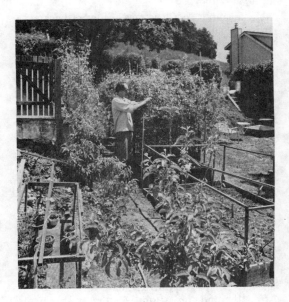

Each December 21, when the vegetable-vitalizing sun began to rise in the sky, after sinking to its nadir, we were ready to celebrate the return of light to the world. This enduring thread of primitive tradition gave an unassail-

(continued on p. 324)

raise all their vegetables. "The average person may require as much as 3,000 gallons of water per day if you include the water to raise his food," said Javits. "We cut down on that water requirement substantially."

The house has no drains. All the water used in the house is piped to the garden through a gray-water system. This includes water from the shower, kitchen sink, and urinal. The residents of the house hold human urine in high regard because it is rich in nitrogen and normally free of pathogens. No water is required for the toilet, a dry composting toilet called the Clivus Multrum and made in Sweden. Human wastes and kitchen scraps enter the toilet and come out two years later thoroughly composted and usable in the garden. Drip irrigation also cuts down the water requirements for the vegetables.

"All these resource-saving techniques are important," said Javits. "But the most important of all is raising our own food. That's where we save the most energy."

Along with raising all their own vegetables by cultivating 2,500 feet of their 6,000-square-foot space, they compost all vegetable and animal wastes, creating new soil in which they can grow more vegetables. Some crops, such as winter squash, are stored on drying racks in the basement.

In the backyard I met Helga Olkowski squashing aphids on the cabbage by hand. She and her husband William are well known in the field of biological control of insect pests. They have also authored the bible of urban self-reliant food raising, *The City People's Book of Raising Food.* "We think of the garden as a zoo," she said. "We keep the little animals diversified,

(continued from p. 323)

able meaning to Christmas. Flowers became a helpful adjunct of our vegetable gardening effort, because small control insects, called miniwasps, which help us keep the aphid population in check, need constant blooms to keep their own population up.

Several observations can be offered for kindred spirits who would like to join us in urban farming.

First, discover your space for growing. You have more space than you think. The landless apartment dweller can manage container beds or a greenhouse window. Sprouting seeds, eating the seeds as a sprouted vegetable, requires no space beyond that in a mason jar. Use vertical as well as horizontal space for climbing peas and beans. Community gardens are increasing in number and size for city people who have no land.

Second, utilize your sunlight and seasonal warmth. Grow spinach, lettuce, and chard in partial shade. Your climate has peculiar strengths and limitations. I store fresh carrots and beets in the ground by bringing them to maturity as the cool of winter approaches.

Third, build your soil gradually but steadily. Good soil requires proper structure and adequate nutriments. Add as much organic material as possible. When you commence gardening, all the organic wastes from your kitchen become valuable resources for your compost pile or for direct burial in your ground, where worms process the material.

Fourth, plan your time daily for gardening. Get into the satisfying rhythm of food growing: 15 minutes a day will be worth more to the garden than three hours on the weekend. Start small, handling only what you can manage. As you meet success, you'll be prompted to develop more ground.

Finally, what should you plant? Start with the vegetables you like to consume. If you've never eaten kohlrabi, don't grow it. Begin with productive plants, such as Swiss chard, that maximize yields from small spaces. In warm weather a square meter of Swiss chard, about nine vigorous plants, can support one person nicely. If I were limited to only a few seeds to start with, I would choose: a zuccini squash, six Swiss chard, a cherry tomato (Sweet 100), and six Black Seeded Simpson lettuce. All these plants are cut-and-come again. You can eat from them for a longish time.

With vegetable self-reliance behind us, we still have much to learn. Maintaining our production, improving our strategies, and advancing our timing to make the land more productive require skills that invite further refinement.

so they can keep each other in check. We control insects directly by hand picking and by physical barriers. Seldom do the insects cause intolerable damage to our food."

She shared with me some of the many techniques used to control common pests, such as aphids. "We leave some flowering herbs in the garden at all times," she said. "The herb flowers are needed for the life cycle of miniwasps. The wasps, in turn, lay their eggs in the soft bodies of aphids and caterpillars, helping to keep down the insect population."

The benevolent Bay Area climate, with a 12-month growing season for vegetables, makes the task of food self-reliance easier than elsewhere.

Tom Javits explained why they concentrate on vegetables and fruits rather than grains and dairy products. "Vegetables are about 20 per cent of our nutritional needs, but 50 per cent of our grocery bill for the average family," he said, "because of the high energy inputs required to grow, fertilize, pick, and transport the vegetables to us. These costs are bound to rise. Grains, by contrast, can be grown for relatively lower energy costs. Grains can be stored and transported relatively economically. Dairy products would not be possible in this limited urban space."

Every bit of space in the house is used, including the roof area off the kitchen, above the greenhouse. Salad vegetables and herbs grow in container boxes filled with compost, which is only 50 per cent of the weight of regular soil. Drip irrigation to the containers further minimizes the weight that the walls of the house need to bear. "We call this agriculture 'detritus' or waste-based agriculture," said Javits. "We contrast it with the usual fossil-fuel agriculture commonly practiced."

Stalk and leaf parts of vegetables not succulent enough to interest humans are fed to chickens in their cages on the shaded north side of the house.

Beehives at the back of the lot produce about a hundred pounds of honey per year. "The bees are our

New varieties of vegetables wait to be tried, such as Sugar Snap Peas, first offered to gardeners in 1979. Beyond vegetables, what can be done toward fruit self-reliance? We have one established plum tree that bears nicely on our property. I have added a dwarf apple, pear, and peach. Strawberries are another good fruit choice for the urban food garden. I have 110 plants scattered over our land. Could we raise small animals, chickens for eggs and rabbits for meat? Could we produce honey? Could I utilize our flat roof? These questions will be answered in the coming years.

An intent urban food producer will probably become absorbed also in processing foods upward from basics. My wife Anke makes our yogurt from bulk powdered milk three times a week. I buy grains in bulk, cracking them for cereal and grinding them for pancakes and breads. We juice carrots, apples, tomatoes, and plums. To cut energy waste in cooking, we use a parabolic solar cooker when possible.

For most of us, the notion of escaping the city to live in the country is a misguided ideal, fraught with illusion and littered with examples of failure. But bringing the country into the city, healing this artificial split in our sensibility between the farm and the urban center, can stimulate a more joyous and environmentally sound lifestyle in America.

SUGGESTIONS FOR FURTHER READING

Walter L. Doty, *All About Vegetables*. Ortho, 1973.

Sunset Magazine Editors. *Vegetable Gardening.*

Joan Lee Faust, *Book of Vegetable Gardening*. New York Times-Quadrangle, 1975.

John Bryan, *Small World Vegetable Gardening*. 101 Productions, 1977.

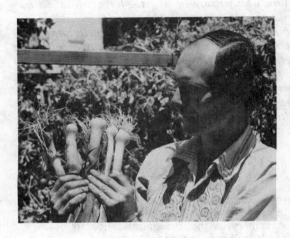

goodwill ambassadors to the neighborhood," said another house resident, Tom Fricke. "They pollinate everyone's flowers, trees, and vegetables."

On the back deck I saw the *pièce de résistance* of the system: a parabolic solar disc boiling a whistling kettle of water that would be used to make tea for lunch. The house residents also use a large solar reflective oven for baking.

The longer I stayed at the Integral Urban House, the more ideas emerged. All the concepts had been carefully worked out in this practical environment by competent realists rather than utopian dreamers. If there is an antidote to environmental pessimism about our ability to adapt and survive, this is it.

"We always favor the term self-reliance rather than self-sufficiency," said Javits. "Here we try to be self-reliant, depending on ourselves. Self-sufficiency suggests that we are little islands, but we are in fact closely related to each other and interdependent on each other."

SUGGESTIONS FOR FURTHER READING

Helga Olkowski, *Self-Guided Tour of the Integral Urban House*. Integral Urban House, 1979.

Helga and William Olkowski, *The City People's Book of Raising Food*. Rodale Press, 1975.

Tom Javits, *How To Raise Rabbits and Chickens in an Urban Area*. Integral Urban House, 1975.

Tom Javits *et al.*, *Integral Urban House: Self-Reliant Living in the City*. Sierra Club Books, 1979.

John Seymour, *The Self-Sufficient Gardener*. Doubleday, 1979.

Lee Foster is a veteran writer-photographer with a special interest in urban self-reliance. Educated at Notre Dame and Stanford, he has published five books and contributes to magazines here, in Europe, and in Japan. Besides writing on innovative lifestyles, such as urban self-reliance, he also writes on travel and natural history.

Establishing Relationships with Plants

Julie Fuchs

The following material describes an attitude toward nature which many of us have forgotten or perhaps never had the opportunity to experience. Little do we think of the treasury of our natural environment outside of its use as an industrial resource or private recreational site. However, along with the sustenance we glean from her bounty, the kingdom of nature has many teachings to convey, if we will only listen. These secrets are freely shared as we increasingly cultivate a sense of reverence and joy in our new-found education.

"Perhaps the reason gardening is so healing to modern man, who is speeded up almost beyond endurance by the pulsing beat of machinery, is that it requires deliberate, loving hands, and cannot be done in a hurry."

Helen Morgenthau Fox,
*Gardening with Herbs for
Flavor and Fragrance* (1933)

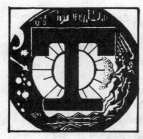

Today we are seeking to rediscover the healing properties of plants. Our ancestors knew the importance of being in harmony with the cycles of nature, and that this balanced interdependence of human, plant, and animal elements was the basis of health. When an individual lost this natural equilibrium, local plants were called on for help.

The Cherokee people have an old story about the origin of disease and medicine. "In the old day," they say, "the beasts, birds, fishes, insects, and plants could all talk, and they and the people lived together in peace and friendship." But as time went on, the people took over more and more space, and killed many of the animals without offering them proper respect. The animals held their counsel and decided to curse humankind with various diseases to limit the destructive actions of the humans. The plants, upon hearing the news of this decision, held their counsel and decided to assist the people by becoming medicine. "Each Tree, Shrub, and Herb—down even to the Grasses and Mosses—agreed to furnish a cure for some one of the diseases."[1]

This Native American "myth" shows conscious understanding of the fundamental interrelationship and communication between all life forms sharing the Earth, what today might be called a holistic viewpoint.

Many people begin the search for knowledge about herbs by reading books, and buying dried, packaged herbs. This is a good beginning, but in order to discover the deeper healing qualities of herbs, we must augment our intellectual understanding with a physical and spiritual connection. Healing energy is most available when these three levels of consciousness are in balanced, active relationship.

THE PHYSICAL RELATIONSHIP

The physical qualities of herbs are the most obvious; and by observing the growth patterns and life cycles of the plants, we can learn a great deal about their healing properties. Perhaps the most basic observation is of the changes in the physical energy of plants with the seasons. In the spring, we can see the life energy being born in the young plants "springing" up. The urge to grow is at a peak. This is the time to gather tender shoots and leaves. At this time young dandelion leaves, raspberry and blackberry leaves, and the unopened shoots of horsetail grass (*Equisetum*) are rich sources of minerals. Next, in summer, nature is at the zenith of her productive bounty, and the flowers and fruits are created. Delicious teas can be made from flowers of the hollyhock, hybiscus, borage, and chamomile in this season. Such fruits as raspberry, blackberry, and elderberry are further signs of summer's cycle of abundance. The fall is a time of harvest or reseeding. The culinary spices, celery, dill, anise, and fennel seeds may be gathered at this time. Winter allows a time for rest and rebuilding of the vital energy needed to start a new cycle. During this rest period, the plants' energies descend to the roots, and a dormant cycle occurs. This is the appropriate time for gathering the roots of plants such as dandelion, blackberry, burdock, and comfrey.

In addition, many subcycles of change take place in plants. The monthly cycles based on lunar forces (gravitation) have long been of interest to farmers and other people in close relationship with the plant world. For instance, the new moon is a time for sprouting seeds, making tinctures (extractions of herbs), and new beginning in general: the energy is increasing. The full moon marks the greatest amount of energy available and signifies a period of release, followed by a decrease in energy. During the waning (decreasing) moon, root crops are planted, and weeding is most effective.

Even within the 24 hours of each day there are cycles. For example, 10 A.M. to 3 P.M. is the time period most favorable for picking leaves and flowers to be used for healing. After 3 P.M. the vital energy of the plant begins to descend toward the roots; so roots are harvested at night.

This clearly observable, unending pattern of the seasons and subcycles gives us insights on how we can best balance our energies at certain times of the year. Assuming that our human energies are subject to the same universal forces of the sun, moon, and seasons, to mention only a few, we begin to see ourselves as part of a consistent, balanced world. In Chinese medicine the influence of the seasons on human activities receives serious consideration. The *Nei Ching,* or *Classic of Internal Medicine,* gives advice on harmonizing the human spirit with the seasons. In spring we are advised to get up early, loosen the hair, and slow down body movements. It is a time to give freely. Summer is a period of luxurious growth. We are en-

couraged to develop physical abilities and positive communications with the outside world. The fall is seen as a time to begin gathering in our personal energies. An atmosphere of clearness and tranquility prevails. Finally, winter is called the period of "closing and storing." Ideally, we would retire early and rise later, as does the sun. These changes in our energy levels are part of the flow of nature, and require an appropriate time for expression. This viewpoint is in itself healing, especially at a time when we are subject to so many artificial and chaotic circumstances.

Historically, plants were named for their color, shape, odor, etc., which were said to reflect their specific healing virtues. This concept became known as the Doctrine of Signatures. Its legacy lives on today in the common names of many plants: birthroot, bloodroot, eyebright, horsetongue, lungwort, and bladderpod, to name a few. Observing the growth patterns of a plant will also often reveal its healing properties. Comfrey (*Symphytum officinale*) is a good example of this principle. Famous for its ability to mend broken bones, comfrey heals by speedily (internally and/or externally) rebuilding tissue. Its high mineral content and a substance known as allantoin make comfrey a powerful "cell proliferant," accelerating the formation of new cells. If you watch comfrey grow, its fast rate of proliferation is reflected by an amazing ability to regenerate itself. You can pick all the leaves of a comfrey plant, and it will grow a whole new plant in 21 days during its active growth season. Comfrey also reproduces itslef quickly by root divisions. Start with one plant, and soon you will have many.

The location where a plant grows can also give clues to its uses. For example, Horsetail (*Equisetum arvense*) and watercress (*Nasturtium officinale*) both grow near water. They are useful in treating kidney

(Text continued on p. 330)

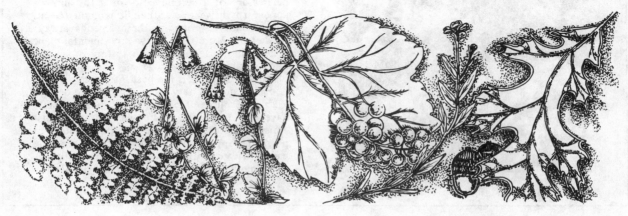

Plant Walking:
A Healing Ritual
Alan Siegel

In Beauty may I walk.
All day long may I walk.
Through the returning seasons may I walk.

Navajo Prayer, "Night Way"

At your doorstep, in meadows and parklands and deep woods, are weeds and seeds and roots and fruits that have been used as food and medicine for centuries.

There is renewed interest in the art of plant walking. Some people want to learn how to forage for survival foods. Others want to learn how to harvest the plentiful nutrients, to experience the new tastes, or to know the powerful medicinal properties of local wild plants. The preservation and expansion of this knowledge is vital, but the true medicine power of

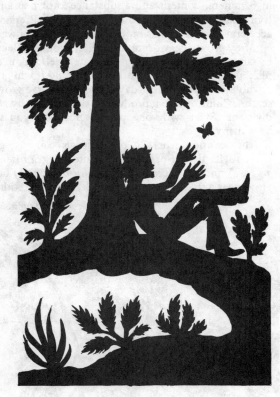

plant walking goes far beyond their curative, nutritional, or economic power.

Plant walking restores a sense of reverence for nature and a feeling of connectedness to all living beings. For too long our culture has sought to control nature without caring for her. It is like controlling the wild and fertile part of our own imagination instead of letting it flourish.

Opening all our senses and being in the presence of a living plant is a soothing and balancing experience. To touch the fuzzy leaf of the hazelnut tree, to taste the sweetness of the wild strawberry, or to rest in the peace of a hidden pine grove is to feel a simple yet profound joy. Perhaps it is an ancestral memory of a time when we all lived in closer harmony with nature.

Native Americans ventured into wilderness on vision quests, to seek visions and to pray for guidance for themselves and their tribe. As we walk our own hills, greenbelts, and forests, we too become more grounded and more open to creative inspiration, more ready to receive a vision that may heal ourselves, our community, or our planetary tribe.

When I go plant walking, the hills come alive. I allow myself to imagine animated relationships with certain plants or areas. Sometimes I imagine that I am a shaman picking elder flower on a clear May morning, or a Miwok woman gathering black oak acorns for my clan, or a young boy of a thousand years ago wandering through the woods singing a different song to every herb, listening to the monkey flowers laugh at me.

LEARNING PLANTS

It is essential to identify a plant positively before even tasting a tiny amount of it. Some legends say that if a plant tastes sweet, or the berries are of a certain color or if the animals appear to thrive on it, then it is good to eat. Unfortunately, none of these legends always holds true. More than a few experimental plant tasters have perished in the testing of an unknown plant! Knowledge of the poisonous plants in your area is the best insurance.

Please do not harvest near a roadside or near a known source of pollutants. Roadside plants have not only picked up lead from exhaust emissions but often have been subjected to pesticide applications meant to kill roadside weeds. If you notice wilted roadside foliage, you may want to investigate and bring any chemical abuses to the awareness of your community and your fellow plant walkers.

Getting involved is important. We can renew the oral plant tradition by playfully making up our own common names and legends about the plants we learn. A plant that you learn on the solstice can become solstice herb, or mugwort, with its dream-inspiring qualities, may become dreamwort. Latin names stay the same and are universal. An example is the Latin name for yarrow, *Achillea.* It is named for Achilles, who used its wound-healing qualities as medicine for his soldiers. The oracle nature of the yarrow plant was also known to the ancient Chinese, who used the stalks for consulting the *I Ching.*

In the classes and walks I lead, I suggest looking at a plant with acute vision, as if you were a camera; photographing in your mind's eye the lattice shape of the leaf veins, the exquisite colors of the flower petals, or the deeply grooved geometry of the tree bark. Always observe the structure and habitat. As you relax and become absorbed in the details, images may arise that will aid your memory and give you valuable information about the nature and uses of a plant.

CONSCIOUS FORAGING

In urban areas we now need more nibbling Plant Guardians than wholesale plant eaters. Conservation is far superior to careless or large-scale harvesting. Learn to forage with a camera or a sketch pad. Harvest the energy of a plant by writing a poem or a song about it.

The Algonquins of New England would thrice chant before plucking any herb: "Nikomo, Mother Earth, I put my hands into thy side to get this herb." They would then utter the plant's intended use three times. You too may want to develop your own ritual of herb-gathering. Harvesting a fresh medicine plant for an ailment or for a friend can be a very rewarding experience. Your direct involvement in the harvesting will enhance the healing process.

A conscious forager will pick only plants that are very abundant. If possible, always harvest as if you were pruning a plant. Always leave the root intact unless you plan to use it or transplant it to your garden. Gathering seed or cuttings for your garden is an excellent way to learn about native plants. Native-plant cultivation not only saves water, but helps to preserve and spread knowledge about native plants.

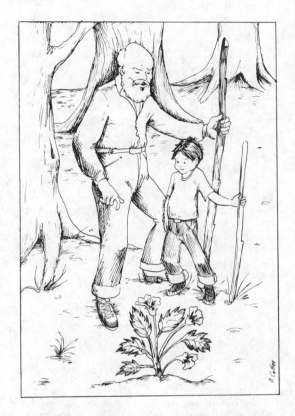

A native food garden will add variety to your diet and beauty to your yard.

Often the most common weeds that we think of as a nuisance can be weeded right into the salad bowl or the sauce pan. Weeds such as chickweed (*Stellaria*), curly dock (*Rumex crispus*), and purslane (*Portulaca oleracea*) are often more nutritious than the vegetables you have chosen to grow.

Picking a wild salad or potherb gets you in touch with the source of your nutrition in a way that your food market never will. There are many incredible new tastes and textures in wild plants, and there are potentially many wild foods that could contribute significantly to the world food crisis if cultivated.

Plants are essential to the survival of our Spaceship Earth. They recycle the oxygen that we need to breath. Yet if you look around, you see condominiums planted on once green hills, forests clearcut for newsprint, and pesticides and radioactive waste senselessly polluting the

(continued on p. 330)

(continued from p. 329)

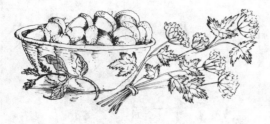

Earth. We have chosen economics and profit over caring for and regenerating our environment.

Any holistic approach to health must include changing the environmental and cultural climate that spawns imbalance and disease. Learning to know and use and care for the plants around us is like learning to care for something precious within ourselves.

In his poem entitled *For the Children,* Gary Snyder put it this way:

> "Stay together
>   Go lightly
>   Learn the Flowers."

When you go plant walking, you find the nourishment not only for your body, but for your spirit as well. With this comes the vision to balance our culture and restore a more loving connection with nature. That is important survival food!

SUGGESTIONS FOR FURTHER READING

Charlotte B. Clark, *Edible and Useful Plants of California.* University of California Press, 1977.

Alma Hutchens, *Indian Herbalogy of North America.* Merco, 1969.

Gary Snyder, *Turtle Island.* New Directions, 1974.

Alan Siegel, M.A., L.M.F.C.C., is on the faculty of Vista College in Berkeley and The Holistic Life University in San Francisco, where he teaches Wilderness Psychology and Dream Psychology. He has spent seven years studying wild plants and being nourished by their energy. He has led walks on edible, medicinal, and survival plants of Northern California for plant-walkers of all ages, and has guided Wilderness Therapy Experiences in Community Mental Health and Holistic Health Centers throughout the San Francisco Bay Area. He is the Training Coordinator for the City of Berkeley Mental Health Adult Clinic.

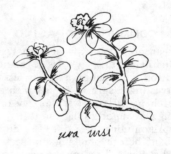

uva ursi

(continued from p. 327)

problems and in cleansing the urinary tract where the flow of liquids is blocked.

Observing colors in plants can also suggest ways to use them. The dark-green leaves of stinging nettles (*Urtica dioica*), parsley (*Petroselinum crispum*), and watercress reveal their high mineral content, making them an excellent tonic for building up and cleansing the blood. The yellow-gold flowers of chamomile (*Matricaris chamomilla*), yarrow (*Achillea millefolium*), and elderberry (*Sambucus canedensis*) are indicative of their diaphoretic or warming (like the sun) properties. In the rich brown category are burdock root (*Artium lappa*), dandelion root (*Taraxacum officinale*), and licorice root (*Glycyrrhiza glabra*). These herbs may be useful in cases where a person needs to feel more connected with the Earth energy, that is, more "rooted."

THE SPIRITUAL RELATIONSHIP

How we think about plants is also important. Do we see them as inanimate "botanicals" to be plugged into a formula, or as conscious co-workers and allies in the process of healing? An attitude of receptivity

(Text continued on p. 334)

Practical Plant Usage
Rob Menzies

Here are some plants to look for when you are out in the countryside.

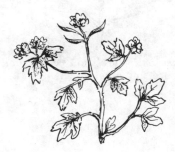

MUSTARD

This ancient plant is geographically widespread and has a wide variety of uses. Most important is its purifying and strengthening effect on the blood, liver, stomach, bowels, skin, and heart muscles, and its decongesting effect (because of the heat it produces) on the lungs and rheumatic joints. Pioneers and Indians made a plaster from ground seeds and water, which brought relief when placed on the chest. A syrup for coughs can be made from the fresh juice of the leaf, honey, and lemon. This syrup will even restore a lost voice. For a mustard condiment spread, brown some whole wheat flour till golden; add equal parts of ground mustard seeds; moisten with a mixture of apple cider, vinegar, and water. Add a dash of kelp powder, honey, oil, dill.

Mustard is an excellent source of vitamins A, E1, E2, and C, and of some trace elements. The tenderest greens make an excellent salad. The bloom buds contain even more nutrients than the leaves, plus protein from the developing nitrogenous pollen (steam for only three minutes). The bright yellow flowers are delicious on soups, added at the last minute like sprouts, or in salads for an appetizing, nutritious digestive aid. The seeds form plentifully, and can be parched and ground into meal suitable for seed cakes (the Pomo Indians used it with corn meal). Also, a delicious gravy can be made with the seeds, a dash of miso, tamari, and arrowroot flour.

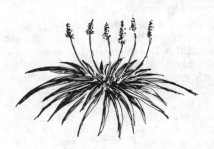

PLANTAIN

Another universal plant, easy to find and to use, is common plantain (*plantago major* and related species, also called buckhorn). The Indians called plantain White Man's Foot because it arrived as a weed with the first settlers. The leaves are good in salads (the broad-leaved, tender kind is best). Steamed, they make a delicious potherb. If the variety you have is very strong, drain off some liquid and cook a little with more water. There will be some loss of vitamins and minerals, but they will still have more than most mass-produced vegetables on the market. Medicinally plantain has many uses, in the form of poultices of crushed leaves to soothe insect and nettle stings, cuts, and other skin irritations. Just bruise a leaf to release the green sap, and rub it on. The seeds were an important source of Pinole for Indians and for many settlers. They are good eaten raw from the seedhead; or dried, parched (slightly browned in a skillet), and made into mush; or added to cornmeal in soups, etc. To use the seeds, first place them between your palms and rub to release the hulls, then blow the chaff away.

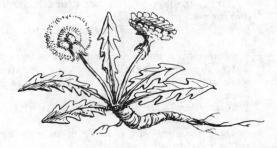

DANDELION

This nutritious healing plant has been widely used since ancient times as food and medicine.

(continued on p. 332)

(continued from p. 331)

The spring greens are delicious in salad; the leaves, available later on, are best when steamed five minutes like spinach. The crowns (whitish base, where the stem stalks come together) are a perfect salad vegetable or steamed potherb. The almost-developed blossomhead tastes like artichokes.

Dandelion roots can be dug any time of the year; cook them like parsnips. You can use them as a coffee substitute: roast the roots in a 150° to 200° oven for 4 hours, until brown and crisp, then grind. They also make a delicious wine.

Nutritionally, dandelions are a highly therapeutic food: an almost unequaled natural source of Vitamin A, most beneficial in repairing damaged mucous membranes, especially in the throat, for bronchitic children. The properties of the dandelion flush and stimulate the liver, kidneys, stomach, female organs, pancreas, and spleen. They relieve jaundice, diabetes, anemia, scurvy, lymphatic inflammation, rheumatic accumulation in the joints, toxins in the blood. There is even enough protein in dandelions to sustain life, as was found during the famine of Minorca.

OTHER USEFUL PLANTS

Acorns (white oak): grind, boil, and drain bitter water; repeat, dry, and use as cornmeal.

Aniseed is a digestive aid.

Carob pods provide protein, minerals, and vitamins, and are a good chocolate substitute.

Fennel tea is good for upset stomach, aids in digestion of beans and cabbage.

Fig seeds cure constipation. Chew completely.

Mosses hold up to 20 times their weight in water; they make excellent beds for sprouting seeds and beans, and for protecting perishable food.

Nasturtium seeds were an Indian favorite, an excellent antibiotic.

Okra, roasted and ground, is an excellent coffee substitute.

Sesame seeds are high in calcium, complete protein, minerals, vitamins.

Watermelon seeds stimulate the kidneys, and are reputedly very nutritious.

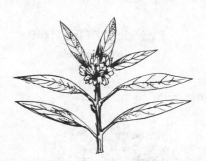

California bay laurel and *wormwood* will repel fleas, lice, and other insects.

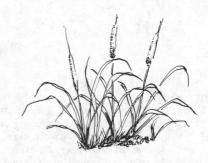

Cattail down is excellent stuffing for mattresses, pillows, quilts. Miners put it in their boots for warmth and water repellency. The Indians used it for diaper material. Life jackets often contain this down. Toast the seeds over coals, then drop in ashes; winnow the ashes and husks out. They make an excellent mush.

Manzanita berry juice is available all year round in California. In winter, collect the dry berries. They make a fine sweet/sour sugar, high in Vitamin C, which, when added to water, makes a refreshing drink.

Yerba Santa ("Holy Herb") is a tobacco substitute, and good for coughs and colds; use in a light tea for stomach pains. Crush the leaves for poultices to use on wounds. Mild psychic energizer.

Elderberry (blue-black) shoots make bows, arrows, fire spindles, flutes, flower tea for fevers, antiseptic wash. Crushed leaves are good for poison oak and wounds.

Indian soap plant (Amole) is both food and medicine. Cook bulb (in emergencies only). Juice is good glue; for soap, crush leaves, add to water, shake. Cook young leaves.

Yarrow's crushed leaves stop bleeding.

Mullein has many uses, including bandages, seed food, "tobacco" for colds; fuzzy stems can be dipped in grease for lamp wicks.

POISON OAK REMEDIES

Manzanita and Madrone berries, either crushed or made into a skin wash, as well as their root bark, are excellent remedies, as are elderberry juice, aloe vera, and soap plant root. For the latter, dig carefully to preserve the plant: dig on one side, push the brown husks aside, but do not break off. Peel petals off the lily bulb to reach the white, mucilaginous ones that can be used for application to the rash, which heals fast if caught early. Take another petal or two for a later treatment, then replace bulb cover carefully, and stamp the ground well around it. The plant will regenerate for other users.

EDIBLE, NUTRITIOUS FLOWERS

Dandelion, elderberry, squash, borage, madrone, nasturtium, marigold (soup flower), calendula, rose petals, violets.

SNAKEBITE REMEDIES

Milkweed juice and seeds (boiled), yellow dock, sunflower roots.

PAIN REMEDY

Boiled, mashed roots of thistle (also reported to be used for gonorrhea and for hastening parturition). For menstrual pains, clover tea (made by Oregon Indians).

NATURAL TOOTHBRUSHES

Used frayed dry root of cow parsnip, scouring rush, dandelion root, barks, licorice root, or reeds.

NATURAL ANTISEPTICS AND ANTIBIOTICS

Bark of sumac, valerian leaves, tobacco leaves, yarrow root, banana skins, natural unboiled honey, juniper berries, slippery elm bark, comfrey, mallow, muskmelon, jewelweed, garlic, parsley, pine pitch (lodge-pole pine), amole (soap plant).

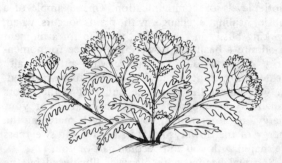

SUGGESTIONS FOR FURTHER READING

Euell Gibbons, *Stalking the Healthful Herbs.* McKay, 1966.

Maude Grieve, *A Modern Herbal.* Dover, two vols., 1972.

Ben Charles Harris, *Eat the Weeds.* Barre, 1971.

Alma Hutchens, *Indian Herbalogy of North America.* Merco, 1969.

Oliver Medsger, *Edible Wild Plants.* MacMillan, 1963.

Virginia Scully, *Treasury of American Indian Herbs.* Crown, 1970.

Maida Silverman, *A City Herbal.* Knopf, 1977.

Gary Snyder, *Turtle Island.* New Directions, 1974.

Some Useful Wild Plants, Vancouver, B.C.: Talon Books, 1972.

Muriel Sweet, *Common Edible and Useful Plants of the West.* Naturegraph, 1962.

Rob Menzies has traveled around the world, gathering information about plant uses and is an authoritative speaker on the subject. He is author of The Herbal Dinner.

(continued from p. 330)

is very important for healing; simply sitting with plants is one way to begin to understand their powers. The healing forces of nature will communicate with us, if we choose to listen; however, our "normal" everyday consciousness is not usually tuned in to such subtle levels of communication. One example of a subtle healing exchange with plants occurs when, working busily in the garden, we stop for a moment to admire a beautiful flower. The choice to momentarily suspend our mental activity automatically creates an opening for healing energy to be received. As you inhale the fragrance and absorb the colors visually, you experience a transformation of your energy. In other words, your energy is matching the energy of the flower, so that its beauty and sweetness are shared with you and become part of you.

Spiritual healing with plants is illustrated by the customary gift of flowers brought to persons who are sick. Hospital patients are always getting flowers. This is more than a social gesture of concern; it is a traditional means of offering the person's spirit assistance in healing. The terms "uplifting" and "lifts our spirits" indicate how we respond to the beauty of a fresh bouquet.

At Findhorn Garden in Scotland, the power of spiritual communication with plants has been explored extensively. By meditation, contact has been established with many plant spirits called "devas." The devas help slove practical questions about how to grow the garden as well as providing spiritual guidance. The amazing results of these "cooperatively" grown vegetables is documented in several books and recorded on film. This garden serves as a living testimony of what is possible when humankind transcends its exploitation of nature.

Traditional Native Americans express their spiritual relationship with all the inhabitants of nature by following a lifestyle that validates and respects the power of plants, animals, and humans. Many of the sacred plants used by Native American healers were common "weeds," growing in abundance in their own locale. This practice arises from the belief that the Earth is our Mother, and that she provides us with plants for nurturance and healing where we live. Therefore, our immediate environment can be a sacred spot, and local plants our medicine.

CONCLUSION

Learning to use plants for healing requires an integration of many ideas. The uniqueness of each person's energy and that of each plant must be honored. The choice of an herb for healing is as complex as the study of human psychology, and as simple as feeling yourself and the world around you.

NOTES

[1] James Mooney, *Myths of the Cherokee.* Nineteenth Annual Report of the Bureau of American Ethnology, 1900.

Julie Fuchs has taught classes through the Berkeley Holistic Health Center on the power of herbs. She leads herb walks in the East Bay, where she has been a professional gardener for the past six years.

Ecotopia Now

Sim Van der Ryn

"We have the means right now to design a sustainable, ecologically sound pattern into the compact urban context." With this statement the former state architect of California launches us on a journey into the very real possibilities for a new urban structure based on principles such as energy-efficient alternative technology and decentralization.

Mr. Van der Ryn suggests a merging of the architect's and biologist's points of view in order to achieve an environmentally sound community. The solutions he puts forth are persuasive in light of the problems of our cities. This article, however, is not so much a critique of city life as a positive approach to a more human and ecologically stable community. His down-to-Earth recommendations are drawn from rich personal experience and active small-scale operations which successfully demonstrate the value of alternative approaches. Mr. Van der Ryn and his colleagues offer a practical vision which can be accomplished now.

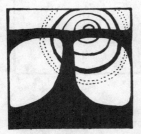

he image of a self-sufficient way of life in balance with nature has always been presented as an alternative that can only be realized in the country and by means of a rural economy. But we have the means right now to design a sustainable, ecologically sound pattern into our cities. We can build new communities that integrate available technologies with ecological principles to produce a high quality of urban life that is sustainable without the use of the nonrenewable resources.

Realizing this goal will require some important shifts in how we live and in the design of our urban life-support systems. The values that are inherent in

such shifts are steadily gaining ground in this country. In the long run, our choice will be to adapt our cities and suburbs toward ecological stability or to abandon them. First, we need to build some models from scratch to show that the goal can be realized, and that it is worth doing. The major features of the Ecotopian city include the following.

1. Bringing home and workplace closer together, in a decentralized mode, thus reducing the need for private autos to a fraction of today's use and cutting down not only energy use, but also the insatiable demand of the autoculture for space (30 to 50 per cent of the land area in our cities and suburbs is given over to cars). Reducing cars and streets makes possible a compact, human-scale environment where much of what is today asphalt can be used productively.

2. Bringing food production and processing into the home, neighborhood, and region, thus reducing dependency on an energy-intensive, land-exploitative food system.

3. Generating electricity locally from the sun and from biomass, and employing it selectively for its best uses: mechanical energy and lighting.

4. Bringing water use into balance with locally available, sustainable supplies, by means of conservation and recycling.

5. Returning all organic wastes to the soil.

6. Designing all buildings so that they are integrally heated and cooled by the action of sun and local climate (this is feasible in most parts of the country year-round).

By incorporating these features, we could forge a pattern that retains the best of the high-technological, urban, information-oriented culture, and yet renew people's sense of place and their connection to the basic rituals involved in an active participation in the natural cycles of the Earth.

Traditionally, cities have always been thought of and designed as dense human settlements that require a vast hinterland for their support. In the orthodox view, the city is seen as a transformer where the vast bounty of natural systems is converted into the capital savings of civilization, in the form of cultural

A SYSTEMS SPECTRUM

Linear System

- Energy flows in straight lines.
- Made up of components with separate, specialized functions
- High entropy, low information
- Memory stored in centralized, specialized components
- High rate of energy flow and material loss
- Single channels for energy flow
- High waste and pollution: resources out of place

Ecological System

- Energy flows in loops
- Made up of components with overlapping functions
- Low entropy, high information
- Memory stored in all components
- Low rate of energy flow and material loss
- Multiple channels for energy flow
- No waste: the output of one channel is input for another

Cycled Energy Flow in the Urban Village

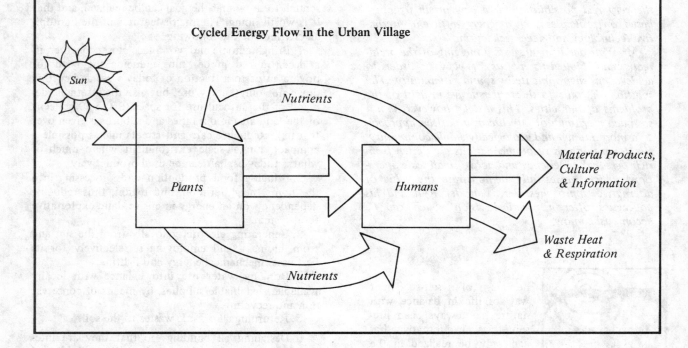

information and material products. In other words, cities are conceived of as machines—indeed, inefficient and inelegant machines for living. Raw materials move through them as quickly as possible. Some fuel the machine itself; some are transformed into products and information; and most are wasted.

In contrast is the natural system, in which materials flow in a continuous cycle or loop, and energy is extracted at each level. The result is a balanced system, driven by the energy of the sun and transformed by the diverse strategies devised by evolution.

The idea of designing a city around ecological balance is not new. Seventy years ago, Britain's Ebenezer Howard diagramed "garden cities" ringed by agricultural and open-space zones. The garden cities were linked together with mass transit, and movement within the city was by foot or bicycle, with a maximum travel time to workplace of fifteen minutes. In the 1930s Frank Lloyd Wright presented his utopian plan, called "Broadacre City": the dense center of the megalopolis was dismantled into a horizontal city, where each family had its own home and space to grow food—an organic version of the suburbs that were to follow.

These and other earlier utopian proposals were visionary responses to the growing tide of urbanization. High population density was seen as a destabilizing force, because it would lead to domination by large, alienating institutions and to the loss of a direct connection with the land, nature, and the food supply.

Even more significant than population density today is energy density, or the quantity of resources—per unit area—that must be imported to maintain the life of any community. Chances are, the greater the quantity of imported resources needed to support life, the greater the ecological damage and social instability in the community.

Urban cultures will probably survive as long as humanity survives. The challenge, then, is to design ecologically balanced communities—ideally, where little or no nonrenewable resources need to be imported into the community for its maintenance and survival. Since most of the technologies and systems that now maintain modern urban life are dependent on one-time-use fossil fuels, the trick will be to merge the built environment with nature; to design new systems that will harmonize with, amplify, and harvest the products of natural cycles in the environment; and to transform solar energy into forms capable of powering modern society. This task will require both scientific and aesthetic understanding, if not wisdom—which is, after all, an understanding of events in their total context.

Our understanding of how to translate ecological principles into the design of buildings, neighborhoods, cities, and towns is only just beginning, and creative solutions will depend on the fruitful marriage of disciplines—biology and ecology on one side, architecture and engineering on the other—that today rarely communicate with one another. Architects and planners are not expected to know anything about ecology, and biologists—with the rare exception of activists such as Barry Commoner or Paul Ehrlich—stay in the laboratories, or in the field. Those people who actually shape our cities and our futures—the politicians, senior bureaucrats, business people, developers, financiers—come out of law and business schools, speaking another language. Yet it is their decisions and visions—or lack of vision—that will decide our future.

TRANSLATING LINEAR TO ECOLOGICAL

A brief comparison of the differences between an ecological system and the linear, machinelike system that is typical of today's urban pattern might be useful. The properties of a linear system, and their ecological equivalents, exist along a continuum. We

The New Aesthetics
Sim Van der Ryn

Without aesthetics, neither economy nor efficiency of energy have any meaning. Aesthetics is conceptual information and varies from culture to culture: it is the meaning that we find in form. The meaning that we derive from any environment is limited by the form of that environment. Our interactions with complex and diverse living systems increase our awareness and add to the meaning that we derive from life.

Our spirits are enriched and constantly recharged by our functional and ritualistic connections to the natural world. The preindustrial aesthetic was always based on that kind of connection. Whether evidenced in the miniature garden found in each home in a dense Japanese neighborhood, or the simple Arab courtyard fountain, or the shade elms of New England commons, the whole picturesque "architecture without architects" of the earlier world adapted habitat to local materials, site, climate, and ecosystem.

The importance of aesthetics is the kind of participation that it brings about with natural systems. It is from this relationship that the new aesthetics must be derived. For the most part, however, Americans have lost that intimate connection and an awareness of their place in the natural world. The "natural" aspect has been reduced to empty symbols, such as the tract house lawn, which started out as a sheep meadow—the lawn was there for sheep to crop. Ecosystems have become dim landscapes to be appreciated out of car windows—low-information media like TV screens.

The task, then, of ecological design, is to begin to recreate the opportunities for people to derive meaning and satisfaction from their experience with natural cycles.

need to get a feeling for when a particular design approaches the linear and when it approaches the ecological.

In brief, ecological systems incorporate four basic principles:

1. Materials and energy are processed through closed loops and webs of multiple channels.

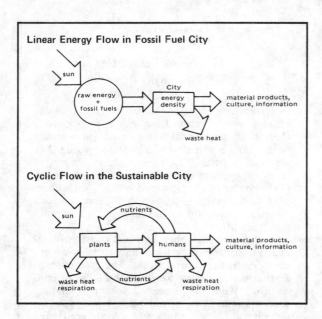

Linear Energy Flow in Fossil Fuel City

sun

raw energy + fossil fuels → City energy density → material products, culture, information

waste heat

Cyclic Flow in the Sustainable City

sun

nutrients

plants → humans → material products, culture, information

waste heat respiration   nutrients   waste heat respiration

2. Energy is released within the system, in small increments.

3. A steady rate is maintained by means of information passed through the permeable boundaries between systems.

4. Information is stored in a decentralized, genetic memory.

Some of these principles are illustrated in the Farallones Integral Urban House. In the Integral House, each major functional system employs multiple pathways for material and energy flow. The heating system, for example, includes direct solar gain through windows, a solar air space-heating system, and a woodstove heater for cloudy cold days. Organic waste can be shunted in a variety of ways. Human fecal matter decomposes in a composting toilet and, when fully decomposed, is used as a soil amendment for ornamental plants. Urine is collected and used as a nitrogen-rich fertilizer. Kitchen scraps are fed to the chickens and thus converted into edible protein; the chicken manure is recycled in the garden. Garbage can also be composted or fed into worm cultures to make a nutrient-rich casting for garden use; the worms are then fed to the chickens or the fish in the pond. Duckweed in the pond absorbs toxic fish waste and in turn is dried and fed to the chickens. These are all examples of multiple loops.

An important feature of the multiple pathway is that each component in such a system tends to perform overlapping functions. Thus, one test of the

integral quality of any system is the extent to which components are integrated into multiple functions. An electric heater can only be an electric heater. A garbage truck can only be a garbage truck. However, windows admit light, provide a view, and can also act as a solar collector. An attached greenhouse can be a solar collector and a storage system, a place to grow seedlings and winter vegetables, or a location for a hot tub. A planting box, however small, together with composting buckets, can take the place of a smelly garbage can and noisy garbage truck; besides processing waste nutrients, it provides a source of beauty, foods, and flowers, and can be the focus for many pleasant leisure hours.

The system of multiple pathways is closely linked to the idea of the diversity and stability of healthy, natural systems, and the multiple pathway is an interactive process within any food or nutrient chain. For example, in a healthy garden, a diversity of plants will ensure that there is going to be a diversity in insect life associated with those plants; thus, one insect population is not likely to get out of control and become a pest. The use of pesticides, on the other hand, is a positive feedback cycle: to devote the entire Midwest to one crop, such as corn, is to foster a predator that gets totally out of control; then pesticide is used, but the insects become resistant, and it becomes necessary to continue to apply more and more pesticide. Slowly, learning from its mistakes, agriculture is beginning to take the principle of diversity into account.

The linear mode is particularly inefficient in dealing with waste and garbage. Waste is simply hauled to land-fills, and most urban areas are running out of available land-fill areas: cities are being forced to haul garbage to remote locations hundreds of miles away. Human waste is diluted in the ratio of 100 to 1 with potable water and piped to large sewage factories, where the solids are removed through mechanical and bacterial action; the nutrient-rich effluent that remains is dumped into rivers or the ocean, where it overloads the ability of natural systems to provide oxygen needed by the organisms in the effluent. There results a condition known as eutrophication, and a surge of microbiological and algae growth depletes the oxygen and fouls up the water. (For a more complete description of the modern sewage scandal and some alternatives, see my book *The Toilet Papers*.)

The concept of flow is crucial. Ecological design tends to rely on smaller, more decentralized units, to reduce the over-all flow, and thus to reduce energy use. As a rule, in any ecologically designed system,

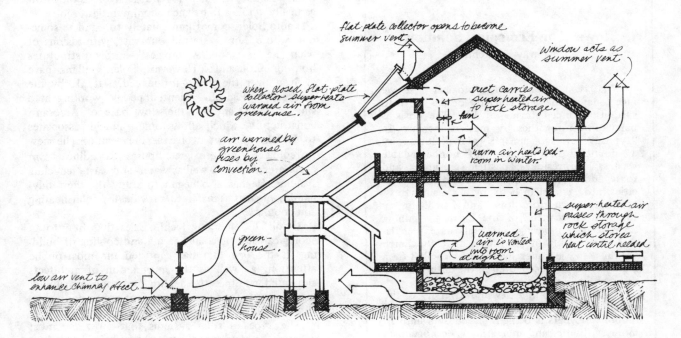

flat plate collector opens to become summer vent

window acts as summer vent

When closed, flat plate collector super-heats warmed air from greenhouse.

duct carries super-heated air to rock storage.

fan

air warmed by greenhouse rises by convection.

warm air heats bedroom in winter.

green-house.

warmed air is vented into room at night.

super-heated air passes through rock storage which stores heat until needed

low air vent to enhance chimney effect.

Integral solar heating for this home incorporates greenhouse and rock storage for heating and food production.

the total energy flow required will be less than that in the linear system. In linear systems, energy pulses through in order to achieve maximum product flow, with a high rate of waste. The use of electricity to heat a house is a prime example: much more high-quality fuel is consumed than will finally result in useful heat in the home. The way we heat our homes with electricity—particularly that provided by nuclear power—is equivalent to "using a chainsaw to cut butter." Moreover, the economic costs are not borne by the immediate user but get buried in the increasing entropy of larger systems. With nuclear electricity, the costs are buried in the entire rate base, and consumers generally don't know what they're paying for.

Modern agriculture is another energy sink: it uses far more energy to produce food than it takes out. In traditional agriculture, that ratio is reversed. In the U.S. it takes 20 to 30 calories of energy to produce 1 calorie of food; in China it takes 1 calorie of energy (mostly human) to produce 30 calories of food. The agribusiness approach is rationalized on the basis that the total productivity of energy-intensive agriculture is far higher than traditional methods, and that we would starve without it: if the fossil-fuel subsidy were removed, food prices would be astronomical. With

our food system so dependent on energy waste, that claim is all too sadly true.

PROTOTYPES AND PROGRESS

By careful orchestration of food and nutrient chains integrated with land use and the design of human space, we can begin to create systems with multiple functions, each using the products of the other, wasting nothing; we can make sure that functions overlap, so that if one system fails, others may take its place. This type of design is distinctly unlinear and nonstatic: its aesthetic grows, not out of the arbitrary and increasingly foolish dictates of architectural fashion, but out of the dynamic and functional interplay of living systems in harmony with human needs.

The concept of designing and constructing new communities around the principles of ecological stability and energy efficiency is slowly gaining ground. Most of the innovation I'm familiar with has come from committed individuals and small struggling groups, rather than from the corporation or established research factories. Beginning in the early '70s, a number of groups began to design, construct,

Toward an Ecological Solution
Murray Bookchin

What is at stake in the ecological crisis we face today is the very capacity of the Earth to sustain advanced forms of life. The crisis is being drawn together by massive increases in "typical" forms of air and water pollution; by a mounting accumulation of nondegradable wastes, lead residues, pesticide residues, and toxic additives in food; by the expansion of cities into vast urban belts; by increasing stresses due to congestion, noise, and mass living; by the wanton scarring of the Earth by mining operations, lumbering, and real-estate speculation. The result of all this is that the Earth within a few decades has been despoiled on a scale that is unprecedented in the entire history of human habitation on the planet.

Finally, the complexity and diversity of life which marked biological evolution during many millions of years is being replaced by a simpler, more synthetic, and increasingly homogenized environment. Aside from any esthetic considerations, the elimination of this complexity and diversity may prove to be the most serious loss of all. Modern society is literally undoing the work of organic evolution. If this process continues unabated, the Earth may be reduced to a level of biotic simplicity where humanity— whose welfare depends profoundly upon the complex food chains in the soil, on the land surface, and in the oceans—will no longer be able to sustain itself as a viable animal species.

This passage is excerpted from *Towards an Ecological Solution, Ecology Center Reprint No. 6.* Available from Ecology Center, 2701 College Avenue, Berkeley, CA 94705.

and experiment with various forms of habitation. The significance of these experiments is their focus on the connections among the systems that make up a house, and their insistence on seeing the design of habitation as fundamentally a question of biological design. These rudimentary projects started on a small scale, not only because limited funding has a way of keeping things small, but because the individual habitation is an obvious place to start. Those very modest beginnings, however, have been conceived from the outset as the first step toward a larger vision of organically whole and balanced communities.

Paolo Soleri comes immediately to mind as someone whose canvas started out vast, with visions of what he termed "Arcologies"—massive structures housing thousands. However, Soleri's plans have evolved over the years—influenced, I think, by the work of biologically oriented people working at a smaller scale, and by the slow pace of Arcosanti construction, which allows Soleri and his associates to let the concept evolve as they build. The new "Arcologies" feature greenhouses cascading down austere canyons, as well as water- and waste-recycling systems. He has also begun to study the thermodynamics of heat transfer to provide for solar heating and cooling.

Of all the emerging technologies that fit into an ecological design, solar heating and cooling of buildings is the one that has captured the most public attention, as well as the imagination of architects and builders. Since the heating and cooling of buildings accounts for some 40 per cent of our nonrenewable energy use, that interest is well-placed.

The type of solar systems that show the most promise so far are those misleadingly labeled as "passive"; that is, the system is designed as part of the building and its functions, as opposed to "active" systems, which involve solar machinery added on to the structure. Integral solar design makes use of, and combines, many commonsense design principles, such as proper orientation, shading and placement of landscaping, and especially the use of the building's mass as a thermal battery to store heat or "coolth."

In the past several years, solar greenhouses have gained favor, since they can be added onto existing buildings as well as designed as part of new structures. In this concept, a south-facing greenhouse, combined with storage mass in its walls or in a sunken rockbed, catches and stores heat, which is then distributed to the rest of the building. And, of course, the greenhouse serves not only as part of the solar system, but also as a place to grow plants, and as a usable room. In locations such as the Midwest, with its dry winters, a greenhouse equipped with a hot tub, woodstove, and planting area could not only serve as part of a heating system (with the hot tub contributing to the heat-storage system), but could also change the whole interior climate and psychology of the house, providing needed humidity, winter salads, and pleasurable space.

Experiments that try to create biologically stable habitats by integrating various technologies on a small scale can, of course, be only part of the answer. I have never liked the bomb-shelter mentality behind some people's idea of self-sufficiency. The goal is to reduce dependency and centralization where possible, but in the end our well-being is tied to the local networks that we create.

Accordingly, many people are now working hard to develop and test specific technologies that can come together to form an integrated life-support system at the community scale. A balanced community should be able to grow most of its own food in its backyards and on the block, with the rest coming from the immediate region; any organic wastes generated by food production and use can be returned to the soil to maintain fertility. Thus, the basic building block in designing biologically stable human settlements may be the development of simple, small-scale, intensive agricultural techniques that can be used by the average urban person and small farmers.

In a garden covering several acres in a Palo Alto industrial park, former Yale systems analyst John Jeavons has for some years been quietly and methodically developing what he calls a "minifarm": plots of one-tenth of an acre, which, he calculates, could produce $10,000 to $20,000 worth of vegetables with one person working a forty-hour week eight months of the year. Each 2,800-square-foot plot should, he estimates, provide a balanced year-round diet for one person, including grain (wheat was heading up on the December day we visited), vegetables, and fruit (dwarf fruit trees are interplanted in the beds). Jeavons claims that one person could tend such a plot in a half-hour per day, using one-hundredth of the fossil fuel that today's agriculture would devote to that area, and one-eighth the water.

A shift from massive monoculture-type agriculture to local intensive agriculture would result in substantial water savings across the board, since agribusiness uses 90 per cent of our water (often with federal subsidy) and uses it extremely wastefully.

High-quality water is rapidly becoming a scarce resource in many parts of the country. At its price, though, it is still a best buy: what else can you purchase, delivered in your home, for pennies per ton? In parts of the country, particularly the western Sunbelt, water is being mined and used up much like any other nonrenewable resource, and natural underground reservoirs, which take hundreds of years to build up, are being depleted at alarming rates.

When we were planning the Farallones Rural Center, one of our goals was to demonstrate the potential for low water use in water-short rural areas. The authorities in the county initially refused us permits on the basis that we must be able to supply and

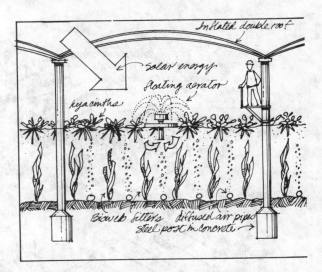

The Solar Aquacell System produces recreational quality water out of sewage using water hyacinths and the sun to convert waste nutrients into plant material.

dispose of 150 gallons per person per day, which is the accepted standard for water use. We were able to get by with about a tenth of that for domestic use. Since then, necessity—in the form of recurrent droughts in California—has spurred an interest in water-conserving technologies, and even the affluent folks in Marin County were able to reduce their water consumption by 60 per cent without any change in technology.

The prevalent suburban pattern in the United States could be easily adapted to save even more energy, by being converted to intensive garden production of the sort promoted by Jeavons. The 19 million acres of suburban lawns in this country are major consumers of pesticides and fertilizers; if they were converted to mini-farms, they could, according to Jeavon's productivity figures, feed this country!

Removing redundant streets would add many millions more of farmable acres in our spread-out cities. Most of our cities and suburbs are built on flat, alluvial plains, and the soil is often the best there is. Many agriculturists seem skeptical of Jeavon's figures, but it is clear from his work and that of others—including the Farallones gardeners—that the intensively planted, raised-bed approach to urban farming is capable of producing year-round crops in limited space with far greater yields and less care than conventional methods. For most Americans, tending a small intensive garden would mean one less TV show a day and some more time off their duff—not a bad tradeoff.

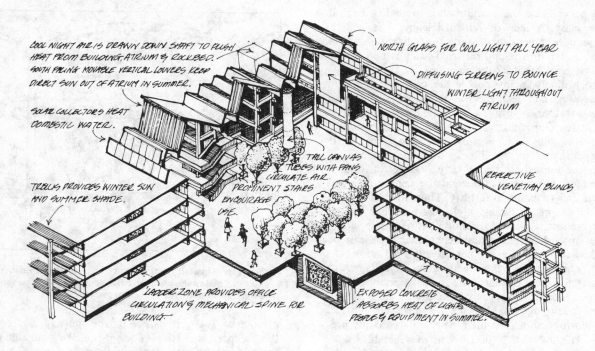

COOL NIGHT AIR IS DRAWN DOWN SHAFT TO FLUSH
HEAT FROM BUILDING, ATRIUM & ROCKBED.
SOUTH FACING MOVABLE VERTICAL LOUVERS KEEP
DIRECT SUN OUT OF ATRIUM IN SUMMER.

SOLAR COLLECTORS HEAT
DOMESTIC WATER.

TRELLIS PROVIDES WINTER SUN
AND SUMMER SHADE.

TALL CANVAS
TUBES WITH FANS
CIRCULATE AIR.
PROMINENT STAIRS
ENCOURAGE
USE.

LADDER ZONE PROVIDES OFFICE
CIRCULATION & MECHANICAL SPINE FOR
BUILDING.

NORTH GLASS FOR COOL LIGHT ALL YEAR

DIFFUSING SCREENS TO BOUNCE
WINTER LIGHT THROUGHOUT
ATRIUM

REFLECTIVE
VENETIAN BLINDS

EXPOSED CONCRETE
ABSORBS HEAT OF LIGHTS,
PEOPLE & EQUIPMENT IN SUMMER.

Cutaway drawing of energy-efficient features in a state office building. These features will reduce energy consumption to 20 percent of that used by standard design office buildings in the same city.

When food and home are brought closer together, the cycle of waste is reduced. Kitchen garbage can be composted and returned to the soil. Collecting human wastes in waterless composting toilets allows us to return these otherwise wasted nutrients to the soil, and so the cycle of water waste and sewage pollution can be broken.

There are many other technologies that might be used in an Ecotopian community. The Solar Aquacell system, developed by a group of young San Diego marine biologists, removes the nutrients from sewage in closed greenhouses, using water hyacinths—a rapidly growing plant whose floating root system soaks up nutrients. Edible seafood, such as giant prawns, can also be cultivated. Composted or dried, the hyacinths make an excellent cattle feed.

During my time in Sacramento, I introduced this innovative and cost-effective technology to bureaucrats and engineers building new energy-intensive mega-sewage plants. Even without the support of state or federal funds, the town of Hercules, California, has decided to build a four-million-gallon-a-day Solar Aquacell plant. The main drawback of this biologically sound system is that more space is required for the plant, since sewage is retained for a

week instead of a few hours. The greatest asset of the Aquacell system is that water purified by this fully biological process is of such high quality that it can be used for recreation or irrigation.

Left to its own devices, standard development intensifies water problems. In the typical suburb, more than half the surface area is covered with streets, driveways, and roofs that do not retain water. The result is a massive runoff that overpowers the holding capacity of native streams, which then become the subject of concrete "stabilization" programs. Now communities such as Monterey County, California, are considering requiring that homes install old-fashioned cisterns to contain runoff and to store rain water for use in the dry season.

All the technologies discussed so far could be implemented in our existing communities without causing major social disruption and change. They are transitional technologies; they create the basis for a sustainable society. However, one radical, obvious, and difficult change remains: the segregation in time and space of workplace from homeplace, and our total dependence on the automobile—the production, care, and feeding of which consumes around 40 per cent of our natural resources and the lion's share of the world's depletable energy supplies.

Fly low over any major city and suburban area, and you will begin to get a full picture of how the automobile dominates the use of the land. Not until people can see an alternative that works is the pattern likely to change. In the Ecotopian community, the road system must be designed so that cars cannot be used for short trips, and work locations must be scattered throughout the community, to reduce auto commuting.

Some people seem to think that our unique purpose as a species is to release all the hydrocarbons from underneath the Earth's surface and then go the way of the dinosaur. If this is the case, then the internal combustion engine and the automobile fill an important ecological niche toward our own destruction.

CONSCIOUS COMMUNITY

The Ecotopian city need not be built in a radically different way from how communities get planned and built today. The critical aspect is the disposition of land, building guidelines, and the design of life-support systems.

The Bible tells us that "Without vision the people perish." Today people seem to be without a shared positive vision of what the future could be; indeed, the polls continually tell us that the future looks bleak to most Americans. Everything seems to have become unmanageable. Thus, a concern for the collective environment, outside of neighbors and friends, has been replaced by the urge for self-improvement, if not plain self-indulgence. The future is nowhere to be found.

Meanwhile, every eight weeks the equivalent of a new city for 400,000 people gets built in this country —an extension of the existing pattern. The cities continue to rot, essential services deteriorate, and the thin mantle of soil, water, air, and biotic life that is the true basis for our affluence continues to be assaulted, out of ignorance and greed.

The over-all picture is not so unremittingly grim as current trends might seem to suggest. Ecotopian com-munities are possible *right now,* and the construction of some modest first examples might help to restore some of our lost hope. Visionary eco-designers need to join forces with number-crunching analysts and can-do engineers to create prototypes. Our more enlightened entrepreneurs and politicians need to commit themselves to an idea that could bring some much-needed credit to a system whose concern for human and environmental values seems to be at a cynical new low point.

The seeds of ecological design *are* beginning to sprout, however, and many of the hardware components to create an ecologically stable urban community have already been developed and are working. What we have yet to do is bring together all the threads and weave them into a single coherent design for a new community.

SUGGESTIONS FOR FURTHER READING

Farallones Institute, *The Integral Urban House.* Sierra Club Books, 1979.

Sim Van der Ryn, *The Toilet Papers.* Capra Press, 1978.

E. F. Schumacher, *Small Is Beautiful.* Harper and Row, 1975.

Sim Van der Ryn, a native of the Netherlands, has been active in the San Francisco Bay Area for twenty years as an architect, teacher, writer, and environmentalist. While serving as California State Architect from 1975 to 1978, he developed successful administration initiatives and legislation for alternative energy and solar design. He also established and was the first director of the Office of Appropriate Technology in the Governor's Office, and was later appointed Chairman of the State Solarcal Council. He is now president of the Farallones Institute, a research and educational center for the design of ecologically sound forms of community which he founded in 1970.

He is the author of several articles, monographs, and books, the latest being The Toilet Papers, *an exposé of modern sewage-treatment practices.*

Nuclear Morality
Margaret Mead

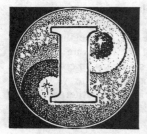

In the summer of 1945, I had a book on the post-war world about half-finished, when we got the news that the Bomb had gone off. I simply took the manuscript and tore it right straight across. There wasn't a single sentence that would have been right any more. The world had changed for good. It would never be the same world again.

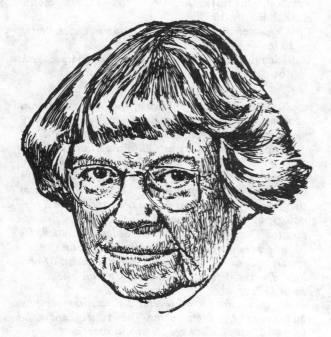

From then on, the human race had the power to destroy itself, and the responsibility to see that it didn't destroy itself, and could continue on this planet. For the meantime, we were first preoccupied

This article is taken from the transcript of a talk given by Dr. Mead in June 1976 at the U.N. Habitat Conference on Human Settlements. It originally appeared in *New Directions,* No. 15 (Sept. 1976), and is reprinted here by kind permission.

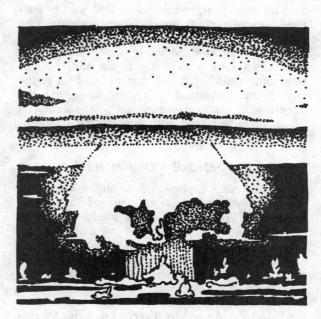

When the Bomb dropped in 1945, the world was changed— and changed for good.

with trying to reduce the dangers of the existence of the Bomb. Many people felt that bombs were like warships—if you had a lot of them, you were more likely to have a war—and if you could get rid of them, then you wouldn't have a war. That's the way they felt after World War I. There was a great deal of emphasis on *getting rid of the Bomb* by older people that had been in favour of sinking warships. They didn't understand that *you cannot get rid of the Bomb;* you can get rid of bombs, but not of the Bomb. There is no possible way, in the present-day world, that we will get rid of the knowledge of how to make bombs. The knowledge is there, and we cannot get rid of it. The only problem for us is how we're going to use it.

Now, at the time that the Atoms for Peace declarations were made, there was a tremendous, very strong hope, particularly among the nuclear scientists themselves, that this monster that they'd loosed on the world could somehow be tamed and used for peace-

Nuclear Madness
Helen Caldicott, M.D.

The growing controversy surrounding nuclear fission is the most important issue that American society and the world at large has ever faced. A national and international debate on this subject is long overdue, and the participation of each individual will determine its outcome. We must begin today by first of all learning as much as we can about the critical health hazards involved, because what we don't know about these dangers may kill us.

Item: The world's major military powers have built tens of thousands of atomic bombs powerful enough to kill the world's inhabitants several times over.

Item: Each 1,000-megawatt nuclear reactor contains as much radioactive material ("fallout") as would be produced by one thousand Hiroshima-sized bombs. A "meltdown" (in which fissioning nuclear fuel and the steel and concrete structures that encase it overheat and melt) could release a reactor's radioactive contents into the atmosphere, killing 50,000 people or more, and contaminating thousands of square miles.

Item: Each reactor daily leaks carcinogenic and mutagenic effluent. These radioactive materials increase the amount of background radiation to which we are constantly exposed, increasing our risk of developing cancer and genetic disease.

Item: Each reactor annually produces tons

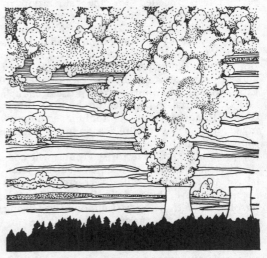

A commercial nuclear reactor annually produces 400 to 500 pounds of plutonium that will remain hazardous to life for 500,000 years.

of radioactive waste, some of which remains dangerous for more than 50,000 years. No permanent fail-safe method of disposal or storage has yet been found for them, despite millions of dollars spent during three decades of research. Despite recent proposals, there is good reason to suspect that we may never develop safe methods of disposal and longterm storage.

Item: Each commercial nuclear reactor produces approximately 400 to 500 pounds of plutonium a year. Dangerous for at least 500,000 years, this toxic substance poses a threat to public health which cannot be overemphasized. Present in nature in only minute amounts, plutonium is one of the deadliest substances known. In addition, it is the basic

(continued on p. 346)

ful purposes. It was thought that somehow, if we could use nuclear energy for peaceful purposes, then we would make up for the iniquity of having made the Bomb. I suppose this was felt more strongly in the United States than anywhere else, especially by the nuclear physicists. And we still have a lot of them around, who have commited themselves very strongly to the hope that nuclear energy would be *good* for the human race; they simply cannot face the fact that it may not, which is one reason you will find nuclear

physicists on both sides of the argument. There are undoubtedly people that are in the employ of the industry, or in very particular positions, but there is also a very large number of nuclear physicists who have testified in favour of nuclear energy because they so very much *want* it to be true that it could benefit the human race.

One of the things we thought about in those days was that if there were countries in the Third World that were short of oil, short of coal, we could give

(continued from p. 345)

raw material needed for the fabrication of atomic bombs, and each reactor yearly produces enough to make forty such weapons. Thus, "peaceful" nuclear power production is synonymous with nuclear-weapons proliferation: American sales of reactor technology abroad guarantee that, by the end of the century, dozens of countries will possess enough nuclear material to manufacture bombs of their own. Moreover, the "plutonium economy" urged upon us by the nuclear industry and its supporters in government presents the disturbing probability that terrorist groups will construct atomic bombs from stolen nuclear materials or that criminals will divert such materials for radioactive blackmail. Because of this terrorist threat, we may find ourselves living in a police state designed to minimize unauthorized access to such nuclear materials.

Most early developers of nuclear energy explored its potential forty years ago to produce bombs that would inflict unprecedented damage. Seven years after the United States tested two such weapons on the populations of Hiroshima and Nagasaki, the collective guilt generated by the deaths of some 200,000 Japanese civilians prompted the American government to advocate a new policy: the "peaceful use of atomic energy" to produce "safe, clean" electricity, a form of power touted as being "too cheap to meter." Together, industry and government leaders decided that nuclear power would become the energy source of the future. Today, 25 years later, that prospect threatens the well-being of our nation and the world.

I believe it imperative that the American public understand that nuclear-power generation is neither safe, nor clean, nor cheap; that new initiatives are urgently required if we are to avoid nuclear catastrophe in a world armed to the teeth with atomic weapons; and that these initiatives must begin with awareness, concern, and action by individual citizens.

One need not be a scientist or a nuclear engineer to take part in this emerging debate; in fact, an overspecialized approach tends to confuse the issue. The basic questions go beyond the technical problems of reactor safety and radioactive waste management. Even if the present state of nuclear technology were to be judged fail-safe, for example, we must ask ourselves how much faith we would be willing to invest in the infallibility of the human beings who must administer that technology. Granted, we may someday be able to isolate nuclear waste from the environment: how confident can we be in our ability to control the actions of fanatics or criminals? How can we assure the longevity of the social institutions responsible for perpetuating that isolation? And what moral right have we to burden our progeny with this poisonous legacy? Finally, we must confront the philosophical issue at the heart of the crisis: do we, as a species, possess the wisdom that the intelligent use of nuclear energy demands? If not, are we courting disaster by continuing to exploit it?

From a purely medical point of view, there is no controversy: the commercial and military technologies we have developed to release the energy of the nucleus impose unacceptable risks to health and life. As a physician I consider it my responsibility to preserve and further life. Thus, as a doctor, as well as a mother and world citizen, I wish to practice the ultimate form of preventive medicine by ridding the earth of these technologies which propagate suffering, disease, and death.

them nice nuclear reactors, make up for it, and close many of the economic gaps that worried us. That argument is still hanging around, and there are still people who think, although they're against nuclear power in the affluent world, somehow it would do the Third World good. Unfortunately, they are joined by people who'd like to *sell* nuclear reactors to the Third World.

So, we're now having arguments like, "The United States and Canada have topped off the best customers; so there's nothing left for Germany and France except the Third World; so they should have a right to sell them reactors." The general public came to believe that nuclear power would solve our energy problems, and although it went in little spurts of people who didn't like it, or didn't want it downwind, or something of the sort, it went on and on.

It wasn't until the Energy Crisis, with people's tensions getting directed to the big power companies, and getting annoyed with the power companies on all

An Alternative to Atoms
The Abalone Alliance

Renewable forms of energy and energy conservation stand as immediate alternatives to electricity generated from nuclear fission. Alternative energy requires less capital per unit of energy delivered than nuclear power, but provides enough energy for a prosperous economy.

The amount of solar energy that reaches the United States in twelve hours is equal to the nation's yearly energy consumption. Solar heating and cooling involves the use of collectors on site which absorb the sun's energy. This method of heating buildings and water is not new. In fact, it has been employed in this and other countries for many years.

Wind energy has been used to pump water, compress air, and generate electricity since the mid-nineteenth century. A federally sponsored report by Project Independence estimates that 23 per cent of our electricity could be generated with wind power by the year 1990. The National Science Foundation concluded that electricity produced by wind power could become cost-competitive with conventional diesel-fuel electrical generating plants, by the end of 1979.

Biomass conversion involves the changing of organic matter into useful fuels, or directly into heat. The various biomass techniques include utilizing urban and industrial wastes, agricultural and forest residues, and farming on land or in the ocean. About 80 per cent of the total annual municipal waste is combustible and could be used to generate energy equivalent to more than half the 1970 oil imports from the Middle East. Harvest and bioconversion of ocean kelp into methane gas would generate 23 trillion cubic feet of gas per year. (This is equal to the current national annual gas demand.) Land plantations could generate 8-11 trillion cubic feet of gas per year. As with all renewable energy sources, biomass conversion has a minimal impact on the environment.

Solar photovoltaic cells convert sunlight directly into electricity. The primary impediment to solar-cell development has been the inability to develop a cost-efficient means of mass production. Their efficiency has been going up, and their price going down, despite limited federal and industrial interest. By the early 1970s the cost had dropped to $100/watt. By 1973, it was $30/watt; and in 1975, $17/watt. Recent estimates indicate that the price of photovoltaic cells will drop below $1/watt within five or ten years.

Energy conservation is a technology of common sense. By adopting energy-conservation principles, we would eliminate wasteful forms of energy production and consumption. A study released by Senator Edward Kennedy reported the possibility of reducing the growth rate of our energy consumption to zero by the combined application of alternative energy generation and energy conservation.

Co-generation, a form of energy conservation, is the process by which the waste heat from industries is converted into electricity or rechanneled for direct space heating. In many cases there would be excess electricity that could be sold back to the power company. Co-generation is employed now and will be utilized more as the price of conventional electricity continues to rise.

This is a partial list of the USA's viable alternatives to nuclear power. Implicit in all the alternative technologies available is our ability to influence policy makers to reorder the nation's priorities and our willingness to seek creative solutions to *our* energy problems.

For further information on alternative energy sources and antinuclear activities, please contact the Abalone Alliance, 944 Market St., Room 307, San Francisco, California 94102.

SUGGESTIONS FOR FURTHER READING

Anna Gyorgy and Friends, *No Nukes: Everyone's Guide to Nuclear Power.* South End Press, 1979.

Helen Caldicott, *Nuclear Madness: What You Can Do.* Autumn Press, 1978.

Barry Commoner, *The Politics of Energy.* Knopf, 1979.

Ralph Nader and John Abbotts, *The Menace of Atomic Energy.* Norton, 1979.

John W. Gofman, *An Irreverent, Illustrated View of Nuclear Power.* Committee for Nuclear Responsibility, 1979.

This article first appeared in the *Radioactive Times,* published by the Abalone Alliance, and is reprinted here by permission.

sorts of counts, that people began to pay attention to the dangers of building up more and more nuclear plants.

The most important reason, I think, why we are facing so much discussion today, all around the world, is because we're on the verge of taking another step in devoting ourselves and our future to nuclear power that is at least as drastic as when we moved from the atom bomb to the hydrogen bomb. One of the ways that you can measure what that step meant is this: when there was only the atom bomb, the theory in New York City was that if you could get thirty miles out, when the bomb hit New York, it wouldn't hit you. And the cost of real estate went way up over thirty miles from New York (laughter) and way down near New York. Once the hydrogen bomb was there,

nobody talked anymore about getting any real estate that would save them. We still have old signs up, saying Air Raid Shelter, that are utterly and completely meaningless.

This is a point in history that is at least as momentous as the step between the atom and the hydrogen bomb, and it has some of the characteristics of the step when we invented the Bomb in the first place, because it means that we are going to fasten tons and tons of artificial, terribly poisonous material on this planet, for thousands of years. For our children, and our children's children and for generations of people that we are incapable of thinking about imaginatively, plutonium in large quantities—loose, free, leaking, wandering around—will be there. Now, this is the moment at which we've got to stop and say *no!*

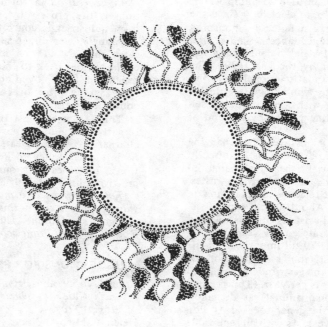

Section VI:
Evolution of Holistic Health
Concepts, Networking, Legal Issues, The Future

"We are going to be here on this planet a while. We've got to think and act holistically. Putting the holistic concept into effect would have profound social and political implications."

George Leonard

"Many medicines, few cures."
Poor Richard

"While some of its roots go back hundreds or thousands of years in history, the current holistic health movement in the U.S.A. is, at best, at the stage of a two-year-old, just learning to walk among a bustling world of older kids and adults."

John Travis, M.D.

"I see our biggest need as being a method for motivating people to want to be healthy and to accept the major requirements for health as worthwhile."
C. Norm Shealy

"In a holistic approach that integrates techniques ranging from meditation to the most modern medical technology lies a new medicine that seeks a balance within ourselves and with our environment."
Kenneth R. Pelletier

[We have] "nothing but politics and bank holidays to satisfy the eternal human need of living in ritual adjustment to the cosmos in its revolutions . . . The human race is like a great uprooted tree, with its roots in the air. We must plant ourselves again in the universe."

D.H. Lawrence

Introduction
EVOLUTION OF HOLISTIC HEALTH:
Concepts, Networking, Legal Issues, The Future

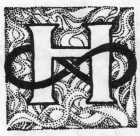olistic health is steadily expanding, from a set of practices and techniques used to enhance one's health, to include a whole way of living one's life. A primary concept of holistic health, that of personal responsibility for our lives, has propelled many people into action. People are now more willing to accept the challenges that this responsibility sometimes represents. In this last section of the book, we present articles that celebrate this growth and discuss some of the obstacles that remain to be worked through.

Holistic health centers are now serving many needs all across the country. The Berkeley Holistic Health Center is one of the original centers, and has served its community for several years. It is an excellent model of what can be done when people put their talents together. Its services range from a spiritual healing circle, to an extensive referral file, to a program that can lead to a master's degree in holistic education. The article featuring the Health Center in this section further illustrates the services and learning opportunities that are available at many health centers.

Another article in this section explains how you can find holistic-minded people in your community, and how to start a center of your own if one is not available already. People everywhere are ready to get together and share knowledge and learning experiences that lead to happier, healthier lives.

Our country's need for a national health plan is becoming increasingly evident. We have presented information on the leading bills now being discussed in Congress. These bills are certainly not a definitive statement of an ideal national health-delivery plan, but they do show the importance of the issue. Now is the time for all holistic advocates to express their desires to their politicians; what has not been communicated cannot be incorporated into public policy.

We are witnessing a strong surge toward more humanistic health care. Many medical professionals are responding to this demand. Continuing education is now available to doctors and nurses at the Berkeley Holistic Health Center, and at many other centers around the country. An organization represented in this section, the American Holistic Medical Association, is a growing group of medical professionals working together to sponsor excellent holistic-health conferences and to integrate holistic principles into traditional medical education.

The holistic health movement is gathering momentum. The concept of holism has begun to make sense to many people as an answer to several of our present social problems. Susan Koenig, an administrator at the Berkeley Holistic Health Center, says, "As people re-educate themselves about healthier lifestyles, they question all aspects of their lives: food, jobs, insurance, relationships, everything. Holistic health is broadening people's concepts of what is happening in the world. You can take any area—ecology, education, medicine, sexuality, foreign policy—and find that it overlaps and connects with all other areas. A holistic perspective allows you to see everything in a bigger way."

We are proud and excited to be representing the tangible growth and progress that is taking place, and we are enthusiastic about where the continued public response to the principles of holistic health will take us in creating a social structure that fits our needs and aspirations.

Evolution Survey
How well does each statement describe your patterns
of thought and action?

1. I would like to know more about holistic health.
2. I am aware of the holistic health centers in my community and the services they offer.
3. I would like to pursue a career in holistic health.
4. I enjoy participating in groups, and feel capable of finding groups whose interests and needs are similar to mine.
5. I feel this country needs a new medical-delivery system.
6. I cannot always afford medical treatment under the present system.
7. I feel medical costs are excessive.
8. I am informed about the present proposals for a National Health Policy.
9. I know who my local, state, and federal representatives are, and how they affect my life.
10. I feel that holistic methods of healing and traditional medical technology can be interrelated.
11. My doctor is open to holistic thinking.
12. My doctor supports preventative methods and lifestyle health habits.
13. I understand the legal issues about holistic health.
14. I feel informed enough about my choices in health care to make the best decisions for myself and my family.

Holistic Health: Will the Promise Be Realized?
Rick J. Carlson, J.D.

In part I of this article, we see why "holism" may be the most important idea to hit the health field in a long time. This swiftly growing movement will have even greater impact—and create less anxiety among policy makers, practitioners, and consumers—when certain distinctions are clearly understood.

In part II some social, political, and economic barriers to the growth of holistic health are realistically discussed, along with some strategies for dealing with them. Mr. Carlson makes a strong point in suggesting that, if holistic health is going to have broad influence, it must be promoted in a way which doesn't overly threaten the existing system, avoids parochialism, and maintains "the critical balance between exploration and avoidance of consumer fraud." Holistic health must also be made available to all consumers, not just to those who can afford "luxurious" treatment.

I. HOLISTIC HEALTH: CONCEPT, MOVEMENT, MODALITY

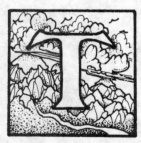 here are three important ways to look at "holistic health": first, as a concept; second, as a movement; third, as a mode of practicing the healing arts. Both the significance and the implications of holism—today, at least—depend on these distinctions. Unfortunately, they are rarely made. The "holistic" field is young, even embryonic. It has many of the characteristics of a new field, over-enthusiasm being one. That's why some distinctions are crucial.

This article is part of a report made to the National Institute of Health by the Center for Integral Medicine, Los Angeles, California. Part I first appeared in the *Holistic Health Review*, Vol. 1, No. 1 (Sept. 1977), and the entire article first appeared in the *Holistic Health Review*, Vol. 3, No. 1 (Fall 1979).

Holism has made its most significant mark as a concept. The practice of modern medicine—and, indeed, almost all of our policy made about it—is based on older notions. Holism as a concept can be clearly distinguished from the animating premises of the current medical model. At a minimum, holism, as applied to the health of individuals, requires us to recognize that they are whole people, with cognitive, physiological, emotional, and spiritual qualities. Furthermore, individuals and populations must be understood in their social, economic, political, and philosophical contexts. This point of view is dramatically different from the premises underlying the existing medical model. (For further development of these premises, see accompanying feature.)

The concept of holism is being accepted as public policy in the United States. Today, people in some key positions recognize the need for a more comprehensive, integrative approach to the health of our population. Nonetheless, as a movement "holistic health" has caused some policy makers and practitioners real anxieties, even though its threat is often seen largely in economic terms.

Much of this anxiety about the movement stems from an incomplete understanding of the concept, and, often, a real concern about some of the practices associated with it. This anxiety and fear are not large, however, simply because only a few of those who run the health and medical game in the United States have even heard of holistic health. This may be hard for ardent holistic-health advocates to believe, but a trip to the eastern seaboard will sober them up quickly. This isn't to say that the concept of holism hasn't had its impact—it has. But policy makers are rarely as glib with the term as people on the west coast, and perhaps that's fortunate, given how loosely the term is being used. The holistic-health movement has made a dent—but not one that would be worth taking to the body shop.

In practice, holism suffers the most. When hard evidence is sought, the field often turns soft. There simply isn't much hard empirical work examining the effectiveness of many of the modalities which people

The Five Major Premises Underlying the Modern Medical-Care System

Rick J. Carlson, J.D.

The modern medical care system rests on the following five major premises.

1. Modern medical care applies *specific approaches to individual disease processes*. In other words, the therapeutic approach to the patient is specific and targeted on the primary problem presented by the patient.

2. Most but not all therapies *intervene* in bodily processes, by either pharmacological or surgical techniques. Such interventions, of course, are made in concert with other modalities such as bed rest, quiet, dietary restrictions, etc.

3. Specific interventions and all treatment approaches generally assume that the body can be conceived in *mechanistic* terms, meaning that disease is presumed to respond to a specific intervention in a causal manner, and that both the intervention and the response are largely independent of emotional, psychosocial, and (in many instances) psychophysiological factors.

4. The appropriate approach to the health of the population is one which addresses the identification of *disease* and its *management* and/or extirpation, rather than the prevention of disease or programs designed to enhance health and well-being. This premise is more related to the medical-care system.

5. Medicine is best provided by a *professional* physician who bears the responsibility for both therapeutics and management. Again, this relates more to the medical-care system.

Modern medicine has a history of successes. The practice of medicine, and biomedical research generally, have given us an impressive amount of knowledge about human biology. Moreover, medical care is very effective in the treatment of emergency and acute conditions, and achieved much in rehabilitation and in prevention of some diseases as well. These achievements can be traced directly to the power of the model upon which it is premised. But at the same time this model can lead to relative neglect of other health problems, of prevention generally, and of approaches to the health of the population which do not depend on therapeutic intervention. Despite medicine's achievements, its fidelity to the model upon which it is based contributes to the "crisis" in modern medicine. For example, the "specific" nature of treatment, and the professionalism of medical practice, has led to impersonality in relationships between providers and patients, and this, among other things, is a major cause of medical malpractice litigation. In addition, the emphasis on specific interventions, on a mechanistic premise, has led to the development of costly (even though effective) programs such as kidney dialysis. Kidney disease is theoretically preventable, but in recent years almost all the resources available to deal with that disorder have been spent on the development and elaboration of dialysis technology, which neither cures nor prevents. Its cost—estimated to reach about two billion dollars by the next fiscal year—has led many to wonder whether or not the program is cost-effective. Is it the wisest investment of increasingly scarce public resources?

associate with holistic health. I recently undertook a project for the Office of Technology Assessment, which is a research arm of the U.S. Congress. I was asked by OTA to find out whether or not there was enough literature on what they called "new technologies for health" to justify an assessment of efficacy, safety, and effectiveness. What I found in my preliminary review, with the help of the staff of Commonweal, Inc., in Bolinas, California, was that, except for biofeedback, relaxation, some aspects of therapeutic suggestion and autogenic training, acupuncture, and Chinese medicine (if one accepts the vast literature on the latter, most of which is not in En-

glish), very few of the so-called new technologies in health have been adequately researched, at least by the standards that OTA was applying.

Part of the problem, of course, is a problem of proof. Some of the approaches to patients that holistic practitioners take do not lend themselves to replicable clinical observation. Often the healing process is idiosyncratic, and cannot always be reproduced time and time again with a variety of patients. Nonetheless, for public policy purposes, current standards of scientific measurements have been and will be applied to the holistic movement. And thus far, when they have been applied, the yield has been small. This may not be fair, and in the long run may prove to be far too limiting to innovation. But that is the way it is.

In sum, the holistic field today is an amalgam. For policy purposes, holism as a concept is expanding the way some key health policy makers perceive both the problem and the solution. Even Senator Kennedy, long the most ardent advocate of national health insurance, is beginning to realize the need for a more comprehensive approach to the health of our population.

As a movement, holism seems to be gaining momentum, but its potential is critically dependent on at least three things.

First, it must relate conceptually (even in the interests of acceptance alone) to those ideas, programs, and practices which are thematically consistent with it and which have led the way. Holism may be a larger, richer, and riper concept than its predecessors in the history of ideas, but it is not wholly novel. The health literature contains many antecedents, principally the work of Thomas McKeown, George Engel, Rene Dubos, and McFarland Burnett. Perhaps more importantly, the most "holistic" practitioner is probably the small-town general practitioner, crotchety or not, who has no choice but to relate to patients as whole persons. The same might be said of many nurses. The term cannot honestly be said, however, to apply to the masseuse or masseur who does what he or she has always done, but now blissfully claims to be a holistic practitioner.

Second, it must maintain a critical balance between exploration and avoidance of consumer fraud. The history of the healing arts is a history of guilds. The holistic movement isn't likely to deviate much from this historical pattern. Accordingly, the holistic movement runs two grave risks. The first is that the fear of ostracism may force it to close its ranks before we learn enough. One can easily imagine another overcredentialed professional group called the Holistic Health Guild setting up shop at high fees, even leasing space from the Mayo Clinic. Ultimately there may be nothing wrong with this, but if calcification sets in too soon, we will have lost the opportunity to learn more. The other risk is injudicious acceptance. A thousand flowers should bloom, but a few of those flowers may be Venus flytraps. If too many health-hungry consumers are ripped off by holistic health practitioners, the whole movement, and indeed the concept itself, will be degraded. Admittedly, this is a very delicate balance to strike, but ignoring the need to strike it doesn't help.

Third, it must avoid parochialism. The holistic-health movement has not grown in isolation; it is part of a larger movement concerned with human values, stewardship of the Earth, and restoration of liveable communities. As a movement it will suffer if it assumes the role of an "alternative" to doctors and hospitals. It may be that for some, but it shares deeply in larger issues and communities of concern. It can gain strength from them, and in turn can nourish those movements as well.

If the concept and the movement are in peril, the practice of the holistic healing arts is in downright jeopardy. It is one thing for a band of hardy practitioners to develop new modes and techniques to apply to patient problems. Practitioners like John Travis at the Wellness Resource Center in Mill Valley, California, and a host of others are performing good and valuable services in meeting the needs of many patients and clients. These activities can and should continue. Nevertheless, they will only be available to those with the twin luxuries of time and money. For the vast majority of the population, the real question is whether or not some of the holistic healing arts will become more generally available, as much to the patient in Moline, Illinois, as in Mill Valley. And this has not yet occurred.

At the same time, an old ghost hangs around. In the past what has often been referred to as the fringe practice of medicine remained at the fringe because of the more than occassional fraud of many of the practitioners. Many conventional physicians trained in the allopathic tradition commit what approximates fraud when they oversell the high technologies of modern medicine to cure-hungry patients. But existing practitioners and programs have the benefit of widespread consumer belief, and operate in a safe and accepting political and economic climate. This is not true for new approaches. Consequently, charges of fraud are not only more likely to be lodged, but more likely to be perceived as accurate. This is often unfair, both to individual practitioners and to the movement as a whole; but it is a fact, and spokespersons for the holistic movement must always distinguish the very best of what is being offered from what still remains snake oil.

In short, the concept of holism may be the most important new idea to hit the health field in a long time. But the task of translating the idea into practice has barely begun. This job cannot be undertaken naively. There are a number of major obstacles to the translation job, which if recognized clearly, can usually be overcome.

II. SOME SOCIAL, POLITICAL, AND ECONOMIC OBSTACLES

The crisis in modern medicine *is* real. Costs continue to soar, and patients continue to complain about impersonality and lack of access. Many factors contribute to the crisis, but no doubt the very model on which modern medicine is based is implicated. A major question which arises, then, is how that model might be transformed to incorporate some new ideas, concepts, programs and practices, without risking the loss of the benefits which flow from its application. At a minimum, this will require a shift in emphasis away from the existing model toward a model which retains what is efficacious in our current approach but stresses other considerations. These will necessarily include an emphasis on the psychophysiology of health, holistic approaches to balance the "specificity" of the current model, more reverence for human life in lieu of indiscriminate invasions of the body, more local control and community involvement, and a lessening of the professional stranglehold on the provision of care.

A fundamental restructuring of our approach to health will not be swift. A great deal must be known before society might confidently retool its approach to health. A few of the problems and obstacles to be anticipated are the following.

1. The economic incentives sustaining our excessive reliance on medical care are so strong, and the disincentives to more holistic approaches so equally strong, that rapid change to a more holistic approach will not be possible without a realignment of incentives.

2. The medical-care services system is a major employer, and has absorbed many workers who lost their jobs with the contraction of the industrial sector. Accordingly, any attempt to reduce the size of the system—and correspondingly the capacity of the system to provide jobs—will meet fierce resistance.

3. The medical-care system serves many social objectives other than the production of health, such as employment and the legitimation of malingering, to name a few. Accordingly, any reformulation of the objectives of medicine must take these other objectives into consideration.

4. The continued development of sophisticated and expensive medical technology (however effective) will continue to "drive" the system toward provision of sophisticated and specialized services, making more holistic approaches difficult.

5. Arguments about the "limits" of medicine might be captured by those political actors in the United States who are interested solely in curbing medical-care costs and not in improving the health of the population.

6. In spite of the validity of the arguments about the limits of medicine and the promise of various holistic approaches, the political, economic, and social pressures for rapid passage of a national health insurance program—one which might "freeze" our societal approach to health through medicine—are great.

7. The danger exists that many promising approaches and techniques might be "oversold" as so much "snake oil," and the concept of holism tarnished as a result.

8. Many of the programs and practices parading under the banner of holism neither can nor should be incorporated into a national health strategy, since they are essentially local and idiosyncratic in their design and operation.

9. The danger exists that the government might design programs and interventions to affect the health of the population that would compromise the freedom of individuals to live their lives as they choose.

10. Although concepts of holism do show promise, unless the ways in which health scientists are educated can be better related to holistic concepts and approaches, the people who will provide and administer medical care and health programs in the future will still be trained in the conventional manner.

11. It will be difficult to realign the research priorities of the National Institutes of Health and other medical-research funding agencies to accelerate and increase the flow of funding to new and promising programs which don't necessarily fit into categorical grant programs.

12. Despite the evidence of how much an individual can affect his or her health, there is little solid evidence that health education of both providers and consumers and behavioral-change programs have had much impact.

13. Perhaps most frustrating of all, consumers of medical care and health may continue to know and care less than some of the more enlightened observers of health affairs about the relative importance of the individual, and the relative lack of importance of medical care, in the achievement of health.

These obstacles are not insurmountable. I am optimistic, but usually a prerequisite to change is a clear and practical assessment of the barriers to be encountered.

SOME STRATEGIES

In a modern building in Berkeley, California, a group of physicians and psychologists have put together a psychosomatic medicine center. The clinic is formally associated with the Gladman Memorial Hospital and Alta Bates Hospital, also in Berkeley. It looks a lot like other offices on the outside, but inside things are a little different: a new kind of medicine is being practiced. Dr. Ken Pelletier emphasizes the importance of "playing the game."

The same philosophy prevails in Yonkers, New York, of all places. There, in a somewhat less-modern building, a group of health professionals and their associates has created a family medical practice. But it too is different on the inside. Patients are treated as whole people; families, school, and police all get involved in patient-care problems; drugs and hospital stays are deemphasized; and physicians, unlike in almost all other settings, work cooperatively with others with different trainings and orientations.

In downtown Manhattan it's still the same. Ruth Lubic, a nurse and midwife, along with her associates, is convinced that many healthy expectant mothers can and should have their babies at home if they want to do so. But she knows the importance of setting up the program right: "If you want to get approval of everyone that you need to consult to do the job legally, you've got to get professional support, and you have to avoid appearing to be too far out."

The idea that the founders of these programs had in mind was that if you were going to affect the existing system—and, indeed, if you were going to convince Blue Cross to pay for the work that you want to do—you have to do it in a manner not too unlike what has always been done. This lesson is almost always forgotten in the holistic-health movement.

In the Berkeley group I mentioned, for example, a range of holistic services is provided, and the providers of those services are fully convinced of the philosophical merits of holism, but all the work is done in a professional and polished manner. The organizers of the clinic recognize that if you want to do something different, you have to do it in a manner which doesn't unnecessarily antagonize the existing system. The ultimate question, then, is one of integration. The existing medical-care system is not going to roll over and play dead. Too much is at stake for medicine to relinquish its monoploy; opposition will be

fierce. Yet, unless some holistic thinking and practice "sticks," medical care will soon be available only to the very rich. If holistic health practices are available only to those with the twin luxuries of time and money, then the movement itself will remain faddish and peripheral. And much of it will; for example, consider artisans in massage who claim that their techniques can cure everything from hives to hepatitis. But if holism as a concept has real value, and if at least some of the new programs and techniques which are holistic are to compete with allopathic medical care, they must be made available to most consumers of health care; and so they must be integrated into major federal, state, and private health-care programs. In other words, Blue Cross must eventually agree to reimburse holistic practitioners for what they do, just as Dr. X gets paid for overdosing his patients with drugs.

A lot of what has been called holistic health simply isn't going to meet this test. Filipino psychic surgeons can hardly be expected to fill out Blue Cross forms for reimbursement. Moreover, programs like those offered at health spas, like the Renaissance Revitalization Center in the Bahamas, however effective they may be, are limited to pampering the very wealthy, and are therefore unlikely to be the wave of the future. On the other hand, solid and proven techniques, taking patients in context, looking at them holistically in terms of their life experiences, biofeedback, acupuncture, cancer counseling, humanistic approaches to health and healing, recognition of the vital roles the family and workplace play in human health, will and should "stick." The question is whether those who argue in favor of holistic health are willing to set aside their rhetoric and get to work to make the best of it available to as many as want it. Only then will the revolution occur!

Rick J. Carlson, J.D., is a Senior Program Associate for Commonweal, Inc., Bolinas, California, and a Senior Associate of the Institute of Noetic Sciences, San Francisco, California. He has recently organized a consulting firm, Health Resources Group. He has also authored numerous books and articles. Additionally, he has done extensive consulting for the Institute of Medicine of the National Academy of Sciences, Blue Cross/Blue Shield, American Hospital Association, and various foundations including the Rockefeller Foundation.

Networking Within the Holistic Health Community

Steven Jay Markell and Jerry Yanuck

The holistic-health movement has now found its way to every major city in the country. People are getting together everywhere to share the experience of holistic living. The following article gives some clear, practical suggestions about how you can find holistic-minded people and practitioners in your community. The article also outlines some beginning procedures for creating a healing community if one does not already exist.

The emphasis here is on personal involvement in creating the group or health center that best suits your needs and the needs of the community you are in. The possibilities for what a determined person or group can accomplish are endless.

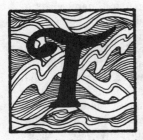
he human animal is a social beast. It needs the help of other members of the species to survive the rigors of modern society. The human finds that tasks are easier, projects get completed in less time, and the results of labor are multiplied when individuals cooperate. Yet many facets of life work to separate people from each other. Personal transportation vehicles and Sunday drives have replaced the neighborhood stroll and meeting the neighbors. (The gasoline games currently in vogue promise to diminish this form of isolation.) Offices are cubicles. Telephones separate people from face-to-face contact. These technological tradeoffs have seeded an alienation, a loneliness, a longing for belonging, and a striving for identity. The marketing industry preys on this human need incessantly, subtly implanting these images in virtually every commercial or advertisement.

GETTING IN TOUCH

How people get in contact with other like-minded souls in this huge, separated, alienating, multifaceted society is sometimes a complete mystery to me. People are often wafted together like two leaves tumbling before an autumn breeze, seemingly by chance. Yet there also seems to be some guiding force directing the most crucial steps in each of our lives, if we know how to look for such influences. We can also consciously direct our steps by exercising our free will and self-responsibility.

If we choose to pursue our interest in holistic health, for example, how might we go about seeking out people who are studying acupressure, practicing their sensitivity to subtle energies, experimenting with herbal gardens and treatments, or looking for people with similar physical sensations, symptoms, or diseases to share hopes, fears, struggles, and successes with? The solutions to this dilemma are as varied as the seekers.

WHERE TO TURN?

Some people turn to their families for support. Others reach to the church, civic groups, hobby clubs, sports teams, and a myraid of other ways to connect and to receive and give encouragement. Urban life offers a selection of resources for networking different from those in rural environs, but the process of initiating contact is similar no matter where one lives. Establishing a relationship almost always involves taking a bit of a risk. If I reach out, will someone take my hand? Will I like that person? Will they get along with me? The bulk of the time, the answer to all of these questions is a resounding yes!

"What does networking have to do with holistic health?" the astute reader must be musing by now. A holistic approach to health encompasses not only an analysis of a person's biochemistry, health, medical history, family history, and current health needs, but also an in-depth inquiry into that person's social environment and relationship to job, family and community. This approach includes the economic and political aspects of lifestyle, abode, air quality, and food sources, and their impact on health and symptomology.

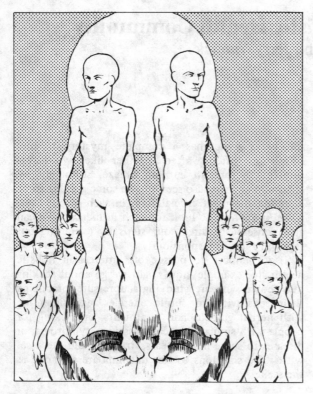

How people get in contact with other like-minded souls in this huge, alienating, multi-faceted society is a mystery.

When a loved one dies, or when the wage-earner must move the family for better working conditions, support networks are shattered. People who once shared innermost thoughts and feelings are no longer available. Emotions are pent up, unreleased. Stress accumulates on emotional, physical, and spiritual levels; symptoms and physical sensations appear. The holistically oriented health practitioner takes into account this need for support, and will help clients reestablish themselves in a community, or will work toward the resolution of family rifts as part and parcel of a holistic solution to health problems. The research is incomplete, but reconnecting people to support networks helps balance psychology as well as biochemistry. This is obvious from the psychosomatic literature flooding the journals and popular literature.

MAKING CONNECTIONS

Within the holistic health community, making connections can sometimes be difficult. Professional associations are not yet fully developed. The Chamber of Commerce rarely lists unorthodox health prac-

titioners. Individual practitioners are difficult to ferret out, especially since many states have no laws regulating holistic practice. If you are new to town, how do you find a holistically oriented physician? How do you find a good masseur for that once-a-week rubdown of your tired bones? How can you find a midwife to assist you in the home birth you've chosen? Where can you get organic vegetables that you *know* aren't sprayed with toxic pesticides, herbicides, or fumigants? How can you check the credentials of an unlicensed iridologist, uncertified holistic-health educator, or psychic healer?

Unfortunately, the holistic-health field has expanded so greatly in the last few years that there are no established national bodies universally accepted as the spokespeople for the holistic field (except for a few specific modality associations). The accompanying feature lists the major holistic-health associations that have emerged to further the networking in many areas of the country.

THERE IS NO SUCH THING AS A FREE LUNCH

Many of the techniques used by holistically oriented practitioners cannot be learned in formal training programs; they are based on many years of empirical observations, clinical practice, oral tradition, and old texts. Some of the health practices undergoing an American revival are widespread in other parts of the world, but are not too well-known here yet. We are cautioned by the government that quacks abound in the health-care bushes, that valium may be hazardous to your health, and that some plants that have been used medicinally for centuries could be harmful if used incorrectly. How can we find out who the best practitioners are? Where can we go to find out about the Alexander technique, rolfing, or hair analysis? How can I be assured of quality care, an honest professional, and my money's worth?

There are no magic potions to cure all your ails that you can take and have all of your troubles vanish. There are no guarantees of finding a "perfect" health practitioner. Each person must answer the questions we have posed for himself or herself. Use any advice from friends, relatives, "people-in-the-know," and your professional health consultants (or practitioners) that you can generate. One must be assertive and ask questions in order to get the basic information needed to make informed choices. *There is no such thing as a dumb question. If you do not know the answer, then it is a good question.* Then, based on all the evidence and information, check your inner feelings about the choice; ask your conscience/inner self/ guides/higher power for the best direction. When you ask honestly and humbly, you can usually trust the answer. Then, take the chance, in the same way you initiate social relationships. There is always a bit of a risk; again, don't wait for the sure bet, or you'll wait a long time.

TRIED AND TRUE METHODS

If a holistic-health association does not exist yet in your area, consider forming one. Any of the existing groups will be happy to support you in the ways that they can. Minutes from early meetings, organization charters, statements of purpose and goals,

Groups and Associations Concerned with Holistic-Health Issues
Steven Jay Markell and Jerry Yanuck

The Alacer Vitamin Corporation has a directory of nutrition-minded doctors available: The Alacer Corp., 7425 C Orangethorpe Avenue, Buena Park, CA 90622. (714) 522-3904. $.50.

Alternative Medical Association, 7916 S.E. Stark, Portland, OR 97215. (502) 254-7555.

American Healing Association, 6311 Yucca Street, Los Angeles, CA 90028. (213) 320-2907.

American Holistic Medical Association, 6932 Little River Turnpike, Annandale, VA 22003.

Association for Holistic Health, P.O. Box 33202, San Diego, CA 92103. (714) 298-5965.

Austin Area Holistic Health Association, P.O. Box 13281, Austin, TX 78711. (512) 441-1297.

California Health Action Coalition, P.O. Box 1315, Oakland, CA 94604.

The Canadian Holistic Healing Association, 308 E. 234d, Vancouver, B.C. Canada V5V 1X5. (604) 876-5955.

Colorado Holistic Health Network, Suite 526 South, Mercy Hospital, E. 16th Street at Milwaukee, Denver, CO 80218. (303) 399-1840.

Council of Nurse Healers, P.O. Box 31211, San Francisco, CA 94131.

Eastern Holistic Health Association, 50 Maple Place, Manhasset, NY 11030. (516) 627-0395.

The Feldenkrais Guild, 1776 Union Street, San Francisco, CA 94123.

Holistic Health Practitioner's Association, 1030 Merced Street, Berkeley, CA 94707. (415) 526-2000.

The International Academy of Biological Medicine, P.O. Box 31313, Phoenix, AZ 85046.

The International Academy of Preventive Medicine, 10409 Town and Country Way, Houston, TX 77024. (713) 468-7851.

The National Council on Wholistic Therapeutics and Medicine, GPO Box H, Brooklyn, NY 11202.

Princeton Area Holistic Health Association, 360 Nassau, Princeton, NJ 08540. (609) 924-8580.

Rolf Institute, P.O. Box 1868, Boulder, CO 80306. (303) 449-5903.

Sacramento Holistic Health Association, 1616 21st Street, Sacramento, CA 95814. (916) 442-6425.

Self-Help and Mutual Aid Association, Dr. Alfred Katz, UCLA, Los Angeles, CA 90024.

Tucson Holistic Health Association, 300 East River Road, Tucson, AZ 85704. (602) 888-6473.

Washington Association for Holistic Health, P.O. Box 7123, Olympia, WA 98507.

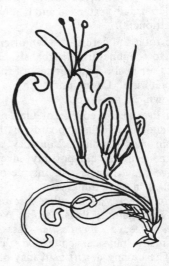

by-laws and other materials can be useful in starting your own association. Make sure to send a self-addressed, stamped envelope and a small donation with your inquiry; many of these associations are volunteer-staffed, low-budget operations, in their initial stages of development. You can ask them for names of people or practitioners in your area that may be on their mailing list or referral file.

If you are looking for practitioners, classes, study, self-help, growth or support groups, or conferences, or want to quietly pursue your own inquiries, you can make contact with the holistic community by the following tried and true methods.

1. Sit down and get clear about what your interest is. Set a goal based on your interest. Make a list of your own strategies for entering the field. Devise a big-picture strategy. Now and again, check back into your self-developed and self-directed strategy list and goals to see if changes are called for by recent turns of events. Also look to see if you are still purposeful by moving toward achieving your initial goal.

2. Ask family members, friends, business associates, or clergy for leads or referrals.

3. Go to a health-food store and ask employees if they know of any of these activities or holistic practitioners.

4. Look in the Yellow Pages of the telephone directory under holistic health, wholistic health, alternative medicine, health-food stores, drugless practitioners, acupuncturists, natural-food stores and restaurants, colon therapy, registered physical therapists, massage, naturopathic, osteopathic, or chiropractic physicians, herb, vitamin, or health-aid distributors (this last group usually caters to and is referred to by holistic practitioners).

5. Ethnic food and herb stores can often be useful for referrals to acupuncturists/herbalists, curanderos, native healers, or health practitioners of that particular tradition/culture. Community centers in ethnic sections of town can assist you.

6. If you live near a college or university, go to the campus and read bulletin boards in the student building or in class buildings. You may see posters for classes and centers, and possibly advertisements for alternative practitioners. An instructor may be offering a class in something you are interested in, or be able to direct you to other resources in the community. For example, yoga, aerobic exercise, jogging, modern dance, or *Tai chi chuan* classes are being offered in many physical education departments these days. The botany department may offer classes on wild plant identification, cultivation, history of plant use, etc. The psychology department may offer courses in parapsychology, psychosomatic roots of disease, counseling, family therapy, etc. Curricula may be offered on a seasonal or regular basis, or may appear in continuing education or adult education programs and bulletins. Survival, self-help, first-aid, and medical terminology classes can also provide leads into the holistic community. Alternative-energy groups are often in contact with other parts of the alternative community in their area.

7. Call your local medical society for listings of local M.D.-acupuncturists.

8. Any city with a population over 250,000 has *someone* (and usually more than one) doing at least an alternative modality. Every major city in the U.S. has holistic practitioners; help is certainly available if you can travel.

9. If nothing at all is available in your town, go to a town with a health-food store or book store that carries health books and browse. Buy a couple of books that interest you and read them. Strike up conversations with fellow browsers, and ask your questions. Share books that you've read with friends, doctors, nurses, and other health professionals that you know back home. With friends and health professionals (if they will join you), form a study group. Read material and discuss it. Share your experiences and experiments. Invite practitioners and health educators from larger towns to come and speak with your group. Offer to pay their transportation costs.

10. In a small town, when your study group feels confident, call a town meeting, or put it on the agenda of the city council, to create interest for enticing a holistic practitioner to move to your area, or to a place where a few small towns could share the practitioner. If your community would support this person, you can advertise in various publications for a holistic practitioner to come and settle in your area. (See list of journals in accompanying feature.) There are numerous government agencies that are concerned with getting professional health care into rural locations. Contact the Department of Health, Education, and Welfare in Washington, D.C., for health manpower distribution information, and for assistance in attracting health personnel to your area.

11. Tell local traditional, orthodox practitioners that they can receive continuing education credit by attending holistic-health conferences and seminars in many parts of the country. The practitioners must get a certain number of continuing-education units per year to maintain their licenses. Give them any brochures of these events that you have received by

being on the mailing list of groups or associations listed here. The practitioners can meet peers from their area or from around the country at such events, and acquire new skills which will benefit their practice and the community.

12. Contact your state and federal government representatives, and tell them they should support legislation that encourages holistic practices and freedom of choice. Contact local medical societies and state regulatory agencies, and encourage them to offer holistic classes to the state's health professionals. Public demand is often the most powerful influence on slow-moving bureaucracies.

13. Put a notice in the personals section of your local newpaper's classified section, soliciting interest in holistic health. Put a notice in the church calendar for an informal meeting or discussion group. Place notices for the formation of a study group on natural-health approaches in the public library, laundromat, grocery store, town meeting hall, school, and hospital, and in doctors', naturopaths', chiropractors', or dentists' offices. Write letters to the editors of your local paper, regional magazines, or national health magazines asking for interested people to contact you. Study groups can create their own correspondence courses, using tapes and letters, if people are very isolated.

14. Send postcards to centers and associations requesting that your name be placed on their mailing list. Send a small donation, too. Many holistic-health groups share their mailing lists; before you know it, you will be receiving numerous notices from around the country.

15. Be persistent. You may get the runaround for a while, but in the long run, the search will be worth it.

WHAT TO DO WHEN YOU FIND A HOLISTIC PRACTITIONER

Beware! Many practitioners use the word "holistic" these days; it is a popular label. When you make an inquiry, ask practitioners what services they offer and what techniques they use. Ask questions over the telephone or visit them in their office casually, prior to an appointment and professional consultation. If you feel the need, ask the practitioner for references from patients they have worked with. Ask to see testimonials, letters of recommendation, resumés, curriculum vitae, and any certificates of course completion or licenses he or she may have earned. If you do not feel comfortable with this person, or if he or she does not offer the services you desire, ask for a referral to someone who may.

Publications Concerned with Holistic Health and Related Areas
Steven Jay Markell and Jerry Yanuck

Alternatives, P.O. Box 330139, Miami, Fl 33133.
Applewood Journal, P.O. Box 1781, San Francisco, CA 94101.
Common Knowledge, P.O. Box 316, Bolinas, CA 94924.
East/West Journal, P.O. Box 305, Dover, NJ 07801.
Health Science, 1920 Irving Park Road, Chicago, IL 60613.
The Herb Quarterly, P.O. Box 576, Wilmington, VT 05363.
Herbalist. P.O. Box 62, Provo, UT 84601.
Holistic Health Review, P.O. Box 166, Berkeley, CA 94701.
National Journal of the Nutritional Academy, 1238 Hayes, Eugene, OR 97402.
Natural Life, P.O. Box 4564, Buffalo, NY 14240.
New Age, P.O. Box 4921, Manchester, NH 03103.
New Realities, P.O. Box 26289, San Francisco, CA 94126.
Organic Gardening, 33 East Minor Street, Emmaus, PA 18049.
Prevention, 33 East Minor Street, Emmaus, PA 18049.
Well-Being, P.O. Box 1829, Santa Cruz, CA 95061.
Whole Foods, 2219 Marin Ave., Berkeley, CA 94707.
Yoga Journal, 2054 University Avenue, Berkeley, CA 94704.

Within the next ten years, the professional aspects of holistic care should mature, especially with pressure from the public. It is best, though, that the practitioners themselves, with public input, develop the standards and guidelines to assure quality. The traditional medical societies and associations are *not* the ones qualified to judge this emerging field, though some of the same procedures they went through in their own professionalization may prove to be useful for and applicable to the holistic community's situation.

In any case, the changes and challenges facing the interested seeker/student are a growth process themselves, and hold much potential for opening one's attitudes, perceptions, and biases toward oneself and one's community. The search is as important as what one is searching for. Good travels!

Steven Jay Markell, B.A., Biochemistry, is editor-in-chief of the Holistic Health Review, *co-director of the Holistic Health Organizing Committee, and a founding member of the Holistic Health Practitioners' Association. He is an advisory board member of the Health Policy Council, Des Plaines, Illinois. He is a very active member of the holistically oriented political community and is in private practice in Berkeley, California, as a Life Choice Awareness Counsultant, incorporating an academic background in biochemistry with holistically oriented philosophies and modalities.*

Jerry Yanuck is a holistic-health educator and consultant in private practice in Marin County, California. He incorporates bodywork, movement, herbs, nutrition, iridology, vision training, and western research techniques into his practice. He is a certified instructor of Ortho-Bionomy/Phased Reflex Techniques. Jerry leads seminars at universities, colleges, and health and community centers throughout the country and Canada.

National Health Service:
A New Concept in Health-Care Delivery

Deborah Dilloway, L.V.N.,
and Patricia Ann Kenny, R.N., M.P.H.

The question of a National Health Service is fast becoming one of the most important issues of our time. There is no doubt that our present health-care delivery system falls drastically short of the needs of a vast majority of people. Spiraling costs of specialized medical technology have created an aura of catastrophe around the prospect of any hospitalization. There are several health-insurance bills now up for discussion in Congress. We have presented here a description of the four major bills, the Long, Carter, Kennedy, and Dellums proposals.

In this article the Dellums proposal is strongly supported, because it is the only one that would give consumers a voice in how health care will be provided in their community. We encourage you to become as fully informed on these proposals as possible, because whichever bill is finally adopted will greatly affect all our lives.

n this paper we will talk about a new concept in health-care delivery and financing, and briefly contrast it to other mechanisms which are currently being debated in congress. With 24 million Americans having no health insurance at all, and 18 million having inadequate insurance, it is clear that there needs to be a new approach to health-care delivery and payment in this country. We pose this question: what would happen if people in a federally funded health-care delivery system plan were able to decide regionally the kinds of health-care services provided to them?

We will briefly describe the Long, Carter, Kennedy, and Dellums proposals, focusing mainly on the Kennedy and Dellums bills. First we will cover the bill sponsored by Senator Long. This bill would cover expenses only for catastrophic illnesses. After a person has spent $2,000 or has been 60 days in the hospital, he or she would then be covered for the rest of the expenses of that illness or accident. This plan would be financed by a 1 percent payroll tax on employers, with the Federal government paying for the poor.

The Carter proposal is to "phase in" coverage, starting with catastrophic coverage after a person has spent $2,500, and making Medicaid totally federally administered (it is now both state and federally funded). Although details are not spelled out, ultimately the coverage would be "comprehensive," phased in by different legislative proposals when economically feasible. This bill would be financed by general tax revenues as well as by employer and employees.

These two "catastrophic" bills cover what are considered to be the most expensive aspects of medical care, but ignore the less-expensive areas of prevention and routine medical care. By ignoring these daily health and medical needs of people, it creates the situation in which they enter the health-care system in a more serious state of illness, which in turn, increases

> "We have in this country today a health delivery system where the quality of health care received is determined by race, language, national origin, or income level. Health is viewed as a commodity to be bought and sold in the marketplace; it is not viewed as a right of the people, a service to be provided by the Government. However, financing is not the only problem facing the people when it comes to the delivery of health care. Other equally important problems are the maldistribution of health manpower, the unequal access to services, the unreliable quality of care, and the lack of public control over health care."
>
> Congressman Ronald Dellums,
> speaking in Congress, March 19, 1979

the cost of treatment. Clearly there are inflationary components built into this approach.

The bill sponsored by Kennedy, "Health Care For All Americans," would offer the following: full coverage for all U.S. residents for hospital, physician, and lab bills; limited drug and nursing-home costs; physician and hospital fees set by negotiation at state level; Medicare expanded to include all people over 65 and many disabled under 65. It would also cover X-rays, prosthesis, mental-health treatment, and drugs for chronically ill seniors. To improve access to care, neighborhood health centers would be "encouraged," as would home care for the chronically ill. The plan would be financed by having employers buy coverage from private insurance companies, with employees paying up to 35 per cent of the premium. Based on income, the premium could be a maximum of $800 per year for a single person, and $1950 for a family of four. People who are unemployed and retired people would be covered by funds from a pool of employee-employer premiums. All people would have the same coverage, regardless of which of the three different plans they belonged to.

Both Carter and Kennedy stress the need for preventive services; however, their proposals lack a clearly defined mechanism to promote these services. Carter suggests a "pilot project" to study how to implement such services, and Kennedy "encourages" Health Maintenance Organizations (HMOs) where such services are included into the plans.

A major change in the present Kennedy bill from the former Kennedy-Corman bill is the role given to the insurance companies. Because of this change, Corman, and number of important national support groups such as labor and senior organizations, have firmly denounced this new position. The foundation of the original bill had been built on the concept of public administration, which the current bill negates.

In contrast to a strict insurance mechanism, the Dellums bill, a National Health Service Plan, not only has public financial administration at its core, but also changes the structure of the present delivery system.

The crucial feature of the concept of a National Health Service as proposed by Dellums is that all health workers would be government employees, and all care would be provided in government hospitals and health centers. The entire population of the United States would be included in this national health service at no additional cost after an individual's tax contribution had been made. It would be a free service without hidden costs. All health services for prevention, diagnosis, treatment, and rehabilitation would be phased into the program in an orderly fashion. Considerable emphasis would be placed on preventive, dental, mental, and long-term services in order to make up for the deficiences caused by past and present neglect in these areas.

Care would be given primarily in community health centers providing team practice by salaried general and specialist physicians, dentists, nurses, laboratory workers, nutritionists, psychologists, public health nurses, and other members of the health-care team. These centers would be established in all communities and neighborhoods, with first priorities going to underserved rural and urban areas. They would be linked to hospitals and medical schools in regional networks which would provide not only for referrals of patients to major medical centers but also for extensive educational and technical assistance by the latter to the smaller centers. Regionalization would become a reality.

Administration throughout would be by federal, regional, and district health departments, each having specific responsibilities for all preventive and therapeutic services. Democratic control of health services would be implemented by the provision that every health department and health facility be responsible to a governing board on which two thirds of the members represent the people being served, and one third represent the health workers. The quality of services would be greatly improved by team practice, regional coordination, peer review, a vast expansion of continuing education, and the development of a spirit of service to the people of the community and responsibility for maintaining their health. The keystones of this plan for national health service are the promotion of health and the prevention of disease.[1]

The Dellums bill puts strong emphasis on the need to address and attack the problems and diseases which are environmentally and occupationally induced. Specifically, in addition to screening, diagnosis, and treatment, there would be occupational and safety councils, and national guidelines in health and safety.

Funds to run the health service would come from a Health Service Trust Fund containing receipts from the special health-service tax, from individuals and employers, and from general federal revenues. The individual health service tax would rise with increased income. Dellums has proposed that there would be a 20 per cent savings over-all, by cutting out the administration costs of the private insurance companies, and by the elimination of fee-for-service billing.[2]

Our bias is that only the Dellums bill, because of its new financial and service approach, will adequately meet the health needs of Americans who are presently with or without insurance. This bias is based on our own personal experience as health professionals, and on the experience of the Canadian and British people with their health-care delivery systems.[3] The Canadian government, by public administration of its health insurance, pays 2.5¢ per $1.00 for administrative costs, where Americans pay 15 to 16¢ per $1.00. Only one province, Ontario, chose to go with private insurance companies, but changed to public administration within the second year, because their administrative costs were similar to America's. Thus, Americans lose 12.5 to 13.5¢ per dollar in order to pay for competing advertisement and "overhead" charges of private insurance companies.

Many people wonder why "fee for service" is now such an issue for health care. The reason is that the fee-for-service pattern encourages doctors to do unnecessary treatments. Attempts have been made to contain costs within this system; however, it has been shown that limiting the amount which can be charged merely inspires providers to do more treatments in order to make up for the loss of revenues. Marketplace economics does not work in this situation, because doctors can create their own demand. An example of this occurred in Canada, where the supply of physicians rose, and the number of patients available per physician therefore decreased but the incomes of the doctors continued to rise. Investigation showed that various types of surgeries, such as tonsilectomies, hysterectomies, and venous ligations (vein stripping), were performed more frequently, and, in addition such ancillary services as laboratory tests were being prescribed more often.

In contrast, lower rates of utilization, particularly for the above-mentioned surgical procedures, have been documented where there are prepaid plans or doctors on salaries, as is the situation with Kaiser or the British health system. Critics have proposed that these lower rates may be detrimental, in that people may not be getting the services they need. They often point to the long waiting list for elective surgery in England. In the British system, there are three categories for people having surgery: acute, urgent, and elective. Acute cases are seen immediately; urgent cases are seen within one to three months, and can be moved up to acute upon professional recommendation. Elective cases are anywhere from three months up to a year, and may be moved up to urgent. Clients are called regularly to assess their need and move them up the list, so that they can have a sense of the amount of time that they can plan on before going to the hospital. What has happened during this waiting period is that a good many clients have

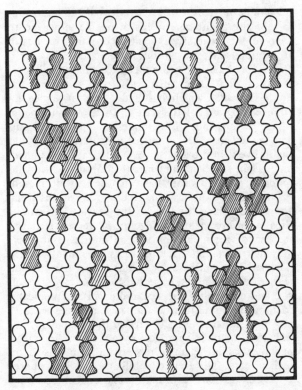

At least 24 million Americans currently have no health insurance at all, and 18 million have inadequate health coverage.

decided that the proposed surgery is not necessary. This must be seen as a benefit to their health, since they are not exposed to the hazards of surgery and prolonged hospital stay.

A more dramatic anecdote is the report in the *Los Angeles Times* that, during the doctor's strike around the malpractice crisis in 1974, the death rate in the city of Los Angeles decreased significantly. Such findings suggest that all "medical care" may be not only unnecessary, but one cause of morbidity and mortality.

Currently, money paid to doctors for fees is generally paid to surgeons, radiologists, pathologists, anesthesiologists, and other hospital-based physicians. The consumer pays 39 to 93 per cent for the services of pediatricians, obstetricians, family doctors, ear, nose, and throat specialists, eye doctors, and others who maintain out-of-hospital offices. This has perpetuated consumers receiving the more costly and high risk type of medical services.

Built into the fee-for-service/insurance mechanism is the greater emphasis on the medical aspects of deliverable services. Medical services are an important part of the health-care needs of people; however, to focus on them exclusively, leaving no funds for health promotion and prevention, undercuts the opportunity for Americans to experience the over-all level of health that they might otherwise have. For example, Canada, which has had a fee-for-service insurance program for the past 15 to 20 years (depending on the province), is now questioning whether putting money into predominantly medical services has qualitatively improved the over-all health of Canadians. Even though the infant mortality rate and maternal mortality rate have significantly decreased, the morbidity rate has not. One reason for this situation is that, since the turn of the century, infectious diseases have been on the decline in western societies because of innoculations and antibiotics, but stress and environmental-related diseases have made a sharp increase. These diseases or conditions, which include heart disease, cancers, hypertension, anxiety, alcoholism, and depression, are not addressed in a medically oriented system until after they have become acute.

Americans can benefit from the Canadians re-evaluation of their approach, by not depending on an insurance billing plan whose main emphasis is on medical care. The Kennedy bill, though it proposes to be comprehensive in nature and concerned about health, will continue to feed money into a system which does not alter the health of the nation anywhere near as much as it should for the amount of money and technology at its disposal.

Can any health or medical system be instrumental in determining whether health *will* exist? Other factors, such as adequate housing, food, and job security, play a much greater roll than the medical system in determining a person's health. We maintain that the Dellums proposal, because of its demand for community decisions on services to be rendered, and its verbalization of the issues important for the community's well-being, will create a greater opportunity for people's real needs to be addressed and met. This approach may even improve the health status of particular populations. In addition to this positive outcome, this plan emphasizes the social responsibility we all share in creating a better life and livelihood for all people, understanding that basic needs must be met before people can go on to greater self-actualization and sense of well-being.

The Dellums proposal would legislate for community-based and consumer-controlled health centers, whereas the Kennedy proposal only "encourages" the establishment of neighborhood health centers. This emphasis, along with a multidisciplinary, team approach to health-care delivery, would create a way for consumers and professionals to work together to construct a rational and meaningful health system. It would also open the door for many previously discounted health workers. There would be much greater incentive to make good use of the very real skills which people have developed, but which they cannot now use in the conventional system of delivery and financing. The Kennedy bill would maintain the predominance of services delivered by physicians and other traditional health professionals because it promotes self-interest and reimbursement policies.

In Canada a growing number of salaried-staff clinics are using a multidisciplinary professional and consumer team approach that incorporates the concept of psychosocial and psychosomatic components of illness. This approach has been shown to have a positive outcome for the professional and consumer. Both have experienced increased satisfaction in their interactions, and have a greater sense that "quality care" is being delivered; there was both a subsequent decrease in consumer utilization and improved health.

The goals and objectives of any plan must speak to the needs of the particular regions and people they propose to serve. We feel that only the Dellums bill takes these considerations into serious account, since it not only makes provisions for consumer voices to be heard, but bases the very success of the plan on their continual input *and participation* locally, regionally, and federally. Then and only then can the well-being of all peoples be realized.

NOTES

[1] M. Terris, P. Cornely, H. Daniels, and L. Kerr, "The Case for a National Health Service," *American Journal of Public Health,* 67: 1183-1185 (Dec. 1977).

[2] Taken from the August 6, 1978, Congressional speech made by Assemblyman Ronald Dellums when he introduced the bill.

[3] Information regarding the Canadian and British experiences come from unpublished interviews with Canadian and British health care officials. These interviews took place during Tisha Kenny's two-year MPH program, at which time she visited Canada and England.

Deborah Dilloway, L.V.N., has been active in nursing for several years. Currently she is a nurse at Mount Zion Hospital in San Francisco, California.

Patricia Ann Kenny has been active in the community of nursing and health care for many years. Her contributions are too many to list here. Currently she is Director of Health Services Administration Graduate Program and coordinator of the Holistic Health Bachelor of Arts Degree at Antioch University in San Francisco.

The Place of the Holistic Health Center in Urban Communities

Bruce Gorman, M.C.R.P.

In our current "life in the fast lane" urban condition, it is often very difficult to find a place where meaningful, nurturing, wholesome activities occur. Our neighborhoods, for the most part, have become sprawling highways, or so crowded and overstimulating that it is necessary to become isolated to find some peace.

The community health center can serve as a wonderful meeting place for people who want to share common interests and learning experiences. People have always needed a community gathering place. The following article begins with a history of what these meeting places have been to people, from the baroque castles in early Europe to our modern suburban malls of today. The community health center is born from a human need for a place to go to strive for "high-level wellness," a state of self-fulfillment that is reflected back into the community by happy, healthy, contributing individuals.

"Living thus, year in and year out, at second hand, remote from the nature that is outside them and no less remote from the nature within, handicapped as lovers and as parents by the routine of the metropolis and by the constant specter of insecurity and death that hovers over its bold towers and shadowed streets—living thus, the mass of inhabitants remain in a state bordering on the pathological."

Lewis Mumford, *The Culture of Cities.*

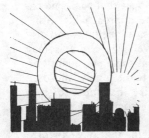

ne of the basic principles followed by mankind in creating settlements has been the need for contact with other people, the elements of nature, and the works of man. Paradoxically, since the industrial revolution, this primary social need for which we created cities and metropolises—that is, the need for social contact, support, and interchange—has been rendered nearly impossible in our massive, inhumanly scaled, commerce-oriented urban areas.

In 1938, Mumford was fully aware that urban dwellers were being robbed of this need when he wrote:

"Beyond a certain point, density even obstructs association; if friendship requires a degree of isolated communion, so does neighborliness. There is less chance of knowing your neighbors on a block with a thousand people than on one that holds a hundred; for all association, even that in primary groups, has a selective aspect: it rests on the existence of recognizable faces and repeatable opportunities. Distance has an effect similar to density in breaking down associated life."

Anyone who lives in a modern metropolis is all too aware that this isolation and lack of social connection is even more prevalent in today's masses of urban sprawl. Modern post-industrial cities and their suburbs are designed almost solely on the priorities of economic growth and development; the social needs of people who choose to or, for economic purposes, must live in or near the cities are rarely considered. The most recent census estimates illustrate that ours is becoming almost an exclusive urban society. In 1977, approximately 72 per cent of us lived in Standard Metropolitan Statistical Areas (does this sound like a place where people would want to live?), up from 69 per cent in 1970 and 63 per cent in 1960. Much of this increase represents growth in the strangely ambiguous, characterless suburbs, communities which seem designed to minimize any opportunity for group support or neighborhood contact.

As we enter the last decades of the twentieth century, it is likely that this trend toward social dehumanization of our cities and urban areas will continue. One need just visit one of our newer cities, such as Dallas, Phoenix, or Los Angeles, to see that they have developed in a vacuum of social and human contact. The growth of monotonous subdivisions and shopping malls, based geographically on the population's ability to transport itself in automobiles (a mode that in itself encourages social isolation and neighborhood dispersal), exacerbates the problem. The rapid disappearance of the urban sidewalk, which used to provide an impromptu source of casual human interaction and a means of neighborhood identification, further isolates the individual from the community. This increasing lack of social intercourse and support, accompanied by the diminishing control of our environment, has a devastating effect on the physical, mental, emotional, and spiritual health of our overwhelmingly urban society.

The need for social association and man's attempt to facilitate human interaction is exemplified by the planned (or *de facto*) development of common meeting places throughout history. These community focal points provide an opportunity for people to play out their need for social interdependency—a place, building, or group of buildings reflecting the cultural, spiritual, and social life of the human settlement in which it was located. Now more than ever, as the urban dweller's psyche is barraged by a rapidly deteriorating social and physical environment, as his isolation and loneliness are magnified by increasingly anonymous, dehumanizing, and unfamiliar people and buildings, it is essential that we recognize the need for a place to develop and nurture human interaction and community growth in a healthy and supportive manner.

HISTORICAL PERSPECTIVE

After the fall of the Roman Empire, medieval cities began to blossom in western Europe. The development of these cities, usually contained within stone walls, reflected the need for protection, economic interchange, and social intercourse. During these middle ages the church was the one universal institution. Membership and involvement in that organization provided people with a constant source of communion and support. The church or cathedral, sometimes abutted by the marketplace or other community areas, definitively served as the spiritual and social focal point of insulated human settlements. The church was the social nucleus of the medieval city, dominating all other institutions. Its powers were so pervasive that one could hardly be unaffected by its presence and unifying force.

By the seventeenth century the church, although still an imposing physical entity, had begun to lose its function as a unifying social and cultural force. In the baroque city the palace served as the community focal point, with the city's marketplace, theaters, concert halls, parks, and art galleries being considered part of the palace complex.

With the advent of the industrial revolution, the major elements and meeting places of the new urban configuration were the factories and the low-income neighborhoods where the industrial workers lived. Although there were settlement houses in many communities in the United States, these usually served not as a gathering place but more as a service center for European immigrants during the latter half of the nineteenth century and the early part of the twentieth. The factories, like the medieval churches and baroque palaces, were bordered by bustling marketplaces.

In today's post-industrial metropolis, the market in all its varied forms tends to be the nucleus of social and economic functions. The downtown business and office centers, suburban malls, neighborhood shopping districts in older neighborhoods, and highway strip developments dominated by fast-food chains and service stations are the environments in which we modern metropolitan dwellers meet our friends and neighbors and attempt to fulfill our need for community dialogue and social interaction.

These new metropolises, by the nature of land use and economic priorities, are even more devastating to cultural development and social exchange than their industrial predecessors. Even in the oppressive conditions of the slums and working-class neighborhoods of the industrial-era cities, there were opportunities for human exchange and interaction on the city's sidewalks, parks, and neighborhood taverns. Today, with few exceptions, even these opportunities rarely exist. We seek to develop human interactions by frequenting uncomfortable, sterile singles bars and computerized dating services, joining traditional churches (even if we find the doctrines and rituals somewhat archaic), driving to the local shopping center or regional mall hoping to chance upon someone with whom we can share some of ourselves, and traveling to faraway places in hopes that someone on an airplane or tour bus may be approachable. Still, we somehow feel that all-pervasive loneliness and disassociation from the world. We believe that something is lacking in ourselves, that some personality or character deficiency forces us to be lonely, morose, and introverted. We don't realize that much of this condition is the result of our social and physical environment, of a grotesque imbalance by those powerbrokers, factors, and systems that have distorted the priorities of our habitations, denying us the human and community contact which we must have to lead happy, fulfilled, and meaningful lives. The

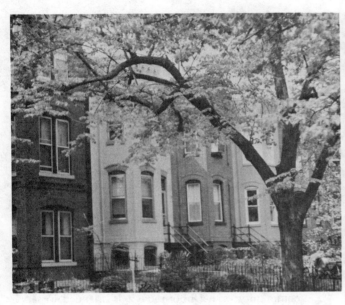
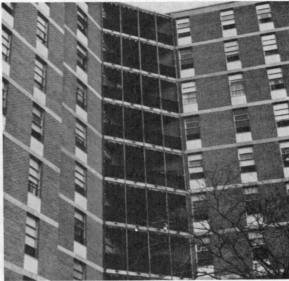

Cities provide choices. They are the centers of culture, art, progress, and development of civilization. To realize the potential of our modern society, we must make our metropolises humane and civilized places in which to live.

implication of this social isolation, along with the accompanying denial of aesthetic and natural amenities experienced by the urban dweller, is staggering to consider.

It can be argued that many of our current anxieties and social pathologies are largely a result of this modern-day perversity of environment. Stress, pollution, alcoholism, drug abuse, depression, mental disorders, violence, heart disease, cancer, apathy, emotional insecurity—the list of modern dysfunctions which can be attributed to the human condition in the urban environment is endless. We are the victims of what our short-sighted pursuit of power and wealth has wrought. We must put humanity back into our environments and lives if we are to survive as a civilization.

THE COMMUNITY-BASED HOLISTIC HEALTH CENTER AS A RESPONSE TO THESE CONDITIONS

I do not intend here to advocate abandoning the cities for the pastoral life of the country. Even if we chose this alternative, within the next twenty to fifty years probably not much inhabitable countryside will remain. As modern economies become more service-oriented and interdependent, all except a very small proportion of us will probably live in "standard metropolitan statistical areas." The only open space

to survive will likely be in the hands of governments (in the form of parks, reserves, and protected lands), agribusiness concerns, and the wealthy few who can afford to hold at bay the onslaught of real-estate development emanating from the overcrowded cities and suburbs.

Cities provide choices. Given all their problems, they are the centers of culture, art, progress, and development of civilization. The Western rebirth of intellectual thought and culture, the Renaissance, began in the cities of western Europe. In order to realize the potential of our modern society, we must make our metropolises humane and civilized places in which to live.

The church, the baroque palace area, and the factory all served as community centers. At the beginning of the twentieth century, specifically planned community centers were established in several communities in the United States. These community centers provided a place for group discussion and interchange, serving the function of establishing local initiative, control, and human contact. They formed the center of spiritual and cultural life of the community, as the church had once done. When this movement began to dissolve after the 1920s, many communities in the United States planned schools intended to serve the community at large. Unfortunately, in many urban neighborhoods, schools have evolved into reflections of municipal or school-board bureaucracies rarely soliciting input from the neighborhoods they serve. It is difficult to realize "ownership" and to use the facilities of the school under these conditions. Furthermore the lack of physical and aesthetic amenities at most schools, combined with the lack of a unifying philosophy by which to attract people and encourage social interchange, make it difficult to consider local schools a unifying community nucleus.

The community-based holistic health center, rather, is a responsive, meaningful, and likely place to carry on the role of the community center, a focal point for the reawakening of much needed social interaction in our post-industrial metropolitan areas. The unifying philosophies of holistic health, those of "high-level wellness," and integration of mind, body, and spirit, must include a natural extension to the community, social structure, and environment. That is, high-level wellness is as much a function of external social and physical factors as it is of internal, individual consideration. Striving toward high-level wellness is a means of promoting a collective spirit that could enrich and enhance community social life. Purposeful group life is essential to the renaissance of meaning, fulfillment, and humanity currently lacking in our urban lives and culture.

The community-based holistic health center is and will be a place in which the individual strives to achieve maximum health. The term "health" is used here generically to mean over-all integrated health rather than an absence of disease. It does not necessarily imply treatment; on the contrary, it necessitates responsibility for one's own health. The pursuit of health is not a doctrine but a philosophy by which an individual, with the social support of friends, family, and neighbors, can achieve his or her own potential.

Visiting and participating in the activities of the holistic health center does not include commitment to any doctrine, as might be the case in a neighborhood church. It does not force us to feed into an unfeeling, product-oriented sector as we must when we frequent bars, shopping malls, and other endeavors which play on our need for human contact in order to sell us products and services which often are unnecessary or unhealthy. The holistic health center will be a place for people to join together to strive toward self-fulfillment, human interaction, and social and environmental improvement on their own terms, in their own modes of expression, and in fulfillment of their own needs in a healthy and supportive atmosphere.

The community-based holistic health center will

serve as a nucleus of social contact among the heterogeneous groups who reside in our metropolises. Churches tend to follow socioeconomic and ethnic lines; rarely do congregations accept new members and worshippers who do not share their beliefs and lifestyles. Commercial enterprises that function as gathering places often exclude the "less desirable" in order to protect entrepreneurial financial investment. Most of the community centers that do exist are usually social service centers that feel like cold bureaucracies. Schools rarely attract use or attention during the evening hours when they are available, remaining empty and unused. There are day-care centers, youth centers, and senior service centers, mostly in lower-income neighborhoods, that separate people along age and socioeconomic lines. The intention of the holistic center, based on health and mutual support, would be to encourage and nurture human communication and social interaction along cross-cultural and heterogeneous lines based on the community or neighborhood it is intended to serve. This type of approach can only result in the improved health of people, communities, and social and physical environments.

The development of the holistic health center as the social and cultural nucleus of urban communities would promote local control of neighborhoods and environments, and, by extension, control over our individual and collective destinies. The quest for health and well-being is strongly associated with the pursuit of constructive and positive power. The social contact and human interaction promoted by the existence of the community holistic health center would extend this pursuit of health and power to the community. The residents, by understanding and harnessing this power, could make strides toward neighborhood self-government in its broadest sense, that is, control and management of the community's own affairs. One of the major consequences of being isolated in one's own city or community is that the decisions affecting our homes and surroundings are left in the hands of anonymous bureaucrats and capitalists who don't take into consideration the needs and desires of residents. Social and group action is one way of reversing this system, to give the power and control of the environment back to the people. If this can be accomplished in a supportive, healthy manner, it will promote a greater humanity and community spirit.

Perhaps most importantly, the advent of holistic health centers as community nuclei would be a major factor in improving the personal health of the metropolitan dwellers whom it attracts. It is a sobering fact that, throughout modern post-industrial history, life expectancy has usually been greater in the countryside than in the city, and the disabling effects of disease have been less. One of the original impetuses for the holistic health movement in the United States and Europe was that the debilitating effects of living in a stress-ridden metropolitan environment could not be solved totally by treatment of pathologies or public-health methods. Many of the holistic health disciplines are directly related to modern society's problems of stress management, anxiety reduction, and healthy living in a basically unhealthy environment. Promoting the holistic health center as a community focal point will expose people to its disciplines and attitudes. There is evidence that mere exposure to and education in holistic health attitudes and practices has a positive effect on people. The degree to which people may wish to become more directly involved in these practices and disciplines is, of course, an individual decision.

DEVELOPMENT OF COMMUNITY-BASED HOLISTIC HEALTH CENTERS

The development of community holistic health centers must be based on the initiative and actions of grassroots organization. These efforts must be local in conception, design, and implementation to reflect local needs. Information about the attributes and shortcomings of holistic health and holistic health centers must be made available to community groups, neighborhood clubs, and other interested parties.

Architecturally, holistic health centers should be consistent with the tastes of the community residents whom it serves. They should also be aesthetically appealing, with much thought given to noise levels, light, ventilation, and the development of a pleasant ambiance. One of the major problems with our metropolitan environments is that little consideration is given to the tastes of the community when public buildings and homes are designed.

The holistic health center should be located near the geographic center of the community. It should be small and local enough to allow repeated opportunities for face-to-face contact. The community must feel that it owns the center, so that it can reflect their needs and desires, and the social and cultural nature of the neighborhoods. The center should be easily accessible and located on public transportation lines. It should be near exisitng community gathering places and other public places, such as shops, schools, and other community and municipal facilities. Open-space park land should be close by. Most importantly, the holistic health center should be a physical focal point, compatible with its function as a social and cultural nucleus.

The holistic health center should be large and varied enough to accommodate a multitude of uses. The physical layout might include facilities for the healing arts, small group discussions, individual meditation and sanctuary, theaters, visual arts, community meetings, social events such as dances, parties, and dinners, recreational and natural park lands, libraries, and classrooms. Some of the programs that communities might wish to implement and support in their center include a holistic health clinic, classes in health maintenance and stress management, group travel to nature areas, health and emotional counseling services, group discussions, healing circles, neighborhood schools and art programs, lifestyle evaluation, publications, group support sessions, entertainment, and political action groups.

Financing for the development of holistic health centers could emanate from a combination of community support drives, local, state, and federal government revenues, and private and community foundations. Once a center has been developed, maintenance financing would be the responsibility of the local community through memberships, government funds earmarked for local use and development, and other sources of local support, such as business and civic groups. Individual programs and projects could be financed by special drives and appeals, sale of items and services at affordable prices (preferably on a sliding scale), and appropriate government and philanthropic sources.

CONCLUSIONS

The development of the community-based holistic health center in metropolitan communities can be viewed as a part of the various movements and actions by which people are attempting to take control of their lives, communities, destinies, and world. Many of the problems, inequities, and feelings of isolation we face are due to our own lack of initiative, our complacency, and our acceptance of being controlled by people, forces, and institutions perceived to be beyond our comprehension and ability to influence. By providing a means for people to change some of these ostensibly given facts of life, we can begin to rebuild our society and world, by starting with our own bodies, minds, spirits, communities, and environments. A renaissance of health and humanity must evolve to ensure a meaningful and worthy legacy for our civilization.

SUGGESTIONS FOR FURTHER READING

Robert Adams. *The Rise of Urban Civilization.* Aldine, 1977.

Leonardo Benevolo. *The Origins of Modern Town Planning.* Routledge and Kegan Paul, 1967.

C. A. Doxiados. "Ekistics, the Science of Human Settlements," in *Systems Approach and the City,* ed. by Mesarovic and Reisman (American Elsevier, 1972), pp. 8-42.

Clifford C. Ham. *The Neighborhood Church in Urban Extension.* Action Housing, 1964.

Jane Jacobs. *The Death and Life of Great American Cities.* Random House, 1961.

Lewis Mumford. *The City in History.* Harcourt, Brace, and World, 1961.

_____. *The Culture of Cities.* Harcourt, Brace and World, 1938.

U.S. Department of Commerce, Bureau of the Census. *Social and Economic Characteristics of the Metropolitan and Non-Metropolitan Population.* Washington, D.C.: 1977.

Bruce Gorman is the executive director of the Berkeley Holistic Health Center. He received his Master's degree in City and Regional Planning from Rutgers University in New Brunswick, New Jersey. He has worked in health planning, economic development, and community services planning in Washington, D.C., and San Francisco, California. Bruce is interested in creating a means by which holisitc health services and philosophies are integrated into community health and social services.

Making Legal Contracts with Your Doctor
Jerry A. Green, J.D.

Clear agreements which define responsibilities are beneficial to any situation where people are trying to accomplish something together. In this article, Jerry Green talks about making contracts or agreements between doctors and clients (or patients). These agreements help in clearing up any unrealistic expectations on the part of each person involved and help in creating a healing program that is suited to the needs of the client and the skill of the doctor.

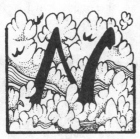

ot long ago a malpractice suit was brought by a patient who failed to recover her hearing after difficult and expensive surgery. The physician argued that he had performed the surgical procedure correctly, but that excessive scar tissue had blocked recovery. The doctor won. Why? Because he had performed his role in the treatment of pathology according to established medical practice. The problem was that the patient failed to heal properly.

This case illustrates a common misunderstanding about the role of the physician in health care. As the science of medicine has developed, its practice has been mystified to the extent that people no longer understand what they can and cannot expect from their doctors. In my opinion, the medical malpractice crisis is the result of this lack of understanding.

People tend to expect health as a product of medical care. In another malpractice case, suit was brought by the relatives of a woman who had died of skin cancer. Two years before her death she had visited a physician and had him remove a wart. Her family sought to hold the doctor responsible for her death. The negligence alleged was failure to diagnose a disease, which may or may not have existed at the time of the wart removal, but the thrust of the lawsuit was

This article first appeared in *New Realities,* Vol. 2, No. 1, and is reprinted here by permission of the author.

to establish medical responsibility for the patient's failing health. In other words, the doctor was blamed for the woman's having contracted cancer. Yet the patient had never asked him to examine her for possible illnesses or diseases.

CAN WE DEFINE THE PHYSICIAN'S RESPONSIBILITY?

It would greatly clarify the doctor-patient relationship if people had a better understanding of what they legitimately can expect from their physicians. Medicine, as it is currently defined and practiced, is actually a science of pathology, developed to diagnose and treat illness, injury, and disease. Doctors study the dynamics of health primarily to discover the origin and treatment of pathology. The treatment of pathology is far different from the maintenance of health.

In his three-volume *Divided Legacy,* medical historian Harris L. Coulter traces back for 2,000 years the parallel development of two opposing schools of thought about healing—the Empirics and the Rationalists. The Empirics studied the interaction of the life force with threatening influences in the environment and discovered practices which facilitated healing. They considered observation and experience to be the only source of knowledge. The Rationalists, on the other hand, placed a premium on logical analysis, disapproved of the "vitalist" viewpoint, and sought to classify diseases based upon "common symptoms." The Empirics focused on the "peculiar symptoms" which identified the individuality of each patient, and sought to facilitate the organism's interaction with its natural environment.

The rational viewpoint, with its focus on pathology, has dominated our medical education and practice for the last 200 years. Standards of medical practice which form the basis for our laws governing health professions have developed according to rational methodology. We have come to believe that medicine and health are synonymous and have grown to expect health from our doctors. This assumption has led to unrealistic expectations which go unful-filled and lead to litigation. This misunderstanding, not medical negligence, was the common denomina-tor in most of the malpractice cases I was exposed to.

THE DOCTOR-PATIENT RELATIONSHIP

How can we promote better communication be-tween doctor and patient? One way is to clarify responsibility by making agreements. The doctor-patient relationship is basically one of contract. How-ever, the terms of the contract, which include the specific identification of the roles of both parties, have remained largely unspoken. Consequently, in the eyes of the law, the relationship has been one of *implied* contract. This means if litigation occurs, the rules of tort law are applied in the absence of a con-tractual relationship. If for example you pick up a hitchhiker, crash the car, and hurt him, he can sue you for not driving within the established standard of care. However, if you and a friend agree to split the gasoline on a trip and you have an accident, you have a contract and a different standard applies.

WHAT MAKES A CONTRACT LEGAL?

Courts will recognize private agreements as con-tracts if they are reasonable and not contrary to exist-ing law or public policy.

A contract for professional health-care services need not be written to be legal. In fact, a writing which purports to be a contract may be used to invalidate the agreement if it suggest inappropriate terms. A written contract also suggests that the parties may anticipate litigation. Verbal statements, notes of conversations, correspondence, or the behav-ior of the parties all evidence a contract. The con-tract exists in the minds of the parties.

The essential elements of a contract include af-firmative obligations of both parties, a mutual or common purpose, and a term or length of time. For example, a woman I'll call Carol was diagnosed by her physician as suffering from pelvic inflammatory disease. This is a serious infection which normally requires hospitalization. However, Carol did not want to go to the hospital. She and her physician discussed alternative possibilities and hammered out the follow-ing plan. For the period of one month Carol would attempt to fight the infection naturally by working with a nonmedical holistic practitioner. However, if at the end of one month, the infection had failed to clear up, she would enter the hospital for tradi-tional treatment with antibiotics. Carol and her doc-tor had a contract. A contract is simply a plan. Each person identifies his or her specific responsibilities, decisions, and skills which are necessary to the fulfill-ment of the plan.

Since we are not used to making contracts in health-care relationships, go easy at first. Make simple agreements which will help make the relationship work better. Use contracts as tools for clarifying expectations, keep time periods short, and anticipate renewing and modifying your plan as you discover elements which need to be included.

Many physicians are asking their patients to sign arbitration agreements before treating them. Arbitra-tion agreements simply shift the forum of resolving disputes from courts to private arenas. They do little to minimize the chance of malpractice. And they may increase the likelihood of breakdown in the relation-ship by focusing attention on the anticipation of fail-ure at an early stage. Arbitration provisions should be considered in the context of an agreement which helps make the relationship work by allocating responsibility between the parties.

MIXING RATIONAL AND EMPIRICAL APPROACHES

The holistic health movement is today's expression of the Empirical tradition. The growing popularity of holistic perspectives has encouraged many physi-cians to explore incorporating them into their medical practices.

Can holistic practices be mixed with traditional medicine?

Physicians are not trained in holistic practices. Holistic practices will often be contrary to standards of medical practice which physicians are legally re-quired to respect. If your doctor offers services other than the diagnosis and treatment of disease, you should recognize that this is beyond the scope of his medical education, and satisfy yourself about his training and experience in the service offered.

Considerable confusion has been generated by our temptation to see holistic practices as an alternative form of treatment. This wrongfully encourages prac-titioners to offer what their work cannot provide, and promotes as much public misunderstanding as do our assumptions that medicine is a comprehensive health science. Holistic practices should be seen as tools for stimulating the body's own healing energies, by reducing stress, evoking balance, and encouraging more efficient interaction with the environment. The allo-cation of responsibility in a holistic relationship also requires clarification by agreement. Holistic practitioners should discuss with you what service, experience, and expertise you can expect from them. Misunderstandings can result in your failure to appreciate the area of individual responsibility for health and may give rise to criminal liability for practicing medicine without a license.

Not too long ago, Dana Ullman, a lay practitioner of homeopathy in the San Francisco Bay Area, was charged with practicing medicine without a license. Ullman had been set up by an "agent" who visited him complaining of a chronic cold. We were able to reach an agreement with the district attorney and the court to dismiss the case because Ullman had, by the time of trial, established a practice of making agreements with clients which clarified a nonmedical role in health care.

His case has been misinterpreted as legitimizing holistic practices by unlicensed persons if they tell their clients that they are not doctors. This is not so. The court-approved disposition simply recognized the potential area within which a nonmedical health practice might be created and acknowledged private contracts as a means for defining responsibility. Its reasoning will apply to others who structure their relationships by agreement in a manner which properly allocates responsibility for decision making about health services. Agreements which may be interpreted as providing for the diagnosis and treatment of pathological conditions will be considered void for illegal purpose. It should also be remembered that Ullman's situation involved the dismissal of a criminal case. purpose. It should also be remembered that Ullman's situation involved the dismissal of a criminal case. This disposition may be influential in a similar case, but other courts are not bound by precedent to follow it.

YOUR INDIVIDUAL RESPONSIBILITY

Remember, your health is your own responsibility.

If all your doctor can tell you is that you have no condition amenable to medical treatment, you have received a valuable service helping you to define the limits of medical responsibility. Rather than expecting the doctor to "Do something!" you may begin to examine what you might do for yourself, and how nonmedical health services might assist your efforts.

Decide for yourself the direction of growth which you would like to further with the aid of holistic practices. View with care the promise that a practice will correct your condition by pushing your magic button. Holistic practices encourage the growth of awareness. Their effectiveness depends on remaining centered in your own experience.

SUGGESTIONS FOR FURTHER READING

Coulter, H., *Divided Legacy: A History of Schism in Medical Thought.* Wehawhen Books, 3 vols., 1975.

Green, J. A., "Legal Issues in a Health Revolution," in *The Holistic Health Handbook,* (And/Or Press, 1978).

———. "Responsibility for Health," in *Journal of Holistic Health,* no. 1 (1976), p. 76.

Green, J. A., with S. Markell, "The Health-Care Contract: A Model for Sharing Responsibility," in *Holistic Health Review,* vol. 4, no. 1 (Fall 1980).

The author is an attorney in Mill Valley, California, who specializes in medicine and holistic health. He conducts seminars in structuring health-care relationships by contract at the offices of the Institute for the Study of Conscious Evolution, 2418 Clement St., San Francisco, CA 94121. A collection of his earlier writings and additional material relevant to allocating responsibility in health-care relationships is available from the author at this address.

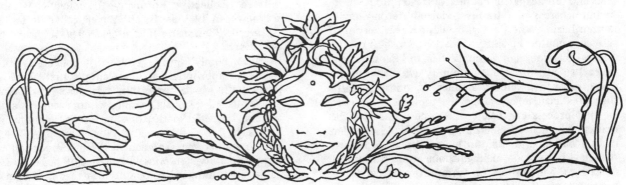

The Berkeley Holistic Health Center

Mary Ann Dosch

The Berkeley Holistic Health Center has evolved and expanded right along with the rest of the Holistic Health Movement. We have seen many wonderful people and experiences come and go, all of which have contributed to the growth and life of the Center. Our programs and services are very well-received and reflect the needs and interests of the community the Center serves. In this article we give you an update on the activities of one of the first health centers of its kind in this country.

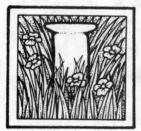 n facilitating health holistically, practitioners often use a kind of "double vision," with one eye on the acute symptom and one eye on the long-term reality. When someone is in pain, that pain must be dealt with, but the immediate cure has to fit in as part of the person's over-all health program.

Similarly, the Berkeley Holistic Health Center (BHHC) functions like a practitioner. The staff handles immediate needs: answering phones and visitor's questions, scheduling classes, paying the rent. At the same time, it keeps the whole picture in focus, from evaluating the health referral file to organizing volunteers and proposing community outreach programs.

But whereas practitioners concentrate on individualized healing, the Center, by design, reaches out to the community at large. This relationship to the population around it is implicit in the Center's purpose: "to provide the community with the philosophy, practices, and disciplines of holistic health through a creative and supportive process."

That process can begin when one walks into the Center, which is located in a beautiful, old, wooden church building. A bulletin board displaying numerous health services highlights one wall, pamphlets, magazines, and posters on various alternative health programs are easily accessible on other walls and tables. Natural light comes in through tall windows to nourish plants or a bouquet of fresh flowers. "We want people to feel healed when they walk in that door; it's a healing experience," says Joanne Tupper, an acupuncturist who works as the Center's office manager.

The Center's current home covers most of the upper floor in the church building, which also houses a theater, a dance studio, and other community groups. The Center has come a long way from its beginnings in the office of a Berkeley chiropractor in 1975. At that time, the seeds of the holistic health movement were just taking root. Individuals had begun looking for natural ways of healing themselves, but their searches were often isolated, without a community base.

One event which catalyzed the gathering of these individuals into a group was the arrest of Dr. John R. Christopher, a well-known iridologist and natural healer who was arrested in 1975 for practicing medicine without a license. A weekend healing retreat was organized as a benefit for his defense, and a surprising, overflow crowd of more than 300 people showed up.

Armand Brint and others in Berkeley drew inspiration from the overwhelming response to the retreat, and made plans for a permanent holistic health center. Sprouting from announcements distributed through a small mailing list and leaflets posted around the community, the Berkeley Holistic Health Center grew into a large group of workers and volunteers who formed a collective. For many, the collective became a "new family," as Isaiah Meyer called it in the Spring, 1978 *Holistic Health Quarterly* published by the Center.

This "family" group and small collective work force was appropriate to the Center's first phase of growth. "It was a supportive, safe place to develop our skills as teachers, administrators, and practitioners," Amelia Wright, one of the founding members, says.

The Center mushroomed in direct proportion to the community's response to it, and it began to include larger numbers of people. But that growth put strain on the collective structure. "The Center has always been an honest attempt to create a structure that is meaningful and inspiring to the workers," BHHC founder Armand Brint says, "But it was difficult to carry off a collective. There wasn't a feeling of shared responsibility, except for a core group. Everybody wanted to have a say, but not everybody was willing to work. That became too hard on the core group."

Besides the fluctuating nature of collective energy, the sheer volume of the Center's growth prompted a change in the structure. The *Holistic Health Quarterly,* which began as a mimeographed sheet listing a few classes, grew into a 16-page newspaper filled with notices about natural healing, workshops, and services. The first *Holistic Health Handbook* sold 50,000 copies. More people began calling into the Center, and visitors from all over the United States, as well as New Zealand, Canada, Great Britain, and India, dropped in to find out more about holistic health.

Responding to the expanding needs of the Center, Bruce Gorman was hired as Executive Director in 1979. He brought in his training as a city and regional planner and experience as a consultant to community groups. "The handbook was a real catalyst when I came in, because it showed we can be a lot more," Gorman says. "Now, we've started planning sessions, because if the organization wanted to stand pat, it could probably do it with an office manager. But if it wants to be different, it has to grow. You always need to be two steps ahead. If you stand pat, you'll be finished eventually."

Also, the Center moved to enlarge its Board of Directors to include more of a cross section of the community. Nancy Snow, an aide to Congressman Ron Dellums, Dan Liebson of the Berkeley City Planning Commission, and Bob Broudy, a real estate agent, joined the Board in early 1980. Dr. Robert Picker, who has done health counseling at the BHHC since 1977, has been joined on the staff by Marc Sanders, an M.D. trained in psychiatry, and Helena Weil, a biofeedback and stress-management practitioner.

Initially, the Center scheduled classes for teachers and advertised them in the *Holistic Health Quarterly.* Now, Instructors like Gayna Uransky, a hatha yoga teacher; Patrick Woods, who does deep-tissue bodywork; and Ethan Nabelkoff, an herbalist, function more as independent contractors to the Center, renting space, buying ads in the *Quarterly,* and splitting a percentage of their class income with the BHHC. "Having teachers put their own ads in the paper and renting space has really freed up the Center," Isaiah Meyer says. "And it's made the teachers more responsible."

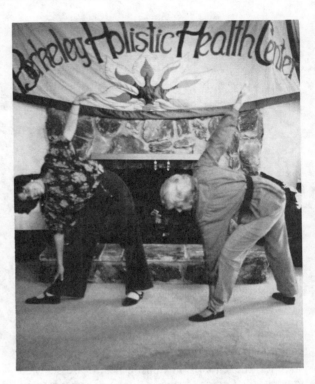

Structural changes in the operation have taken place, but the guiding force of the Center has remained constant. "Perhaps the most important thing about the Center is that we have never sold out our feeling for what we were doing," Armand Brint says. "We're still basically coming from the same place, still a group of people who realize there's a better way to work with health. We're still dedicated to serving people and developing a healing relationship with the community."

The work of serving the community in a healing relationship takes many forms through the various programs and services offered by the Center. One of the most direct contacts with the community occurs with referrals, either on the phone or in person. The referral file includes a broad range of practitioners. including acupuncturists, naturopaths, midwives, nutrition counselors, iridologists, and herbalists. Established doctors and dentists with a holistic outlook are also included.

"There are all different levels of awareness when people call," says Robert Patten, a volunteer who answers the phone one morning a week. "Some people have had contact with alternative health and want a specialist; others may be dissatisfied with their present medical situation and searching for an alternative."

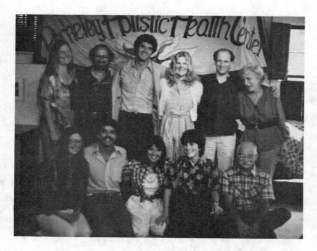

The whole spectrum of health problems and questions are reflected in the referral calls, including a teenager with acne who wishes to avoid using tetracycline; a probations officer who wants nutritional treatments for behavioral problems; or someone with cancer looking for an alternative to radiation or chemotherapy treatments.

Since the choices in holistic health are so wide-ranging, the Center's manager Joanne Tupper is working to pare down the referral file and channel people with questions to health educators who are available at the Center most afternoons. "We want to make sure people get the best referrals possible," she says. "With volunteers, its hard to teach them enough about holistic health to answer questions, and there's always a turnover in volunteers. So we are channeling calls to the health educators; we want to use them as much as possible."

Health educators like Susan Koenig and Eddie Bauman, who have both worked at the Center several years, play a role in broadening the vision of treatment possibilities. "If we can spend five or ten minutes with someone instead of 15 seconds on the phone, we can perhaps open up the possibility of things they hadn't thought about," Susan Koenig says. "We want people to realize the choices they have. We're broadening the choices, but we also want to have an integrating effect. We're not a shopping center. We want to integrate pieces of information into the picture of a person's whole life."

One service of the Center which typified this integrative approach is the Lifestyle Education and Referral Network (L.E.A.R.N.) program. The basis of the program is an extensive questionnaire which explores a person's medical history, nutritional habits,

emotional health, relaxation awareness, and environmental stresses. After completing the questionnaire, a person can then choose to have a counseling session, a computerized dietary analysis, hair analysis, hypoglycemia testing, or other blood tests. The information from the questionnaire and the various tests can then be coordinated to create a specialized health program for each individual. Nutritional supplements (which can be purchased at the Center) might be appropriate for one person, whereas another may need an exercise regimen.

It is the individualized nature of L.E.A.R.N. that Baba Silberzweig, who helped formulate the questionnaire, finds valuable. "There are so many different nuances," she says. "One food that goes with you might be impossible for someone else. The service is very powerful. It is meant for people who really want to examine themselves and work at making the necessary changes."

Another special service of the Center is the Nurse's Continuing Education (CE) program. These classes provide credits for nurses who are renewing or maintaining their licenses. Besides Center classes, workshops for nurses, such as Touch for Health, are also available.

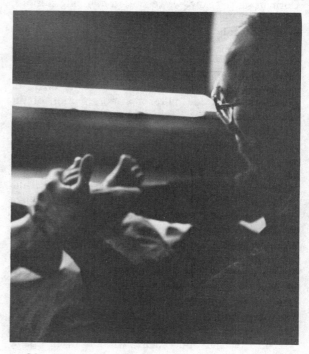

Many activities on the Center's agenda involve individual work. Group energies, however, are fostered in a special service called the Healing Circle. Using guided meditations and a gentle laying on of hands, the Circle channels spiritual energy for healings during weekly gatherings at the Center. "It's a wonderful, heartening experience," Isaiah Meyer says, "People get up from the healings with stars in their eyes."

A complement to the many services offered at the Center are the numerous projects which branch out from it. The *Holistic Health Quarterly,* which Baba Silberzwieg edited and developed during its first four years, provides general information on holistic health as well as the Center's classes and activities. The current editor, Ruth Gendler, now supervises a press run of 50,000 copies which are available free through subscriptions in health-food stores and in schools. The Speaker's Bureau connects the Center's health educators with community groups ranging from senior citizens and church organizations to halfway houses and high-school classes.

All the programs and services at the Center evolved out of real health needs in the community. Dissatisfaction with standard medical treatment has increased as health care in this country has grown more expensive, technological, and specialized. That dissatisfaction has caused many people to seek out alternatives and assume more responsibility for their own health.

One expression of this discontent which has shown up at the Center is the increase in calls from people with serious illnesses. Recalling her experience with

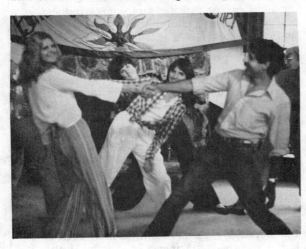

such calls, Susan Koenig said, "People call and say 'The doctor has told me I must get a cancer operation, and I must have chemotherapy and radiation treatment. I'm scared.' They're calling to see what holistic health has to offer."

"One of the first things we do is have people see past the fear," she added. "Then we look at their

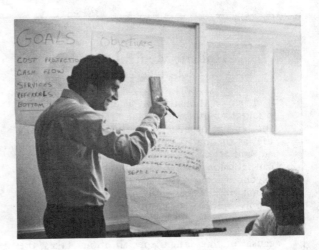

real needs and the parameters in their lives. We might suggest an individualized nutritional evaluation or other methods that promote healthy lifestyle changes."

Because the Berkeley Holistic Health Center is a forerunner in the alternative health field, it is not surprising that its vision of the future reaches into uncharted territory. As part of its ambitious plans, the Center is working to include low-income groups and others—such as people in institutions—who would not normally have access to holistic health information and techniques. Besides health service consumers, the Center intends to increase its role in providing holistic health education to medical professionals.

"We want to work with health professionals, to work with doctors," Eddie Bauman says. "There's no point in pretending we can replace them, because we can't. It's so easy to lock horns; then what happens is that alternative healing groups pretend they can do stuff that they can't."

Workshops, for professionals and consumers alike, will be the main vehicle for accomplishing the proposed outreach. The workshops are part of the Holistic Health and Health Enhancement Program, a comprehensive proposal by the BHHC which outlines its plans for the future.

Perhaps the most ambitious part of the plan is the idea for a Healing Arts Center. Such a center would not only enhance holistic education, but it would also include such services as a bookstore, a health-foods restaurant, a vitamin-herb store, saunas, and other amenities.

Executive Director Gorman sees all such goals as part of the over-all purpose of "getting holistic health education to a much greater part of the population."

(Text continued on p. 385)

Holistic Medical Practice
Robert Picker, M.D.

I am a holistic physician. My "holistic" orientation attempts to take into consideration the entire broad-view picture of a patient's life, as the matrix out of which dis-ease is created, and often subsequently manifested as physical pathology. When assaulted by stress, such as psychological pressures, physical trauma, nutritional imbalances, environmental toxins, or simply spiritual disharmony, the subtle forces maintaining health and vitality may be disrupted. All too often, traditional medicine, because of increasing specialization, takes the narrow view in attempting to cure physical symptoms without addressing the psychospiritual malaise out of which they arise. Surely, Western medicine has become highly technical and complex, and most patients are awed into submissive acquiescence to its authoritative pronouncements. That situation, however, appears to be changing.

The public today is increasingly realizing its power through consumer advocacy. Individuals are becoming better informed about health matters, and appear to be more ready than ever to take more responsibility for their well-being, rather than giving their power up to a parental authority figure. The old "Please fix me, doc" attitude is changing to "Please show me how I can help myself." Sure, technology can be helpful, and I use it myself in my practice, with laboratory testing, biofeedback instruments, computerized dietary analysis, and audiovisual aids. However, when it comes to potentiating the life force, neither technology nor any healer can do it for us. Symptom removal is important, of course, but until the creative force within achieves harmony and equilibrium, the relief will be temporary. Becoming truly healthy involves growing up, in the sense that we realize the healer lies within, and that we can and will use this healing power.

My practice, therefore, does not focus solely on the removal of symptoms. As part of my history taking with patients, I use a lifestyle questionnaire which I helped to develop at the Berkeley Holistic Health Center. This questionnaire is part of our L.E.A.R.N. program (Lifestyle Education and Referral Network). By means of this questionnaire, I can pinpoint lifestyle factors which may be contributing to disease, in such diverse areas as relaxation habits, exercise, diet, environmental exposure, and social and sexual life. After evaluating these factors, I help the person set up a wellness program which addresses his or her particular resources and needs. I might suggest a massage practitioner or chiropractor to help realign physical energies, or perhaps acupressure or acupuncture for correction of more subtle energy imbalances. In some cases, I personally provide psychotherapy, utilizing philosophy and techniques borrowed from Gestalt, transactional analysis, Psychosynthesis, dreamwork, autogenics, and creative visualization. Bioenergetics and Reichian therapy can help release psychophysical barriers to the free flow of life energy, and I refer to therapists who do this work. I have been conducting dance therapy groups for more than seven years now, with excellent results. I believe dance/movement therapy is a very effective holistic therapy which can be used for a wide variety of problems. With almost all patients, I feel that relaxation training is valuable. I teach meditation, autogenics, and self-hypnosis by both live and pre-recorded sessions, and I give clients training tapes to take home for practice. I often refer them to an associate for biofeedback training, which uses muscle tension, finger temperature, and sweat-gland activity as indices of relaxation.

A major aspect of my practice is nutritional counseling. I use hair analysis, computerized dietary analysis, and various blood tests to help evaluate an individual's nutritional/metabolic status. I often suggest a five-hour glucose-tolerance test to check for blood-sugar abnormalities, such as hypoglycemia (low blood sugar) or diabetes. A full third of the patients I see turn out to have symptomatic hypoglycemia, and I am convinced that many medical and psychiatric patients are hidden cases of hypoglycemia. I often suggest dietary changes and supplements to help correct imbalances which are discovered, and I refer clients to classes at the Berkeley Holistic Health Center, such as our health-food cooking class and the Health Awareness Class.

I also make specific suggestions for developing a physical exercise program, and may suggest running, dance, and "aerobics" groups. Sometimes my therapy sessions take place running in the hills with a client. I have seen cases of depression alleviated by running.

Last, but by no means least, is my role as social advisor. Loneliness is as deadly as any chronic stress I know. Many people simply don't know where to go to meet people, besides bars. I have seen "cures" when clients discover more gratifying social resources, such as local outings, clubs, social groups, and non-partner-oriented "dance-free" groups. Educational classes are recommended, and I keep a reference file of reading materials at the health center for clients, which is also a friendly and warm place to meet others interested in improving their well-being.

The following case history illustrates this holistic approach. Mary is a 45-year-old woman who presented me with a chief complaint of depression, anxiety, and general dissatisfaction with life. She was unhappy about her relationship with her husband and children, and bored by her secretarial job. For several months prior to seeing me, she had suffered from insomnia and stomach pains when she was nervous. She had been losing her zest for life for several years, and was beginning to feel desperate, finally seeking out my help. The L.E.A.R.N. questionnaire spotlighted several trouble areas. She rarely took time to relax, and used alcohol and tranquilizers to calm herself. Although not yet addicted, these habits were leading into dependency. She was not getting adequate physical exercise, and felt very restless and agitated at times. Her sexual needs were not being met, and she had rather poor communication with her husband and children. She had a tendency to feel victimized by the housewife role her family expected of her, and she felt trapped by their expectations.

Nutritional analysis indicated inadequate dietary intake of B vitamins, and hair analysis revealed low tissue concentrations of magnesium, magnanese, and zinc. A five-hour glucose-tolerance test revealed a borderline case of hypoglycemia, with anxiety symptoms aggravated when blood sugar fell.

A treatment plan was devised that took into account the different factors contributing to this woman's problems, and that provided her with adequate resources and time to deal with each problem area. Since she was primarily bothered by her unrelenting insomnia, we dealt with that problem first. I taught her autogenic relaxation exercises, and gave her a sleep-induction tape to further help her relax. I urged her to start a gradually increasing exercise program, and she reluctantly agreed to try jogging. She felt it was somewhat inappropriate for a woman of her age to be "running through the streets"; so she ran at a local track, still feeling rather embarassed to be out there with "real athletes." At first, one or two miles was all she could manage at a time, but with encouragement she persisted. To assist her sleep, I gave her L-Tryptophan to replace the sleeping pills she had been using. Tryptophan is a naturally occurring essential amino acid which is effective in treating sleep disorders and depression. We reviewed her diet, eliminating as many refined and processed foods as possible, emphasizing raw fruits and vegetables, whole grains, and high-quality proteins, with frequent wholesome snacks, and avoidance of coffee, alcohol, and sugar. We replaced alcohol and valium with Tryptophan, calcium-magnesium mineral tranquilizers, B-complex, and a good general vitamin and mineral supplement. Within a few weeks, her insomnia disappeared. Mary was beginning to enjoy her daily runs, and felt that this, more than anything, was helping her sleep.

We next focused on her family problems, involving her husband and children in family counseling sessions. I continued individual counseling with Mary, supporting her desire to get more out of life. I urged her to join my dance-therapy group, and after some initial resistance because of shyness and fear, she attended a session and "felt like a playful child again." She became a regular member and began to be more vivacious and energetic than she had been in recent memory.

Within six months, the transformation was indeed impressive. She was now running more than 40 miles a week, and was preparing to run her first 26-mile marathon race. She had won several races in her age division, was an active member of a local running club, and was quite proud now to be "running in the streets." She felt strong and healthy, and had achieved a good measure of new self-confidence. She found the courage to quit her job, and ventured out to find something more interesting and challenging. She pursued political interests, and began working as an administrative assistant to a local congressman. In addition, she seemed increasingly to feel that her marriage was unsalvagable, and decided to separate, trying out single life again for the first time since she was

(continued on p. 384)

(continued from p. 383)

a teenager. As of this writing, she is enjoying it greatly. Now, whenever she gets down, or feels nervous, she repeats her self-healing affirmations, together with a visualization of herself in her ideal environment. She has told me, "It's pretty hard to get seriously depressed now when I know it will disappear when I go for my run later. I don't feel trapped by my emotions any longer. Now I've got the tools to let the light in when it gets dark."

Certainly, no one approach is right for everyone, nor totally effective for any one individual. The more tools and resources I have available for clients, the more appropriate and comprehensive can be the individualized wellness plan. I feel extremely fortunate in having so many excellent allied healing-arts practitioners as co-workers. I am not grandiose enough to believe I alone can provide all the guidance that my clients need, and I would strongly urge other physicians, holistic or otherwise, to utilize paraprofessional practitioners and health counselors. Patients know they are being short-changed by quick fifteen-minute examinations, and welcome the opportunity for more in-depth sharing and attention. Developing a network of allied health counselors is one way to satisfy this need, using the physician's time most effectively, yet providing in-depth care and attention to the problems and stresses underlying individual symptoms. Quality medical care will, I believe, be enhanced by such an approach. Ultimately, in truth, we are all healers. I believe the holistic health movement will help us join together to heal ourselves and our planet.

SUGGESTIONS FOR FURTHER READING

Paavo Airola, *Are You Confused?* Health Plus Publishers, 1971. A good overview of nutrition.

————, *How to Get Well.* Health Plus Publishers, 1974. Outstanding collection of nutritional regimes for treatment of a wide variety of maladies.

————, *Hypoglycemia: A Better Approach.* Health Plus Publishers, 1977. The best book available on the causes and cures for low blood sugar.

Don Ardell, *High-Level Wellness.* Rodale Press, 1977. A highly readable description of numerous complimentary paths to optimal health.

Mark Bricklin, ed., *The Practical Encyclopedia of Natural Healing.* Rodale Press, 1976. A collection of articles on natural treatments for various medical problems. A good reference book.

David Hawkins and Linus Pauling. *Orthomolecular Psychiatry.* W. H. Freeman and Co., 1973. A rather technical textbook aimed at the professional wishing to understand and incorporate orthomolecular medicine.

Thaddeus Kostrubala, *The Joy of Running.* Pocket Books, 1976. A deeply moving personal account of an overweight, out-of-shape physician's physical and psychological journeys into the joy of running.

Andrew Michaels, *Why Do You Think They Call It A Deadline? A Wholistic Stress-Management Workbook.* Andrew Michaels, 1979. A concise yet comprehensive self-help guide for personal stress management. (Available through the Berkeley Holistic Health Center).

Ken Pelletier, *Mind as Healer, Mind as Slayer.* Delta, 1977. A review of the effects of stress on health, pertinent research in psychosomatic medicine, and various therapeutic approaches to stress reduction.

Robert Picker, "On the Path: A Moving Experience." In the *Holistic Health Handbook* (And/Or Press, 1978). This article discusses my approach to dance therapy.

Carl Pfeiffer, *Mental and Elemental Nutrients.* Keats, 1975. An excellent text revealing current thinking on a variety of nutritional subjects. Highly readable; appropriate for both layman and professional.

Chris Popenoe, *Wellness.* Yes!, 1977. An extensive bibliography of books on a wide variety of health-related subjects.

Ram Dass, *The Only Dance There Is.* Anchor-Doubleday, 1974. A collection of talks and essays by the most popular new-age spiritual leader in America. Inspiring.

Norman Shealy, *90 Days to Self-Health.* Bantam, 1976. A review and guidebook for the improvement of one's mental and physical health. Packed full of holistic jewels.

Robert Picker, M.D., is a psychiatrist and holistic physician, and is the clinical director of the Berkeley Holistic Health Center. Dr. Picker is a founding member of the American Holistic Medical Association.

(continued from p. 381)

"That's something we're committed to," he says, "And everything we do is going in that direction."

Enlarging the circle of holistic health to encompass as many people as possible is not just an aspiration for the future of the Center; rather, it is a process that has been in the works since the beginning. "It seems the Center has entered a phase of real acceptance in the community," Armand Brint says. "Instead of being an esoteric organization, our goals and what we're doing are not so far from the average person. We've had to come down to earth in some ways, and in some ways the community has had to catch up."

The BHHC has also contributed to the widening holistic health world in the form of healers who studied at the Center and then went on to establish centers in the Northwest and New Mexico. In California, the BHHC has also tied in to other centers in Santa Rosa, Santa Cruz, and Palo Alto.

In recent years, holistic health has become more and more intertwined with the general culture. The *Holistic Health Review,* a magazine published by the Holistic Health Organizing Committee covering political, social, and legal aspects of holistic health, now reaches a national audience. Alternative health approaches are the subject of television talk shows and newspaper articles.

It is in providing health education to the culture at large that holistic health can play its greatest transformational role. "There's so much new consciousness coming in now," Eddie Bauman says, "that people getting angry about the lack of medical attention have to shift some of that energy to find out what kind of health practices they can do for themselves and others. In fact, there's a new culture forming. We've got to do it and we've got to do it together."

As the best of the established and alternative medical worlds begin to mesh, there is no question that the Berkeley Holistic Health Center will continue its role in the front and center of this growing health movement.

Service
Gabriella Mistral

All of Nature is a place of Service.
The clouds serve, the wind serves, the fields too.
When there is a tree to be planted,
You plant it.
When there is an obstacle in the road
Or hate in a heart,
You attempt to remove it.

There is the joy of being healthy
And of being just.
But, above all, there is the beautiful
And immense happiness of serving.

How sad the world would be
If everything was already done,
If there was not a rosebush to plant
Or a project to begin.

It is not only the great works that count,
But the small services as well,
Like setting a good table
Or putting books in order.

To serve is not to be inferior.
God, who gives the fruit and the light
Serves.
He has eyes, fixed on our hands,
and asks us each day,
How have you served?

Gabriella Mistral
(translated by Edward Bauman)

Mary Ann Dosch is a writer and associate editor for Pacific News Service. She graduated with a bachelor's degree in journalism from the University of North Carolina at Chapel Hill in 1974. Her articles on health have appeared in newspapers throughout the United States.

Making Holistic Health Accessible to All
Margo Adair

Traditional medicine is increasingly missing the boat about the health-care needs of the country. "More than $100 out of every $500 we spend on health care is wasted on unnecessary hospitalization, needless surgery, and duplication of facilities. More than money is involved: about two million needless operations are performed each year, killing as many as 24,000 people, according to some estimates."[1] With the rising cost of medicine and the astronomical cost of hospitalization, more and more people will be turning to holistic health to meet their needs. It is imperative that holistic health practitioners be there for them.

In order for this to occur, we must understand some of the social realities in this country. To be fully holistic, we must take into account the economic context of people's lives. It is necessary once and for all to dispel the myth that if someone wants it bad enough, they'll get the money together, that there is equal access to economic resources.

"Paul Samuelson, Nodel laureate in economics, has warned against thinking that America's wealth is broadly shared by the majority. Displaying his special sense for graphic illustration, he observed of the present income structure: 'If we made an income pyramid out of children's blocks, with each layer portraying $1,000 of income, the peak would be far higher than the Eiffel Tower, but almost all of us would be within a yard of the ground.' . . . America today is still, despite all our hopes, all our efforts, and all our dreams, a vastly unequal society. The most affluent third of Americans receive each year two times the income of the other two-thirds. One half of America lives on less money than the richest 10%, the poverty of the grim, soul-breaking kind endures for nearly one out of three of our countrymen."[2]

Richard Parker, in the preceding quotation, is speaking only of dire poverty. Felix Greene said in 1970 that "at least 105 million persons, or more than 50 percent of the population, live below the poverty line (as defined by Sargent Shriver, the Director of the Office of Economic Opportunity in the Kennedy and Johnson Administration)."[3]

With the rising of unemployment rolls and inflation, we can only conclude that the situation has gotten even worse, as indeed it has. Between 1970 and 1975 alone, the number of persons living in poverty increased by half a million.[4]

Some would like to believe that the civil rights and women's liberation movements are changing this. In fact, since the rise of these movements, things have gotten worse. The disparity between black and white worker's median weekly income in 1967 was $34, but by 1976 it had risen to $52.[5] The picture for women is all too similar: in 1955 women made 64¢ to every dollar men earned, but in 1975 women made only 57¢ for every dollar men earned.[6]

We all feel it. The price of every necessity has skyrocketed in the last five years.

To take into account these economic factors, we must arrive at reasonable policies in charging fees for services. The following is the formula I have arrived at during years of working with my clients. I've come to it by continually asking for feedback. I have come to the conclusion that sliding scales and barters are the only viable methods to use for accessibility. Scholarships are condescending, and perpetuate unequal power relationships (although they are certainly better than nothing).

Sliding scale for fees and barter.

Service	Percent of monthly income	Barter
Individual session (1-2 hours)	4%	5 hours
One-evening workshop	2%	2½ hours
Eight-hour workshop	4%	5 hours
Twenty-hour workshop	10%	16 hours

I find using percentages of people's incomes the best tool for working through this maze. When I give people the formula, I ask that they take into account assets and debts. If several people are living on one income, I have the person divide the income by the number of those living on it (including themselves) to come up with their own personal income. The percentages in the following table are based on monthly income. If the person needs to barter, I use the same percentage, but I base it on the total number of monthly hours worked by a full-time worker, which is 160 hours per month.

These figures represent my formula, but I am always open to negotiation. If someone has no regular monthly income (living off savings or making money irregularly, etc.), I average the amount of money spent each month during the last six months to get a monthly income figure.

When I use percentages in this way, all my clients are in fact paying equally, for they are using the same proportion of their total resources. There is another factor: the less money one has, the more each dollar counts. For this reason, some practitioners increase the percentage as the client's income level increases.

Using a sliding scale in this manner is better than charging low, set fees to make oneself accessible; the practitioner who charges low fees across the board loses the money that she or he rightly deserves from more affluent clients.

NOTES

1 *Why Do We Spend So Much Money?* (Popular Economics Press, 1977), p. 34.
2 Richard Parker, *The Myth of the Middle Class.* Liveright, 1972), pp. 6 and 165.
3 Felix Greene, *The Enemy.* (Vintage Books, 1970), p. 252.

4 *U.S. Capitalism in Crisis.* (Economics Education Project of The Union for Radical Economics, 1978).
5 *Ibid.*
6 Research Group One, *Women and Men: A Socioeconomic Factbook.* (Vacant Lots Press, 1975). p. 3.

Margo Adair is a socialist-feminist working to develop a materialist theory and practice of spirituality. Over the last seven years she has developed Applied Meditation, using the meditative state for practical problem solving. She works to make these kinds of techniques available to all people by charging on a sliding scale. She has also worked with people in halfway houses, drug-treatment programs, and jails. For several years she has conducted forums addressing the contradictions between politics and spirituality. Much of her focus has been teaching on Applied Meditation skills to activists to enable them to work more effectively to create change. She maintains a practice in the Bay Area, conducting support groups, working individually, and teaching. She travels around the country holding workshops and consulting. She also makes and distributes problem-solving meditation tapes dealing with particular issues. She is now writing a book on her work.

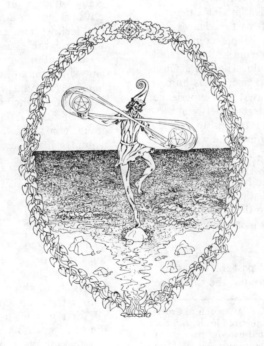

Medical Care at a Holistic Health Center:
Treating the Whole Person
Donald A. Tubesing, Ph.D.

The experience of being cared for in a community of committed people is perhaps the principal ingredient lacking in our health-delivery system. Dr. Tubesing and his associates strive to make this kind of contact accessible to their clients. This integrated approach to health problems is enhanced by a sensitivity to the real emotional and spiritual needs of the person along with attention to the physical complaints. The innovations implemented in these Chicago-based Holistic Health Clinics offers a promising new direction in health care.

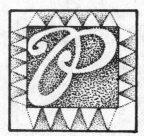

People need the experience of care. I need it; I trust that you need it; I know that lots of people who are sick need it. The problem with the present medical model is that for the most part it leaves out the care. People come to us for help, but they seem to be leaving not integrated and warm, but dissembled and cold. There is a sense among patients that they aren't respected as human beings, and it's not just incidental that that experience does not promote health. The interface between provider and patient forms a human relationship. It does not form a technological vending machine where you put in a quarter and get an aspirin.

I think it is possible to build bridges and try to combine the best of medicine and holistic care. What we are trying to do in the Wholistic Health Centers in Chicago is respond creatively to the person and the person's needs that are not being met by many medical facilities today.

The Centers are "family practice" medical centers located in church buildings with a pastoral counselor, a nurse, and a secretary who surround the physician

This article is adapted from "A Practical Approach to Creating Wholistic Health Centers," which appeared in the *Journal of Holistic Health,* vol. 3. It is reprinted here by permission of the Mandala Society and the Association for Holistic Health.

and form a team focused on delivering care for the whole person. Because we're located in churches and try to do things a bit differently, people often get the impression we don't do real medicine. We do. Our physician is licensed; he is on the local hospital staff; we hospitalize people. People come to us with sore throats, financial worries, broken bones, headaches, inability to concentrate, flu, ulcers, fear of failure, all sorts of doubts. They come to the centers for help with the full range of personal needs into which we as human beings seem to be so good at getting ourselves trapped. Whatever people need, we try to listen carefully and then plan with them what they need to do.

If you were to come into one of our centers for your first visit, we'd ask you to complete "The Initial Health Planning Conference Inventory," where we briefly ask about the kinds of things that have been going on in your life. We also ask "What are the physical symptoms you're concerned about; what are the feelings and emotions you're concerned about; what are the goals you'd like to begin moving toward; what are your strong points and special abilities; and what kind of help do you want from these people here?" Next you would talk to the nurse. She would take your height, weight, blood pressure, and a short medical history, and also make physical and emotional contact with you, which is kind of nice when you're a little nervous. Then you would go into the Initial Health-Planning Conference, a twenty-minute conference with the pastoral counselor (that's me), the physician, and the nurse. Somebody like me would say, "We believe that health really relates to all of you, and that you don't look just at the body or just at your relationship with your spouse, or whatever," and that's why we all sit down with you the first time you come in. We try to hear your concerns. We'd like to be able to react with you about the kinds of things that might be helpful. We want you to come up with a plan for taking care of yourself that you want to implement. We'll give you all the ideas we think of for helping you do that. We are not making plans only to take pills once or twice a day, but plans for all kinds of things about your life.

I'll give you a couple of examples of how the conference usually works. One woman who was very alive, very alert, complained that she felt tired all the time, and had headaches. She wanted a blood test. When we looked at her inventory, we saw that she'd moved recently to Chicago. She hadn't wanted to move. Her grandmother had died. When she and her husband drove to the funeral, her apartment and furniture had burned up while they were gone. She had a demanding little child, and so on. We said to her, "Hey, do you make any connection between all these changes you've been through and your physical symptoms?" Her immediate response was "Yes." We gave her a choice of a blood test or a couple of counseling appointments to try to get a handle on her stress. She took the latter choice, and when she came back for her first counseling appointment, she'd already made three friends, painted her bedroom, and joined a class at the YMCA. She was coming "alive" again—she didn't need us at all anymore, and that was super.

Another example shows the crisscross of the team approach. A woman had a chest tightness. She was kind of choking. She described long emotional hassles with her daughter-in-law, and how angry she was. "Aha!" I thought, "it's a counseling case." However, the physician asked her a few more questions and very shortly put her in the hospital, because she had a serious heart ailment that I would have missed.

Many times people come in and draw their picture of woe; as they describe their situation, there's just no way out of the box they're in. So we just throw it back at them, and say "What would it mean for you to take care of yourself?" If we hang with this question long enough, people start to move into a position that will allow them to actually begin taking care of themselves. Often people are stuck; they've tried everything they can think of. Often just redefining the problem works like a treatment, and they can figure out some way to care for themselves they hadn't thought of before. There are times when people just aren't able to talk about what's bothering them, but usually it takes only 30 seconds for them to relax, and at the end of the conference they say, "I can't believe it! What a neat feeling to have all you people listening to me. I never had this before." Then they go home and say, "Hey, Sam! Hey, Martha! Why don't you listen to me like that?"

Almost always the nonverbal message of the conference comes through more clearly than the verbal. There's no way to miss the message of a holistic approach while sitting around the table with three other people all trained in different professions.

There's a wholeness within you, and people sense this truth in the experience.

As a therapist, if I think people are caught in a head trip, it's my job to ask, "What are your feelings? What's your gut saying to you?" I need to help people get in touch with their feelings if that's where they are stuck. As a pastoral counselor, if people aren't talking about their beliefs and values at all, and if it looks to me like that's where they are tangled up, it's my job to poke around in the area of faith and ask them what they value. Ours is a non-denominational approach. We don't try to convert or evangelize. It's not my job to tell people what to believe and what their "spirit" conflicts are doing to them.

Let's take as an example, a man who's 45 years old and has made it. He's made a ton of money, but he doesn't have any time to spend it, because he's going too fast. He has a $180,000 house, and that's great, but last month somebody next door dropped dead from a heart attack. So he comes to us concerned about his heart. We can tell him to stop smoking, start exercising, and lose a little weight, but why stop there? There is more going on in his life than just his physical heart. If we ask him "What do you believe?" most likely he'll say, "I don't know. What do you mean?" He probably hasn't stopped to think about beliefs for ten or twenty years. Well, I can tell him what he appears to believe. I'd say, "You believe that you alone can make it, that you need to be perfect, that no God will forgive you, that no person will love you if you're not perfect. You must succeed all by yourself, and your need to prove that is killing you." He might be angry at us for confronting him with this, but that's the only way to get at the health problem this man is experiencing. I don't think professionals should sit by and say, "Well, it's none of my business." It sure is our business. The valueless, faceless approach to helping and healing is about as potent in this sort of case as a yeastless, sugar-filled loaf of bread: it just doesn't do much.

There are some other programmatic aspects to our clinics. Since we are committed to prevention and education, we offer health seminars focused on behavioral changes, not merely on dispensing information. Some of them are "Creative Management of Stress," "Healthy Living," "Taking Care of Yourself," and "Living with Chronic Illness." We foster support groups for weight control, stopping smoking, and assertiveness training, and if something isn't available in our area, we'll do it. We've done community health fairs, heartbeat programs, and screening programs. We do annual health-planning conferences for people whether they're sick or not. If you were our patient, in the month of your birth you would get a call saying, "It's time for your annual health-planning conference." I had one recently, and as a result made some major lifestyle decisions. Things really became clear to me when I had to fill out a form asking me to state in so many words just where I've been this year, what I've done right, what I've done wrong for my health, what I need to do to take care of myself better. We also keep a resource list of every kind of service we can find in the community. We helped one woman find a group that played the flute every Sunday afternoon, because that was the only thing she could think of that she liked to do.

We'll do almost anything to get patients in contact with other patients. If you come in as a depressed housewife (a stereotype again) because your kids are gone and you're sitting around, the best person to help you is someone with similar problems. If the two of you have coffee, you can get much more accomplished a lot more cheaply and make a friend at the same time.

It seems to me that if professionals can follow the three principles I want to lay out here, they will become living examples of better ways to care for people.

The first of these principles is that *the medical model of the future, if it is to promote the health of people, must offer the experience of being treated as a whole person.* It's the whole person and the whole picture that's essential. I get nervous when medical doctors push one kind of treatment for one kind of disease, that is, physical medicine for physical disease. But I also get nervous when Gestalt therapists push one kind of treatment: awareness, and when clergy push prayer and worship and reading the Bible to the exclusion of everything else, and when holistic practitioners push acupuncture, biofeedback, whatever they happen to be into. Do you get the idea that I'm a nervous person?

Well, I'm not excluding myself from the pushers. It's normal to be tempted to push something that you're excited about. But my point is that to treat the whole person you can't treat by digitals and X-ray alone. Those are effective medical tools, but we need to add other, equally effective treatments, like, "How about making a friend this week?" "Why don't you find a hobby?" "Why don't you learn to meditate?" "Have you thought about going back to worship again?"

The second principle is that *the medical model of the future must offer the experience of personal responsibility.* There is something wrong when a patient says, "You take care of me. I promise I won't gripe, I'll be good if you only promise to heal me without making it hurt." That deal just doesn't work. Sick people have lost control over part of their lives. Professionals need to help the person get some of that control back, and take it and run. Patients' ideas should also be taken seriously and carefully listened to. They should get to read the information on their chart, add their own notes, and scratch out what they don't like. Finally, a new form of diagnostic questioning should go along with the old. To the old questions like "How long have you had it?" "When does it hurt?" professionals should add new questions, like, "What do you think is wrong with you?" "Why did you get this disease now?" "What does it mean in your life?" "What would you have to give up to get rid of it?" These kinds of questions affirm that people don't pick up the disease, they earn it.

The third, and to me the most important principle of the medical model of the future is *to promote health by means of the experience of being cared for in a community of committed people.* I have yet to see it substantiated by research, but I believe that to be loved and cared for is the most effective promoter of health, and that being alone, isolated, and out of touch is the most potent distroyer of health. The health care of the future will hold forth a firm belief in the power of the healing effects of care and of the exchange of love between people. I'm not speaking about professional care. I'm talking about the caring of daily living. Professionals need to encourage sick people to get out among their friends and, if they haven't found care, to help them get some from the people they live with.

All of us, professionals and patients, need to redefine our concepts of health and illness in a way that puts people—care and love for whole people—back into the center of our life style. I believe that we will not begin to experience the best of the medical model of the future until a person is no longer seen as an assemblage of varied parts which can be fully discovered through minute scrutiny, piece by piece, but is again seen as a whole to be cared for with and contacted with awe.

Donald A. Tubesing, M. Div., Ph.D., is Clinical Associate Professor at the University of Illinois Medical Center in Chicago. For the past six years he has been helping to develop working model wholistic Health Centers in the Chicago area that synchronize the different aspects of the holistic approach and has recently published Wholistic Health: A Whole Person Approach to Primary Health Care.

A New Voice for Medicine:
The American Holistic Medical Association
Dean Challes

The American Holistic Medical Association is composed of medical professionals who are concerned with the present trends in American medical care, and who are working together to integrate holistic principles into the education of future physicians. The association hosts three major regional programs during the year, presenting outstanding authorities on the various aspects of healing. In this article, Dean Chellas tells about his first A.H.M.A. conference. The American Holistic Medical Association is a positive force working toward the renaissance of medicine and the integration of the art of healing.

"Many alternative techniques offer a safe approach to psychosomatic or stress illness, a far superior, and more truly scientific approach than tranquilizers, which are so commonly used.

"We have demonstrated that persons with serious illness have 85 per cent less medical expense when they are treated holistically. Think what such an approach could do when applied to all aspects of medical health care."

C. Norman Shealy

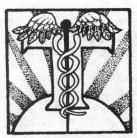 his pronouncement was voiced by C. Norman Shealy, M.D., Ph.D., early in 1979 in Denver, Colorado. This statement rings true also for the hundreds of other physicians across the country who have joined with Dr. Shealy in developing the American Holistic Medical Association (AHMA).

Principal mover and former president of the AHMA, Dr. Shealy is a neurosurgeon, founder and Director of the Pain and Health Rehabilitation Center in La Crosse, Wisconsin, a Clinical Associate in Psychology at the University of Wisconsin, and the author of several books on his specialities, the treatment of chronic pain and holistic health training.

The AHMA was founded by Dr. Shealy in 1978 in response to the need for holistic education for physicians. The major activities of the organization currently focus on presentation of three major regional programs during the year, ranging from four to six days each. Through these programs the AHMA offers a valuable education to health professionals in the principles of "medicine of the whole person."

I attended one of the Western Regional Programs, which featured outstanding authorities in the physical, emotional, nutritional, environmental, and spiritual aspects of healing. In all my previous exposure to holistic-health programs, conferences, seminars, etc., I cannot recall having been more inspired and encouraged about the prospects of responsive change in the manner of medical delivery in this country.

I was witness to a "call to consciousness" by the new breed of medical physicians to their counterparts in the orthodox medical profession. The movement toward and the practice of "new medicine" posts many basic questions about the precepts of modern medical care, including the following.

What is the role of the practitioner?

What is the responsibility of the patient?

What is effective application of drugs and invasive techniques?

What is the value and limitation of the reductionistic and atomistic philosophy in medical science?

What is the nature of disease and stress?

What is the definition of health?

What are the origins and processes of healing?

What are the relevance of nonconventional and "nonscientific" methods, and where do they integrate?

It was difficult for me to realize that what I heard being propounded with unwavering conviction was not something emanating from another fringe sub-

391

culture group, where most new thought tends to originate. Rather, here were distinguished physicians from the professional medical world all chanting to the same vibration, a chant heralding a renaissance in medicine. It was coming from those who were actually conducting their practices according to their new prescriptions. This realization was exciting; it showed me that the beliefs I've been advocating to countless others during the past few years were not spurious but a reality for our future. For these reasons, I would like to summarize here some highlights of the thoughts, perceptions, and approaches covered in the presentations of the initial AHMA conferences.

HOLISTIC HEALTH AND MEDICINE

The tendency in the past to employ the terms "holistic health" and "holistic medicine" interchangably has concerned me, because confusing these terms would inevitably lead to the erosion of the significance of each. The AHMA has distinguished the two terms as follows.

Holistic health: a state of well-being in which an individual's body, mind, emotions, and spirit are in tune with the natural, cosmic, and social environment.

Holistic medicine: a system of health care which emphasizes personal responsibility, and fosters a cooperative relationship among all those involved, leading toward optimal attunement of body, mind, emotions, and spirit.

Holistic medicine encompases all safe modalities of diagnosis and treatment, including appropriate use of drugs and surgery, emphasizing the necessity of looking at the whole person, including analysis of physical, nutritional, environmental, emotional, spiritual, and lifestyle values. Holistic medicine particularly focuses on patient education and patient responsibility for personal efforts to achieve balance.

Holistic health, according to the founders of the AHMA, is a state of well-being. It *can* be achieved, and physicians can play an important facilitating role with individuals motivated to assume the responsibility for achieving it. Most people enter this world with this state, but lose it because of a lack of proper upbringing, education, and example, leading to poor habits and stressful lifestyles. Poor nutrition, lack of physical exercise, and emotional anguish are overwhelming contributors to disease. The AHMA physicians see one of their major goals to be teaching the principles of good health: nutrition, physical exercise, mental attitude, and attunement with spiritual ideals.

THE NEW MEDICINE

In Dr. Shealy's keynote address to the founding membership meeting of the AHMA in May 1978 in Denver, he portrayed the path of medicine leading to the current dilemma. He stressed the excesses of today's practice of medicine, the overuse of drugs and surgery, and the accompanying high costs. In the face of this, only fifteen to twenty per cent of all illnesses representing acute or life-threatening situations actually require medical or surgical intervention to prevent serious harm or death.

He indicated it was recognized as early as 1952 that overspecialization was reducing the ability of the physician to look beyond the acute problem and to become humanely involved with the patient. Along with this decreased ability to deal with the patient in a systems manner, the products of society—smoking, alcohol, pollution, lack of physical exercise, processed diets, excess calories, etc.—added further complication to the problems of effectively dealing with the illness problems of the patient.

The medical response to this condition has been overspecialization and prescription of excessive amounts of tranquilizers (they are now the most-prescribed drugs) in all shapes, sizes, and forms. The result is suppression of symptoms and treatment of patients as diseased organs rather than as organically complex human beings.

Dr. Shealy clearly pointed out that a medicine that treats the whole person has never been needed more, and that holistic health and holistic medicine can effectively fill this void and contribute to the "next great advance in the health of the American people."

TREATING THE PATIENT, NOT THE DISEASE

The AHMA is addressing (attacking may be more descriptive) the issue of the scientific practice of modern medicine. A debate has been precipatated by AHMA with deans of several medical schools to define what scientific medicine is and what the criteria are for proving a technique scientific. This dialogue could develop into an issue of national medical significance if what many of AHMA members contend, that 20 per cent of modern medical techniques are scientific, is borne out. Yet the loudest criticism of new medicine by conventional institutions, such as the AMA, is that most of it is unscientific.

Dr. Eugene A. Stead, Jr., M.D., Professor of Medicine at Duke University, remarked in an address before an AHMA membership audience that, "Many forms of treatment are helpful that are not based on Western scientific medicine. The American-trained doctor believes these forms are irrational methods and rejects them. . . . I do not believe that a given therapy has to have a scientific rationale. One needs to determine that the therapy helps and does not cause harm."

Dr. Stead talked about how doctors can be educated to function in an environment where science can only partially support the premises of their techniques and approaches. Basically, physicians must integrate what they have been taught about the scientific treatment of illnesses with a clear understanding of the role of the healer in those areas where science has not been brought to bear. The medical professional and student must appreciate the difference between tightly structured knowledge that can accurately predict the sequence of events and the knowledge of the potentiality of biological systems, which does not allow for long-range accurate predictions.

Dr. Stead testified to his own propensity to proceed with his patients on an experiential basis rather than according to scientific methodology and rationale. He is confident in his knowledge of the capabilities of biological systems and the range of possibilities, although he admits he does not know what may happen next. He is able to move with this because of his willingness to go and look in the absence of understanding, and to watch and listen closely to the patient.

The lack of a simple frame of reference for the study of behavior is the greatest disadvantage of the scientifically trained doctor. Most doctors have no frame of reference for handling behavior comparable to the one they have for discovering the structure and function of organs. Behavior seems something mystical, and the patients' perceptions of themselves, the role of the nervous system in transferring information from one person to another, and the changes in patients' brains which allow them to "pick up their beds and walk" in defiance of the apparent physical facts are among the many nonscientific factors which must be recognized and sensitively dealt with in the care of a patient.

Dr. Warren M. Ross of the University of Maryland enlarged upon the need to become involved with the patient's experience. He argued that the holistic approach recognizes the need to understand patients' beliefs concerning their disease, the experience of their illnesses, and the experience of a certain level of health within them. When there is such an understanding, meaningful communication about the personal, family, and community issues surrounding illness can take place.

HOLISTIC DIAGNOSIS

A call for revision of the diagnostic approaches to states of health and disease was made by Robert Leichtman, M.D., an internist and noted clairvoyant diagnostician. Before the AHMA assembly in Denver, he related that traditional views of the human body and mind have emphasized the physical components of the human body and its relations to the physical environment. Psychological and spiritual factors have been given small roles; they are seen too often as interesting, perhaps fascinating, factors that are largely beyond the physician's control.

Dr. Leichtman feels that the expanded view of the human condition, one that sees man as a multidimensional being living in a multidimensional world, allows for a more complete assessment of matters of health and disease. The innermost care of our human status is seen as both healthy and a source of healing for the mind, emotions, and body. In this approach, mind and emotions are not passive victims of the physical environment, but are full participants in the healing process. The holistic physician should understand how the mind and emotions facilitate healing, and should be able to instruct the patient in psychological techniques that will enhance healing and health. This should be adjunctive to whatever physical changes, treatment, medication, etc. might be useful to the patient's total care.

Patient education is needed to help patients cooperate more fully with the healing centers in themselves that can enrich and heal their own minds, emotions, and bodies. Specifically, Dr. Leichtman encouraged exercises of the mind and emotions to facilitate health by the constructive use of imagery and the positive direction of ideas and energies toward altering attitudes, self-image, and physiology.

These self-healing activities help patients share in their own treatment, and facilitate the conventional modes of treatment.

The view of holistic diagnosis presented by Dr. Leichtman emphasized that disease and distress can be seen as the results of a deficiency. The missing healthy factors may be even more important than the elements of disease present.

In this regard, a holistic approach to diagnosis would look for:

(1) a lack of harmony and cooperation within the personality;

(2) a lack of competence in the personality;

(3) a lack of attunement by the body and personality to the inner life and healing centers of consciousness; and

(4) a lack of positive self-expression.

Such an approach views all the vital health factors that may be important to healing in any one individual, and points the way to the kind of training for the patient that will facilitate healing.

HOLISTIC MEDICAL EDUCATION

Are the medical colleges around the country responding to educating future physicians for the coming age of "new medicine?" Although it would be nice to think so, the curricula are still mired in the old mold. The training that students receive in school is almost totally technologically oriented, and not adequate to prepare students for a holistic practice. Student representative Doug Outcalt, President of the American Medical Student Association, has spent a year away from his studies to tour campuses on behalf of the Association. His concern is substantiated everywhere he goes; the system supports those who are highly technologically or scientifically oriented, but students who are people and humanistically oriented have a hard time getting into or making it through the system. Behavior such as bookworming, sealing oneself up to study to the exclusion of all social interactive activity, is rewarded with better grades. With competition for entrance into medical schools so fierce, the bookwormiest who have managed the top grades succeed in making it in and staying there.

Student Outcalt suggested that probably 80 per cent of the first two years of study in the basic sciences in medical school is irrelevant to medical practice. Only a fraction of course time is spent on the things for which probably 90 per cent of people seek advice when they visit physicians' offices: psychosomatic illnesses, nutrition, obesity, alcohol abuse, sexual disorders, etc. When students pass on to clinical study they are taught the technical side of patient care. The future physician is not taught how to talk to patients in order to see how they feel and how to delve into personal backgrounds. In short, the *art* of medicine is not respected.

The AHMA can be an instumental in challenging the current educational concepts firmly imbedded in the teaching institutions. This young organization is already well-represented by physicians with university affiliations, and its effort to bring the "What is scientific medicine?" question directly to the deans of medical colleges is sure to begin having good effects.

Mr. Outcalt concluded his remarks with recommendations on six visionary roles that those in the holistic health-care movement can assume to ensure the future success and growth of holism in the American medical-care system. They are as follows.

1. To set standards in a way that will ensure legitimacy, but will not prevent innovation and new thought.

2. To further the good of humankind by organizations such as the AHMA, and to discourage those who would make it a narrow, self-serving, special-interest group.

3. To publish research articles under rigid standards of excellence and verification of theories.

4. To work on health-care-delivery models and to try to find ways for holistic principles to be applied on a day-to-day basis by professionals whose primary orientation is not toward holism.

5. To demand representation on admission committees of medical schools, curriculum committees, and clinical faculties, in addition to establishing separate teaching facilities.

6. To work with medical students, who represent an untapped resource for creating institutional change.

The thoughts summarized above represent a small portion of the wealth of perspectives and approaches offered during the first year's programs of the AHMA. Those involved are highly enthusiastic about their organization, and will not be discouraged when confronted with resistance. My own feeling is that the AHMA is here to stay, to grow, and to prosper; its future success will herald a new age for medicine.

For further information on the AHMA, *write Jean Ann Caywood, Executive Director, AHMA, 6932 Little River Turnpike, Annandale, VA 22003.*

Dean Challes is an editor of the Holistic Health Review. *In addition to his broad interests in the holistic health field, Mr. Challes is a Project and Business Management consultant in a variety of fields.*

Conclusion

This book has been compiled in a spirit of hope and of great urgency. We have attempted to recreate a picture of wholeness out of the fragmented images of contemporary life. Some of the suggestions within these pages arise from ordinary common sense and the wisdom gained from living close to the fabric of life. Others arise as a direct response to the massive devaluation of existence in the technological world; still other material stands as a vision of a world yet to come. All contribute in one way or another to the formation of an integrated life. The diversity of its content is a measure of the highly transitional times in which we live.

We, as a species, are evolving at a tremendous rate. That which prompts our advance along the evolutionary ladder is no longer a changing biological nature, but rather the transformation of our consciousness. Many can already feel the dawning of a new age. Indeed, the violence and alienation that assails us daily may be seen as one last great gasp of the passing era before the new paradigm slips neatly into place. This book is a statement of hope that we will tenaciously move forward. We believe the emergence of holistic health represents the leading edge of this movement.

Although holistic health is not a new invention, it is a new name for that which has always preserved our innate relationship to one another, nature, and the cosmos. The forms adopted to express this understanding differ according to the needs of the time; yet the essential feeling that binds all of life together remains forever the same.

This book is devoted to an unyielding faith in the human spirit and its eternal quest to reflect itself within the great circle of life.

Everything the Power of
the World does is done in a circle. The
sky is round, and I have heard that the earth
is round like a ball, and so are all the stars. The wind,
in its greatest power, whirls. Birds make their nests in
circles, for theirs is the same religion as ours. The sun comes
forth and goes down again in a circle. The moon does the same,
and both are round. Even the seasons form a great circle in their
changing, and always come back again to where they were. The life
of a man is a circle from childhood to childhood, and so it is in everything where power moves. Our tepees were round like the nests of birds,
and these were always set in a circle, the nation's hoop, a nest of many
nests, where the Great Spirit meant for us to hatch our children.
Black Elk,
Black Elk Speaks

From *Black Elk Speaks* by John G. Neihardt, copyright 1932, 1961, published by Simon & Schuster Pocket Books and by the University of Nebraska Press.

From and About the Contributing Editors

We, the four persons who have been the editorial committee for the *Holistic Health Handbook* and this *Holistic Health Lifebook*, would like to emphasize that we have functioned as editors on behalf of the Berkeley Holistic Health Center as a whole. We here also want to acknowledge and thank each other, as well as all the many other persons who have helped make these books possible.

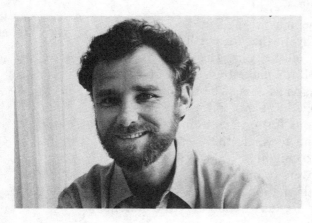

Edward Mann Bauman

Student, teacher, counselor, and advocate of natural healing therapies. In a gradual, integral way, he is learning the inner teaching of holistic health. Awareness and education of self, in all aspects, physical and metaphysical, have been the core of his self-healing experience. This understanding and conviction expresses itself in the way he lives and in the work that he does.

He teaches Health Awareness, Nutrition, and Natural Food Cooking classes, and does private health and nutritional consulting. He is a long-standing member of the Healing Circle, and of the Board of Directors of the Berkeley Holistic Health Center.

He received a B.A. in Political Science from Syracuse University in 1968, and a master's in Education from the University of Massachusetts in 1971. He was born in Washington, D.C. on September 22, 1946.

For their help in this book, he wishes to thank Armand Brint; Julie Fuchs; Kesa Kivel; John McClain; Dr. Bernard Jensen; Dr. Hazel Parcells; Mildred Jackson; Steve Markell; Leslie Strauss; The Lucius Trust; The Healing Circle; Jean Erlbaum; David Guss; Jane and Paul Bauman; his Guides and Masters; his mother, his father, and God—not necessarily in that order.

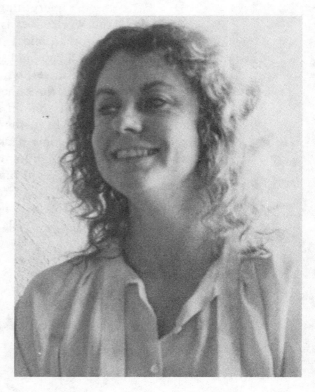

Lorin Piper

Lorin's vision of a holistic life has led her to develop many aspects of herself. These have included being a published author, world traveler, masseuse, flamenco dancer, and metaphysical practitioner and seeker. She is currently living in southern Spain, immersing herself in gypsy flamenco and writing fiction.

For their help during the editing of this book, she extends grateful thanks to Eleanor, Kate, and Ruth Adams; Heig Back; Peter Beren; Henry Miller; Sebastian Orfali; Patricia Parker; Joya and Maya Pope; Augustine Totten, Theresa, Pepito, and Victoria Rios; Barry Taxman; and Layla Viking.

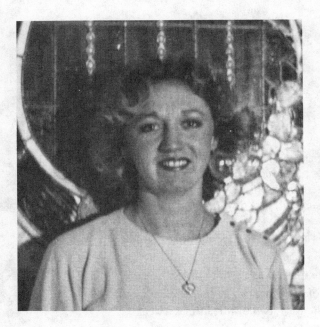

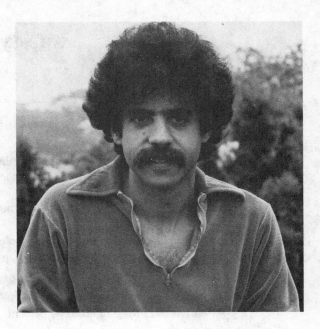

Amelia Sol Wright

Amelia aspires to achieve her full potential as a human being. Work on these books and as a former administrator at the Berkeley Holistic Health Center has been an integral part of this process. She sees her work in the future as being involved with creating and organizing healing environments and communities. As an expression of her long-term interest in all aspects of health, she has lectured and taught introductory classes in holistic health, and is now a minister with the healing Church of the Gentle Brothers and Sisters in San Francisco. In other facets of her life, she enjoys raising her ten-year-old son, belly-dancing, organic gardening, and working with children and the elderly. She describes her work on this book as a rewarding effort which brings together information important to everyone.

For their help and loving inspiration during work on this book, she wishes to offer her thanks and appreciation to Justin Orwat; Wiley H. Reed; Elizabeth Dostal; Christine Wright; Bonnie and Greg Gay; Aerin Land; Baba Silberzweig; Peggy Hughes; her mother and father; Fern and Joseph Orwat; The Gentle Brothers and Sisters; Cecelia Turconi; Billy Wright; Sean and Melanie Wright; the Church of the Star; Marge and Bill Moore, Leslie Strauss; Sebastian Orfali; Alta Kelly; all those who wrote articles for the book that could not be used; Eddie, Lorin and Armand; My Tarot Deck!!!!! and all of my guides. One With The Light.

Armand Ian Brint

Armand has worked for several years toward the establishment of a new direction in health care. In 1975 he founded the Berkeley Holistic Health Center (BHHC) as a permanent home for education in the healing arts. Since its inception, he has acted in numerous capacities with the BHHC cooperative, and currently serves on its Board of Directors. Armand teaches and writes on holistic health and derives much inspiration for his poetry from the integral spirit expressed in holistic health.

For their help on this book, Armand is pleased to thank Harold L. Brint; Elaine Brint; his brothers, Steven and Michael; Melissa, Chuck, and Rachel; Shirl Brint; Seth, Caroline, and Dharma; Susan Koenig; Daniel Leibsohn; Patricia Parker; Mrs. Ida Markus; Linnea; STAR; Dr. Max Wu; Drs. Edward Ogden and Alice Francis; Dr. Edward Bach; The Gentle Brothers and Sisters; and Shandor and Laughingbird.

He extends special thanks to the staff, members and friends of the Berkeley Holistic Health Center: Barbara (Baba) Silberzweig; Dovid Ent; Patrick Woods, Gayna Uransky-Woods, and Rainbow; Bruce Gorman; Robert Picker; Isaiah Mayer; Sunny Prism Robero; Susan Stone; Sally Madden; Michelle Martin; Juanita De Sanz; and Judy Jackl.

Finally, he extends extraordinary thanks to Steven Markell and Dana Ullman for serving as research consultants for this book.

Lifestyle Survey

In conjunction with a fairly standard medical history, the staff at the Berkeley Holistic Health Center uses a Lifestyle Survey similar to the one that appears here, which has been adapted for self-administration. This Survey, while incomplete by itself, may give you some indication of what areas in your life could stand some improvement, and of what your overall trend toward wellness or illness is like.

Mark your response in one of the five columns according to the following key:

1 = **Rarely or never true**: less than three times a year.

2 = **Seldom true**: roughly 1 to 5 percent of the time; once a month or less.

3 = **Sometimes true**: roughly 5 to 30 percent of the time; two to four times a month.

4 = **Often true**: roughly 30 to 60 percent of the time; two or three times a week.

5 = **Usually or always true**: roughly 60 to 99 percent of the time; every day or every other day.

Notice that all the statements in the test have been adjusted so that answers which tend toward poorer health will produce higher numbers. For this reason, be sure you are marking your answers at the correct end of the scale. For example, consider a statement like, "I do not eat wholesome food." If you take care to eat wholesome food, then this statement is *rarely true,* so you need to mark the number 1 as your response.

A numerical key is provided at the end of the survey to give you a rough guide to interpreting your responses in terms of your own health risks.

Please check the column reflecting your general state for the past few months. Keep in mind that we are measuring *frequency.*

I. Relaxation Awareness and Habits

	Rarely (1)	Seldom (2)	Sometimes (3)	Often (4)	Usually (5)
1. I do not feel relaxed.	☐	☐	☐	☐	☐
2. I am "keyed up."	☐	☐	☐	☐	☐
3. I have difficulty relaxing.	☐	☐	☐	☐	☐
4. I am aware of inner stress/tension.	☐	☐	☐	☐	☐
5. I an aware of *painful* tension in my body.	☐	☐	☐	☐	☐
6. I have a "nervous stomach."	☐	☐	☐	☐	☐
7. I bit my nails, have a tic or other nervous habit.	☐	☐	☐	☐	☐
8. I grind my teeth.	☐	☐	☐	☐	☐
9. I sigh frequently.	☐	☐	☐	☐	☐
10. I do not breathe fully (shallow breathing).	☐	☐	☐	☐	☐
11. I have a hard time getting a deep breath.	☐	☐	☐	☐	☐
12. I do not use breathing exercises to relax.	☐	☐	☐	☐	☐
13. I have a feeling of time-urgency (feeling rushed.	☐	☐	☐	☐	☐
14. I feel unjustifiable fatigue.	☐	☐	☐	☐	☐
15. I fill up all my time with work.	☐	☐	☐	☐	☐
16. I am overactive.	☐	☐	☐	☐	☐
17. I am underactive.	☐	☐	☐	☐	☐
18. I sleep too little.	☐	☐	☐	☐	☐
19. I sleep too much.	☐	☐	☐	☐	☐
20. I feel sleepy during the daytime.	☐	☐	☐	☐	☐
21. My sleep during the night is broken or restless.	☐	☐	☐	☐	☐
22. I wake up early and don't fall back to sleep.	☐	☐	☐	☐	☐

Rarely (1) Seldom (2) Sometimes (3) Often (4) Usually (5)

23. I have difficulty falling asleep. ☐ ☐ ☐ ☐ ☐
24. I have trouble coping with the stresses of life. ☐ ☐ ☐ ☐ ☐
25. I prefer to spend time away from where I live. ☐ ☐ ☐ ☐ ☐
26. I have little time for rest and/or meditation. ☐ ☐ ☐ ☐ ☐
27. I don't like to waste time on leisure activities. ☐ ☐ ☐ ☐ ☐
28. It makes my nervous to spend time without planned or structured activities. ☐ ☐ ☐ ☐ ☐
29. I smoke tobacco. ☐ ☐ ☐ ☐ ☐
30. I drink alcohol. ☐ ☐ ☐ ☐ ☐
31. I use tranquilizers. ☐ ☐ ☐ ☐ ☐
32. I use "uppers" and/or diet pills. ☐ ☐ ☐ ☐ ☐
33. I use other drugs not mentioned above. ☐ ☐ ☐ ☐ ☐
34. Drugs interfere with my daily life activities. ☐ ☐ ☐ ☐ ☐
35. I have not personally used:
    (a) autosuggestion (self-hypnosis). ☐ ☐ ☐ ☐ ☐
    (b) progressive relaxation. ☐ ☐ ☐ ☐ ☐
    (c) diaphragmatic breathing. ☐ ☐ ☐ ☐ ☐
    (d) guided visualizations. ☐ ☐ ☐ ☐ ☐
    (e) affirmations. ☐ ☐ ☐ ☐ ☐
    (f) meditation. ☐ ☐ ☐ ☐ ☐

SUBTOTAL __ __ __ __ __

II. Exercise

36. I do not exercise. ☐ ☐ ☐ ☐ ☐
37. Exercise is work to avoid. ☐ ☐ ☐ ☐ ☐
38. My exercise does not include some form of breathing. ☐ ☐ ☐ ☐ ☐
39. I avoid regular vigorous exercise that is good for the circulation. ☐ ☐ ☐ ☐ ☐
40. I participate in creative movement such as dance, sports, etc. ☐ ☐ ☐ ☐ ☐
41. I do not include grounding and centering exercises for energy balance (e.g. Tai Chi, Aikido, Yoga, etc.) ☐ ☐ ☐ ☐ ☐
42. I have not considered the effects of exercise on my posture. ☐ ☐ ☐ ☐ ☐

SUBTOTAL __ __ __ __ __

III. Food, Nutrition, and Mealtime Habits

43. Meals are time out from real life. ☐ ☐ ☐ ☐ ☐
44. I eat very rapidly. ☐ ☐ ☐ ☐ ☐
45. After mealtime I resume activity immediately. ☐ ☐ ☐ ☐ ☐
46. Mealtimes are times of tension, conflicts, disagreements, and distractions (including reading). ☐ ☐ ☐ ☐ ☐
47. I eat on the run. ☐ ☐ ☐ ☐ ☐
48. I sneak or hide foods. ☐ ☐ ☐ ☐ ☐
49. I use food for reward, escape, punishment. ☐ ☐ ☐ ☐ ☐
50. Emotions alter my eating habits (overeat, undereat, etc.). ☐ ☐ ☐ ☐ ☐

Rarely (1) Seldom (2) Sometimes (3) Often (4) Usually (5)

51. I eat solid food when emotionally upset. ☐ ☐ ☐ ☐ ☐
52. I ignore labels on canned or packaged foods. ☐ ☐ ☐ ☐ ☐
53. I eat within an hour of retiring. ☐ ☐ ☐ ☐ ☐
54. I don't think about my diet. ☐ ☐ ☐ ☐ ☐
55. I eat foods I know are bad for me. ☐ ☐ ☐ ☐ ☐
56. My meals do *not* include:
    (a) fresh fruits. ☐ ☐ ☐ ☐ ☐
    (b) fresh vegetables. ☐ ☐ ☐ ☐ ☐
    (c) raw vegetables. ☐ ☐ ☐ ☐ ☐
    (d) high-fiber foods (nuts, seeds, fruits, vegetables, bran, etc.). ☐ ☐ ☐ ☐ ☐
    (e) whole grains and cereals (millet, brown rice, etc.). ☐ ☐ ☐ ☐ ☐
    (f) protein-rich foods. ☐ ☐ ☐ ☐ ☐
    (g) cold-pressed oil. ☐ ☐ ☐ ☐ ☐
    (h) dairy products. ☐ ☐ ☐ ☐ ☐
    (i) fish. ☐ ☐ ☐ ☐ ☐
    (j) poultry. ☐ ☐ ☐ ☐ ☐
    (k) raw foods. ☐ ☐ ☐ ☐ ☐
    (l) vitamins. ☐ ☐ ☐ ☐ ☐
    (m) minerals. ☐ ☐ ☐ ☐ ☐
    (n) food suplements (i.e. yeast, kelp, protein powder). ☐ ☐ ☐ ☐ ☐
    (o) beans and legumes. ☐ ☐ ☐ ☐ ☐
    (p) unsaturated fats and oils (which remain liquid at room temperature). ☐ ☐ ☐ ☐ ☐
57. My meals include:
    (a) red meat. ☐ ☐ ☐ ☐ ☐
    (b) sweets (honey, molasses, sugar, etc.). ☐ ☐ ☐ ☐ ☐
    (c) salt (table salt, sea salt, soy sauce, tamari, etc.). ☐ ☐ ☐ ☐ ☐
    (d) refined foods (processed oil, white sugar, white rice, white flour, etc.). ☐ ☐ ☐ ☐ ☐
    (e) quick-preparation foods. ☐ ☐ ☐ ☐ ☐
    (f) fried foods. ☐ ☐ ☐ ☐ ☐
    (g) saturated fats and oils (which remain hard at room temperature). ☐ ☐ ☐ ☐ ☐
58. My fluid intake includes:
    (a) tap water. ☐ ☐ ☐ ☐ ☐
    (b) non-herbal tea. ☐ ☐ ☐ ☐ ☐
    (c) coffee. ☐ ☐ ☐ ☐ ☐
    (d) soft drinks. ☐ ☐ ☐ ☐ ☐
    (e) alcohol. ☐ ☐ ☐ ☐ ☐
59. My fluid intake does not include:
    (a) spring water. ☐ ☐ ☐ ☐ ☐
    (b) distilled water. ☐ ☐ ☐ ☐ ☐
    (c) vegetable juice. ☐ ☐ ☐ ☐ ☐
    (d) fruit juice. ☐ ☐ ☐ ☐ ☐
    (e) milk. ☐ ☐ ☐ ☐ ☐
    (f) herbal tea. ☐ ☐ ☐ ☐ ☐
60. I fear weight gain. ☐ ☐ ☐ ☐ ☐
61. I have not had a specialized diet or fast in the last year. ☐ ☐ ☐ ☐ ☐

	Rarely (1)	Seldom (2)	Sometimes (3)	Often (4)	Usually (5)
62. I stuff myself.	☐	☐	☐	☐	☐
63. I diet to lose weight.	☐	☐	☐	☐	☐
64. I have eating binges.	☐	☐	☐	☐	☐
65. I have not noticed the relationship of food habits to what constitutes healthy bowel and urin elimination (i.e. consistency, color, frequency, odor, etc.).	☐	☐	☐	☐	☐
66. I experience discomfort from gas.	☐	☐	☐	☐	☐

SUBTOTAL __ __ __ __ __

IV. Mental and Emotional Health

	Rarely (1)	Seldom (2)	Sometimes (3)	Often (4)	Usually (5)
67. My work gives me neither satisfaction nor a feeling of accomplishment.	☐	☐	☐	☐	☐
68. I do not have a sense of contributing and being useful.	☐	☐	☐	☐	☐
69. I do not experience self-expression creativity.	☐	☐	☐	☐	☐
70. I am a "workaholic" (compulsive worker).	☐	☐	☐	☐	☐
71. I work more than 10 hours a day.	☐	☐	☐	☐	☐
72. I work on my days off.	☐	☐	☐	☐	☐
73. I don't waste time on things I consider "fun."	☐	☐	☐	☐	☐
74. I feel anxious, worried.	☐	☐	☐	☐	☐
75. I feel like crying.	☐	☐	☐	☐	☐
76. I have difficulty allowing myself to cry.	☐	☐	☐	☐	☐
77. I have difficulty making decisions.	☐	☐	☐	☐	☐
78. I experience little peace of mind.	☐	☐	☐	☐	☐
79. I feel emotionally insecure.	☐	☐	☐	☐	☐
80. I lack initiative.	☐	☐	☐	☐	☐
81. I feel unenthusiastic and negative about my life.	☐	☐	☐	☐	☐
82. I feel fragmentation in my life.	☐	☐	☐	☐	☐
83. I feel absentminded/loss of memory.	☐	☐	☐	☐	☐
84. I feel lonely.	☐	☐	☐	☐	☐
85. I am extremely introspective.	☐	☐	☐	☐	☐
86. I have feelings of being in the midst of struggle.	☐	☐	☐	☐	☐
87. What I get in my life is beyond my control.	☐	☐	☐	☐	☐
88. I lack confidence.	☐	☐	☐	☐	☐
89. I feel bored.	☐	☐	☐	☐	☐
90. I feel ugly.	☐	☐	☐	☐	☐
91. I hate my body.	☐	☐	☐	☐	☐
92. I do not enjoy myself.	☐	☐	☐	☐	☐
93. I deny my feelings (ange, fear, joy, pleasure).	☐	☐	☐	☐	☐
94. I have feelings of being rushed or a sense of time-urgency.	☐	☐	☐	☐	☐
95. I feel my emotions run me.	☐	☐	☐	☐	☐
96. I am aware of and feel helpless to control waves of anger, hostility, violence.	☐	☐	☐	☐	☐
97. I feel depressed, melancholy, get the "blues."	☐	☐	☐	☐	☐
98. I have difficulty expressing anger and hold grudges.	☐	☐	☐	☐	☐
99. I have a quick temper.	☐	☐	☐	☐	☐

	Rarely (1)	Seldom (2)	Sometimes (3)	Often (4)	Usually (5)
100. I have crisis in my life.	☐	☐	☐	☐	☐
101. I express my feelings in destructive ways.	☐	☐	☐	☐	☐
102. I have trouble letting go, trouble forgetting the past.	☐	☐	☐	☐	☐
103. I have not tried to use my dreams for self-growth.	☐	☐	☐	☐	☐
104. I am irritable, annoyed by little things.	☐	☐	☐	☐	☐
105. I am "hard on myself," hold unrealistically high standards for myself.	☐	☐	☐	☐	☐
106. I consider suicide.	☐	☐	☐	☐	☐
107. I feel asking for help would reveal my weakness.	☐	☐	☐	☐	☐
108. I feel unhappy.	☐	☐	☐	☐	☐
109. I feel that all "spiritual" talk is nonsense.	☐	☐	☐	☐	☐
110. I have a poor image of myself.	☐	☐	☐	☐	☐
111. I have no sense of humor.	☐	☐	☐	☐	☐
112. I feel critcized.	☐	☐	☐	☐	☐
113. I feel threatened by criticism.	☐	☐	☐	☐	☐
114. It is hard for me to:					
(a) cry.	☐	☐	☐	☐	☐
(b) smile.	☐	☐	☐	☐	☐
(c) laugh.	☐	☐	☐	☐	☐
(d) say no without feeling guilty.	☐	☐	☐	☐	☐
(e) accept compliments and recognition.	☐	☐	☐	☐	☐
115. I have an indistinct voice.	☐	☐	☐	☐	☐
116. I sap the energy of others.	☐	☐	☐	☐	☐
117. I feel others say my energy.	☐	☐	☐	☐	☐
118. I feel an imbalance in giving and receiving energy.	☐	☐	☐	☐	☐
119. I am impatient.	☐	☐	☐	☐	☐
120. I am extremely talkative.	☐	☐	☐	☐	☐
121. I am fearful of death.	☐	☐	☐	☐	☐
122. I have no sense of self-direction.	☐	☐	☐	☐	☐
123. I avoid responsibility as much as possible.	☐	☐	☐	☐	☐
124. I am unclear about goals and purpose of my life.	☐	☐	☐	☐	☐
125. I am not interested in lifelong learning.	☐	☐	☐	☐	☐
126. I seek the service of a health-care practitioner (e.g. minister, masseuse, nutritionist, physician, etc.) only when forced to.	☐	☐	☐	☐	☐

SUBTOTAL __ __ __ __ __

V. Social Values and Relationships

	Rarely (1)	Seldom (2)	Sometimes (3)	Often (4)	Usually (5)
127. I do not enjoy being alone.	☐	☐	☐	☐	☐
128. I have no close friends.	☐	☐	☐	☐	☐
129. I do not feel acceptance and support from my family and relations.	☐	☐	☐	☐	☐
130. I do not feel a sense of belonging and nurturing from my community.	☐	☐	☐	☐	☐
131. I feel uncomfortable in large groups (i.e., parties, crowds, etc.).	☐	☐	☐	☐	☐
132. I do not think children are my equals.	☐	☐	☐	☐	☐

	Rarely (1)	Seldom (2)	Sometimes (3)	Often (4)	Usually (5)
133. I do not enjoy relating to children.	☐	☐	☐	☐	☐
134. Touching and being touched (even by children in the family) makes me uncomfortable).	☐	☐	☐	☐	☐
135. I feel uncomfortable being nude with a doctor, body-worker, therapist, masseuse, etc.	☐	☐	☐	☐	☐
136. I feel uncomfortable being nude with other nude people.	☐	☐	☐	☐	☐
137. I find it difficult to initiate a new friendship.	☐	☐	☐	☐	☐
138. I prefer to express sex only with a casual partner.	☐	☐	☐	☐	☐
139. I find it difficult to sustain friendships.	☐	☐	☐	☐	☐
140. I feel that I do not express love well.	☐	☐	☐	☐	☐
141. I do not work well with others.	☐	☐	☐	☐	☐
142. Participating in groups makes me uncomfortable.	☐	☐	☐	☐	☐
143. I cannot go outside the traditional family model to develop family-like relations.	☐	☐	☐	☐	☐

SUBTOTAL __ __ __ __ __

VI. Environmental Health

	Rarely (1)	Seldom (2)	Sometimes (3)	Often (4)	Usually (5)
144. I feel apprehensive alone on the streets or at home at night.	☐	☐	☐	☐	☐
145. It's hard to earn enough to pay for shelter, food and clothing.	☐	☐	☐	☐	☐
146. Excessive noise, pollution, and overcrowded conditions have a negative influence on my health.	☐	☐	☐	☐	☐
147. My job has a negative influence on my health (i.e., boss, poor working conditions, alienating, etc.)	☐	☐	☐	☐	☐
148. I throw away newspapers, cans, bottles, and other things that could be recycled.	☐	☐	☐	☐	☐
149. I feel my personal health has nothing to do with the health of the planet.	☐	☐	☐	☐	☐
150. I feel personally discriminated against because of my race, religion, ethnic origins, age, sex, sexual preferences.	☐	☐	☐	☐	☐
151. I prefer to live somewhere else.	☐	☐	☐	☐	☐
152. I do not get much sunshine and fresh air.	☐	☐	☐	☐	☐

SUBTOTAL __ __ __ __ __

VII. Sexual Health

	Rarely (1)	Seldom (2)	Sometimes (3)	Often (4)	Usually (5)
153. Sexual pleasure is not important to me.	☐	☐	☐	☐	☐
154. I am celibate for reasons beyond my control.	☐	☐	☐	☐	☐
155. I feel uncomfortable expressing my sexual needs and desires.	☐	☐	☐	☐	☐
156. Sex is an inhibited and fearful area of my life.	☐	☐	☐	☐	☐
157. My sex life is heavily influenced by "outside" pressures and anxieties.	☐	☐	☐	☐	☐
158. My sexual activity is not what I really desire.	☐	☐	☐	☐	☐
159. I am not satisfied with the frequency of my sexual activity.	☐	☐	☐	☐	☐
160. I feel sexually uninformed.	☐	☐	☐	☐	☐
161. I feel guilty when I masturbate.	☐	☐	☐	☐	☐
162. I believe the primary goal of sex is orgasm.	☐	☐	☐	☐	☐
163. I do not experience orgasm.	☐	☐	☐	☐	☐
164. I cannot enjoy sex without orgasm.	☐	☐	☐	☐	☐
165. I feel unloved and rejected if I am denied sexually.	☐	☐	☐	☐	☐
166. I am disappointed when my partner and I do not have simultaneous orgasm.	☐	☐	☐	☐	☐
167. I feel used and resentful after a sexual experience.	☐	☐	☐	☐	☐
168. I experience jealousy.	☐	☐	☐	☐	☐
169. I feel emotionally unsatisfied after having sex.	☐	☐	☐	☐	☐
170. I am not satisfied with the quality and quantity of foreplay before intercourse.	☐	☐	☐	☐	☐
171. The following influence my sexual expression:					
(a) roles or stereotypes.	☐	☐	☐	☐	☐
(b) fantasies.	☐	☐	☐	☐	☐
(c) contraception.	☐	☐	☐	☐	☐
(d) religion.	☐	☐	☐	☐	☐
(e) having been raped, forced, or coerced into sexual activity.	☐	☐	☐	☐	☐
(f) having raped, forced, or coerced another into sexual activity.	☐	☐	☐	☐	☐
172. I feel frustrated after sex.	☐	☐	☐	☐	☐
173. I am aware of holding tension in an area of my body that I feel relates to sex.	☐	☐	☐	☐	☐

SUBTOTAL __ __ __ __ __

TOTAL ═══════

A Rough Guide for Interpreting Survey Responses

For a multitude of reasons, such a survey cannot be considered to have any significant diagnostic value. However, it can be an insightful tool for self-analysis, and the numbers here can be useful if understood in this way.

In evaluating your responses, look at each section separately, and at the survey as a whole. The numerical range in which your responses fall could reasonably be interpreted about as follows:

A = Your lifestyle on these issues is probably in fairly good shape; but some significant improvements may still be possible.

B = Your lifestyle in these areas is not especially problematic, but many significant improvements are cleatly possible.

C = Your lifestyle in these areas may be putting your health in some risk; great improvement, and perhaps professional help, should be seriously pursued.

Section		A	B	C
I.	Relaxation	40- 80	100-140	160- 200
II.	Exercise	7- 14	18- 24	28- 35
III.	Food, Nutrition, and Meals	53-106	132-186	212- 265
IV.	Mental and Emotional Health	64-128	160-224	256- 320
V.	Social Values and Relationships	17- 34	43- 59	68- 85
VI.	Environmental Health	9- 18	22- 31	36- 45
VII.	Sexual Health	26- 52	65- 91	104- 130
Total Survey		216-432	540-756	864-1080

Contributing Journals

Bestways, a health and nutrition magazine, with an international readership, is published monthly, at $1.25 per copy, from its editorial offices at Box 2028, 400 Hot Springs Rd., Carson City, NV 89701. The president of *Bestways* is Norman W. Bassett, who founded the magazine in 1973. Its editor and publisher is Barbara Bassett.

The Holistic Health Review is a journal covering the growing holistic health movement. In response to increasing health-care costs, the rise of chronic degenerative disease, and growing awareness of the limits of technological medicine, people are seeking ways to optimize wellness as well as to control disease.

The *Review* documents the search for solutions via study of prevention, environmental and social toxicity, and the developing concepts of self-care and self-responsibility. Articles come from, and are addressed to, all parts of the holistic health movement nationwide: providers, consumers, policy-makers, government, medical societies, students, clinicians and researchers, and they cover public policy development, legality, major conferences, interviews with notable practitioners, and more.

For subscription informaiton write to The Holistic Health Review, P.O. Box 166, Berkeley, CA 94701 or The Holistic Health Review, Human Sciences Press, 72 Fifth Avenue, New York, NY 10011. Articles, letters and other contributions are welcome.

An Integral View: Emerging Currents in Modern Thought. The purpose of this biannual journal is to contribute to the welfare of humanity by presenting writings and artwork which point to the emergence of an integral world view, one which is holistic, nondual, and evolutionary. It explores the unifying wisdom generated throughout the ages within varied cultures, as well as an interdisciplinary convergence of views leading to a true integration of knowledge and experience.

Basic to an integral view are four interwoven dimensions to which the journal relates: Individual Transformation, Societal Transformation, Cultural Integration, and Human Unity. Individual transformation implies the harmonious development of all aspects of our being. Through this process we become motivated to serve and work with others for the welfare of the human community. Therefore, societal transformation implies facilitating creative, qualitative developments in values and approaches to action throughout the different domains of our collective structure. As we continue to expand our boundaries of interrelationship, cultures are brought together to experience cross-fertilization and a vital sense of integration. Finally, through an awareness of the unity-in-diversity within the human family, our world may become a fully harmonized whole: physically, economically, politically, socially, and spiritually, ingredients necessary for the goal and practical application of human unity.

The journal is sponsored by the California Institute of Asian Studies under the editorship of Dionne Marx. Subscriptions are $7 a year or $12 for two years. Write to *An Integral View,* 3494 - 21st St., San Francisco, CA 94110.

It's About Time. The Abalone Alliance is a decentralized coalition of more than 60 antinuclear groups across the state of California. They publish a newsletter called *It's About Time.* They also give workshops covering such diverse issues as skill-sharing, public speaking, media, organizing, fund-raising, issues analysis, labor outreach, and ecumenical outreach, as well as workshops in nonviolent demonstrations. For information about the Abalone Alliance and any of their workshops and services, write to The Abalone Alliance, 944 Market St., Room 307, San Francisco, CA 94102; phone (415) 543-3910.

For a year's subscription to *It's About Time* (10 issues), send $5.00 to the above address; sponsoring membership in the Abalone Alliance is $25.00.

The Journal of Holistic Health is an annual publication chronicling the evolution of the holistic health movement. The text of the *Journal* is compiled from speeches presented at the Mandala Society's summer

405

conferences, plus additional papers from the fore-front of research and practise. *The Journal of Holistic Health* has six volumes in print, with a seventh to be published in 1981. The price of the *Journal* is $10.00 per issue; a complete set of all seven issues can be ordered at a discount. For a detailed brochure, write to Mandala, Box 1233, Del Mar, CA 92014.

New Age magazine is a monthly forum for emerging ideas and holistic approaches to living which focus on health, ecology, antinuclear action, learning, appropriate technology, simple living, body/mind work, birth, death and relationships. Columnist Peter Barry Chowka keeps up-to-date with the frontiers of health care and medical freedom of choice. Brian Van der Horst keeps an eye on the California consciousness scene. Other regular columns cover music, film, books, upcoming events, ecological products, self-healing, spirituality/consciousness, and more. Subscriptions are $12 a year; $1.50 a copy on the newsstand. Contact *New Age* magazine, 32 Station St., Brookline, MA 02146, (617) 734-3155.

Vegetarian Times is an informative magazine with an emphasis on nutrition and healthy diets. Its articles contain information on how to get the highest nutritional value from foods as well as many tasty recipes. It is an excellent source of information for those interested in alternatives to meat in their diets. Mailing address: Vegetarian Times, 41 East 42nd Street, Suite 921, New York, NY 10017. Subscription rates for one year (12 issues) are $19.95; for two years (24 issues) are $36.00; for three years (36 issues) are $50.00.

We would also like to thank *Well-Being* magazine, which is now a part of the *Vegetarian Times*.

Yoga Journal. This bimonthly magazine concerns itself with transforming consciousness through Hatha Yoga and related spiritual practices. The *Yoga Journal* promotes yoga for health, stressing physical and emotional benefits and therapeutic uses. With objective reporting, personal experience stories, interviews with teachers from diverse backgrounds, instructional articles, graphics, photography, and occasional poetry, the magazine synthesizes Eastern and Western approaches to the healing arts and holistic living. Writers include scholars, psychologists, doctors, nutritionists, physical therapists, yoga teachers, and students, who practice yoga personally and professionally. By publishing material of both scientific and philosophical interest, the magazine attempts to bridge the schism between body and mind that is manifested in the stress, disease, and aggression prevalent during our times. The *Yoga Journal* is published by the nonprofit, nonsectarian California Yoga Teachers Association, under the editorship of Deena Brown, and is available by subscription and at newsstands, natural food stores, and bookstores throughout the U.S. and Canada. For information about all facets of the Yoga Journal, write: 2054 University Avenue, Berkeley, CA 94704.

And we would also like to thank the magazines *New Directions* and *Alternatives*. These magazines offered articles about alternative health and healing practices, diet, nutrition, and spiritual awareness. Both magazines are no longer in circulation.

National Directory of Holistic Health Centers

Compiled by Steven Markell and Wendy Worsley
(with Bebe Bertolét and Sayre Van Young)
Sponsored by:
Holistic Health Organizing Committee
P.O. Box 166
Berkeley, CA 94701

The inclusion of any center is not to be considered endorsement of the services offered by the group listed. We intend to provide access to these groups only. Please be very careful in your consideration and thorough in your investigation before engaging any services or payment of fees. There are no standards of practice for these facilities . . . yet.

Additional copies of this Directory may be obtained at the above address. Please remit $5.00 and a self-addressed stamped envelope.

National directories of *Schools: Healing and Alternative* and of holistic health-related organizations are also available. Please remit $5.00 and a self-addressed stamped envelope for each directory to the above address.

ARIZONA

- **The A.R.E. Clinic, Inc.**
  4018 North 40th St
  Phoenix, AZ 85018
  (602) 955-0551

- **Healing Waters**
  Indian Hot Springs
  P.O. Box 847
  Eden, AZ 85535
  (602) 485-2008

- **International Holistic Center, Inc.**
  P.O. Box 15103
  Phoenix, AZ 85060
  (602) 957-2181

- **Lukats Prevention & Regeneration Resort**
  Route 1, Box 955
  Safford, AZ 85546
  (602) 428-2881

- **Southwestern Center of Light and Truth**
  P.O. Box 3695
  Tucson, AZ 85722
  (602) 293-3712

CALIFORNIA

- **Actualism Wholistic Health Center**
  739 E. Pennsylvania, Suite D
  Escondido, CA 92026
  (714) 741-7827

- **Alternative Medicine Foundation**
  (Office)
  4145 Via Marina Way, #320
  Marina Del Ray, CA 90291
  (213) 823-6355

- **Alternative Medicine Foundation**
  (Clinic)
  801 Seventh St
  Santa Rosa, CA 95404
  (707) 527-9134

- **Alternative Therapies Unit**
  San Francisco General Hospital Medical Center
  2550 - 23rd St (Bldg 9) Room 130
  San Francisco, CA 94110
  (415) 821-5139

- **Androgyny Center**
  P.O. Box 7429
  San Diego, CA 92107
  (714) 297-4733

- **Astara**
  800 West Arrow Highway
  Upland, CA 91786
  (714) 981-4941

- **Berkeley Holistic Health Center**
  3099 Telegraph Ave
  Berkeley, CA 94705
  (415) 845-4430

- **Berkeley Massage Studio**
  1962 University Ave
  Berkeley, CA 94704
  (415) 845-5998

- **Berkeley Women's Center**
  2955 Telegraph Ave
  Berkeley, CA 94705
  (415) 548-4343

- **Biofeedback and Family Therapy**
  2236 Derby St
  Berkeley, CA 94705
  (415) 841-7227

- **Biofeedback & Psychosomatic Medicine Center**
  400 - 34 th St
  Oakland, CA 94609
  (415) 536-1440

- **Body and Mind Clinic**
  165 O'Farrell, No. 610
  San Francisco, CA 94108
  (415) 956-7527
  (415) 956-7546

- **Buena Vista Women's Services**
  2000 Van Ness Ave
  San Francisco, CA 94109
  (415) 771-5000

- **California School of Herbal Studies**
  Box 350
  Guerneville, CA 95446
  (707) 887-9932

- **The Center for Attitudinal Healing**
  19 E. Main St
  Tiburon, CA 94920
  (415) 435-4130

- **Center for Chinese Medicine**
  230 South Garfield Ave
  Monterey Park, CA 91754
  (213) 573-4141
  (213) 572-0424

- **Center for Counseling & Psychotherapy**
  3017 Santa Monica Blvd
  Santa Monica, CA 90404
  (213) 829-7407

- **The Center for Existential Counseling & Therapies**
  166 Lombard St
  San Francisco, CA 94118
  (415) 928-3022 (San Francisco)
  (415) 932-4682 (Walnut Creek)
  (415) 525-3375 (Berkeley)

- **Center for Family Growth**
  555 Highland Ave
  Penngrove, CA 94951
  (707) 795-5155

- **The Center for Healing Arts**
  2312 Woolsey St
  Berkeley, CA 94705

- **Center for the Healing Arts**
  11081 Missouri Ave
  Los Angeles, CA 90025
  (213) 477-3981

- **Center for Health and Healing**
  Cedars-Sinai Medical Office Towers
  8631 West Third St, #1140E
  Los Angeles, CA 90048
  (213) 652-2101

- **Center for Integral Medicine**
  1515 Palisades Dr
  Pacific Palisades, CA 90272
  (213) 459-3373

- **Center for Metabolic Research**
  Pacific Institute for Advanced Studies
  1312 North Stanley Ave
  Los Angeles, CA 90046
  (213) 876-0474

- **Center for Release & Integration**
  1057 Steiner St
  San Francisco, CA 94115
  (415) 929-0119

- **Cooperation Corporation**
  P.O. Box 5039
  Berkeley, CA 94705

- **Cooperative Healing Center**
  1201 Parducci Rd
  Ukiah, CA 95482
  (707) 462-9473

- **Cotati Holistic Health Center**
  65 W. Cotati Ave
  Cotati, CA 94928
  (707) 795-8584

- **Creating Our Life**
  P.O. Box 374
  Venice, CA 90291
  (213) 397-9692
  (213) 823-6393

- **Dovetail Institute**
  160 Bret Harte Rd
  San Rafael, CA 94901
  (415) 461-9521

- **Dynamic Nutrition Analysis**
  3340 Kemper St, #205
  San Diego, CA 92110
  (714) 225-1489

- **East West Academy of Healing Arts**
  P.O. Box 31211
  San Francisco, CA 94131
  (415) 285-9400

- **East West Health Center**
  61 Camino Alto, #103
  Mill Valley, CA 94941
  (415) 388-0646
  (415) 383-1585

- **The Habitat Center**
  P.O. Box 2363
  Berkeley, CA 94702
  (415) 526-0869

- **Health Enhancement Center**
  930 Mission St, #3
  Santa Cruz, CA 95060
  (408) 429-8161

- **Health Evaluations, Inc.**
  P.O. Box 187
  Hayward, CA 94543
  (415) 582-0286

- **Health Integration Center**
  1625 Olympic Blvd
  Santa Monica, CA 90404
  (213) 450-9998

- **Health Sharing, Inc.**
  317 Spruce St, Sect. E
  Santa Cruz, CA 95060
  (408) 425-1828

- **Health Training Center**
  420 Walnut St
  San Diego, CA 92103
  (714) 296-2178

- **High Point Foundation**
  5337 N. Millbrook
  Fresno, CA 93710
  (209) 222-5695

- **Hippocrates**
  Health Institute of San Diego
  2176 Valley View Blvd
  El Cajon, CA 92021
  (714) 444-9900
  (714) 440-9413

- **Holistic Healing Arts Clinic**
  312 South Cedros
  Solano Beach, CA 92075
  (714) 755-6681

- **Holistic Family Service Health Clinic**
  Encino Medical Towers
  16260 Ventura Blvd, #630
  Encino, CA 91436
  (213) 990-1190

- **Holistic Medical Group Inc.**
  3031 Tisch Way, Drawer 106
  San Jose, CA 95128
  (408) 249-1991

- **The Holmes Center**
  3251 West Sixth St
  P.O. Box 75127
  Los Angeles, CA 90075
  (213) 380-6176

- **Humboldt Open Door Clinic**
  P.O. Box 367, 10th and "H" Sts
  Arcata, CA 95521
  (707) 822-2957

- **Hypnosis Clearing House, Inc.**
  370 Fifteenth St
  Oakland, CA 94612
  (415) 451-6440

- **The Institute of Colonic Hygiene**
  803 Fourth St, Suite 8
  San Rafael, CA 94901
  (415) 453-4852

- **Institute for Creative Aging**
  P.O. Box 142
  Malibu, CA 90265
  (213) 456-6297
  (213) 456-8907

- **Integral Health Center**
  905 Sir Francis Drake Blvd
  Kentfield, CA 94904
  (415) 454-9690

- **Julian Preventive Medical Clinic**
  1654 Cahuenga at Hollywood Blvd
  Hollywood, CA 90028
  (213) 466-0126
  (213) 467-5555

- **Kairos**
  P.O. Box 111
  Encinitas, CA 92024
  (714) 753-9018

- **King Harbor Wellness Institute**
  P.O. Box 524
  Redondo Beach, CA 90277

- **Learning for Health**
  1314 Westwood Blvd, #107
  Los Angeles, CA 90024
  (213) 474-6929
  (213) 475-2990

- **Meadowlark**
  c/o Friendly Hills Fellowship
  26126 Fairview Ave
  Hemet, CA 92343
  (714) 927-1343

- **Mid-Peninsula Health Service**
  704 Webster
  Palo Alto, CA 94301
  (415) 324-1940

- **Min An Health Center**
  1144 Pacific Ave
  San Francisco, CA 94133
  (415) 771-4040

- **Natural Environmental Health Center**
  Hwy 9 — Adjacent to Brookdale Lodge
  P.O. Box 11
  Brookdale, CA 95007
  (408) 338-2363

- **The New Age School of Massage**
  P.O. Box 958
  Sebastopol, CA 95472
  (707) 823-1212

- **New Ways of Consciousness**
  3118 Washington St
  San Francisco, CA 94115
  (415) 346-5671

- **Northern Pines**
  October—April
  21050 Waveview Dr
  Topanga, CA 90290
  (213) 455-1222

- **Nurse Consultants & Health Counselors**
  Healing Center of San Francisco
  465 Brussels
  San Francisco, CA 94134
  (415) 468-4680

- **Nyingma Institute**
  1815 Highland Pl
  Berkeley, CA 94709
  (415) 843-6812

- **Orthomolecular Research Institute**
  P.O. Box 1484
  Santa Cruz, CA 95061
  (408) 425-7787

- **Pilgrams Way**
  945 N. Sutter St
  Stockton, CA 95202
  (209) 466-0388

- **Price-Pottenger Nutrition Foundation, Inc.**
  P.O. Box 2614
  La Mesa, CA 92041
  (714) 582-4168

- **Psychosomatic Medicine Clinic**
  2510 Webster St
  Berkeley, CA 94705
  (415) 548-1115

- **Riverwinds Holistic Health Center**
  1545 Franklin near Pine
  San Francisco, CA 94109
  (415) 673-3462

- **Rockridge Health Care Plan**
  430 - 40th St
  Oakland, CA 94609
  (415) 658-8517

- **Round Valley Indian Health Center**
  P.O. Box 247
  Covelo, CA 95428
  (707) 983-2981

- **Sacramento Holistic Health Institute**
  1822 - 21st St
  Sacramento, CA 95814
  (916) 454-4470 (10am - 3pm)

- **San Andreas Health Council**
  531 Cowper St
  Palo Alto, CA 94301
  (415) 324-9350

- **Sandweiss Biofeedback Institute, Inc.**
  5406 Village Road
  Long Beach, CA 90808
  (213) 851-2720

- **San Francisco Women's Health Center**
  3789 Twenty-fourth St
  San Francisco, CA 94114
  (415) 282-6999

- **The Self Center**
  555 - 2nd Ave (at Balboa)
  San Francisco, CA 94118
  (415) 386-7027

- **Self-Realization Fellowship**
  3880 San Rafael Ave
  Los Angeles, CA 90065
  (213) 225-2471

- **Sequoia Institute EDJ**
  Nurse Consultants and Health Counselors
  1820 Union St at Octavia
  San Francisco, CA 94123
  (415) 346-1526

- **Shanti Nilaya**
  P.O. Box 2396
  Escondido, CA 92025
  (714) 749-2008

- **Sonoma County Women's Health Collective**
  P.O. Box 907
  Cotati, CA 94928

- **S. S. Vallejo**
  Gate Five Rd
  Sausalito, CA 94965
  (415) 924-0406

- **St. George Homes Inc.**
  1515 Arch St
  Berkeley, CA 94708
  (415) 848-2393

- **Sufi Islamia Ruhaniat Society**
  410 Precita Ave
  San Francisco, CA 94110
  (415) 285-5208

- **S.Y.D.A. Foundation**
  1107 Stanford
  Oakland, CA 94608
  (415) 655-8677

- **Theta Seminars**
  301 Lyon Street
  San Francisco, CA 94117
  (415) 929-1743

- **University of the Trees**
  P.O. Box 644R
  Boulder Creek, CA 95006
  (408) 338-3855

- **The Village Oz**
  P.O. Box 147
  Point Arena, CA 95468
  (707) 882-2449

- **Vista Center**
  2651 E. Chapman
  Fullerton, CA 92631
  (714) 524-8679
  (714) 996-1800 (ans. service)

- **Well Being Community Center**
  788 Ferguson Rd
  Sebastopol, CA 95472
  (707) 823-1489

- **Wholistic Medicine & Counseling Center**
  1703 Wilshire Blvd
  Santa Monica, CA 90403
  (213) 451-9997

- **Wholistic Health & Nutrition Institute**
  150 Shoreline Hwy
  Mill Valley, CA 94941
  (415) 332-2933

- **The Whole Life Center**
  3437 Alma St, #28
  Palo Alto, CA 94306
  (415) 493-0561

- **William A. Jones & Associates**
  35 Quail Court, Suite 200
  Walnut Creek, CA 94596
  (415) 932-8018

- **Willow**
  6517 Dry Creek Rd
  Napa, CA 94558
  (707) 944-8173

- **Women's Community Clinic**
  696 East Santa Clara St
  San Jose, CA 95112
  (408) 287-4322

- **World University in Ojai Health Program**
  P.O. Box 5096
  Ojai, CA 93023
  (805) 646-1444 (office)
  (805) 646-5222 (res.)

- **Yoga Society of San Francisco**
  2872 Folsom St
  San Francisco, CA 94110
  (415) 285-5537

- **Youth Projects Inc.**
  1696 Haight St
  San Francisco, CA 94117
  (415) 864-6090

COLORADO

- **Colorado Health Center, Inc.**
  1640 Welton
  Denver, CO 80202
  (303) 623-3166

- **Denver Pain & Health Rehabilitation Center**
  3005 E. 16th Ave
  Denver, CO 80201
  (303) 377-9619

- **Whole Life Learning Center**
  1912 W. Colorado Ave
  Colorado Springs, CO 80904
  (303) 475-7322

- **Whole Life Learning Center**
  4601 E. Kentucky, #1A
  Denver, CO 80222
  (303) 758-1314

FLORIDA

- **International New-Life Center**
  P.O. Box 7006
  Miami, FL 33155
  (305) 541-4546

- **Shangri-la Natural Hygiene Institute**
  Bonita Springs, FL 33923
  (813) 992-3811

GEORGIA

- **Chrysalis at Kingswood**
  P.O. Box 725
  Clayton, GA 30525
  (404) 782-4278

ILLINOIS

- **Society for Wholistic Medicine**
  Wholistic Health Centers, Inc.
  137 S. Garfield St
  Hinsdale, IL 60521
  (312) 323-1920

IOWA

- **The Clearing**
  1107 Clark Court
  Iowa City, IA 52240
  (319) 337-5405

KANSAS

- **Cross-Cultural Studies Program**
  P.O. Box 4234
  Topeka, KS 66604
  (913) 233-0532

LOUISIANA

- **Longevity Therapy**
  1765 Coliseum Place, #315
  New Orleans, LA 70130
  (504) 568-1201

MAINE

- **Northern Pines**
  Rt. 85, Box 279
  Raymond, ME 04071
  (207) 655-7624

MARYLAND

- **Koinonia**
  1400 Greenspring Valley Rd
  Stevenson, MD 21153
  (301) 486-6262

MASSACHUSSETS

- **Accupuncture Center of Cambridge**
  380 Green Street
  Cambridge, MA 02139
  (617) 864-4600

- **Beacon Hill Health Associates**
  14 Beacon St., Suite 620
  Boston, MA 02108
  (617) 523-8017

- **Biofeedback Institute of Boston**
  110 Francis St, Suite 7E
  Boston, MA 02215
  (617) 734-7181

- **The Center of The Light**
  P.O. Box 540
  Great Barrington, MA 01230

- **East-West Medical**
  51 Brattle St, Suite 1A
  Cambridge, MA 02138
  (617) 661-0700

- **Heartspring Health Center**
  52 Hampstead Rd
  Jamaica Plain, MA 02130
  (617) 738-4366

- **Interface, Inc.**
  63 Chapel St
  Newton, MA 02158
  (617) 964-7140

- **New England Health Foundations**
  2 Nutting Rd
  Cambridge, MA 02138
  (617) 661-6225

MINNESOTA

- **The Center for Health Promotion**
  601 Brookdale Towers
  2810 - 57th Ave North
  Minneapolis, MN 55430
  (612) 574-7800

MISSOURI

- **Natural Health Institute**
  7624 S. Broadway
  St. Louis, MO 63111
  (314) 631-4514
  (314) 631-4839

NEW MEXICO

- **Healing Arts of Santa Fe**
  P.O. Box 1445
  Santa Fe, NM 87501
  (505) 988-4122

NEW YORK

- **Health Associates**
  13 E. 71st, #2A
  New York City, NY 10021
  (212) 298-1295

- **Institute of Behavioral Kinesiology**
  P.O. Drawer 37
  Valley Cottage, NY 10989

- **Institute for Self Development**
  Wholistic Health Center
  50 Maple Place
  Manhasset, NY 11030
  (516) 627-0309

- **Omega Institute for Holistic Studies**
  Box 396
  New Lebanon, NY 12125
  (518) 794-8850

- **Rochester Center for the Healing Arts, Inc.**
  Human Dimensions Center for Health Awareness
  8 Prince St
  Rochester, NY 14607
  (716) 271-4515

- **Wholistic Health Education Center**
  715 Monroe Ave
  Rochester, NY 14607
  (716) 442-5480

NORTH CAROLINA

- **Ruth Carter Stapleton (Behold)**
  P.O. Box 53757
  Fayetteville, NC 28305

OREGON

- **Academy of Predictive Cell Health Research**
  8 State St, Lakeside Plaza
  Lake Oswego, OR 97034
  (503) 636-8167

- **Aletheia Foundation**
  515 N.E. 8th
  Grants Pass, OR 87526
  (503) 479-4855

- **Atlantis Rising Educational Center**
  7909/7915 S.E. Stark St
  Portland, OR 97215
  (503) 253-4031

- **Eugene Center for the Healing Arts**
  82644 N. Howe Lane
  Creswell, OR 97426
  (503) 895-4967

- **The Institute of Preventive Medicine**
  6171 S.W. Capitol Hwy
  Portland, OR 97201
  (503) 246-7616

- **Mahonia Holistic Health Community**
  219 N.W. E St
  Grants Pass, OR 97526

- **National College of Naturopathic Medicine**
  510 S.W. Third Ave
  Portland, OR 97204
  (503) 226-3717

- **White Bird Sociomedical Aid Station**
  341 E. 12th
  Eugene, OR 97401
  (503) 342-8255

PENNSYLVANNIA

- **Himalaya International Institute**
  P.O. Box 88
  Honesdale, PA 18431

- **Kripalu Center for Holistic Health**
  Box 120
  Summit Station, PA 17979
  (717) 754-3051

VIRGINIA

- **Association for Research & Enlightenment Inc.**
  P.O. Box 595
  Virginia Beach, VA 23451

WASHINGTON

- **Polarity Health Institute**
  Box 68
  Olga, WA 98279
  (206) 376-2291
  (206) 376-4755

WISCONSIN

- **Pain & Health Rehabilitation Center**
  Route 2, Welsh Coulee
  La Crosse, WI 54601
  (608) 786-0611

INTERNATIONAL

- **Centro Medico del Mar**
  Paseo de Tijuana 1-A
  Apdo. Postal 179
  Playas de Tijuana, B.C. Mexico
  Mailing Address: P.O. Box 3793
                          San Ysidro, CA 92073
  (908) 38-7-18-50 to 55

- **Leamington Spa**
  10A Beauchamp Ave
  Warwickshire, England

- **Renaissance Revitilazation Spa**
  Cable Beach, P.O. Box N4854
  Nassau, Bahamas
  (809) 32-78441-2
  Cable Address: RENASSAU

- **Rio Caliente, C.A.**
  Apdo Postal 1-1187
  Guadalajara, Jalisco
  Mexico

- **Sivananda Ashram Yoga Camp**
  8th Ave
  Val Morin P.Q.
  Canada J0T 2R0

Bibliography

Achterberg, Jeanne, and Lawlis, G. Frank. *Bridges of the Bodymind: Behavioral Approaches to Health Care*. Champaign, Ill.: Institute for Personality and Ability Testing, 1980.

_____. *Imagery of Cancer: An Evaluation Tool for the Process of Disease*. Champaign, Ill.: Institute for Personality and Ability Testing, 1978.

Adams, Robert. *The Rise of Urban Civilization*. Chicago: Aldine, 1977.

The Advocate. 1730 S. Amphlett Blvd., San Mateo, CA 94402.

Agel, Jerome. *The Radical Therapist*. New York: Ballantine, 1972.

_____. *Rough Times*. New York: Ballantine, 1973.

Airola, Paavo. *Cancer: Causes, Prevention, and Treatment—The Total Approach*. Phoenix: Health Plus Publishers, 1972.

_____. *Everywoman's Book*. Phoenix: Health Plus Publishers, 1979.

_____. *Hypoglycemia: A Better Approach*. Phoenix: Health Plus Publishers, 1977.

_____. *The Miracle of Garlic*. Phoenix: Health Plus Publishers, 1978.

_____. *Stop Hair Loss*. Phoenix: Health Plus Publishers, 1965.

_____. *Swedish Beauty Secrets*. Phoenix: Health Plus Publishers, 1972.

Alberta, R. E., and Emmons, M. L. *Your Perfect Right: A Guide to Assertive Behavior*. San Luis Obispo, Calif.: Impact, 1979.

Albright, Peter, and Albright, Bets Parker, eds. *Body, Mind, and Spirit*. Brattleboro, Vt.: Stephen Greene Press, 1980.

Altman, Dennis. *Homosexual; Oppression and Liberation*. New York: Outerbridge and Dienstfrey, 1971.

Andersen, Dick. *Holistic Medicine Bibliography*. Berkeley: University of California Extension Media Center, n.d.

Anderson, Bob. *Stretching*. New York: Random House, 1980.

Antonovsky, A. *Health, Stress, and Coping*. San Francisco: Jossey-Bass, 1979.

Applewood Journal. Box 1781, San Francisco, CA 94101.

Arguelles, Jose, and Arguelles, Miriam. *The Feminine: Spacious as the Sky*. Boulder, Colo.: Shambhala, 1977.

_____. *Mandala*. Berkeley, Calif.: Shambhala, 1972.

Auerbach, S., ed. *Child Care: A Comprehensive Guide Series*. 4 vols. New York: Human Sciences Press, 1979.

_____. *Confronting the Child Care Crisis*. Boston: Beacon, 1979.

Austin, Mary. *Acupuncture Therapy*. London: Turnstone Books, 1972.

Bach, George, and Goldberg, Herb. *Creative Aggression*. New York: Avon, 1974.

Bach, George, and Wyden, Peter. *The Intimate Enemy: How to Fight Fair in Love and Marriage*. New York: Avon, 1970.

Baerlein, E., and Dower, A. L. G. *Healing With Radionics*. Northamptonshire, England: Thorsons, 1980.

Baker, Elizabeth, and Baker, Elton. *The Uncook Book: Raw Food Adventures to a New Health High*. Portland, Ore.: Drelwood Publications, 1981.

Ballentine, Rudolph. *Diet and Nutrition*. Honesdale, Pa.: Himalayan International Institute, 1978.

Barbach, Lonnie Garfield. *For Yourself: The Fullfillment of Female Sexuality*. New York: Doubleday, 1975.

Bateson, Gregory. *Mind and Nature*. New York: Dutton, 1979.

Bauer, Cathy, and Andersen, Juel. *The Tofu Cookbook*. Emmaus, Pa.: Rodale Press, 1979.

Baulch, Evelyn. *Home Care*. Millbrae, Calif.: Celestial Arts, 1980.

Beauvoir, Simone de. *The Coming of Age*. New York: Warner, 1973.

Benevolo, Leonardo. *The Origins of Modern Town Planning*. London: Routledge and Kegan Paul, 1967.

Bennett, S. J., and Parker, R. A. *Health Source—1979*. Cambridge: Bennett and Parker, 1979.

Berezin, N. *The Gentle Birth Book*. New York: Simon and Schuster, 1980.

Berg, Peter, ed. *Reinhabiting a Separate Country: A Bioregional Anthology of Northern California.* San Francisco: Planet Drum Books, 1978.

Berk, W. *Chinese Healing Arts.* Culver City, Calif.: Peace Press, 1979.

Bernstein, Anne. *Flight of the Stork.* New York: Dell, 1980.

Berzon, Betty. *Positively Gay.* Millbrae, Calif.: Celestial Arts, 1979.

Bestways. Box 2028, 400 Hot Springs Rd., Carson City, NV 89701.

Bethards, Betty. *Sex and Psychic Energy.* Inner Light Foundation, 1977.

Bicycling Magazine Editors. *Get Fit with Bicycling.* Emmaus, Pa.: Rodale, 1979.

Biermann, J., and Toohey, B. *The Woman's Holistic Headache Relief Book.* Los Angeles: J. P. Tarcher, 1979.

Black Elk. *Black Elk Speaks.* Lincoln: University of Nebraska Press, 1979.

Borelli, Marianne, and Heidt, Patricia. *Therapeutic Touch.* New York: Springer, 1981.

Bolles, Richard N. *What Color Is Your Parachute?* Berkeley, Calif.: Ten Speed Press, 1972.

Brain/Mind Bulletin. Box 42211, Los Angeles, CA 90042.

Braverman, Jordan. *Crisis in Health Care.* Washington, D.C.: Acropolis Books, 1980.

Brenner, Summer. *Everyone Came Dressed as Water.* Berkeley, Calif.: Small Press Distribution, 1973.

———. *From the Heart to the Center.* Berkeley, Calif.: Small Press Distribution, 1977.

———. *The Soft Room.* Berkeley, Calif.: Small Press Distribution, 1978.

Bresler, D. E., and Trubo, R. *Free Yourself from Chronic Pain.* New York: Simon and Schuster, 1979.

Breslow, L., ed. *How to Get the Best Health Care for Your Money.* Emmaus, Pa.: Rodale, 1979.

Brown, E. R. *Rockefeller Medicine Men: Medicine and Capitalism in America.* Berkeley: University of California Press, 1979.

Brown, Rita Mae. *Rubyfruit Jungle.* Plainfield, Vt.: Daughters, 1973.

Bruner, J. *Knowing: Essays for Left Hand.* Cambridge: Harvard University Press, 1965.

Bryan, John. *Small World Vegetable Gardening.* San Francisco: 101 Productions, 1977.

Bubba Free John. *Conscious Exercise and the Transcendental Sun.* Middletown, Calif.: Dawn Horse Press, 1979.

———. *The Eating Gorilla Comes in Peace.* Clearlake Highlands, Calif.: Dawn Horse Press, 1979.

Bucke, Richard. *Cosmic Consciousness.* Rev. ed. New York: Dutton, 1969.

Butler, Robert. *Why Survive? Being Old in America.* New York: Harper and Row, 1975.

Buzan, Tony. *Use Both Sides of Your Brain.* New York: Dutton, 1976.

Caldicott, Helen. *Nuclear Madness: What You Can Do.* Brookline, Mass.: Autumn Press, 1978.

California Institute for Rural Studies. *Research for Action.* Davis: California Institute for Rural Studies, n.d.

California. Office of Health Planning and Development. *California State Health Plan, 1980-1985.* Sacramento: Statewide Office of Health Planning and Development, 1979.

Callen, Anthea. *Women Artists of the Arts and Crafts Movement.* New York: Pantheon Books, 1979.

Campbell, J. *The Portable Jung.* Baltimore: Penguin, 1977.

Canfield, Jack. *A Guide to Resources in Humanistic and Transpersonal Education.* Saratoga Springs, N.Y.: National Humanistic Education Center, n.d.

———. *The Inner Classroom: Teaching with Guided Fantasy.* Englewood Cliffs, N.J.: Prentice-Hall, 1981.

———. *Teaching Students to Love Themselves.* Englewood Cliffs, N.J.: Prentice-Hall, 1981.

Canfield, Jack, and Wells, Harold. *One Hundred Ways to Enhance Self-Concept in the Classroom.* Englewood Cliffs, N.J.: Prentice-Hall, 1976.

Cannon, Minuha. *Sweets Without Guilt: The Fructose Dessert Cookbook.* Charlotte, N.C.: East Woods Press, 1980.

Carter-Scott, Cherie. *The New Species.* San Francisco: Motivation Management Service, Inc., 1978.

Christensen, A., and Rankin, D. *Easy Does It Yoga for Older People.* San Francisco: Harper and Row, 1979.

Chu, M. *A Gentle Approach to Constipation.* Santa Clara, Calif.: M. Chu, 1977.

Citizen's Energy Project. *Self Help Resources.* Washington, D.C.: Citizen's Energy Project, 1980.

Clark, Charlotte B. *Edible and Useful Plants of California.* Berkeley: University of California Press, 1977.

Clark, Don. *Living Gay.* Millbrae, Calif.: Celestial Arts, 1979.

———. *Loving Someone Gay.* Millbrae, Calif.: Celestial Arts, 1976.

Clinebell, Howard. *Contemporary Growth Therapies: Resources for Actualizing Human Wholeness.* Nashville: Abingdon, 1981.

Co-Evolution Quarterly. Box 428, Sausalito, CA 94965.

Cole, John N. Amaranth, From the Past—For the Future. Emmaus, Pa.: Rodale Press, 1979.

Comar, C.L., and Bronner, Felix, eds. Mineral Metabolism. 5 vols. New York: Academic Press, 1960-69.

Comfort, Alex. A Good Age. New York: Crown, 1976.

Common Knowledge. Box 316, Bolinas, CA 94924.

Commoner, Barry. The Politics of Energy. New York: Knopf, 1979.

The Company the Earth Keeps. Skywatch: Annual Celestial Chronicle. San Francisco: The Company the Earth Keeps, 1980.

Coon, Nelson. Using Plants for Healing. Emmaus, Pa.: Rodale Press, 1979.

Cooper, Kenneth. Aerobics. New York: M. Evans, 1968.

Coulter, Harris L. Divided Legacy. 3 vols. Washington, D.C.: Wehawken Book Co., 1973.

Cousins, Norman. Anatomy of an Illness as Perceived by the Patient. New York: Norton, 1979.

Dalton, K. Once a Month. Pomona, Calif.: Hunter House, 1979.

Daniel, E. J. Any Other Song: A Plea for Holistic Communication. Bowie, Md.: Robert J. Brady, 1980.

Darwin, Charles. Autobiography. London: Collins, 1958.

_____. On the Origin of Species: A Facsimile of the First Edition. Cambridge: Harvard University Press, 1975.

D'Asaro, Barbara. Be Young and Vital: The Nutrition/Exercise Plan. Short Hills, N.J.: Enslow Publishers, 1979.

Dass, Ravi, and Aparna. The Marriage and Family Book: A Spiritual Guide. New York: Schocken, 1978.

Davis, A. R., and Rawls, W. C., Jr. The Magnetic Blueprint of Life. Nicksville, N.Y.: Exposition Press, 1979.

Dawson, Adele. Health, Happiness, and the Pursuit of Herbs. Brattleboro, Vt.: Stephen Greene Press, 1980.

Debus, Allen G. The Chemical Philosophy: Paracelsian Science and Medicine in the Sixteenth and Seventeenth Centuries. New York: Science History Publications, 1977.

De Castillejo, Irene. Knowing Women: A Feminine Psychology. New York: Harper and Row, 1973.

Delacato, Carl H. The Diagnosis and Treatment of Speech and Reading Problems. Springfield, Ill.: Charles C. Thomas, 1963.

Deutsch, R. M. Realities of Nutrition. Palo Alto: Bull Publishing, 1979.

Dever, G. E. A. Community Health Analysis: A Holistic Approach. Germantown, Md.: Aspen Systems, 1980.

Diporta, L. Zen Running: Today's Road to Physical and Mental Well-Being. New York: Everest House, 1977.

Donnelly, G., et al. The Nursing System: Issues, Ethics, and Politics. New York: John Wiley and Sons, 1980.

Donsbach, Kurt. The Nutritional Approach to Super Health. International Institute of Natural Health Sciences, 1980.

Doty, Walter L. All About Vegetables. San Francisco: Ortho, 1973.

Doxiados, C. A. "Ekistics, the Science of Human Settlements." In Systems Approach and the City, edited by Mihajlo Mesarovic and Arnold Reisman. New York: American Elsevier, 1972.

Draeger, Donn F., and Smith, Robert W. Asian Fighting Arts. New York: Berkley, 1974.

Dubos, Rene. Man Adapting. New Haven: Yale University Press, 1965.

_____. Mirage of Health. New York: Harper, 1979.

Dychtwald, Ken. The Aging of America. New York: J. P. Tarcher, 1981.

Dychtwald, Ken, with Villoldo, A. Millenium: Glimpses into the 21st Century. New York: J. P. Tarcher, 1980.

East/West Journal. Box 305, Dover, NJ 07801.

Eckstein, Gustav. The Body Has a Head. New York: Bantam, 1980.

Ecology Center Newsletter. Ecology Center, 2701 College Ave., Berkeley, CA 94705.

Edwards, B. Drawing on the Right Side of the Brain. Los Angeles: J. P. Tarcher, 1979.

Einzig, Barbara. Color. Milwaukee: Membrane Press, 1976.

_____. Disappearing Work. Berkeley, Calif.: Small Press Distribution (The Figures), 1979.

Emmons, Michael. The Inner Source: A Guide to Meditative Therapy. San Luis Obispo, Calif.: Impact, 1978.

Erickson, Milton H. A Teaching Seminar with Milton Erickson. Edited by Jeffrey Zeig. New York: Brunner/Mazel, 1980.

Esko, W. Introducing Macrobiotic Cooking. New York: Kodansha International, 1979.

The est Graduate Review. est, 765 California St., San Francisco, CA.

Falk, Ruth. *Women Loving: A Journey Toward Becoming an Independent Woman.* New York: Random House, 1975.

Falls, H., *et al. Essentials of Fitness.* Philadelphia: Saunders College Publications, 1980.

Faust, Joan Lee. *Book of Vegetable Gardening.* New York: Times-Quadrangle, 1975.

Fay, M. *The Dream Guide.* Los Angeles: Center for the Healing Arts, 1979.

Feldenkrais, Moshe. *Body and Mature Behavior.* New York: International Universities Press, 1975.

_____. *The Case of Nora: Body Awareness as Healing Therapy.* New York: Harper and Row, 1977.

Feng, Gia-Fu, and English, Jane (trans.). *Tao Te Ching.* New York: Vintage, 1972.

Ferguson, Marilyn. *The Aquarian Conspriacy: Personal and Social Transformation in the 1980s.* Los Angeles: J. P. Tarcher, 1980.

_____. "Karl Pribram's Changing Reality." *Re-vision,* v. 1, no. 3-4, Summer/Fall 1978.

Fish, S., and Shelf, J. A. *Spiritual Care: The Nurse's Role.* Downers Grove, Ill.: InterVarsity Press, 1979.

Fisher, M. *Palm Leaf Patterns: A New Approach to Clothing Design.* Los Angeles: Panjandrum Press, 1977.

Flower Essence Quarterly. Flower Essence Society, Box 586, Nevada City, CA 95959.

Flynn, Patricia. *The Healing Continuum.* Bowie, Md.: Robert J. Brady, 1980.

_____. *Holistic Health: The Art and Science of Care.* Bowie, Md.: Robert J. Brady, 1980.

Foucault, Michel. *The Birth of the Clinic: An Archaeology of Medical Perception.* New York: Pantheon, 1973.

Fowler, J. S. *Movement Education.* New York: Saunders College Publications, 1981.

Fox, Helen Morgenthau. *Gardening with Herbs for Flavor and Fragrance.* New York: Dover, 1933; 1972.

French, Ruth M. *The Dynamics of Health Care.* New York: McGraw-Hill, 1968.

Friedman, M., and Rosenman, R. H. *Type A Behavior and Your Heart.* New York: Knopf, 1974.

Friendly Shared Powers: Practicing Self-Mastery and Creative Teamwork for Earth's Community. San Diego: Clear Marks, 1979.

Fromm, Erich. *The Art of Loving.* New York: Harper and Row, 1956.

Gadpaille, Warren. *Cycles of Sex.* New York: Scribner's, 1975.

GAIA'S GUIDE. New York: GAIA'S GUIDE, 1981.

Galin, David. "Implications for Psychiatry of Left and Right Cerebral Specialization; A Neurophysiological Context for Unconscious Processes." *Arch. Gen. Psychiatry,* v. 31, Oct. 1974.

Garcia Marquez, Gabriel. *One Hundred Years of Solitude.* Trans. by Gregory Rabassa. New York: Avon, 1970.

Gedlin, E. *Focusing.* New York: Everest House, 1978.

Geiskopf, S. *Putting It Up with Honey.* Ashland, Ore.: Quicksilver Productions, 1979.

Girdano, D., and Everly, G. *Controlling Stress and Tension: A Holistic Approach.* Englewood, N.J.: Prentice-Hall, 1979.

Gofman, John W. *An Irreverent, Illustrated View of Nuclear Power.* San Francisco: Committee for Nuclear Responsibility, 1979.

Gofman, John, and Tamplin, A. *Poisoned Power: The Case Against Nuclear Power Plants Before and After Three Mile Island.* Emmaus, Pa.: Rodale, 1979.

Goldstein, Joseph. *The Experience of Insight.* Santa Cruz, Calif.: Unity Press, 1976.

Goodhart, Robert S., and Shils, Maurice E., eds. *Modern Nutrition in Health and Disease.* 6th ed. Philadelphia: Lea & Febiger, 1980.

Goodheart, George J. *Applied Kinesiology Research Manuals.* 1964-71.

Gordon, Sol. *Let's Make Sex a Household Word: A Guide for Parents and Children.* New York: John Day, 1975.

Grant, L. *The Holistic Revolution.* New York: Crown, 1979.

Green, J. A., with Markell, S. "The Health-Care Contract: A Model for Sharing Responsibility." *Holistic Health Review,* v. 4, no. 1, Fall 1980.

Green, L., *et al. Health Education Planning: A Diagnostic Approach.* Palo Alto: Mayfield Publishing, 1980.

Green, Liz. *Relating.* New York: Weiser, 1978.

Greene, Felix. *The Enemy.* New York: Vintage Books, 1970.

Groch, Judith. *You and Your Brain.* New York: Harper and Row, 1963.

Grof, S. *LSD Therapy: The Principles of LSD Psychotherapy.* Pomona, Calif.: Hunter House, 1979.

Gross, Leonard, and Morehouse, Lawrence. *Total Fitness.* New York: Simon and Schuster, 1975.

Gross, Stanley. "Professional Disclosure: An Alternative to Licensing." *Personnel and Guidance Journal,* v. 55, no. 10, June 1977, pp. 586-88.

Grossinger, R. *Planet Medicine: From Stone-Age Shamanism to Post-Industrial Healing.* New York: Anchor, 1980.

Guay, Terrie. *Personal Fertility Guide: How to Avoid or Achieve Pregnancy.* San Francisco: Harbor, 1980.

Gurtov, Melvin. *Making Changes: The Politics of Self-Liberation.* Oakland: Harvest Moon Books, 1979.

Gussow, J. D. *The Feeding Web: Issues in Nutritional Ecology.* Palo Alto: Bull Publishing, 1978.

Gyorgy, Anna, and Friends. *No Nukes: Everyone's Guide to Nuclear Power.* Boston: South End Press, 1979.

Hall, A., ed. *A Visual Encyclopedia of Unconventional Medicine.* New York: Crown, 1979.

Halpern, S. *Tuning the Human Instrument: An Owner's Manual.* Rev. ed. Palo Alto: SRI, 1978.

Ham, Clifford C. *The Neighborhood Church in Urban Extension.* Pittsburgh: Action Housing, 1964.

Hamilton, M., and Reid, H., eds. *The Hospice Handbook.* Grand Rapids: Eerdmans, 1979.

Hanna, T. *The Body of Life.* New York: Knopf, 1980.

Harman, Willis. *An Incomplete Guide to the Future.* New York: Norton, 1979.

Harris, L., and Meriam, C. *Feeling Good About Feelings.* Palo Alto: Bull Publishing, 1979.

Hastings, Arthur C., Fadiman, James, and Gordon, James S. *Health for the Whole Person.* Boulder, Colo.: Westview Press, 1980.

Hawkins, David, and Pauling, Linus. *Orthomolecular Psychiatry.* San Francisco: W. H. Freeman, 1973.

Hayes, Elizabeth S. *Spices and Herbs: Lore and Cookery.* New York: Dover, 1980.

Health Science. 1920 Irving Park Rd., Chicago, IL 60613.

Henderson, Hazel. *Creating Alternative Futures: An End to Economics.* New York: Berkley, 1978.

Herb Quarterly. Box 576, Wilmington, VT 05363.

Higgins, Ronald. *The Seventh Enemy: The Human Factor in the Global Crisis.* New York: McGraw-Hill, 1978.

Hill, Lewis. *Pruning Simplified.* Emmaus, Pa.: Rodale Press, 1981.

Hills, Christopher. *Nuclear Evolution: Discovery of the Rainbow Body.* Boulder Creek, Calif.: University of the Trees Press, 1977.

————. *The Rise of the Phoenix: Universal Government by Nature's Laws.* Common Ownership Press, 1979.

Hills, Christopher, and Nakamura, H. *Food from Sunlight.* Boulder Creek, Calif.: University of the Trees Press, 1978.

Hills, Christopher, and Rozman, Deborah. *Exploring Inner Space: Awareness Games for All Ages.* Boulder Creek, Calif.: University of the Trees Press, 1975.

Hine, V. *Last Letter to the Pebble People.* Santa Cruz, Calif.: Unity Press, 1979.

Hite, Shere. *The Hite Report: A Nationwide Study of Female Sexuality.* New York: Macmillan, 1976.

Hittleman, Richard. *Be Young with Yoga.* New York: Warner, 1975.

Holistic Health Quarterly. Berkeley Holistic Health Center, 2640 College Ave., Berkeley, CA 94704.

Holistic Health Review. Human Sciences Press, 72 Fifth Ave., New York, NY 10011.

House, Mary Kate. "Home-Style Nursing." *Journal of the American Medical Association,* v. 240, no. 22, Nov. 24, 1978, pp. 2472-74.

Huard, Pierre, and Wong, Ming. *Oriental Methods of Mental and Physical Fitness: The Complete Book of Meditation, Kinesitherapy, and Martial Arts in China, India, and Japan.* New York: Funk & Wagnalls, 1977.

Hulke, M. *The Encyclopedia of Alternative Medicine and Self Help.* New York: Schocken, 1979.

Hulme, W. E. *Let the Spirit In: Practicing Christian Devotional Meditation.* Nashville: Abingdon, 1979.

Human Dimensions Journal. Human Dimensions Institute, Inc., 4612 W. Lake Rd., Canandaigua, NY 14424.

Huxley, Aldous. *The Perennial Philosophy.* New York: Harper and Row, 1970.

I Ching. Trans. by James Legee. New York: Bantam, 1969.

An Integral View: Emerging Currents in Modern Thought. 3494 21st St., San Francisco, CA 94110.

Isherwood, Christopher. *A Single Man.* New York: Avon, 1978.

Jackson, Richard. *Holistic Massage.* New York: Sterling, 1980.

Jackson, Tom. *Guerrilla Tactics in the Job Market.* New York: Bantam, 1978.

Jacobs, Jane. *The Death and Life of Great American Cities.* New York: Random House, 1961.

Jaffee, D. *Healing from Within.* New York: Knopf, 1980.

James, William. *The Varieties of Religious Experience.* New York: Doubleday, 1978.

Javits, Tom. *How to Raise Rabbits and Chickens in an Urban Area.* Berkeley, Calif.: Integral Urban House, 1975.

Javits, Tom, *et al. Integral Urban House: Self-Reliant Living in the City.* San Francisco: Sierra Club Books, 1979.

Jensen, Bernard. *Nature Has a Remedy.* Jensen Publications, 1978.

Journal for the Protection of all Beings. *Co-Evolution Quarterly,* no. 19, Fall 1978 (entire issue).

Journal of Holistic Health. Mandala Society, Box 1233, Del Mar, CA 92014.

Jung, C. G. *Man and His Symbols.* New York: Doubleday, 1976.

———. *Memories, Dreams, Reflections.* New York: Vintage, 1965.

Kaiser, A. *Questioning Techniques.* Pomona, Calif.: Hunter House, 1979.

Kalson, C., and Kalson, S. *Holistic H.E.L.P. Handbook.* Phoenix: International Holistic Center, 1979.

Kaplan, R., Saltzman, B., and Ecker, L. *Wholly Alive!* Millbrae, Calif.: Celestial Arts, 1979.

Karagulla, Shafica. *Breakthrough to Creativity.* Santa Monica, Calif.: DeVorss, 1969.

Kaslow, A., and Miles, R. *Freedom from Chronic Disease.* Los Angeles: J. P. Tarcher, 1979.

Kaslow, L. *Wholistic Dimensions in Healing: A Resource Directory.* New York: Doubleday, 1978.

Katz, D., and Goodwin, M. *Food: Where Nutrition, Politics, and Culture Meet: An Activities Guide for Teachers.* Washington, D.C.: Center for Science in the Public Interest, 1976.

Katz, Jonathan. *Gay American History: Lesbians and Gay Men in the U.S.A.* New York: Crowell, 1976.

Kendall, Henry O., *et al. Muscles: Testing and Function.* 2nd ed. Baltimore: Williams and Wilkins, 1971.

Keyes, Ken, Jr. *The Conscious Person's Guide to Relationships.* St. Mary, Ken.: Living Love Publications, 1979.

Khalsa, R. K. *Healing the Healer.* Los Angeles: Center for Health and Healing, 1978.

Kloss, Jethro. *Back to Eden.* Greenwich, Conn.: Benedict Lust Publications, 1939, 1976.

Kneipp, Fr. *My Water Cure.* Mokelumne Hill, Calif.: Health Research, 1886.

Kostrubala, Thaddeus. *The Joy of Running.* New York: Pocket Books, 1976.

Kropf, William, and Houben, Milton. *Harmful Food Additives: The Eat-Safe Guide.* Port Washington, N.Y.: Ashley Books, 1980.

Kugler, Hans. *Dr. Kugler's Seven Keys to a Longer Life.* New York: Stein and Day, 1978.

Kuhn, Maggie. *Maggie Kuhn on Aging.* Philadelphia: Westminster Press, 1977.

Kuntzleman, Charles T., and the Editors of *Consumer Guide. Rating the Exercises.* New York: William Morrow, 1978.

Kurtz, Ron, and Prestera, Hector. *The Body Reveals.* New York: Bantam, 1977.

Kushi, Michio. *The Book of Macrobiotics.* New York: Japan Publications, 1977.

———. *Macrobiotics: Experience the Miracle of Life.* East West Foundation, 1978.

———. *Natural Healing Through Macrobiotics.* New York: Kodansha International, 1979.

La Chappelle, Dolores. *Earth Wisdom.* Los Angeles: Guild of Tutors Press, 1976.

Lakein, Alan. *How to Get Control of Your Time and Your Life.* New York: McKay, 1973.

Larsen, T. *Trust Yourself!* San Luis Obispo, Calif.: Impact, 1979.

LeMaitre, George. *How to Choose a Good Doctor.* Andover, Mass.: Brick House, 1980.

Leonard, George. *Education and Ecstasy.* New York: Dell, 1969.

———. *The Silent Pulse.* New York: Bantam, 1981.

———. *The Transformation.* New York: Delacorte, 1972.

LeShan, Lawrence. *Alternate Realities.* New York: Evans, 1976.

Levertov, Denise. *Relearning the Alphabet.* New York: New Directions, 1970.

Llewellyn's Moon Sign Book. St. Paul: Llewellyn Publications, 1980.

Longnecker, C. E. *How to Recover from a Stroke and Make a Successful Comeback.* Port Washington, N.Y.: Ashley Books, 1979.

Lowen, Alexander. *The Language of the Body.* New York: Collier Books, 1971.

Luce, Gay. *Your Second Life.* New York: Seymour Lawrence/Delacorte, 1979.

Lunde, D., and Lunde, M. *The Next Generation: A Book on Parenting.* New York: Holt, Rinehart and Winston, 1980.

Luthman, Shirley Gehrke, and Kirchenbaum, Martin. *The Dynamic Family.* Palo Alto: Science and Behavior Books, 1974.

McKim, Robert. *Experiences in Visual Thinking.* Monterey, Calif.: Brooks/Cole, 1972.

Mann, John A. *Secrets of Life Extension.* Berkeley, Calif.: And/Or Press, 1981.

Mao Tse-Tung. *Four Essays on Philosophy.* Peking: Foreign Languages Press, 1968.

Markle, Gerald, and Petersen, James. *Politics, Science, and Cancer: The Laetrile Phenomenon.* Boulder, Colo.: Westview Press, 1980.

Mason, L. John, compiler. *Guide to Stress Reduction.* Culver City, Calif.: Peace Press, 1980.

Masters, William, and Johnson, Virginia. *The Pleasure Bond.* New York: Bantam, 1976.

Maynard, J. *Celestial Calendars.* Ashland, Ore.: Quicksilver Productions, 1980.

Melamed, Barbara, and Siegel, Lawrence J. *Behavioral Medicine* (Springer Series on Behavior Therapy and Behavioral Medicine, vol. 6). New York: Springer, 1980.

Mendelsohn, Robert S. *Male Practice: How Doctors Manipulate Women.* Chicago: Contemporary Books, 1981.

Menzies, Rob. *The Herbal Dinner.* Millbrae, Calif.: Celestial Arts, 1977.

Meyer, Ann, and Meyer, Peter. *Being a Christ.* San Diego: Dawning Publications, 1975.

Michaels, Andrew. *Why Do You Think They Call It a Deadline? A Wholistic Stress-Management Workbook.* Berkeley, Calif.: Andrew Michaels, 1979.

Miller, D. *The New Healthy Trail Food Book.* Rev. ed. Charlotte, N.C.: East Woods Press, 1980.

Miller, Victor, and Dobsen, Terry. *Giving In to Get Your Way.* New York: Delacorte, 1978.

Minuchin, Salvador. *Families and Family Therapy.* Cambridge: Harvard University Press, 1974.

Mitchell, Curtis. *The Perfect Exercise: The Hop, Skip, and Jump Way to Health.* New York: Simon and Schuster, 1976.

Monette, Paul. *Taking Care of Mrs. Carroll.* New York: Avon, 1979.

Mooney, James. *Myths of the Cherokee.* Nineteenth Annual Report of the Bureau of American Ethnology. Reprinted edition. Saint Clair Shores, Mich.: Scholarly Press, 1900, 1970.

The Mouth in Medicine. Minneapolis: Multimedia Education Programs, McGraw-Hill, n.d.

Mumford, Lewis. *The City in History.* New York: Harcourt, Brace, and World, 1961.

———. *The Culture of Cities.* New York: Harcourt, Brace, and World, 1938.

———. *The Transformations of Man.* New York: Harper and Brothers, 1956.

Nader, Ralph, and Abbotts, John. *The Menace of Atomic Energy.* New York: Norton, 1979.

Nasi, A., Rattazzi, I., and Rivetti, F. *The Honey Handbook: An Introduction to New and Exciting Uses for Nature's Most Perfect Food.* New York: Everest House, 1979.

National Journal of the Nutritional Academy. 1238 Hayes, Eugene, OR 97402.

Natural Life. Box 4564, Buffalo, NY 14240.

Needleman, Carla. "Potter's Progress: Self-Understanding and the Lessons of Craft." *Psychology Today,* June 1979, v. 13, no. 1, pp. 78-86.

Needleman, Jacob. *A Sense of the Cosmos.* New York: Dutton, 1976.

Neumann, Erich. Trans. by Eugene Rolf. *Depth Psychology and a New Ethic.* New York: Harper and Row, 1973.

New Age Magazine. New Age Communications, Inc., 32 Station St., Brookline, MA 02146.

New Dimensions Foundation. *The New Healers: Healing the Whole Person.* Berkeley, Calif.: And/Or Press, 1980.

New Games Foundation. *New Games Book.* Garden City, N.J.: Doubleday, 1976.

Nicolaides, Kimon. *The Natural Way to Draw.* Boston: Houghton Mifflin, 1969.

Nin, Anais. *Diaries,* vols. 1-7. New York: Harcourt Brace Jovanovich, 1966-1980.

Nixon, J. E., and Jewett, A. E. *An Introduction to Physical Education.* Philadelphia: W. B. Saunders, 1980.

Nutrition Action Magazine. Center for Science in the Public Interest, 1755 S Street, N.W., Washington, DC 20009.

Nutrition Search Group. *Nutrition Almanac.* New York: McGraw-Hill, 1979.

O'Conner, R. *Choosing for Health.* New York: Holt Rinehart and Winston, 1980.

Ogilvy, James A. *Many-Dimensional Man.* New York: Harper and Row, 1979.

Olkowski, Helga. *Self-guided Tour of the Integral Urban House.* Berkeley, Calif.: Integral Urban House, 1979.

Olkowski, Helga, and Olkowski, William. *The City People's Book of Raising Food.* Emmaus, Pa.: Rodale Press, 1975.

O'Regan, Brendan, and Carlson, Rick J. "Defining Health: The State of the Art." *Holistic Health Review,* v. 3, no. 2, pp. 86-102.

Organic Gardening. 33 East Manor St., Emmaus, PA 18049.

Ornstein, Robert, ed. *The Nature of Human Consciousness.* San Francisco: W. H. Freeman, 1973.

Ostrander, Sheila, and Schroeder, Lynn. *Superlearning.* New York: Delacorte, 1979.

Ouspensky, P. D. *In Search of the Miraculous.* New York: Harcourt, Brace, 1949.

Panos, Maesimund B., and Heimlich, Jane. *Homeopathic Medicine at Home*. Los Angeles: J. P. Tarcher, 1980.

Parent's Magazine. Parent's Magazine Enterprises, Inc., 52 Vanderbilt Ave., New York, NY 10017.

Parker, Richard. *The Myth of the Middle Class*. New York: Liveright, 1972.

Parsons, Talcott. "Definitions of Health and Illness in Light of American Values and Social Structure." In *Patients, Physicians, and Illness*, edited by E. G. Jaco. New York: Free Press, 1959.

Peck, M. S. *The Road Less Traveled*. New York: Simon and Schuster, 1978.

Peck, Stephen Rogers. *Atlas of Human Anatomy for the Artist*. New York: Oxford University Press, 1951.

Pelletier, K. *Holistic Medicine: From Stress to Optimum Health*. New York: Delacorte, 1979.

Peper, E., Ancoli, S., and Quinn, M. *Mind/Body Integration*. New York: Plenum, 1979.

Peper, E., and Kushel, C. "An Holistic Merger of Biofeedback and Family Therapy." *The American Theosophist*, v. 67, no. 5, 1979, pp. 158-68.

Perls, Fritz. *Ego, Hunger, and Aggression*. London: Allen and Unwin, 1947.

———. *The Gestalt Approach and Eye Witness to Therapy*. Palo Alto: Science and Behavior Books, 1973.

———. *Gestalt Therapy Verbatim*. Lafayette, Calif.: Real People Press, 1969.

Perls, Fritz, Hefferline, R., and Goodman, P. *Gestalt Therapy*. New York: Dell, 1951.

Pfeiffer, Carl. *Mental and Elemental Nutrients*. New Canaan, Conn.: Keats, 1975.

Phelan, Nancy, and Volin, Michael. *Sex and Yoga*. New York: Harper and Row, 1967.

Pion, R. *The Last Sex Manual*. Hollywood: Triseme Corporation, 1977.

———. *Rx: Prescription for Wellness*. Hollywood: Triseme Corporation, 1979.

The Plain Truth. Ambassador Publishing Co., Box 111, 300 W. Green St., Pasadena, CA 91123.

Pollard, D. C. *Sprouts for Dieters*. Cobalt, Ontario: Highway Book Shop, 1979.

Polster, E., and Polster, M. *Gestalt Therapy Integrated*. New York: Brunner/Mazel, 1973.

Pomeroy, Wardell. *Your Child and Sex: A Guide for Parents*. New York: Dell, 1975.

Prevention Magazine Editors. *The Prevention Guide to Surgery and its Alternatives*. Emmaus, Pa.: Rodale Press, 1980.

Priessnitz, Vincent. *The Cold Water Cure*. Mokelumne Hill, Calif.: Health Research, 1843.

Putoff and Targ. *Papers on Remote Viewing*. Stanford, Calif.: Stanford Research Institute, n.d.

Radiation on the Job. San Francisco: Coalition for the Medical Rights of Women, 1980.

Radioactive Times. Abalone Alliance, 944 Market St., Rm. 307, San Francisco, CA 94102.

Rajneesh, Bhagwan S. *The Book of the Secrets*. New York: Harper and Row, 1974.

Ram Dass. *Be Here Now*. New York: Crown, 1971.

———. *The Only Dance There Is*. New York: Anchor-Doubleday, 1974.

Rama, Swami, Ballentine, R., and Hynes, A. *The Science of Breath*. Honesdale, Pa.: Himalayan Press, 1979.

Ray, Sondra. *I Deserve Love*. Millbrae, Calif.: Les Femmes, 1976.

Rees, Michael K. *The Complete Family Guide to Living with High Blood Pressure*. Englewood Cliffs, N.J.: Prentice-Hall, 1980.

Research Group One. *Women and Men: A Socioeconomic Factbook*. Baltimore: Vacant Lots Press, 1975.

Revolutionary Health Committee of Hunan Province. *The Barefoot Doctor's Manual*. Seattle: Cloudburst Press, 1977.

Rhodes, Daniel. "Erosion II." *Ceramics Monthly*, v. 20, no. 2, Feb. 1972, p. 27.

Rhyne, Janie. *The Gestalt Art Experience*. Monterey, Calif.: Brooks/Cole, 1973.

Riding, Laura. *Selected Poems: In Five Sets*. New York: Norton, 1970.

Robe, L. B. *Just So It's Healthy*. Minneapolis: Comp Care Publishers, 1977.

Robertson, J. *The Sane Alternative: A Choice of Futures*. St. Paul: River Basin Publishing, 1979.

Robertson, Laurel, Flinders, Carol, and Godfrey, Bronwen. *Laurel's Kitchen*. Petaluma, Calif.: Nilgiri Press, 1976.

Romney, Rodney R. *Journey to Inner Space*. Nashville: Abingdon, 1980.

Rona, L. *Total Glow*. Wilmington, Del.: Enterprise, 1979.

Rose, Jeanne. *Kitchen Cosmetics*. Los Angeles: Panjandrum, 1978.

Ross, Helen S., and Mico, Paul R. *Theory and Practice in Health Education*. Palo Alto: Mayfield, 1980.

Rossman, Michael. *New Age Blues: On the Politics of Consciousness*. New York: Dutton, 1979.

Roszak, Theodore. *The Making of a Counter Culture*. New York: Doubleday, 1969.

———. *Person/Planet: The Creative Disintegration of Industrial Society*. New York: Doubleday, 1978.

_____. *Unfinished Animal*. New York: Harper and Row, 1975.

_____. *Where the Wasteland Ends*. New York: Doubleday, 1973.

Rothstein, William. *American Physicians in the Nineteenth Century: From Sects to Science*. Baltimore: Johns Hopkins University Press, 1972.

Rozman, Deborah. *Meditating with Children: New Age Meditations for Children*. Boulder Creek, Calif.: University of the Trees Press, 1975.

_____. *Meditation for Children*. Millbrae, Calif.: Celestial Arts, 1976.

Rubenfeld, Frank. *Social Gestalt: A Response to Illusions of Freedom and Powerlessness*. Bolinas, Calif.: Psycho-Political Pamphlets, 1978.

Rudhyar, Dane. *Beyond Individualism: The Psychology of Transformation*. Wheaton, Ill.: Quest Books, 1979.

_____. *Culture, Crisis, and Creativity*. Wheaton, Ill.: Quest Books, 1977.

_____. *Occult Preparations for a New Age*. Wheaton, Ill.: Quest Books, 1975.

_____. *The Planetarization of Consciousness*. New York: A.S.I. Publishers, 1977.

_____. *We Can Begin Again—Together*. Garberville, Calif.: Seed Center, 1974.

Sachs, D. *Wonder of Life Coloring Book Series*. Kailua, Hawaii: Moss Publishing, 1979.

Saltoon, Diana. *The Common Book of Consciousness*. San Francisco: Chronicle Books, 1980.

Sappho. *Sappho: A New Translation*. Trans. by Mary Barnard. Berkeley: University of California Press, 1958.

Satin, Mark. *New Age Politics*. New York: Dell, 1979.

Satir, Virginia. *Conjoint Family Therapy*. Palo Alto: Science and Behavior Books, 1967.

_____. *Peoplemaking*. Palo Alto: Science and Behavior Books, 1972.

Satprem. *Sri Aurobindo, or, The Adventure of Consciousness*. New York: Harper and Row, 1974.

Scholl, L., with Selby, J. *Visionetics: The Holistic Way to Better Eyesight*. New York: Doubleday, 1978.

Schutte, Karl H. *The Biology of the Trace Elements*. Philadelphia: Lippincott, 1964.

Schwartz, M. S., and Shockley, E. L. *The Nurse and the Mental Patient: A Study in Interpersonal Relations*. New York: John Wiley and Sons, 1956.

Selzer, Richard. *Mortal Lessons*. New York: Simon and Schuster, 1976.

Seymour, John. *The Self-Sufficient Gardener*. New York: Doubleday, 1979.

Shames, Richard, and Sterin, Chuck. *Healing with Mind Power*. Emmaus, Pa.: Rodale Press, 1980.

Shandler, N., and Shandler, M. *Yoga for Pregnancy and Birth: A Guide for Expectant Parents*. New York: Schocken, 1979.

Sharon, James A. *Holistic Health Inventory*. Greeley, Colo.: James A. Sharon, 1978.

Shedd, C. W. *Time for All Things*. Nashville: Abingdon, 1980.

Shostrum, Everette. *Man the Manipulator*. Nashville: Abingdon, 1967.

Shryock, Richard. *Development of Modern Medicine*. New York: Knopf, 1947.

_____. *Medical Licensing in America, 1650-1965*. Baltimore: Johns Hopkins University Press, 1967.

_____. *Medicine and Society in America, 1660-1860*. New York: New York University Press, 1960.

Silverstein, Charles. *A Family Matter: A Parent's Guide to Homosexuality*. New York: McGraw-Hill, 1977.

Simonton, O. Carl, and Matthews-Simonton, Stephanie. "Belief Systems and Management of Emotional Aspects of Malignancy." *Journal of Transpersonal Psychology*, v. 7, no. 1, 1975, pp. 29-48.

Simonton, O. Carl, Matthews-Simonton, Stephanie, and Creighton, James. *Getting Well Again*. Los Angeles: J. P. Tarcher, 1978.

Singer, Charles. *Science, Medicine, and History*. New York: Arno Press, 1975.

Smith, N. *Food for Sport*. Palo Alto: Bull Publishing, 1976.

Smith, Robert W. *Chinese Boxing: Masters and Methods*. San Francisco: Kodansha, 1974.

Snyder, Gary. *The Old Ways*. San Francisco: City Light Books, 1977.

Sommer, Robert. *The Mind's Eye*. New York: Dell, 1978.

Sorochan, W. *Promoting Your Health*. New York: John Wiley and Sons, 1981.

Spangler, David. *Revelation: Birth of a New Age*. Elgin, Ill.: Lorian Press, 1979.

_____. *Towards a Planetary Vision*. Moray, Scotland: Findhorn, 1978.

Spino, Dyveke. *New Age Training for Fitness and Health*. New York: Grove Press, 1979.

Squyres, Wendy D., ed. *Patient Education: An Inquiry into the State of the Art*. New York: Springer, 1980.

Sri Aurobindo. *The Supramental Manifestation upon Earth*. Pondicherry, India: Sri Aurobindo Ashram Trust, 1973.

Sri Aurobindo, and the Mother. *Conversations*. Pondicherry, India: Sri Aurobindo Ashram Trust, 1973.

_____. *On Physical Education*. Pondicherry, India: Sri Aurobindo Ashram Trust, 1967.

_____. *On Surrender and Grace*. Pondicherry, India: Sri Aurobindo Ashram Trust, 1970.

Stavrianos, L. *The Promise of the Coming Dark Age*. San Francisco: W. H. Freeman, 1976.

Stearn, Jess. *Yoga, Youth, and Reincarnation*. New York: Bantam, 1971.

Steinmetz, Jenny, *et al. Managing Stress Before It Manages You*. Palo Alto: Bull Publishing, 1980.

Stevens, John. *Gestalt Is*. Moab, Utah: Real People Press, 1975.

Stewart, Felicia, *et al. My Body, My Health: The Concerned Woman's Guide to Gynecology*. New York: John Wiley and Sons, 1979.

Sunset Magazine Editors. *Vegetable Gardening*. Menlo Park, Calif.: Lane, 1977.

Suzuki, Daisetz. *Zen and Japanese Culture*. Princeton, N.J.: Princeton University Press, 1970.

Synthesis Magazine. Synthesis Press, Redwood City, CA 94601.

Szasz, Thomas. *The Myth of Mental Illness*. New York: Harper and Row, 1961.

Terris, Milton, Cornely, Paul B., Daniels, Henry, and Kerr, Lorin. "The Case for a National Health Service." *American Journal of Public Health*, v. 67, no. 12, Dec. 1977, pp. 1183-85.

Thie, John F., with Marks, Mary. *Touch for Health*. Santa Monica, Calif.: DeVorss, 1973.

Thompson, William Irwin. *Darkness and Scattered Light*. New York: Harper and Row, 1978.

Thomson, Robert. *The Grosset Encyclopedia of Natural Medicine*. New York: Grosset and Dunlap, 1980.

_____. *Natural Medicine*. New York: McGraw-Hill, 1978.

Tierra, Michael. *The Way of Herbs: Simple Remedies for Health and Healing*. Santa Cruz, Calif.: Unity Press, 1981.

Timms, M., and Zar, Z. *Natural Sources of B-17*. Millbrae, Calif.: Celestial Arts, 1978.

Totman, R. *Social Causes of Illness*. New York: Pantheon, 1980.

Tripp, C. A. *The Homosexual Matrix*. New York: McGraw-Hill, 1975.

Tubesing, D. *Wholistic Health: A Whole-Person Approach to Primary Health Care*. New York: Human Sciences Press, 1979.

Ullman, Dana. "Regulated Freedom of Choice: An Alternative to Licensure." *Holistic Health Review*, v. 4, no. 1, Fall 1980.

U.S. Capitalism in Crisis. Economics Education Project of The Union for Radical Economics, 1978.

U.S. Department of Commerce. Bureau of the Census. *Social and Economic Characteristics of the Metropolitan and Non-Metropolitan Population*. Washington, D.C.: Government Printing Office, 1977.

U.S. Senate Select Committee on Nutrition and Human Needs. *Dietary Goals for the U.S.* Washington, D.C.: Government Printing Office, 1977.

U.S. Surgeon General. *Report on Health and Nutrition*. Washington, D.C.: Government Printing Office, 1979.

University of California Extension Media Center. "Audiotapes and 16mm Films on Medicine and Health Care." *Lifelong Learning*, v. XLV, no. 42, Jan. 16, 1976.

Van der Ryn, Sim. *The Toilet Papers*. Santa Barbara, Calif.: Capra Press, 1978.

Vasconcellos, John. *A Liberating Vision: Politics for Growing Humans*. San Luis Obispo, Calif.: Impact, 1979.

Vida, Ginny. *Our Right to Love: A Lesbian Resource Book*. Englewood Cliffs, N.J.: Prentice-Hall, 1978.

Vincent, Larry. *The Dancer's Book of Health*. New York: Andrews and McMeel, 1978.

Waite, Arthur Edward, ed. and trans. *The Hermetic and Alchemical Writings of Paracelsus*. Berkeley, Calif.: Shambhala, 1976.

Walker, M. *Total Health: The Holistic Alternative to Traditional Medicine*. New York: Everest House, 1979.

Wallerstein, Edward. *Circumcision: An American Health Fallacy*. New York: Springer, 1980.

Ward, M. *The Brilliant Function of Pain*. New York: Optimus, 1977.

Warmbrand, Max. *Encyclopedia of Health and Nutrition*. New York: BJ Publishing Group, 1974.

Warren, Patricia Nell. *The Front Runner*. New York: Bantam, 1975.

Waxman, Stephane. *Growing Up Feeling Good: A Child's Introduction to Sexuality*. Los Angeles: Panjandrum, 1979.

Weininger, Ben, and Menkin, Eva. *Aging Is a Lifelong Affair*. Los Angeles: Guild of Tutors, 1978.

Weinstein, Matt, and Goodman, Joel. *Playfair*. San Luis Obispo, Calif.: Impact, 1980.

Weiss, J. C. *Creative Arts Therapy with Elders: A Pictorial Essay.* San Francisco: Jules Weiss, 1979.

Whitaker, Carl A., and Malone, Thomas P. *The Roots of Psychotherapy.* New York: Brunner/Mazel, 1981.

White, Edmund. *States of Desire: Travels in Gay America.* New York: Dutton, 1980.

Whitman, Walt. *Leaves of Grass* (facsimile edition). New York: Eakins, 1855.

_____. *Whitman Selected by Robert Creeley.* New York: Penguin, 1973.

Whole Foods. 2219 Marin Ave., Berkeley, CA 94707.

Why Do We Spend So Much Money? Somerville, Mass.: Popular Economics Press, 1977.

Whyte, K. *The Original Diet.* San Francisco: Troubador, 1977.

Wickes, F. *Inner World of Choice.* Englewood Cliffs, N.J.: Prentice-Hall, 1963.

Williams, R., and Kalita, D. *A Physician's Handbook on Orthomolecular Medicine.* New Canaan, Conn.: Keats, 1977.

Williams, Strephon Kaplan. *Jungian-Senoi Dreamwork Manual.* Berkeley, Calif.: Journey Press, 1980.

_____. *Transformations—I: Meditations in a New Age.* Berkeley, Calif.: Journey Press, 1980.

Yepsen, Roger B., Jr. *Home Food Systems.* Emmaus, Pa.: Rodale Press, 1981.

Zaffutto, Anthony. *Alphagenics.* New York: Warner, 1974.

Zilbergeld, Bernie. *Male Sexuality.* New York: Bantam, 1978.

Zizmor, Jonathan. *Dr. Zizmor's Guide to Clearer Skin.* Philadelphia: Lippincott, 1980.

Index

The Berkeley Holistic Health Center (BHHC) is a comprehensive healing arts center offering the state of the art care in humanistic/holistic health and medicine.

BHHC currently provides a variety of services and functions. The hands-on clinical practices and health education sessions include: ortho-molecular psychology and nutritional medicine, clinical ecology (allergy testing and treatment), osteopathic medicine and manipulation, biofeedback, stress reduction, Reichian, Gestalt, counseling for the terminally ill, Ericsonian hypnosis, podiatry and reflexology, herbology, and a variety of therapeutic massage and bodywork practices.

A Supporting Membership Plan is now available. Members will get a subscription to our quarterly Holistic Health News, discounts on the special health products and wellness plans, notice of Center and community related special events, and other BHHC publications.

If you have interest in any or all of the above, please mark the appropriate box(es) in the coupon below, cut it out and mail it with a self-addressed stamped envelope to:

Berkeley Holistic Health Center
3099 Telegraph Avenue
Berkeley, CA 94705

or call: (415) 845-4430

Name _____

Address _____

_____ Phone # (_____)_____

☐ **Membership Information**

☐ **Wellness and Health/Life Plans**

☐ **Publications Catalog**

☐ **Testing Services**
    ☐ Allergy Testing
    ☐ Blood Evaluation
    ☐ Cytotoxic Testing
    ☐ Hair Analysis
    ☐ Nutritional Analysis